Oncogenes

2ND Edition

Volume I

Author

Enrique Pimentel, M.D.

Professor and Director
National Center of Genetics
Institute of Experimental Medicine
Central University of Venezuela
Caracas, Venezuela

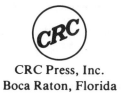

CRC Press, Inc.
Boca Raton, Florida

Library of Congress Cataloging-in-Publication Data

Pimentel, Enrique.
    Oncogenes / author, Enrique Pimentel. — 2nd ed.
      p. cm.
    Includes bibliographical references.
    ISBN 0-8493-6505-8 (v. 1). — ISBN 0-8493-6506-6 (v. 2)
    1. Oncogenes. 2. Oncogenic viruses. 3. Oncogenic Viruses.
I. Title.
    [DNLM: 1. Cell Transformation, Neoplastic. 2. Oncogenes.   QZ 202 P6446]
RC268.42.P56 1989
616.99′4071—dc20
DNLM/DLC
for Library of Congress   89-22100
                                                                       CIP

Direct all inquiries to CRC Press, Inc., 2000 Corporate Blvd., N.W., Boca Raton, Florida, 33431.

©1989 by CRC Press, Inc.

International Standard Book Number 0-8493-6505-8 (v. 1)
International Standard Book Number 0-8493-6506-6 (v. 2)

Library of Congress Number 89-22100

PREFACE

Oncogenes are genes with potential properties for the induction of neoplastic transformation of cells in either natural or experimental conditions. Most oncogenes have been isolated from acute transforming retroviruses, which act as oncogene transducers, although these viruses do not transmit cancer under natural conditions. The viral oncogenes are genes of cellular origin and their normal counterparts, the protooncogenes, are present in the genome of all multicellular animals, including man. Approximately 40 protooncogenes have been detected so far in normal and tumor cells. The normal functions of protooncogenes are related mainly to the transductional mechanisms of cellular signals and to the control of cellular proliferation and differentiation. Structural or functional alterations of protooncogenes are associated with the origin and/or development of malignant diseases. The tumorigenic potential of protooncogenes is counteracted by the effects of tumor suppressor genes or antioncogenes. The available evidence indicates that cancer may be associated with alterations of the normal equilibrium existing between protooncogenes and tumor suppressor genes. The role of protooncogenes and tumor suppressor genes in malignant diseases is at present a subject of very high interest and intensive research work.

Enrique Pimentel, M.D.
May 18, 1989

THE AUTHOR

Enrique Pimentel, M.D., is Professor of General Pathology at the School of Medicine, Central University of Venezuela, Caracas. He was formerly Director of the Institute of Experimental Medicine at the same university and is now Director of the National Center of Genetics in Venezuela.

Born on April 7, 1928 in Caracas, he obtained an M.D. degree from the Universities of Madrid and Caracas. He is a member of the National Academy of Medicine in Venezuela and an honorary, correspondent, or active member of 30 national and international scientific societies. He is Vice President of the International Academy of Tumor Marker Oncology (IATMO).

Dr. Pimentel is the author of more than 100 papers, co-author of 5 books on topics related to endocrinology, genetics, and oncology, and the author of *Hormones, Growth Factors, and Oncogenes* (published by CRC Press, 1987). He is the Editor of a recently created journal (published by CRC Press), *Critical Reviews in Oncogenesis*. On many occasions Dr. Pimentel has been invited to give lectures and seminars at universities and other scientific institutions in North America and Europe. He received several decorations in his country and the Grosse Verdienstkreuz of the Federal Republic of Germany. In 1982, he received the National Award of Science in Venezuela.

TABLE OF CONTENTS

Volume I

Chapter 2
Acute Retroviruses

Chapter 3
Chronic Retroviruses

Chapter 5
DNA Viruses

Chapter 6
Viral and Cellular Oncogenes

Chapter 8
The Rous Sarcoma Virus Oncogene and its Protooncogene Counterpart

Chapter 1

GENERAL BIOLOGICAL ASPECTS OF ONCOGENESIS

I. INTRODUCTION

Neoplasias are pathological processes occurring in multicellular organisms, including animals and plants. They are formed by poorly differentiated cells which have a tendency to continuous, indefinite growth. These cells, termed neoplastic or transformed cells, do not perform useful functions in the host organism and do not respond in an appropriate manner to the regulatory mechanisms controlling the rates of cell proliferation and cell differentiation in the different organs and tissues. Consequently, neoplastic cells can form abnormal growths or tumors, which are potentially dangerous to the health and survival of the organism.

A. TUMORS

Oncology is the branch of biology devoted to the study of tumors and tumorigenic processes. The tumor is the final stage of the process of neoplastic development,[1,2] which usually lasts for a proportionally long period in relation to the average lifetime of the organism. The tumor becomes recognizable by clinical procedures only when the proliferating neoplastic cells have formed a mass of considerable size. According to the biological and clinical behavior in relation to the host, tumors may be classified in two broad groups, i.e., benign and malignant tumors. This classification is useful in spite of the fact that there is a wide and almost continuous spectrum from clear benignancy to extreme malignancy.

1. Benign Tumors

Typical benign tumors have the following characteristics: (1) they are well circumscribed in relation to the surrounding normal tissues and they are limited by a capsule of connective tissue; (2) they grow slowly and according to an expansive pattern, without invasion and destruction of the surrounding normal tissues; (3) they do not produce remote dissemination, i.e., they do not give origin to metastases; (4) they are usually curable and may be frequently controlled by simple surgical excision, and (5) they do not contribute to curtail the average lifetime of the host. However, some benign tumors may produce serious damage to the organism because of their large size or because of their location, which may produce disturbances in the function of neighbor organs and tissues. For example, some benign tumors can produce obstruction in the ways of circulation of body fluids, which may result in serious damage to delicate tissues such as the central nervous system. Benign tumors of the endocrine glands such as functional pituitary adenomas and adenomas of the β cells from the Langerhans islets of the pancreas (insulinomas) can produce severe, life-threatening metabolic derangements.

2. Malignant Tumors

The most important characteristics of malignant tumors, as opposed to those of benign tumors, are the following: (1) they are not well circumscribed in relation to the surrounding normal tissues and do not have a limiting capsule of connective tissue; (2) in the advanced stages of their development, their growth is apparently rapid and is accompanied with an active invasion and destruction of the surrounding normal tissues; (3) they have a tendency to remote dissemination in the form of metastases, whose growth may result in the production of secondary tumors; (4) their total eradication is difficult, even by means of aggressive therapeutic procedures; and (5) they reduce, sometimes markedly, the average lifetime of the host.

Malignancy is only a meaningful concept when applied in relation to the peculiar characteristics of the host. A given type of tumor may have a more malignant behavior in one species than in another species, and the same is valid for different individuals from a given species. Many factors from both the tumor and the host may contribute to the more or less aggressive behavior of tumors. The behavior of a tumor may not be always the same in a given host but it may change, usually in form of increasing aggressiveness and rarely in form of regression. For example, indolent adenocarcinomas of the human thyroid gland, usually characterized by slow growth and a long natural history, may be transformed into anaplastic, undifferentiated tumors with rapid growth and spread, resulting in death.[3] Different host factors, including genotype, age, neuroendocrine influences and immune response, as well as complex interactions between these and other factors, may be of critical importance to determine the fate of a host affected by a given tumor. The term cancer is usually applied to advanced malignant disease with a high degree of malignant behavior.[4]

3. Comparative and Experimental Oncology

Although tumors can occur in most, or perhaps all, multicellular organisms, their incidence is highly variable among different animal and plant species. They may occur in an apparently spontaneous form or may be produced by many different types of environmental influences or experimental manipulations, which suggests that tumorigenic processes are intimately associated with the most essential phenomena of life.[5-7] In fact, the comparative study of tumors occurring in different species may be extremely valuable not only for a better knowledge of the tumors themselves but also understanding physiological phenomena and molecular processes of general biological interest.

Mainly because of practical reasons, rodents (mice, rats, rabbits, hamsters) have been extensively used as model animals for the experimental study of tumors and tumorigenic processes, whereas spontaneous tumors have been observed most frequently in domestic animals (dogs, cats, horses, cattle).[8,9] Obviously, the observations or results obtained in a given species cannot be extrapolated without limitations to another species, or even to different strains or individuals from the same species. However, it is apparent that the study of closely related species would permit more confident extrapolations. Studies in primates, especially higher primates, are most important for a better understanding of the etiopathogenetic processes involved in human cancer but, unfortunately, these studies are limited by factors such as the availability, cost and difficulty of manipulation of the animals. As a consequence, oncological studies on higher primates are scarce.[10] However, it must be recognized that at least some physiological and biochemical changes occurring in tumors from even distantly related species may be similar, if not essentially identical.

In any case, tumorigenic processes are exceedingly complex and multidisciplinary approaches should be more conveniently used for their appropriate study. The comparative analysis of experimental, clinical, and epidemiological studies may be fruitful for appreciating the relative importance of different factors involved in tumorigenic processes. It must be recognized that cancer is not a single nosological entity and that many identified or unidentified genetic and environmental factors, operating in intrincated manners, are almost always involved in the origin and development of spontaneous tumors. As a corollary, the prevention and treatment of cancer in general, or of certain types of cancer in particular, should not be considered with simplistic approaches, which are necessarily unrealistic.

II. NEOPLASTIC CELLS

Neoplastic cells are the result of processes of malignant transformation occurring either spontaneously or by the influence of specific oncogenic agents. In many aspects, these cells are

TABLE 1
Characteristics of Neoplastic Cells as Studied
In Vivo

Altered cell morphology
Increased nucleus/cytoplasm volume ratio
Increased heterochromatin/euchromatin ratio and changes in chromatin composition
Alterations in X chromosome inactivation and changes in X sex chromatin (Barr body)
Abnormalities of mitosis
Aneuploidy with a tendency to hyperdiploidy
Variation in the DNA content of individual cells
Structural chromosome abnormalities
Antigenic changes
Autonomous growth and uncontrolled cell proliferation
Invasion and metastasization

different from their normal counterparts. The characteristics of neoplastic cells can be studied either *in vivo* or *in vitro*.

A. CHARACTERISTICS OF NEOPLASTIC CELLS *IN VIVO*

The characteristics of neoplastic cells, as opposed to those of their normal counterparts, are very numerous and diverse. Moreover, great variation in different phenotypic characteristics may occur among different types of tumors, and even among different cells from a given tumor. Thus, only general rules can be mentioned. A list of the more important, or more useful, characteristics of neoplastic cells as studied *in vivo* appear in Table 1, and a brief description follows.

1. Altered Cell Morphology

The abnormal morphological features of cancer cells were recognized by the pioneer pathologists of the last century.[11] Alterations in cytoskeleton components (microfilaments, microtubules, and intermediate filaments) are importantly involved in cell shape abnormalities occurring in cancer cells.[12] In spite of countless studies on other types of characteristics, the morphological characteristics of cancer cells are still universally used in clinical practice for the diagnosis of malignant diseases.

2. Increased Nucleus/Cytoplasm Volume Ratio

The nucleus/cytoplasm volume ratio is usually increased in neoplastic cells, which may be attributed to the fact that these cells are most frequently hyperdiploid, that is, they have an increased amount of genetic material in comparison to their normal counterparts. In general, there is an excellent correlation between the amount of DNA within the nucleus of different types of normal or tumor cells and their respective nuclear volumes.[13]

3. Increased Heterochromatin/Euchromatin Ratio and Changes in Chromatin Composition

An increased affinity of the chromatin of neoplastic cells for chromatin dyes has been used for almost a century as a valuable criterion for the histological diagnosis of cancer. Heterochromatin corresponds to the repressed, nonfunctional portions of the genome, whereas euchromatin corresponds to the derepressed, actively transcribing portions of the genome. A progressive heterochromatinization occurs in the nuclei of liver cells in the course of liver carcinogenesis induced by chemical agents.[14] These morphological changes partially reflect quantitative and qualitative alterations occurring in the chromatin of liver cells during the sequential events of hepatocarcinogenesis, with appearance of new nonhistone protein species in both eu- and heterochromatin.[15]

4. Alterations in X Chromosome Inactivation and Changes in X Sex Chromatin (Barr Body)

The X sex chromatin, also called Barr body, may be observed in more than 30% of the interphase nuclei of most cells containing two or more X chromosomes, and, consequently, in mammals it is found only in somatic cells of the female. In general, the number of Barr bodies in a given cell is equal to the number of X chromosomes minus one, the latter corresponding to the actively transcribing X chromosome. The inactivation of X chromosomes to form Barr bodies is apparently associated with a process of hypermethylation of DNA sequences,[16] which determines an almost complete transcriptional silence of the whole X chromosome. Barr bodies are difficult to visualize in neoplastic cells due to the aforementioned increase in the heterochromatin fraction and other morphological changes occurring in the nucleus, but there is evidence that their number and/or structure may be abnormal at least in some types of cancer cells whereas no changes are observed in benign tumors.[17-19] However, no correlation exists between the incidence of Barr bodies in malignant tumors and different prognostic factors like the spread and histological grading of the tumor.[20] The measurement of X-linked enzymatic activities in female teratocarcinoma cells, which are malignant cells containing two X chromosomes, give conflictive results as to whether only one or both X chromosomes are active in the tumor cells.[21,22]

5. Abnormalities of Mitosis

The presence of mitotic abnormalities in histological preparations from tumors was also recognized by the turn of the last century and it is still one of the criteria most used by pathologists for the diagnosis of malignancy. The mitotic abnormalities include chromatin bridges, chromosome lagging, multipolar synchronic mitoses, and other alterations reflecting the existence of numerical and/or structural chromosome changes. In some instances acentric fragments may be seen in the equator of the dividing cell.

6. Aneuploidy with a Tendency to Hyperdiploidy

Almost all neoplastically transformed cells are aneuploid, i.e., they have abnormal number of chromosomes.[23-28] Tumor progression may be associated with higher degrees of aneuploidy as observed, for example, in human melanoma.[29] A general tendency to increased chromosome numbers (hyperdiploidy) is observed in tumor cells. Moreover, a large variation in the chromosome number characteristically occurs among different cells from a given tumor and the modal number of chromosomes is almost always elevated. However, in some cells from a tumor the chromosome number may be rather low, even pseudohaploid. Extremely high numbers of chromosomes would correspond to dividing multinuclear cells.

7. Variation in the DNA Content of Individual Cells

In interphase cells the ploidy abnormalities may be studied by methods such as static cytometry and flow cytometry, which allow an approximate determination of the DNA content of individual cells.[30,31] In contrast to normal and reactive histopathologic changes and benign tumors, which are usually diploid, more than 90% of human malignant tumors show aneuploidy when studied with DNA flow cytometry, and most aneuploid tumors are hyperdiploid,[32] which is in accordance with the results obtained by cytogenetic methods. A variety of human tumors show a bimodal distribution of DNA content, with tumors having a near diploid mode or a triploid-tetraploid mode. With few exceptions, tumors exhibit stability of ploidy both spatially and temporally. Tumor ploidy reflects the biological behavior of different tumor types, and the diploid tumors have a general tendency to a relatively good prognosis.[31]

8. Structural Chromosome Abnormalities

The presence of marker chromosomes, i.e., chromosomes that cannot be classified according to the normal idiogram of the species, is also a useful criterion for the diagnosis of neoplastic transformation.[23] Marker chromosomes are generated by deletions, translocations, inversions, and other structural changes. A classic example is the Philadelphia (Ph or Ph[1]) chromosome,[33] which is generally considered as a reliable marker for human chronic myeloid leukemia (CML) and consists of a deleted autosome 22.[34] However, this chromosome abnormality does not represent a simple deletion but is generated by a reciprocal translocation between human chromosomes 9 and 22.[35] Some other marker chromosomes have been described in human and non-human malignancies.[36] In general, the presence of marker chromosomes is highly suggestive of neoplastic transformation.

9. Antigenic Changes

Many different antigenic changes have been described in neoplastic cells but not one of them has been found to represent a universal characteristic of malignancy. In general, natural tumors are much less immunogenic than experimental tumors, especially virus-induced or virus-associated tumors, but it is not known whether this is due to structural differences in the antigens expressed on the cell surface or whether this difference reflects the nature of the different types of tumor cells themselves.[37] In any case, some tumors are able to grow in autologous or syngeneic hosts because of their poor immunogenicity, despite the fact that they express potential tumor-associated rejection antigens.

The hope that monoclonal antibodies would reveal unique cell surface antigens during embryogenesis, differentiation, and oncogenesis has been replaced by the realization that such antigens are mainly determined by carbohydrate structures of glycoproteins and glycolipids occurring in many cell types.[38] Antigenic markers that may distinguish tumor cells from their normal counterparts belong to a family of carbohydrate structures which includes blood group antigens. Some structures which behave as tumor-associated antigens in certain cell types are normal components of others.[39] The oligosaccharide sequences of cell antigenic structures are composed of different sugars (fucose, galactose, *N*-acetylgalactosamine, and sialic acid residues) and are joined to the backbone structures in various positions and linkages by action of specific glycosyltransferases. However, unique antigenic determinants conditioned by abnormal oligosaccharide sequences are usually not found in tumors; in particular, they are not found in human tumors. Since many antibodies may react with the carbohydrate components of tumor-associated proteins, such as mucin glycoproteins expressed in relation to differentiation stages in the normal mammary gland and in breast tumors, antibodies can be conveniently raised, after carbohydrate stripping, against the core protein which may be encoded by a polymorphic gene.[40] Variability in the carbohydrate moieties of plasma membrane proteins may represent an important source for the phenotypic heterogeneity which characterizes tumor cells.[41]

The antigenic changes of neoplastic cells may consist in aberrant expression, deletion, or modulation of normal antigens, expression of fetal antigens, or presence of neoantigens. Some of these changes, as well as other changes observed in neoplastic cells, have been applied as clinically useful markers for the detection and following up of human tumors.[42-44]

Aberrant expression of blood group and histocompatibility antigens may occur in tumors. Different types of altered expression of blood group antigens has been detected in solid human tumors by means of specific monoclonal antibodies.[45] In human prostatic adenocarcinomas and breast carcinomas, A and B structures of blood group isoantigens are frequently lost, but there is a continued expression of both the H and Y antigens in the great majority of these tumors as well as in their metastases.[46,47] A and B blood group isoantigens were also found to be reduced, and occasionally absent, from areas of benign human prostatic hypertrophy as well as from benign human mammary fibrocystic disease and mammary fibroadenomas.[47] Tn and T blood group precursor antigens are present in most normal human tissues but are masked, being covered by covalent linked carbohydrates. These antigens, however, may be unmasked in the cells from human mammary carcinomas and other tumors.[48]

The major histocompatibility complex (MHC) is importantly involved in the recognition and rejection of foreign cells or tissues as well as in the immune responses to cells that have undergone neoplastic transformation. In the human, the MHC is represented by the HLA system, whereas in the mouse it is represented by the H-2 complex.[49] The genetic locus of the human MHC complex has been mapped to the short arm of chromosome 6, at region 6p21.3.[50] Both mouse and human MHCs are constituted by multigene families whose members encode cell surface glycoproteins involved in the recognition and immune response to antigens of either exogenous or endogenous origin. The latter may be exemplified by abnormal MHC antigens present in neoplastically transformed cells. Experimental and clinical investigations have shown that quantitative and qualitative variations in the expression of MHC molecules are important in host-tumor interactions.[51] In murine experimental systems, the anomalous expression of MHC antigens in the tumor cells may be associated with the ability of these cells to evade the immune systems of the host and progress to metastasis.[52,53] Expression of a single MHC class I antigen, introduced by DNA-mediated gene transfer into highly tumorigenic mouse cells transformed with human adenovirus, may be sufficient to abrogate the oncogenicity of these cells.[54] A novel class I MHC molecule isolated from the murine UV light-induced regression tumor 1591 may represent a unique tumor-associated antigen capable of inducing tumor rejection.[55]

Lack of expression of normal antigens may be observed in a diversity of transformed cells *in vitro* and tumors *in vivo*.[56-58] Among 100 primary human colorectal carcinomas and 19 metastases of these tumors, loss of MHC class I antigens (HLA-A, HLA-B, and HLA-C), as determined by monoclonal antibodies and immunohistochemical methods, was inversely correlated to the degree of differentiation.[59] Expression of MHC class II (HLA-D) antigens was observed in 42% of the primary tumors in the same series, irrespective of the tumor grade. About half of the metastases in this series displayed the same staining pattern for class I and class II HLA antigens as the respective primary tumors; the remainder differed from the primary carcinoma by gain of loss of HLA antigens. Findings that are partially similar to those of HLA antigens have been reported for ABH and Lewis blood group antigens in a series of 63 human colon carcinomas.[60] In this series, expression of the ABH and Lewis antigens in the metastases was similar to that of the primary tumors, and alterations in antigen expression were not clinically or histologically distinctive.

Antigen loss from the cell surface of tumor cells may be limited to some classes, whereas other antigens may be preserved even in highly malignant cells. For example, a highly malignant variant of mouse fibrosarcoma 1591 which grew even in immune hosts had lost all known antigens defined by cytotoxic lymphocytes but retained antigens recognized by T helper cells.[61]

The loss of antigens from the surface of tumor cells may be attributed to genome repression or to defective synthesis, including defective glycosylation due to loss or repression of the necessary glycosyl transferases, which would correspond to true antigen deletion. Lack of expression of MHC class I H-2 antigens in murine thymocytes transformed by radiation leukemia virus (Rad-MuLV) is associated with increased methylation and rearrangements of MHC DNA loci.[62] Antigen modulation, on the other hand, would consist of the hiding of normal antigen determinants which are normally present on the cell surface. This hiding may be produced by changes in the structure and biochemical composition of the cell surface. Sialomucins, which are sialic acid-containing glycoproteins, may be abundantly present on the surface of tumor cells and may act as "antirecognition factors", thus contributing to the "masking" of cell surface antigens.[63] Such masking effect may prevent immune destruction of tumor cells. However, it is difficult to distinguish between antigen modulation and true antigen deletion. In any case, a lack of expression of normal antigens on the cell surface may help malignant cells to escape from immune surveillance and to acquire more aggressive properties of invasion and metastasization.

A wide diversity of tumors may produce increased amounts of fetal-type antigens (oncofetal antigens). Production of oncofetal antigens by transformed cells is a frequent phenomenon that can be attributed to alterations in genome regulation with a pattern of gene expression which tends to be similar to that of embryonic and fetal stages.[64-68] This phenomenon has been termed retrodifferentiation; however, a neoplastically transformed cell is probably never identical to its embryonic or fetal cell counterpart. In any case, the expression by neoplastic cells of antigens (and enzymes) specific for particular differentiation stages of the respective cell lineage may be of great importance for the classification of malignancies, especially hematologic malignancies.[69-72] These antigens can be detected by specific monoclonal antibodies and correspond to specific stages of differentiation that are blocked in neoplastically transformed cells.[73]

The study of blood group antigen expression in human endometrial carcinoma indicated that H and Lewis-b antigens can be considered as oncofetal antigens, since they are frequently expressed in fetal and cancer tissues but not in normal adult tissues.[74] Increased expression of Lewis-a antigen might be associated with neoplastic transformation as it was observed only in malignant tissues. Expression of blood group antigens A and B compatible with ABO status of the patient remained the same in normal and endometrial cancer tissue.

Some oncofetal antigens such as the carcinoembryonic antigen (CEA) and α-fetoprotein (AFP) have found a widespread application as markers for the diagnosis, prognosis, and following up of the particular types of malignant diseases. CEA is a complex immunoreactive glycoprotein of 180 kDa comprising 60% carbohydrate found mainly in adenocarcinomas of endodermally derived digestive system epithelia as well as in fetal colon. The gene coding for human CEA has been cloned as a cDNA copy which encodes for a 668-amino acid polypeptide whose first 108 amino-terminal residues are followed by three very homologous repetitive domains of 178 residues each and then by 26 mostly hydrophobic residues which probably comprise a membrane anchor site.[75] Each repetitive domain contains four cysteines at precisely the same positions.

Some neoplastic cells may express antigens that are apparently not present in their normal counterparts.[76-79] These apparently unique, abnormal antigens, are called neoantigens, tumor antigens, tumor-associated antigens (TAAs), or tumor-specific transplantation antigens (TSTAs). Antigens present in tumors such as human melanomas may correspond to modifications of normally occurring proteins.[80] The expression of neoantigens of endogenous origin could be attributed to somatic mechanisms involving mutation, derepression of cellular genes (including endogenous viruses), operation of abnormal biosynthetic pathways, or altered action of enzymes such as glycosyltransferases in certain neoplastic cells. Other possible mechanisms are gene duplication or rearrangement and altered RNA splicing.

Unique tumor antigens have been observed especially in mice, when the tumors are induced with the same carcinogen in the same organ system and in the same strain of mice. However, the expression of such antigens is frequently unpredictable and highly variable, not only among different types of tumors but also among different tumors of the same type and even from one cell to another within a given tumor. Studies with monoclonal antibodies have indicated that most, and perhaps all, of the tumor antigenic markers defined by xenogeneic monoclonal antibodies are not strictly tumor specific but are differentiation antigens shared by tumors and certain normal adult and/or fetal tissues.[81] Only viral antigens constitute an exception to this general rule but such antigens are coded by the genome of viruses that can be associated with the neoplastic transformation of normal cells or that can infect cells transformed by other agents. Notwithstanding, cells transformed by oncogenic retroviruses such as ASV may express cell type-specific antigens which are not encoded by the virus but by the host cell genome.[82] Tumor variants display distinct antigenic properties that may be involved in modulating host immune responses. An inverse relationship may exist between the level of TAA expression and tumorigenicity.[83]

The normal functions of most of the antigens present on the surface of normal or tumor cells are little understood. Two polypeptide isoforms of a mouse TSTA purified from a methylcholan-threne (MC)-induced sarcoma have been identified as phosphoproteins whose amino-terminal sequences are similar or identical to the major 85-kDa murine stress heat shock-related protein, HSP-85.[84] Particular types antigens that can be detected on the cell surface by using specific monoclonal antibodies may be involved in regulating the proliferation of normal or neoplastic cells.[85] Binding of the specific monoclonal antibody to the antigen present on the cell surface may then result in inhibition of cell growth both *in vitro* and *in vivo*.

10. Autonomous Growth and Uncontrolled Cell Proliferation

One of the most important characteristics of neoplastic cells is their relatively autonomous behavior with respect to the intrinsic and extrinsic mechanisms involved in the control of DNA synthesis and cell proliferation, which results in a tendency to indefinite growth. Transformed cells may be able to produce growth factors and may utilize these factors for their own growth in an autocrine manner.[86] For example, rat mammary epithelial cells transformed by chemical carcinogens (DMBA or NMU) display a markedly enhanced growth potential in long-term culture, as compared with the respective normal cells, and a subset of these cells acquire independence of the exogenous supply of specific growth factors and exhibit high neoplastic potential *in vivo*.[87] However, autocrine-stimulated growth is not an exclusive property of malignant cells and can also occur in different types of normal tissues, including human placenta and skin.[88,89] Autocrine growth factors are produced by both normal and immortalized Schwann cells.[90] Normal arterial smooth muscle cells are also able to maintain their own growth in an autocrine or paracrine manner.[91] Moreover, malignant cells may acquire growth factor independency through mechanisms not clearly involving autocrine phenomena. Karyotypic changes are associated, at least in some cases, with the acquisition of nonautocrine, growth factor-independent growth of malignant cells.[92,93] The acquisition of growth factor-independent growth by some transformed cells, e.g., human hematopoietic cells coinfected with two acute retroviruses, is a rare event observed only after crisis of the culture and is apparently due to the occurrence of karyotypic changes. Interestingly, studies with somatic cell hybrids formed by crossing neoplastic mouse cells with normal human fibroblasts indicate that the hybrid cells have a reduced ability to proliferate in growth factor-unsupplemented, serum-free medium relative to the neoplastic cells and that this reduction is associated with the presence of specific chromosome combinations in the hybrid cells.[94] These results suggest a role for chromosomal genes in suppression of growth in serum-free medium.

Neoplastic transformation of cells may be associated with a primary defect in the mechanisms involved in the regulation of specific phases of the cell cycle, which would lead to a loss of the normal control of cell proliferation.[95-97] Uncontrolled nuclear division would represent one of the components in the process leading to the malignant behavior of cells.[98] However, the general validity of this postulate is not readily apparent in all cellular systems. No fundamental differences have been detected in the kinetics of neoplastic hematopoietic progenitor cells and their normal counterparts.[99]

The molecular mechanisms of action of extra- or intracellular factors involved in the control of DNA synthesis and cell proliferation remain little understood. These mechanisms must function in different ways for different tissues, and this should also be true according to the different physiological conditions of the tissue or the whole organism. The rate of cell proliferation in a particular tissue would depend on delicate and tissue-specific equilibria between the action of positive, stimulating factors and negative, inhibiting factors.[100] Exogenous agents such as hormones and peptide growth factors are critically involved in controlling the rate of cell proliferation in their respective target organs and tissues.[86] Hormones and growth factors can act as either stimulators or inhibitors of cell growth. Other humoral influences may exist, although they have not been well characterized. For example, little progress has occurred in the last years on the purification and characterization of chalones, which are defined as tissue-specific factors capable of inhibiting the proliferation of immature cells.[101-108]

11. Invasion and Metastasization

Acquisition of potentialities for the invasion of neighbor normal tissues and for remote dissemination through the production of metastases are among the the most important biological and clinical characteristics of tumor cells. The malignant behavior of tumor cells crucially depend on their properties to invade and metastasize. These characteristics are discussed in detail in a later section of this chapter.

B. CHARACTERISTICS OF NEOPLASTIC CELLS *IN VITRO*

Malignant transformation of cells in culture may occur either spontaneously or, more likely, by the influence of specific environmental factors.[109] The susceptibility of cultured cells to spontaneous or induced transformation *in vitro* is highly variable depending on the species of origin, the type of cell, and other factors. Embryonic or fetal fibroblasts from different rodent species (mouse, rat, hamster, guinea pig) have been utilized in most studies because they are easy to manipulate and are more susceptible to be transformed by a diversity of environmental agents. In general, human cells are resistant to transformation induced *in vitro* and spontaneous transformation of human fibroblasts in culture has not been reported.[110]

Transformed cells cultured *in vitro* are probably not exact replicas of their *in vivo* growing counterparts but they are useful for the study of several properties of neoplastic cells that cannot be analyzed, or are difficult to analyze, under *in vivo* conditions. In any case, the results obtained with cultured cells, such as tumor cell lines of different origins, should be considered with caution and free extrapolation of these results to the respective *in vivo* situation is not justified. Moreover, transformation as defined *in vitro* does not necessarily associate with tumorigenicity *in vivo*.[111-113] Many characteristics have been described in cultured transformed cells, as listed in Table 2, but several of them are not universally present and only selected aspects of this subject are discussed here.

1. Disordered Pattern of Growth

Among the characteristics mentioned in Table 2 the altered pattern of growth of transformed cells is very noticeable, as reflected by a tendency of these cells to grow in the form of multilayer, disordered structures as opposed to the monolayer, ordered growth pattern of normal cells. To the naked eye this abnormality may be observed in plate cultures as dense foci, which are constituted by numerous piled cells. In addition, this alteration is associated with changes in the cell shape and pleomorphism.

2. Decreased Requirement for Serum

Another prominent characteristic of transformed cells maintained in culture is a decreased requirement for serum. This change reflects an autonomous behavior of transformed cells in relation to exogenous regulatory signal molecules, including hormones and peptide growth factors.[86] The decreased dependency from factors contained in serum is due in some, but not all, cases to the endogenous production and utilization of growth factors through autocrine mechanisms.

3. Expression of Extracellular Matrix Molecules

The synthesis and expression of extracellular matrix molecules such as procollagen, fibronectin, and laminin is frequently altered in transformed cells. For example, untransformed mouse embryo fibroblasts AKR-2B express high levels of surface fibronectin and lower levels of laminin.[114] After transformation with 3-methylcholanthrene (MCA), the cells express less fibronectin and greater amounts of laminin. Induction of differentiation of the transformed cells

TABLE 2
Characteristics of Neoplastic Cells as Studied
In Vitro

Disordered pattern of growth
Loss of density-dependent inhibition of growth
Altered cell communication
Reduced requirement for serum in the medium (increased autonomy)
Alterations in cell aggregation
Decreased adhesivity
Increased motility
Alterations of the cyclic AMP content
Changes in plasminogen activator and other protease surface activities
Increased agglutinability by lectins and changes in surface glycoproteins
Changes in the transport of glucose, amino acids, and other nutrients
Changes in membrane transport of ions
Loss of anchorage dependency and growth in semisolid medium (soft agar)
Alterations in the cytoskeletal components
Block in the expression of differentiated functions
Acquisition of an indefinite lifespan (potential immortality)

with *N,N*-dimethylformamide resulted in rapid attachment and spread on the coated dishes, which was associated with restored fibronectin expression and reduced expression of laminin on the cell surface.[114] The synthesis and degradation of extracellular matrix components is regulated by hormones and growth factors as well as by oncogene and protooncogene products.

4. Altered Cell Communication

Cell communication through transmembrane channels, called gap junctions, is important for the exchange between contacting cells of ions and small molecules that may be involved in the regulation of cellular functions, including cell growth and differentiation. A number of studies suggest that altered cell communication may be a common characteristic of transformed cells. For example, studies with microinjection of a dye (Lucifer yellow dye) indicate that transformed cells within foci in culture exhibit only limited communication with each other as well as with surrounding monolayer cells.[115] Lack of communication between transformed and nontransformed cells may contribute to maintain autonomous growth. However, the exact nature of this alteration, as well as its possible role in the origin, development, and maintenance of a transformed phenotype, remain to be elucidated.[116]

5. Loss of Density-Dependent Inhibition of Growth

Normal cells growing *in vitro* put a stop to DNA synthesis and proliferation upon establishing intimate contact with neighbor cells. In contrast, in transformed cells growth is not arrested upon this contact, which determines the afore mentioned disordered pattern of growth with "piling up" of a number of cells.[117-118] The mechanisms involved in loss of density-dependent inhibition of growth (also termed contact inhibition of growth) are not well understood but could depend on structural and/or functional alterations at the level of the cell surface, altered transmission of signals from the cell surface to the nucleus, and/or altered response of the nucleus to these signals. Unfortunately, the cell surface structures and the chemical signals responsible for the phenomenon of density-dependent inhibition of growth have not been identified. However, there is evidence that cell-surface receptors can act as sensors of a complex "cell-surface code" involved in the recognition and transmission of specific signals from the cell surface to the inner structures of the cell. A growing body of evidence supports the hypothesis that particular carbohydrates in form of glycoconjugates can have an important role in acting as cell-cell recognition structures in this system.[120]

The possibility that density-dependent inhibition of growth depends on the release of particular molecules should also be considered. An inhibitory activity, probably represented by a protein of 45 kDa, termed IDF45, acts as an inhibitory factor diffusing from 3T3 mouse fibroblast cells. IDF45 is capable of decreasing DNA synthesis and inhibits growth of chick embryo fibroblasts (FEBs) in a reversible manner.[121-122] The protein product of the v-*src* oncogene of Rous sarcoma virus (RSV) apparently induces loss of sensitivity to IDF45, which would explain why RSV-transformed cells escape to the mechanisms controlling density-dependent inhibition of growth and continue to proliferate up until depletion of the culture medium.

6. Loss of Anchorage Dependency

Whereas normal cells usually require a solid support for growing under *in vitro* conditions, transformed cells display an enhanced ability to grow in suspension in semisolid media, especially in soft agar.[123] Primary human tumors such as ovarian tumors and renal-cell carcinomas show a highly significant correlation between the presence of an abnormal (aneuploid) DNA stemline and the ability of the tumor to form colonies in soft agar.[124] Among the different properties of cultured neoplastic cells, growth in soft agar shows one of the best correlations with tumorigenicity and capacity to metastasization *in vivo*. The remarkable ability of transformed cells to grow in soft agar has constituted the basis for the widespread application of a tumor stem cell clonogenic assay.[125] The growing characteristics of fresh human tumor specimens in soft agar have been extensively used not only for the study of individual patients' response to chemotherapy and for the screening of new chemotherapeutic agents but also for the study of the fundamental biological properties of tumor cell growth *in vitro*.

There are, however, exceptions to the general rule of a close correlation between anchorage independence *in vitro* and tumorigenicity *in vivo*. Not only may many transformed cells retain anchorage dependence but also nontransformed cell lines may grow in soft agar. In fact, there is no single property of transformed cells which correlates perfectly with tumorigenicity.[126] Thus, anchorage independence, although useful for oncological *in vitro* studies, cannot be considered as an exclusive hallmark of tumor cells.

The ability to grow in soft agar may vary from cell to cell, even among related cloned populations of transformed cells, and it cannot be considered as an inherited, stable property of the transformed cells.[127] Rather, this property is phenotypically unstable and cells isolated from different agar colonies may exhibit upon continuous growth *in vitro* an increase, no increase, or loss of their ability to grow in soft agar. Particular types of growth factors (PDGF, FGF, TGF-β) may participate through complex interactions in the induction and modulation of anchorage-independent growth.[128] Moreover, at least one of these factors (PDGF) is able to induce the soft agar growth of several nontransformed cell lines. Human monocytes can secrete factors that enhance growth of epithelial tumor colonies and cloning efficiencies of autologous tumor cells in soft agar.[129] It is thus evident that the humoral microenvironment is of great importance in determining the behavior of either normal or transformed cells in culture.

7. Block in the Expression of Differentiated Functions

A partial or total block in the expression of particular types of differentiated functions is one of the most important characteristics of malignant cells when compared with their normal counterparts. Some specialized functions, however, may be conserved by many kinds of malignant cells. For example, an analysis of clonal variability of derivatives of the rat hepatoma cell line H4IIEC3, adapted to growth *in vitro* from the Reuber H35 hepatoma, has shown that the overwhelming majority of clones express in a stable fashion a number of liver-specific differentiated functions, including secretion of serum albumin, activity of the liver-specific isozymes of alcohol dehydrogenase and aldolase, and high basal activity and hormone inducibility of tyrosine and alanine aminotransferases.[130] However, in some clones of this hepatoma cell line no expression of any of specialized liver functions is detectable, whereas other clones show diminished but significant expression of two or three of the functions.[130] None of the clones shows a total deficiency of only one of the functions and undiminished expression of the others, which suggests that a single change, either genetic or epigenetic, may be responsible for the altered expression of differentiated functions occurring in the hepatoma cells.

8. Potential Immortality

Another important characteristic of transformed cultured cells cultured *in vitro* is an apparently infinite life span, i.e., a potential immortality.[131-134] Cultured normal, diploid cells have limited life spans *in vitro*, which in the case of human diploid cells would correspond to approximately 50 serial passages of the cells. Thereafter, the doubling time increases exponentially and the cultured cells die away even when the environmental conditions are optimal. In contrast, aneuploid, transformed cells have an apparent potential to indefinite growth under adequate environmental conditions (supply of nutrients, renewal of the medium, etc). Of course, the potential immortality of neoplastically transformed cells cannot be expressed *in vivo* because they commit suicide when they kill the host.

Morphologic transformation and immortalization may be separate and distinct steps in the multistage process of neoplastic transformation and they may be dissociated under specific experimental conditions.[135,136] In general, immortalization is a very rare event which is induced at extremely low frequencies in human diploid cell populations, whereas characteristics of morphologic transformation may be induced quite readily in the same cells. This is in contradistinction to the process in rodent cells, in which immortalization is an early and frequent event under similar experimental conditions.

The biological changes responsible for the immortalization of transformed cells have not been characterized but may include genomic changes such as point mutations and/or DNA rearrangements. Particular types of chromosome aberrations may be related to the acquisition of prolonged or indefinite life by cells maintained in culture.[137] This acquisition may be lost by certain transformed cells after prolonged culture *in vitro.* For example, clonal attenuation of the growth potential *in vitro* has been observed in HeLa cells after serial passages in culture,[138] which may represent a consequence of clonal senescence or terminal differentiation. Moreover, immortality is not an exclusive property of transformed cells. Normal mammalian embryonic stem cells, prior to segregation into germinal and somatic elements, can divide indefinitely under appropriate conditions *in vitro* without apparent "crisis" or transformation.[139] Thus, embryonic and malignant cells share the same fundamental characteristic of potential immortality.

9. Summary

Among the characteristics listed in Table 2 no one can be considered as absolutely specific of transformation and they can develop independently of one another.[113] Even immortality can be dissociated from the others. Moreover, many of these characteristics show a rather poor correlation with tumorigenicity *in vivo* when tested by the ability to form a tumor in the animal.[111] Anchorage independence, reflected in the ability of cells to grow in a semisolid medium (soft agar), shows a good but not perfect correlation with tumorigenicity. The transformed phenotype, as studied *in vitro*, should be more conveniently defined by an ensemble of altered cellular characteristics than by the occasional appearance of one or a few of these characteristics. Unfortunately, terms such as "transformation", "transformed phenotype", "malignant transformation", and "oncogenic transformation" are frequently used in a rather loosely manner. Many reported instances of *in vitro* transformation may be laboratory artifacts, not having good correlation with the tumorigenic ability of cells in appropriate hosts.

III. ORIGIN AND DEVELOPMENT OF TUMORS

The development of a tumor is a complex process which occurs through a series of stages

TABLE 3
Etiopathogenic Factors of Neoplasia

Endogenous factors	Exogenous factors
Genetic factors	Radiation
Immunologic factors	Trauma
Hormonal factors	Chemical carcinogens
Metabolic factors	Oncogenic viruses
Etary factors	

starting with certain alterations suffered by apparently normal cells.[140-143] The initial cellular alterations that may lead to the development of a tumor are still poorly understood and may occur either spontaneously or, more likely, by the action of oncogenic factors. Both genetic and environmental factors are involved in the origin and development of neoplasia. The etiopathogenetic factors of neoplasia may be conveniently classified in endogenous and exogenous (Table 3). In the etiologic spectrum of diseases, which spans from purely genetic diseases to purely environmental diseases, cancer should be usually located to the middle part of the spectrum, in the group of common diseases, which are attributable to a complex interaction of genetic and environmental factors, i.e., to multifactoriality.

In general, the tumorigenic process may be divided into two successive stages, i.e., preneoplasia and neoplasia. The fundamental difference between these stages would reside in the possibility of reversion. Whereas preneoplastic changes are potentially reversible, especially under appropriate environmental conditions, neoplastic lesions are essentially irreversible and may progress until formation of the tumor.

A. PRENEOPLASTIC STAGE

The term "precancerous" was coined by the end of the last century for some epidermal changes showing increased liability to subsequent malignant transformation.[144] During the preneoplastic stage normal cells, or cells which are apparently normal, undergo changes that determine in them a predisposition or an enhanced possibility to be transformed into cells with a clear malignant behavior. Preneoplastic cells may have defects in the ability to maintain an integral control of their differentiation and proliferation.[145] These cells may be immortal and aneuploid and may show a proclivity to undergo spontaneous or induced neoplastic transformation.

Sequential alterations in growth control and cell dynamics are observed in rat hepatocytes during early precancerous stages of hepatocarcinogenesis.[146] Foci of altered (atypical) liver cells appear in rats after a combined treatment with a carcinogenic compound (DENA) and partial hepatectomy.[147] However, under natural conditions most cells from preneoplastic lesions are either destroyed or may revert to normalcy. Nodular hepatocellular lesions induced by feeding rats *N*-2-fluorenylacetamide are phenotypically stable and differ from liver carcinomas in their biological behavior, not representing authentic premalignant lesions.[148] In fact, only a small fraction of the cells from preneoplastic lesions, or a minority of preneoplastic lesions in general, will give rise to malignant tumors,[149] and processes of "redifferentiation" or "remodeling" may regularly occur within populations of preneoplastic cells.[150] Host factors, including genetic factors,[151] are critically involved in determining the fate of preneoplastic lesions in particular individuals.

1. Age Dependency of Preneoplastic Changes

Preneoplastic changes may occur either spontaneously or by action of different types of carcinogenic agents (radiation, chemical agents, oncogenic viruses). The appearance of spontaneous preneoplastic changes in different cell populations *in vivo* may be an age-dependent phenomenon. Development of preneoplastic rat tracheal epithelial cells in culture occurs at a constant rate ($7.5 \times 4.1 \times 10^{-6}$), which results in high frequencies of altered cells.[152] These and other observations are consistent with the hypothesis that spontaneous changes play a role in the multistep progression of cells to cancer.

2. Relationship between Hyperplasia, Dysplasia, and Preneoplasia

Hyperplasia, dysplasia, and preneoplasia may be interrelated phenomena. Hyperplasia of the C-cells in the thyroid gland may precede the appearance of medullary thyroid carcinoma in individuals genetically predisposed to this tumor.[153] Cytological screening studies indicate that women with slight dysplasia of the uterine cervix have a risk of cervical carcinoma several times that of women with negative Papanicolaou smears.[154] The age-adjusted death rate from prostate cancer is several times higher in patients with benign prostatic hyperplasia than in controls.[155] However, it is difficult to elucidate whether the hyperplasia and the cancer are interrelated as subsequent stages of the same pathologic process or whether they are independently caused by some common unknown factor(s) resulting in the observed statistical association. Moreover, results from other studies did not demonstrate that patients with benign prostatic hyperplasia are at increased risk for prostatic cancer.[156]

Foci of preneoplastic cells may arise in the liver, after administration of carcinogenic agents, from populations of hyperplastic cells that are contributing to regenerative processes within damaged organs.[157-162] A similar sequence of events, from normalcy to hyperplasia and neoplasia, would occur in the mammary gland of female mice after administration of chemical carcinogens like 7,12-dimethylbenz(a)anthracene (DMBA) and can be mimicked in organ *in vitro* systems.[163] In the stomach of rats, hyperplastic and dysplastic lesions may be observed after administration of N-methyl-N'-nitro-N-nitrosoguanidine (MNNG), and carcinomas may arise in some of these lesions, although most gastric cancers in these animals seem to develop directly from the otherwise unchanged gastric mucosa.[164] In the respiratory tract mucosa of rodents exposed to some chemical carcinogens a high incidence of metaplastic and dysplastic lesions is observed but the ultimate incidence of invasive carcinomas is low and the incidence of lesions diminish with time.[165] Thus, with no further exposure to either carcinogenic or tumor-promoting agents, many preneoplastic lesions of the respiratory tract of these animals, including highly dysplastic ones, may regress. In any case, the question may be raised as to whether the preneoplastic cells in the hyperplastic tissue evolve, by some unknown mechanism, into neoplastic cells or whether both hyperplastic and neoplastic cells coexist in the initial lesion in their respective microenvironment.

3. Phenotypic Alterations of Preneoplastic Cells

Preneoplastic cells may be recognized on the ground of different kinds of alterations, including enzymatic and antigenic changes, chromosome abnormalities, and morphological characteristics.[166,167] The latter are frequently used by the pathologist for the diagnosis of hyperplasia, dysplasia, focal atypia, carcinoma *in situ,* or preneoplasia in lesions occurring in different human organs, such as the uterine cervix, the endometrium, the mammary gland, the prostate, the stomach, and the esophagus.[168-175] Although the diagnosis and grading of such lesions are based on somewhat arbitrary criteria, frequently depending on the experience and criteria of the pathologist, it is generally accepted that dysplastic lesions represent, at least in certain organs, true preneoplastic lesions. In any case, the large majority of lesions of the human uterine cervix or other organs classified as dysplasia, focal atypia, or carcinoma *in situ* will show a spontaneous complete regression and only a small fraction of such preneoplastic lesions will turn eventually into invasive carcinomas.[168]

Hematologic diseases classified as preleukemic or myelodysplastic syndromes are characterized by a variety of structural, biochemical, and cytogenetic abnormalities in the bone marrow and /or the peripheral blood cells. Myelodysplastic syndromes represent a diverse spectrum of disorders ranging from refractory anemia to a preleukemic state with enhanced likelihood of developing ANLL.[176] In patients with suspected preleukemia, the frequency of individual abnormalities is highly variable and, in many patients with suspected preleukemia, leukemia will never develop.[177-184]

Karyometric analysis of liver cell dysplasia and hepatocellular carcinoma yields evidence against a precancerous nature of liver cell dysplasia.[185] Metaplastic lesions occurring in the human intestine are heterogeneous, representing various patterns of differentiation and maturation of the metaplastic glands.[186] Most intestinal metaplasias show small bowel-like properties but may later acquire properties that resemble those of the colonic mucosa along with the increasing age of the patients and the increasing extent of intestinal metaplasia in the stomach. Intestinal metaplasias with colon-like characteristics seem to be linked with the morphogenesis of gastric carcinoma more clearly and more specifically than intestinal metaplasias in general. It seems thus clear that lesions classified as metaplastic or preneoplastic for both solid tumors and leukemias are highly heterogeneous from one case to another and, moreover, that they are constituted by intralesional highly heterogeneous cell populations. Consequently, the biological fate and the evolution of a given preneoplastic cell, or a given preneoplastic lesion, cannot be anticipated.

B. NEOPLASTIC STAGE

In the neoplastic stage, preneoplastic cells, or perhaps also cells that are apparently normal,[187,188] undergo essentially irreversible changes which determine in them the expression of a transformed phenotype, associated with a block of cell differentiation and increased rate of cell proliferation.[95,188,189] Uncontrolled nuclear division may be an important feature distinguishing preneoplastic from neoplastic cells.[190] In general, these alterations are heritable at the cellular level, and a neoplastic cell may give origin to a clone of similarly abnormal cells, whose continuous proliferation in a susceptible host might result in the formation of a tumor recognizable by clinical procedures.

IV. NEOPLASTIC PROCESS

The neoplastic process, as observed *in vivo* under either natural or experimental conditions, is usually a protracted one. Most frequently, a long period of latency exists between the action of a potentially dangerous, oncogenic agent and the clinical manifestation of the disease in form of a tumor. The latency period may represent a considerable proportion of the normal lifespan of the organism and in humans it may range from several years to a few decades. Frequently, more than three fourths of the doublings of neoplastic cells correspond to the preclinical stage of the disease, whereas in the final stage the growth may appear as an almost explosive one, according to the exponential laws of cell growth.[191] The possibility should be considered that certain cancers appearing in children are the late result of a transplacental carcinogenic process due to the exposure of the mother to carcinogenic agents, either chemicals or viruses, during pregnancy.[192]

A diversity of factors, including the rate of death within the population of neoplastic cells, may produce great variation in the rates of tumor growth in different types of tumors and different hosts. In some experimentally implanted tumors, such as Lewis lung carcinoma and Walker carcinoma, the differences between total body weight and carcass weight may be very large after a few days of tumor implantation, which may be attributed to the extremely high rates of growth of these tumors. The causes of host depletion and death in natural or experimental tumors are not always clear. Many factors are involved in this process, including destruction of normal tissues, presence of abnormal routes, decreased absorption of nutrients, anorexia, altered metabolism, and dysfunction of the endocrine glands.[193]

The stages of the neoplastic process are multiple and complex,[143,194-196] and they may be different from one tumor to another, even among tumors of the same type. This statement is especially true for tumors occurring under natural conditions.[197] A simplistic but useful approach for the study of tumorigenic processes has been obtained by the use of defined experimental systems. In classic experiments of carcinogen-induced tumorigenesis in the mouse skin, successive stages of the neoplastic process were defined, namely, initiation and promotion, which lead to the transformation of a normal cell into a malignant cell, and progression, which may lead to the development of a malignant tumor.[198-205]

A. INITIATION

In this stage a normal or, more likely, a preneoplastic cell would undergo a particular change which is essentially irreversible and which would determine its neoplastic transformation. The transformed cell is characterized by the acquisition of an intrinsic capacity for growing in a relatively autonomous manner, although, obviously, an interplay between the transformed cell (acting in a manner similar to a parasite) and the host organism should always be established. In any case, defined or undefined host conditions may be of critical importance for determining the fate of transformed cells. Initiated cells may be destroyed by the host or may remain dormant (nongrowing) during more or less extended periods of time but, under selective conditions in a susceptible host, they may proliferate and may eventually give rise to a tumor. Environmental agents, acting either immediately or a variable period of time after the action of initiating stimuli, may have a critical role as promoters of tumor growth by contributing to the selective proliferation of initiated cells.

1. Clonal Origin of Tumors

In certain experimental systems more than one transformed cell may participate in the formation of a given tumor, which is, consequently, of polyclonal origin. In contrast, most spontaneous tumors derive from a single transformed cell and should be considered as tumors with a simple clonal (monoclonal) or unicellular origin. Many experimental tumors, especially those induced by chemical carcinogens, are also monoclonal.[206] For human tumors, several types of markers have been used for reaching this conclusion, including cell-surface-associated immunoglobulin markers and glucose-6-phosphate dehydrogenase (GPDH) variants.[207-211] More recently, specific rearrangements of the antigen receptor peptide chains have been applied as markers for establishing the monoclonality of a vast majority of human T cell lymphomas.[212-216] The study of a 2.8-kb region, termed major breakpoint region (mbr), on human chromosome 18 that translocates and rearranges with Ig loci on chromosome 14 in the majority of follicular lymphomas has allowed the conclusion that the neoplastic subpopulations observed in these lymphomas arise from a common clonal progenitor cell.[217]

Restriction fragment length polymorphisms (RFLPs) from tumor cells DNA can be used to determine the clonal origin of human tumors.[218-221] Linkage map of the human genome based on the pattern of inheritance of 403 polymorphic loci, including 393 RFLPs distributed among the haploid set of human chromosomes, has been constructed recently.[222] Whereas the analysis of GPDH variants can be applied to only 1 of every 50 tumors, the method based on analysis of RFLP of the hypoxanthine phosphoribosyl transferase (HPRT) gene (an X-linked gene) can be applied in approximately one fourth of female tumors. In the initial report using RFLP of the HPRT gene, each of three human cancers analyzed was monoclonal.[219] Using DNA probes derived from the HPRT gene as well as from the phosphoglycerate kinase gene, clonal analysis could be applied in over 50% of females examined.[223] The X-inactivation patterns observed with the probes used in this study were found to accurately reflect clonality in more than 95% of 92 tumors examined.

Most human tumors are monoclonal in origin. These clinical results are supported by experimental studies indicating that a single tumor cell may be sufficient to determine the development of a potentially lethal tumor upon implantation into a susceptible host.[224-226] However, the possibility should be considered that tumor monoclonality could be a late event

TABLE 4
Comparison between the Biological Properties of Initiator and Promoter Agents

Initiator agents	Promoter agents
Are considered as carcinogens	Are usually not considered carcinogens but as cocarcinogens
Must be administered before the promoter	Must be administered after the initiator
At least in some cases only one exposure could suffice	Prolonged exposure is usually required
Action is irreversible and additive	Action may be reversible and is not additive
No apparent threshold	May have a threshold
Electrophile production and covalent binding to cellular macromolecules	No electrophile production and noncovalent binding to cellular macromolecules
Are usually mutagenic	Are usually not mutagenic

in carcinogenesis.[227] Interestingly, the scarce human tumors of multicellular origin are often hereditary, which indicates that in those cases there is a marked genetic predisposition to malignant transformation of multiple cells. Kaposi's sarcomas occurring in patients with the acquired immune deficiency syndrome (AIDS) appear to be polyclonal even within the same lesion.[228] However, Kaposi's sarcomas in AIDS patients are usually multifocal, occurring as a consequence of immunosuppression, and often follow a benign clinical course.

In tumors associated with virus infection, the site of virus integration into the host cell genome can be used as a criteria for the study of clonality. For example, the site of integration of hepatitis B virus (HBV) DNA into the host cell genome has been used for evaluating the clonal origin of human hepatocellular carcinomas.[229] Most of the tumors studied with this method (13 of 14 tumors), including metastatic tumors, were found to be of monoclonal origin.

B. PROMOTION

The progression of neoplastic cells to form tumors depends on both their intrinsic properties and appropriate environmental conditions. Specific environmental factors favoring tumor progression are considered as tumor promoters or cocarcinogens. In general, the promoter agents are chemical compounds that must act in a repetitive manner for an extended period of time in order to be effective. The promotion of cells initiated by chemical carcinogens or radiation can be favored by agents acting as tumor promoters. Oncogene-induced malignant transformation of rodent cells *in vitro* can be enhanced by chemical promoters such as phorbol ester or teleocidin.[230-232]

Tumor promoters have characteristics that are somewhat different from those of tumor initiators, which are the carcinogenic agents responsible for the malignant transformation of cells.[233,234] The respective characteristics of tumor initiators and tumor promoters may be compared in Table 4. However, there are exceptions to the general characteristics of these agents as indicated in the table. Moreover, certain agents have overlapping characteristics and may act as both initiators and promoters, being properly considered as "complete carcinogens". An important general conclusion suggested by the data appearing in Table 4 is that most initiators are mutagenic or genotoxic agents whereas promoters would probably act through epigenetic or regulatory mechanisms.

Promotion of initiated cells may be a reversible process both *in vivo* and *in vitro*.[235,236] Tumor promoters such as phorbol esters may act, at least in part, by enhancing the expression of particular cellular genes which would contribute to the appearance of morphological alterations in the initiated cells, including changes in the cytoskeleton.[237] Two mouse genes that specify sensitivity to tumor promotion, designated *pro*-1 and *pro*-2, have been isolated and character-ized.[238] The normal function of these genes is unknown. Preliminary results indicated the existence of sequences homologous to mouse *pro*-1 and *pro*-2 in the human genome and suggested that the putative *pro*-1 gene could be involved in the etiology of human tumors that would include nasopharyngeal carcinoma.[239]

Phorbol esters can display important actions on the promotion of tumor cells *in vivo*. Injection of PMA into C57BL/6 mice bearing tumors produced by inoculation of the fibrosarcoma cell line MC1A resulted in the appearance of tumor cells that, unlike the parental tumor cells, were able to grow in animals immunized against the parental tumors.[240] This property was maintained for at least six tumor passages after the initial PMA injections and showed tendency to decrease thereafter. The relatively high frequency of generation of cells with increased tumorigenic potential in the PMA-treated animals, as well as the tendency to reversion of this potential in subsequent tumor cell generations, suggests that generation of these cells occurred by an epigenetic mechanism.

The genetic constitution of the host may be important in relation to the effectivity of tumor promoters. Almost all of the data related to the concept of tumor promotion have been obtained in experimental murine systems. The general validity of the initiation-promotion concept in relation to carcinogenic processes occurring under natural conditions, especially in relation to human cancer, has been questioned recently.[241] There is evidence that the sensitivity for tumor promoting agents may be inherited independently of whether there exists genes activated during the initiation process.[238]

C. PROGRESSION

Progression includes the processes whereby transformed cells develop into a malignant tumor which may eventually become metastatic.[29] Tumor cell progression is characterized by an increasingly higher level of autonomy and independence from the microenvironmental conditions and the exogenous supply of hormones and growth factors.[242] Many complex mechanisms and factors from both the transformed cells and the host are critically involved in determining the growth and development of a tumor. The genetic instability of tumor cells, which can occur at both the cytogenetic and the molecular levels, may have an important role in determining tumor progression.[243]

1. Clonal Expansion vs. Recruitment

In general, the progression of initiated cells to form a tumor occurs by clonal expansion depending on successive cell divisions,[209] but there is evidence that a phenomenon of recruitment of normal neighbor cells by malignant cells may take place at least in some experimental tumor systems.[244-249] The mechanism responsible for this horizontal transmission of malignancy is unknown, but some possibilities are cell fusion, transformation by growth factors, and transfection of DNA containing active transforming genes (oncogenes). The study of premature condensation phenomena gives evidence in favor of the occurrence of *in vivo* cell fusion in human malignant tumors, including leukemias and carcinomas.[250] On the other hand, studies on cell cultures from a human small cell lung carcinoma growing as a xenograft in nude mice indicated the presence of human DNA sequences in mouse cells that became spontaneously transformed in this system, suggesting the occurrence of natural or spontaneous DNA transfection and not cell fusion.[249] The transformed mouse cell lines derived from the human small-cell lung carcinoma xenograft expressed both mouse- and human-specific histocompatibility antigens. In any case, tumor growth depending on recruitment of normal cells by tumor cells would be proportionally very small under natural conditions *in vivo*.

2. Interactions between Tumor Cells and Normal Cells

Diffusible factors, called angiogenic factors, contribute to the capillary proliferation required for tumor growth after the initial, avascular phase of its development.[251,252] Microenvironmental conditions are crucially involved in the progression of transformed cells. The initial sustained

TABLE 5
Heterogeneity Aspects of
Tumor Cell Populations

Morphology
Karyotype
Antigenicity
Immunogenicity
Metabolism
Hormone receptors
Growth patterns
Metastatic potential
Sensitivity to radiation
Sensitivity to drugs

proliferation of myeloid leukemic cells depends on the conditions created from the stroma cell microenvironment until the full acquisition of autonomous growth.[242] Blood cells, especially macrophages, may have a critical role in the regulation of tumor cell growth. Junctional communication between normal cells and transformed cells may also be relevant for the stimulation or inhibition of tumor cell growth.[253] This type of communication would take place by mediation of growth-controlling signals and factors capable of going from one cell to another through specialized channels with a diameter of 16 to 20 Å.

3. Tumor Cell Heterogeneity

One of the most important characteristics of tumor progression is the constitution of a highly heterogeneous population of neoplastic cells which, arising in the earliest stages of tumor development, will critically contribute to the survival of neoplastic cells under different and variable environmental conditions.[254-258] Tumor cell diversification can occur during the process of transformation or soon thereafter and may result in uniqueness of each of the early descendants of the transformed cell.[258-261] Moreover, heterogeneity associated with the malignant transformation of cells may in some cases involve most, if not all, the progeny of the initially transformed cell and extend to many different properties of the cell.[258] This heterogeneity involves not only the primary tumor but also the metastases, whose cellular components exhibit wide phenotypic variation at both the intralesional and interlesional levels.[262]

Many phenotypic characteristics of neoplastic cells are usually involved in the expression of this heterogeneity, including cells with chromosomal and antigenic variants, cells with increased potential to metastasize, cells with decreased or increased sensitivity to radiation or drugs, and cells with lethal changes (Table 5). The phenomenon of intraneoplastic diversity has obvious consequences for the successful treatment of cancer.[263] Tumor cell populations spontaneously develop, for example, heterogeneous response to the cytotoxic effects of tumor necrosis factor α (TNF-α).[264]

The mechanisms responsible for the origin of tumor cell heterogeneization are little understood. In general, tumor cells are characterized by a remarkable genetic instability which may be observed at both the cytogenetic and the molecular levels.[243] Conventional mutations (point mutations) can be ruled out because of their low frequency and their effect on a limited number of characters, an effect that is also coordinate in tumor cell populations.[258] Chromosome aberrations may occur with high frequency in tumors but clones originating from single cells isolated from tumors are karyotypically stable in their early passage.[265]

Inductive processes conditioned by different microenvironments in vivo are probably involved in the generation of a phenotypic diversity within individual tumor cell populations, including the generation of phenotypic variants with high metastatic potential.[266] Many of the induced phenotypic changes may remain stable for successive cell generations but the underlying mechanisms for induction of these changes are unknown. Other phenotypic changes may, however, undergo variation according to the state of differentiation of the neoplastic cells, which may respond in different ways when exposed to appropriate signals from the microenvironment. For example, phenotypic heterogeneity is a characteristic feature of tumor lesions in patients with melanoma and the diversity in the differentiation state of melanoma cells can account for much of the phenotypic heterogeneity observed in melanoma lesions.[267] In turn, some differentiation traits expressed by these cells in a coordinate or isolated manner can be altered, following specific changes in the microenvironment or the general environment of the host.

Epigenetic phenomena, i.e., regulatory changes not primarily involving structural alterations of the genome, would more easily explain the singular characteristics of tumor cell heterogeneity. However, both genetic and epigenetic changes are probably responsible for tumor progression and for the constitution of a heterogeneous population of neoplastic cells within the tumor.[209,268-270] The importance of genetic changes in the generation of tumor heterogeneity is suggested by the loss of polymorphic DNA restriction fragments in cells from tumors like malignant melanoma.[271] The occurrence of random RFLP loss in tumor cells with the resulting homozygosity/heterozygosity at multiple loci, suggests that transpositions and/or rearrangements occurring at the genome level may contribute to the early constitution of the heterogeneous population of tumor cells.

D. INVASION AND METASTASIZATION

The most important biological and clinical characteristics of malignant tumors are invasion and metastasization, which determine the final fate of the host. The normal neighbor tissues may be actively invaded, and progressively replaced, by the growing mass of the tumor. A complex interplay between the tumor cells and the normal surrounding tissues is crucially involved in tumor invasion and metastasization. The microvasculature has a central role in these processes.[272] A combination of properties of the tumor cells, including increased cell locomotion and increased cell proliferation, is involved in tumor invasion.[273-276]

1. Degradation of the Extracellular Matrix

The extracellular (interstitial) matrices of normal tissues are penetrated and degraded during the invasion of tumor cells. These matrices can be divided into two major categories, basement membranes and interstitial connective tissue, which differ with respect to composition, location, and function.[277] Basement membranes are composed of a uniform acellular sheet-like structure which is widely distributed throughout the body, separating organ cells, epithelia, and endothelia from the interstitial connective tissue. The basement membranes provide a substratum for orderly growing cells and are responsible for maintaining the normal tissue architecture. Loss of basement membranes appears to play a crucial role in tumor invasion and hematogenous dissemination.[278] Basement membranes are composed of a number of glycoproteins which include type IV collagen, laminin, heparan sulfate, chondroitin sulfate, and entactin. These components form a highly crosslinked matrix structure. The interstitial tissue is composed of cells (fibroblasts, osteoblasts, chondrocytes, and macrophages) located in a meshwork of collagen fibers and glycoprotein, proteoglycan, and hyaluronic acid ground substance. Interstitial tissue has a major mechanical and supportive function in the body. Their main chemical components are type I, II, and III collagens, fibronectins, proteoglycans, and elastin. The interstitial tissue is invaded and destroyed during tumor progression.

The presence of proteolytic enzymes in tumor invasion-associated matrix degradation processes has been widely documented.[277] Proteinases capable of hydrolyzing peptide bonds, acting as either exopeptidases or endopeptidases, are present in increased amounts in malignant tumor tissues, as compared with the normal control tissues, and can be produced not only by the tumor cells themselves but also by the normal host tissue cells that surround the tumor cells. The most abundant proteinases are plasmin, cathepsins, collagenases, proteoglycanases, and elastase.

Plasminogen activators, a group of serine proteolytic enzymes, are specifically involved in the conversion of plasminogen to the active proteinase plasmin, an enzyme which has a broad substrate specificity and can degrade a variety of tissue proteins including fibrin.[279] There are two types of plasminogen activators, the tissue-specific type and the urokinase-like type. Both types of plasminogen activators may be found in increased quantities in malignant tumor tissues. Cathepsins, particularly cathepsin B, and collagenases, particularly type IV collagenase, are often associated in increased amounts with malignant cells. The activity of proteinases is normally regulated by a delicate balance between biosynthesis, secretion, and degradation, as well as by the action of proteinase inhibitors, and this balance can be disrupted in neoplastic transformation. Transcription of the gene encoding transin, a secreted protease, is stimulated in the mouse skin by a classical initiation-promotion protocol which leads to the appearance of squamous cell carcinomas.[280] Secretion of transin and other proteases may contribute to the progression of benign, encapsulated tumors to malignant, invasive carcinomas.

In general, malignant cells and tissues are characterized by an increase in net proteinase activity. Localization of hydrolytic enzymes in the plasma membrane of tumor cells could result in focal dissolution of the extracellular matrix, thus facilitating invasion and metastasis.[281] Secretion of increased amounts of proteases is associated with the growth and spread of at least certain tumor cells. The production of plasminogen activator, which results in increased generation of the active protease plasmin, may be stimulated in transformed cells by the production of particular factors including transforming growth factors (TGFs).[282]

Interaction of cells with particular components of the extracellular matrix such as the cell adhesion proteins fibronectin and laminin, as well as interaction with collagen, may be of critical importance for tumor cell invasion and metastasization.[283,284] Fibronectins are high molecular weight glycoproteins synthesized by a wide variety of cells and exhibit an affinity for collagen, fibrinogen or fibrin, glycosamineglycans, and surface components of many kinds of cells.[285] The ability of tumor cells to bind fibronectin and related adhesion proteins appears to depend on a short, hydrophilic amino acid sequence, Arg-Gly-Asp-Ser, located in the cell binding domain of the fibronectin molecule. A synthetic pentapeptide which contains this sequence may act as a reversible inhibitor in assays of cellular adhesion and is able to inhibit the formation of metastatic lung colonies of B16-F10 murine melanoma cells in C57BL/6 mice.[286] Transformed cells may be characterized by decreased expression of genes coding for extracellular matrix components, including fibronectin and collagen.[287] Moreover, fibronectin glycosylation may modulate cell adhesion and spreading.[288]

Interaction between extracellular matrix components and cells occurs through membrane receptors for the particular types of extracellular matrix adhesion proteins which include fibronectin, vitronectin, laminin, and collagen receptors. A subset of these adhesion receptors seem to belong to a superfamily of proteins, all in the 100- to 160-kDa range, which mediate a variety of both cell-cell and cell-matrix adhesive responses. The role of adhesion receptors in tumor cell invasion and metastasis is probably important but remains little characterized as yet.

An additional factor favoring tumor invasion is the dedifferentiation of tumor cells, which is associated with the presence of either rudimentary formation of mechanic cell junctions (junctional complexes and desmosomes) or a complete loss of these junctions.[275] Thus, the dedifferentiation-associated dissociation of the organized tumor cell complexes into isolated tumor cells may represent a crucial prerequisite for tumor cell mobilization and tumor invasion. Other possible factors associated with the invasive properties of cancer cells remain poorly characterized.

Both genetic and epigenetic changes occurring in the tumor cells may be responsible for an enhanced potential for invasion and metastasization. There is evidence that amplification of specific gene sequences, which may be or not protooncogenes, can favor the acquisition of higher capability for invasion and metastasization by the tumor cells.[289,290]

2. Angiogenic Factors

Whereas in the first stages of tumor development an adequate supply of oxygen and nutrients may depend only on simple diffusion phenomena, the progressive expansion of the tumor mass depends critically neovascularization (angiogenic) processes. Angiogenic processes of both normal and tumor tissues require a complex interplay between endothelial cells, extracellular matrix components, and soluble growth factors and mitogenic peptides.[291,292] Both normal and malignant cells produce a variety of soluble polypeptides, including hormones and growth factors, that can promote angiogenesis. Angiogenic factors involved in tumor growth include FGFs, TGFs, a factor termed angiogenin, and other factors that remain little characterized.[293] A factor with strong angiogenic properties *in vivo*, designated angiotropin, was isolated and purified to homogeneity from activated monocytes.[294] TNF-α, produced and secreted by macrophages, is also a potent angiogenic factor.[295] Angiogenic factors can act either directly on vascular endothelial cells to stimulate locomotion and mitosis or indirectly by mobilizing host cells (e.g., macrophages) to release endothelial growth factors.[293]

3. Detachment and Circulation of Tumor Cells

Eventually, some cells may be detached from the primary tumor and may be disseminated throughout the body after entering the blood and/or lymph circulation.[296-301] These cells may circulate in form of platelet-tumor cell aggregates,[302] and some of these aggregates may be arrested in remote sites within the vessels and the tumor cells may go across the capillary walls into the extravascular space, where they may be established. In spite of the fact that this complex process is, in general, highly inefficient, some tumor cells may grow on at the distant sites to form metastases and secondary tumors.

4. Role of Immunologic Factors in Tumor Growth, Invasion, and Metastasization

In spite of numerous clinical and experimental studies, the role of the immune system of the host in tumor development, progression, and metastasization is difficult to evaluate.[303] In general, natural tumors are much less immunogenic than experimental tumors, especially virus-induced tumors, but the reason for this difference is not clear.[37] Both antigen structural differences and specific cellular factors may be responsible for the immunogenic differences observed between natural and experimental tumors. In any case, many natural tumors can grow in their autologous hosts because of their poor immunogenicity.

Cancer is much more frequent in immunodeficient or immunosuppressed patients than in people with normally operating immune mechanisms.[304,305] Moreover, there is evidence that certain tumor cells can actively produce immunosuppresive factors which could contribute to cancer invasion and dissemination.[306] Specific cell-mediated immune responses can retard the growth of tumors or can even eradicate metastases.[307] However, in other systems the immune response can facilitate or stimulate oncogenic processes.[308] Thus in some cases the presence of a tumor-specific immune reaction may constitute a positive aid to tumor development, which suggests that cancer may be considered in some way as an autoimmune disease.

It is generally accepted that cell mediated immune responses are more relevant as reactions to tumor cells than humoral responses. Cellular effector mechanisms postulated to be of importance in the host response to malignancy include antigen-specific T lymphocyte cytotoxicity, antibody-dependent cellular cytotoxicity, macrophage cytotoxicity and cytostasis, and natural cell-mediated cytotoxicity.[309] Natural killer (NK) cells and natural cytotoxic (NC) cells are crucially involved in the immune responses of the host against the tumor.

NK cells, which are closely associated with a subpopulation of cells, the large granular lymphocytes,[310-312] may play an important role in resistance to tumor growth and metastasization.[313,314] NK cells originate in the bone marrow and can appear in the absence of prior immunization. Activation of NK cells can be easily achieved in experimental systems by treatment with IFN or IFN inducers as well as with IL-2 and bacterial adjuvants. Precytotoxic or immature cytotoxic T cells as well as NK cells generated in the spleen of tumor-bearing animals may migrate into the circulation and mature cytotoxic cells would then develop at the tumor site.[315] Furthermore, at least in certain experimental systems, the cytotoxic T-lymphocytes and NK cells may be responsible for the inhibition of tumor invasion and metastasis from the primary tumor. The biological effects of NK cells may be mediated by liberation of cytotoxic factors, including a potent cytolytic protein, termed cytolysin, which has been isolated from the granules of large granular lymphocytes. In general, lymphoid and myeloid tumor cells are more sensitive to NK cell-mediated killing than cells from solid tumors.[313] NK cells may play a significant role in host defenses against hematogenous and lymphogenous dissemination of tumors. However, the role of NK cells in oncogenic processes is not totally clear and no major changes in the activity of these cells have been detected, for example, in leukemogenic processes induced in mice by either radiation or chemical carcinogens.[316]

The lytic activity of NC effector cells may be mediated by the production of specific factors, in particular by TNF-α.[317] Cloned cell lines resistant to NC activity exhibit a decrease in TNF-α sensitivity, which suggests that the same resistant mechanism protects tumor cells against both NC cells and TNF-α. Thus, NC and TNF-α lysis of target cells may be exerted through similar, if not identical, mechanisms.

Monocytes/macrophages may be importantly involved in controlling tumor growth, since they can secrete factors with cytolytic effects such as TNF-α.[318] Monocytes circulating in the peripheral blood are apparently not spontaneously cytotoxic for tumor cells but can acquire cytotoxicity upon activation by endotoxin or endotoxin-like agonists, and this acquisition is associated with the production of humoral factors such as TNF-α.[319] Macrophages are referred to as accessory cells in the induction of immune responses because of their participation in the processing of complex antigens and their presentation to T and B lymphocytes. They can also intereact with lymphocytes by way of secreted molecules termed monokines and lymphokines.[309] The available evidence indicates that macrophages are importantly involved in antitumor immunologic responses.[320,321] However, the role of macrophages in destroying or inhibiting nascent tumor cell populations is not well understood.

Facilitation of tumor growth may depend on mechanisms associated with cellular immunity. One of these mechanisms may consist in the development of specific suppressor T cells with concomitant augmentation of tumor growth.[309] Besides T cells, macrophages and B cells may exert suppressor effects, and there is evidence that tumor cells themselves can exert a direct suppressive effect on the immune response.

5. Cellular and Molecular Mechanisms Involved in Tumor Progression

The tendency to remote dissemination is a most important characteristic of malignant tumors. Most cancer patients are killed not by the primary tumor but by the growth of metastases.

The cellular and molecular mechanisms responsible for tumor invasion and/or metastasization are little understood.[322-324] The particular composition and structure of the cell surface is very important for the expression of a metastatic phenotype. Tumor cell surface glycoproteins are involved in the expression of invasive and metastatic capacity of tumor cells. Carbohydrates contained in these proteins, especially certain sialylated asparagine-linked oligosaccharides, are related to the metastatic potentialities of tumor cells.[325]

Expression of proteolytic enzymes may also be important for tumor invasion and metastasization. Increased production of plasmin and other proteolytic enzymes capable of degrading fibrin as well as fibronectin and other extracellular matrix molecules may have a role in the invasion of normal tissues by tumor cells. Conversion of the inactive zymogen plasminogen into plasmin is required for these processes.[326] Plasminogen activator, which is synthesized as a single chain proenzyme and many types of cells, often under hormonal control, can produce specific plasminogen activator inhibitors.[327] The equilibrium between plasminogen activator and its inhibitor could be deranged in tumor tissues, which may favor their aptitude to invade normal tissues.

It has been suggested that metastases arise from special genetically determined cell subpopulations in the primary tumors,[328] but other observations are more compatible with processes occurring at random,[329,330] involving the formation of "transient metastatic compartments",[331] or some kind of "dynamic heterogeneity",[332] which would be more likely generated by epigenetic, regulatory mechanisms. However, there is evidence that some discrete DNA fragments derived from human tumor cells may be capable of conferring a metastatic potential when transfected into transformed mouse fibroblasts,[333] which suggests that certain structural DNA changes may be associated with an enhanced capability of cancer cells for remote dissemination. There is also evidence that sublines derived from cells metastasizing preferentially specific organs, such as the lung and the liver, can maintain the respective affinities to these organs for a period of over 2 years.[334] Unfortunately, the molecular bases of these affinities are unknown.

Activation of particular cellular genes, probably including protooncogenes, may play an important role in tumor invasion and metastasization. As discussed in the last chapter of this volume, overexpression of specific protooncogenes, which could be associated or not with amplification of the protooncogene DNA sequences, may contribute to the progression of certain types of human tumors. Some protooncogenes may be activated by point mutation but the rates of spontaneous conversion of some cells, e.g., established REF cell lines, for the acquisition of invading and metastasizing properties are too large to provide definite evidence that genes with transforming potential are involved in the acquisition of these properties.[335,336] In general, the role of protooncogene activation in the complex processes leading to tumor progression and metastasization is not clear. In addition to protooncogenes, other genes may contribute to these processes.

Somatic cell hybridization studies suggest that one or more dominant genes located on human chromosome 7 may play a key role in invasion and metastasis of T-cell malignancies, and possibly in other types of human cancer.[337] The identity of these genes is unknown. A useful method for the characterization of these genes consists in the screening of cDNA libraries constructed from normal tissues and the respective tumor tissues.[338] This screening may allow the identification of mRNAs that differ significantly in abundance between the normal tissues and the tumor tissues, and the metastases of these tumors. Eventually, the differences detected in such studies may find clinical application as markers related to the progression of particular types of tumors. The screening of cDNA libraries derived from transcripts expressed in normal human stomach and human gastric carcinoma allowed the identification of three genes which were specifically expressed in the tumor tissue.[339] These genes did not exhibit structural homology with known viral oncogenes and the functions of their products are unknown.

The cellular composition of different metastases in the same host may be heterogeneous, both among different metastases (interlesional heterogeneity) and within a single metastasis (intralesional heterogeneity).[262] This heterogeneity reflects two major processes: the selective nature of the metastatic process and the rapid evolution and phenotypic diversification of clonal tumor cell populations during progressive tumor growth resulting from the inherent genetic and epigenetic instability of tumor cell populations. The phenotypic diversity of tumor cell populations represents a major obstacle for the prophylactic and therapeutic control of metastatic processes.

V. GENERAL MECHANISMS OF THE NEOPLASTIC PROCESS

The neoplastic process is usually a long one in relation to the lifetime of the host and comprises multiple steps for its full development. The general stages of this prolonged multistage process include the following aspects.

A. INTERACTION OF AN ONCOGENIC FACTOR WITH A SUSCEPTIBLE CELL

Cells with capability for originating tumors are generally immature, nonterminally differentiated cells. The genetic program that is being expressed in the cell may be of critical importance for the appearance, or the lack of appearance, of neoplastic transformation as well as for the formation, or the lack of formation, of a given tumor. In addition to genetic changes, the hormonal milieu and the immune status of the host may be of paramount importance for the initiation and/or development of particular types of tumors.

1. Etiopathogenetic Factors of Neoplasia

The etiopathogenetic factors associated with neoplastic diseases may be of either endogenous or exogenous origin. (Table 3). Endogenous factors include genetic factors, which may be vertically inherited through the germ line or may be horizontally acquired either before or after birth.[340,341] Whereas genetic factors inherited through the germ line are expected to be present in all the cells from an individual, genetic changes of postzygotic origin may affect only a single cell or a group of cells of the individual. Some rare inherited diseases determine a high risk for malignancy. Examples of such diseases are xeroderma pigmentosum, Bloom's syndrome, Fanconi's anemia, ataxia telangiectasia, familial polyposis coli, and retinoblastoma.[342] The cell to be transformed may be a normal one or, more likely, may already have an intrinsic alteration determining a predisposition to malignant transformation, i.e., it may be a preneoplastic cell. In any case, some specific types of genetic changes, either inherited or acquired, would usually determine a more or less marked predisposition to the development of one or more types of neoplasia rather than determining a direct induction of neoplastic transformation. According to a hypothesis, at least two different genetic changes, either inherited or acquired, would be required for the appearance of tumors such as retinoblastoma,[343] but multiple genetic changes are probably involved in the origin and development of common tumors.

Nongenetic endogenous factors, especially immunological and hormonal factors, are more likely related to the development of tumors than to their origin at the initiation stage. On the other hand, exogenous oncogenic factors such as radiations, chemical carcinogens, and oncogenic viruses may be instrumental etiologic agents for the initiation of neoplastic transformation.[344-345] The available evidence supports the concept that most human tumors are not due to an inherited predisposition to cancer but are predominantly triggered by exposure to specific environmental factors which may act either alone or in combination.[346] From a practical point of view, the multifactorial origin of neoplastic diseases represents the main obstacle to the design and development of effective approaches for their prevention.

B. STRUCTURAL AND/OR REGULATORY ALTERATION OF THE GENOME

At present it is difficult to decide whether or not structural alterations of the genome are a critical prerequisite for the expression of a transformed phenotype. Although most investigators accept that some mutational event(s) should be an essential component of the early stages of the neoplastic process, the evidence on this subject is only circumstantial and specific mutations involved in the initiation of transformation have not been identified. Moreover, there is evidence that at least certain intracellular regulatory changes, apparently not associated with mutational events, may be critically involved in the origin and expression of neoplastic transformation, and some of these regulatory changes would be transmitted to the progeny of a transformed cell in a similar manner as normal differentiation is transmitted to the progeny of normally differentiated cells. Supporting this possibility is the fact that an essential component of the transformed state is frequently, if not always, the existence of a partial or total block in the expression of terminal cell differentiation.

C. ALTERED GENOME EXPRESSION

A wide diversity of genes may be expressed in an altered manner in cancer cells.[347] However, most of these alterations may be a late result of tumor growth and development and they should be preceded by some critical changes, which would be more probably involved in the origin of the transformation phenomenon or, at least, in the early stages of its development.

It could be assumed that whether the initial changes of neoplastic transformation involve structural genomic alterations or regulatory modifications of genome expression, some critical genetic information should be expressed (or derepressed) and perhaps some other should be repressed in order to malignant transformation being expressed. Again, however, it has been a difficult task to identify specific genomic functions whose expression, or lack of expression, are critically involved in the appearance of malignant transformation and its transmission to the cell progeny. Comparison of rat liver gene expression during development, regeneration, and neoplasia indicates that RNA populations from both fetal liver and hepatoma lack sequences expressed in the mature adult liver, but the tumor do not reexpress sequences which are preferentially expressed in the fetal liver.[348] Thus, there are essential differences in the expression of genetic programs between liver tumor cells and liver fetal cells.

The clonal nature of most tumors indicates that some essential changes in genome expression are required for the appearance and maintenance of a transformed phenotype but the early phenotypic diversification of neoplastic cells to form a highly heterogeneous population points to the existence of important additional changes, which must be superimposed to the early ones. As noticed above, this early production of a heterogeneous population of neoplastic cells is probably of utmost importance for tumor development under the different and variable environmental conditions determined by the host. It seems likely that both genetic and nongenetic changes are involved in the formation of a heterogeneous population of neoplastic cells within a tumor.

D. PHENOTYPIC ALTERATION OF THE CELL

As a consequence of the preceding stages, several biochemical, functional, and morphological aspects of the cell will appear as abnormal. The differences between neoplastic cells and normal cells, as described before, are multiple but most of them are of a quantitative, rather than qualitative, nature. In fact, a universal, specific, and essential qualitative biochemical difference between tumor cells and normal cells has never been found. From a practical point of view this fact imposes severe limitations to the application of biochemical changes present in tumor cells for diagnostic purposes as "tumor markers". Most probably, a universal tumor marker will never be found.

E. ALTERATION OF CELL BEHAVIOR AND FORMATION OF THE TUMOR

The most typical alterations of cell behavior in transformed cells consist of poor differentiation, tendency to autonomy and uncontrolled cell proliferation. Such alterations represent an asocial type of behavior in relation to the harmony of the organism. Eventually, the sustained, uncontrolled proliferation of neoplastic cells may result in the formation of a tumor capable of killing the host.

VI. HYPOTHESES ON THE ORIGIN OF NEOPLASTIC TRANSFORMATION

The molecular events responsible for the transformation of a normal cell into a malignant cell are not understood. Two main hypotheses have been postulated to explain the origin of malignant transformation, namely, the genetic hypothesis and the epigenetic or regulatory hypothesis.[349-352] According to the genetic hypothesis neoplasia would be the result of some structural genetic changes occurring in the cell. However, not all of the structural changes occurring at the genomic level should be considered as mutations and, accordingly, the genetic hypothesis may be divided into two variants, namely, the mutational hypothesis and the nonmutational genetic hypothesis. In addition, the possible role of either infection by exogenous viruses or activation of endogenous viruses in the neoplastic transformation of cells should be considered. In contrast to the aforementioned hypotheses, the epigenetic hypothesis postulates that genetic changes are not required for the origin of neoplasia, which would rather result from

TABLE 6
Hypotheses on the Origin of Cancer

Mutational hypothesis
    Point mutations
    Chromosome aberrations
Nonmutational genetic hypothesis
    Changes in DNA methylation
    DNA rearrangement, transposition, or amplification
Viral hypothesis
    Infection by oncogenic DNA viruses
    Infection by oncogenic retroviruses
    Activation of endogenous oncogenic proviruses
Epigenetic hypothesis
    Alteration in regulation of genomic functions
    Alteration in regulation of nongenomic functions

some regulatory changes occurring within the cell. The assumed regulatory changes would alter genomic functions related to the control of cell differentiation and proliferation. The different hypotheses are listed in Table 6 and in the following they are discussed.

A. MUTATIONAL HYPOTHESIS

According to this hypothesis the neoplastic transformation of cells would be the result of some structural genetic changes occurring at either the molecular level or the supramolecular level, i.e., it would be a consequence of point mutations and/or chromosome aberrations.

1. Point Mutations

The possibility that cancer may result from point mutations occurring in somatic cells has been discussed for more than 5 decades.[353-355] An impressive body of experimental and clinical evidence lends support to the validity of the mutational hypothesis of the origin of cancer and most investigators in the field of oncology do accept a direct cause-effect relationship between mutation and cancer. The nature and number of the mutational events required for the neoplastic transformation of cells has remained elusive but recent evidence indicates that specific mutational events occurring early in particular protooncogenes may be involved in the experimental induction of some tumors.[356] Moreover, similar changes may occur in some common human tumors.[357-361] However, more than one mutational event may be required for the expression of a transformed phenotype.[362] In any case, it remains to be critically demonstrated that mutation is a universal and crucial prerequisite for neoplastic transformation and that there is a direct cause-effect relationship between point mutation and neoplasia, especially nonexperimental neoplasia.

The main lines of evidence in favor of the mutational hypothesis of cancer include the following: irreversibility of the process of neoplastic transformation, correlation between mutagenicity and oncogenicity, and relationship between defects in mutation repair mechanisms and cancer. However, a critical analysis of these arguments may show some inconsistencies and weaknesses.

In several studies the frequency of transformation reversion has been estimated as a very low one, falling into an order of magnitude which is similar to that of the rates of spontaneous mutation reversion. However, this fact cannot be considered as a proof in favor of a mutational origin of cancer. The normal processes of cellular differentiation in the organism are also essentially irreversible in spite of the fact that they are not associated with mutational events. Rather, the processes of normal differentiation are generally attributed to regulatory phenomena occurring at the genomic level. The neoplastic transformation being considered as the result of a block of differentiation, an abnormal form of differentiation or a partial process of dedifferentiation or retrodifferentiation could also be generated directly by epigenetic, regulatory mechanisms which are not necessarily nor directly associated with any mutational events.

The existence of a positive correlation between mutagenicity and oncogenicity for a diversity of exogenous agents does also not prove a cause-effect relationship between mutation and cancer. It is true that most chemical carcinogens are also mutagens or may acquire mutagenic properties after being subjected to metabolic activation processes but the correlation between mutagenicity and oncogenicity is not perfect.[349,350,363-365] Many noncarcinogenic substances have clear mutagenic properties, which would lead to the assumption that only certain specific types of mutational events could result in neoplastic transformation. On the other hand, some of the most potent carcinogenic agents have only a weak mutagenic action or may not be mutagens at all. Moreover, many carcinogenic agents produce remarkable alterations in cellular components other than DNA, including nuclear proteins, and these alterations could be important for determining their carcinogenic properties.

Cancer is a relatively frequent complication of human inherited diseases associated with DNA processing abnormalities and defective mechanisms of mutation repair.[342,366-368] In such diseases cancer would occur as a result of an interaction between the endogenous, genetic defect and mutagenic environmental factors, which would lead to an accumulation of unrepaired mutations. A good example of this situation is xeroderma pigmentosum, a disease in which there is an autosomal recessively inherited defect of the mechanisms of excision of pyrimidine dimers produced in the skin by UV radiation.[369-371] Many different pathological changes are observed in the skin of patients with xeroderma pigmentosum, including the frequent appearance of malignant tumors (carcinomas, melanomas). Although one may be tempted to consider these tumors as a direct consequence of the increased amount of unrepaired mutations, it should also be considered that a host of other biochemical abnormalities is present in the same cells and that cancer may possibly be the consequence of some of these secondary changes, which are more or less removed from the primary genetic defect. However, it is apparent that an accumulation of mutational events in somatic cells may lead, through short or long pathways, to neoplastic transformation. Patients with Bloom's syndrome (an inherited disease associated with chromosome rearrangements and increased levels of SCE and point mutations) are also characterized by a greatly increased incidence of cancer, and this syndrome is due to a mutational defect in the structure of DNA ligase I, the major DNA ligase in proliferating human cells.[372] A direct analysis of discrete cellular DNA sequences whose alteration may be relevant to neoplastic transformation may contribute to lend a more secure basis to the knowledge of mutations crucially involved in carcinogenic processes. Such DNA sequences appear to be represented, at least in part, by protooncogenes.

2. Chromosome Aberrations

The existence of chromosome abnormalities in human tumor cells was suggested already by observations dating from the last century and was confirmed several decades later in studies of experimental tumors, like an azo dye-induced Yoshida ascites tumor.[373,374] The results from an immense number of studies performed since that time indicate that numerical and/or structural chromosome abnormalities are almost universally present in malignant cells.[23,25,375-377] Moreover, similar or identical chromosome abnormalities are present in preneoplastic lesions as well. Numerical chromosome abnormalities observed in neoplastic and preneoplastic lesions include hyperdiploidy and, less frequently, polyploidy, pseudodiploidy, and hypodiploidy. Structural aberrations observed in these lesions may consist in terminal or interstitial deletions, reciprocal or nonreciprocal translocations, pericentric of paracentric inversions, centric or acentric rings, duplications, and fragments. Specific translocations and deletions are the most important types of structural chromosome abnormalities associated with malignant diseases. Some of these structural alterations are difficult to recognize even with the use of modern cytogenetic techniques and, in some cases, their proper diagnosis and characterization can be achieved with the aid of methods working at the molecular level (restriction enzymes, DNA probes, or DNA sequentiation).

The origin of tumor-associated chromosome abnormalities is variable. According to the original postulation of the chromosomal hypothesis of the origin of cancer,[378] mistakes may occasionally occur during mitosis and some of the resulting chromosome alterations could result in generation of neoplastic cells. Oncogenic factors such as radiations and chemicals would be capable of inducing neoplastic transformation because they can produce chromosome abnormalities. Many chromosome abnormalities may appear in animals shortly after irradiation or administration of carcinogenic substances,[379] but the pooled data from human and experimental tumors strongly suggest that chromosomal aberrations in spontaneous and experimental tumors, especially in hematologic neoplasms, are not random and that genic material of main importance in tumor development is accumulated not only in a number of specific chromosomes but, more importantly, in specific regions within chromosomes.[23,25,36,380-382] However, it should be recognized that a host of other cellular alterations occur as well in the cells of animals treated with radiation or chemical carcinogenic agents.

Different types of constitutional or acquired chromosome abnormalities are associated with an increased risk for cancer.[383] Leukemia is a relatively frequent disease in children and young people with Down's syndrome, a disease characterized by trisomy of human chromosome 21. Several inherited diseases characterized by chromosome fragility or instability, such as Bloom's syndrome, Fanconi's anemia and ataxia telangiectasia, are cancer-prone diseases.[367,384,385] Chromosome fragility has also been found in patients with multiple endocrine adenomatosis,[386] as well as in children with sporadic unilateral retinoblastoma.[387] Results of cytogenetic studies with cultured human lymphocytes and caffeine as a mutagen enhancer suggest that constitutive fragile sites may represent targets for the action of mutagenic agents.[388] Mutagen-sensitive fragile sites would frequently coincide with the location of specific chromosome breakpoints associated with certain types of malignant diseases as well as with the location of protooncogenes. Whether it can be generalized that constitutional or heritable chromosome fragile sites are a predisposing factor for human cancer is still an open question.[389] The relationship between chromosomal fragile sites and cancer-associated chromosome breakpoints remains controversial.[390]

Chromosomal alterations may result in changes in the expression of genes, including cellular oncogenes (protooncogenes), in the tumor cells.[391] It is difficult, however, to establish a direct cause-effect relationship between chromosome aberrations and cancer. Although chromosome abnormalities are almost universally found in experimental tumors induced with carcinogenic substances or oncogenic viruses, there are some remarkable exceptions to this general rule.[392,393] Early passage diploid rat embryo cells become tumorigenic and acquire metastatic capability in nude mice after transformation with a cloned H-*ras* oncogene of either cellular or viral origin, but no chromosome rearrangements, aneuploidy, or increased rates of SCE are observed in these cells, which remain essentially diploid.[394,395] No increase or decrease in a specific chromosome number and no consistent structural changes in particular chromosomes (marker chromosomes) have been observed in tumors induced by a given chemical agent or virus in different animals from the same species.[396] Normal human foreskin fibroblasts treated *in vitro* with a chemical carcinogen acquire neoplastic properties, including the production of nodules after subcutaneous inoculation into nude mice, but G-banded karyotypic analysis of some (2 of 10) of the cell lines induced by this method showed a normal diploid karyotype.[397] Since the karyotypically normal two cell lines are indistinguishable in their neoplastic characteristics from the others that exhibit chromosome abnormalities, it seems clear that genetic and/or epigenetic changes not necessarily involving chromosome aberrations may be involved in the acquisition of malignant properties by cells exposed to certain carcinogenic agents. Moreover, extensive chromosome alterations induced in particular experimental systems are not always associated with malignancy.

Chromosomes are apparently normal in some patients with acute lymphocytic leukemia (ALL), although when modern cytogenetic banding techniques are used most of these patients would have chromosome abnormalities.[25,398-400] No chromosome aberrations are observed in at least a quarter of patients with chronic lymphocytic leukemia (CLL).[401,402] The vast majority of cells from primary human breast carcinomas maintained in short-term culture are diploid but these cells represent true malignant cells with capability for invasive growth.[403,404] In contrast, most cells of the malignant effusion-derived cultures from these tumors are aneuploid, which suggests that minor subpopulations of viable aneuploid cells may be responsible for malignant effusions.[404] In *Xiphophorus* fishes, chromosome aberrations are present in carcinogen-induced tumors, but are totally absent in heritable tumors.[405]

Structural chromosome aberrations occurring in particular types of tumors are frequently located near the loci of protooncogenes.[28,381,382,406,407] The regularity of this association in certain types of hematopoietic neoplasms lends support to the possibility of a close correlation between the cytogenetic abnormality and the activation of the protooncogene. However, in other tumors, especially in the common solid tumors, the association between protooncogene alteration and tumorigenic process may not be observed consistently and its biological significance remains controversial. Similar associations may be observed in some benign tumors, e.g., in human pleomorphic adenomas.[408] Solid tumors are generally characterized by karyotypic heterogeneity, which may be a consequence of an apparent instability of the chromosome endowment of the tumor cells. Karyotype instability may play an important role in providing cell variants for tumor progression.[409] In any case, multiple chromosome changes may occur early in the evolution of solid tumors.

Deletion of specific genomic sequences may be importantly involved in certain tumorigenic processes, including human cancer. Results from recent studies indicate that some particular types of human tumors are consistently associated with specific deletions of small or large segments of cellular DNA. Such deletions could be causally related to the tumorigenic process if they result in the elimination of genes, called tumor suppressor genes, antioncogenes, or emerogenes, that can inhibit the expression of the tumorigenic phenotype.[410]

B. NONMUTATIONAL GENETIC HYPOTHESIS

According to this hypothesis certain nonmutational genetic changes would be responsible for the neoplastic transformation of cells. Such changes would include altered patterns of DNA methylation and DNA rearrangement, transposition, or amplification. These types of changes could be involved not only in the increased rate of proliferation associated with neoplastic transformation but also in the inhibition of DNA replication which is observed, for example, in cultured cells rendered quiescent by prolonged serum deprivation. Genomic DNA extracted from quiescent human embryo fibroblasts exerts inhibitory effects on cell growth upon its transfer into recipient HeLa cells, and the strongest inhibition is observed with DNA prepared from serum-deprived cells.[411] Most probably, the inhibitory effect of this DNA is controlled by modifications such as rearrangement, amplification, or methylation events, which could result in the activation or inactivation of discrete DNA sequences including protooncogenes and/or other types of genes.

1. Changes in the Patterns of DNA Methylation

Methylation is the only postreplicational modification of DNA occurring in eukaryotes. Analysis of DNA by the nearest neighbor method has shown that in most mammalian species methylation occurs in the 5'-CpG-3' dinucleotide. However, it is known that this dinucleotide is underrepresented in mammalian genomes and a study of the pattern of DNA methylation in human DNA has demonstrated that 54.5% of total genomic methylation occurs in sites other than CpG, i.e., in CpC, CpA, and CpT.[412]

It has been postulated that DNA methylation has an important role in the regulation of gene expression as well as in cell differentiation.[413-416] The patterns of DNA methylation are maintained by enzymatic systems (DNA methylases) and they are heritable at the cellular level.[417] There is much evidence supporting the idea that the patterns of DNA methylation are tissue specific and that they have an important role in the mechanisms of differentiation and in the control of gene expression.

Cancer is generally considered as a disease associated with aberrant cell differentiation and there is overwhelming evidence indicating the existence of abnormal gene expression in transformed cells. Thus, it may be accepted *a priori* that DNA methylation patterns are altered in neoplastic cells, and the results of many studies lend support to this assumption.[418-422] This would open the way to the possibility that oncogenic factors may initiate and maintain cell transformation by altering the normal patterns of DNA methylation. Moreover, changes in DNA methylation could play a central role in the generation of intratumoral heterogeneity and phenotype instability in cancer.[423] However, human tumor cell lines may not differ from normal fibroblasts in the content of 5-methylcytosine,[424] which suggests that the relationship between DNA methylation and neoplastic transformation may not be a simple one. However, these results should be reviewed on the basis of the evidence indicating that in the human genome there is a high proportion of 5-methylcytosine in dinucleotides other than CpG.[412] In cases where the alterations in gene activity seem unrelated to CpG methylation, the important determinants may reside with 5-methylcytosine in other sequences.

DNA alkylation may produce changes in the patterns of DNA-protein interaction, including the function of DNA-methylating enzymes. A single treatment of human cells (Raji lymphoblastic cells) with *N*-methyl-*N*-nitrosourea (NMU) results in inhibition of methylation of internal cytosines at 5'-CCGG-3' sequences of DNA.[420] The consequent aberrant patterns of DNA methylation may be reflected in altered patterns of genome expression, which could eventually lead to a heritable malignant behavior of the cell. A similar phenomenon could be involved in the mechanisms of action of other carcinogens including BP, DMBA, ethionine, aflatoxin B$_1$, and 2-(acetylamino)fluorene (AAF).[425-427] Treatment of RJK92 Chinese hamster fibroblasts with the alkylating carcinogen MNNG can result in activation of the thymidine kinase gene associated with alteration in the focal or general patterns of DNA methylation.[428] It is, however, unlikely that thymidine kinase gene activation is directly involved in the process of neoplasia.

5-Azacytidine is known to inhibit DNA methylation and to activate the expression of cellular or viral genes and it is also capable of inducing a diversity of tumors in rats, acting as a complete carcinogen.[419,429,430] Hypomethylation of total cellular DNA and specific DNA sequences induced by short-term treatment of C3H/10T1/2 mouse embryo fibroblasts with 5-azacytidine may persist in the progeny of the treated cells for at least 50 subsequent passages.[431] Exposure of C3H/10T1/2 fibroblasts to 5-azacytidine for 24 h followed by serially passage in the absence of 5-azacytidine results in changes in cell morphology, saturation density, growth rate, and serum dependence.[432] By the 5th passage the cells acquire the ability to grow in 0.3% agarose medium, and by the 30th passage they give rise to fully transformed foci that grow in agarose, in agar, and in liquid suspension. This progression can be rapidly accelerated if the cultures derived from 5-azacytidine-treated cells are exposed for 48 hours to the carcinogen BP. These results provide convincing evidence that aberrations in DNA methylation patterns "may be one of a series of critical events during the course of multistage carcinogenesis and thus enhance the evolution of tumor cells."[432]

Treatment of human cell lines with 5-azacytidine may also result in profound alterations in the growing characteristics of cells, including clonogenicity and growth rate,[433] probably by activation of gene sets involved in the control of cell proliferation. Progression of virus-transformed cells is associated with changes in the patterns of DNA methylation and can be reversed by treatment with 5-azacytidine.[434] Methylation of cloned oncogene DNA reduce its transforming capacity in susceptible cells upon transfection, and treatment of the transfected cells with 5-azacytidine reverses this inactivation.[435]

Administration of diets deficient in the methyl donors methionine and/or choline to rats enhances the activities of several hepatocarcinogens, promotes liver tumor formation, and can exert complete carcinogenic activity in the rodent liver.[436,437] The chronic feeding of a methyl-deficient, amino acid-defined diet results in decreased levels of S-adenosylmethionine and increased levels of its metabolic inhibitor S-adenosylhomocysteine in the livers of rats.[438] These changes produce a hypomethylating environment in the liver and may result in hypomethylation of DNA, RNA, and phospholipids. The protooncogenes c-H-*ras* and c-K-*ras* are hypomethyl-ated in DNA samples from both neoplastic and preneoplastic livers of rats fed methyl-deficient diets, regardless of whether or not the rats had received an initiating dose of the carcinogen diethylnitrosamine (DENA).[439] However, the relevance of protooncogene hypomethylation to carcinogenic processes is not understood.

Hypomethylation of discrete DNA sequences may occur not only in fully transformed cells but may be associated with the altered gene expression that is observed in premalignant cells, for example, in hepatocyte nodules occurring in rats treated with carcinogenic agents such as ethionine.[440] In general, hypomethylation distinguishes genes of cancer cells from the respective genes of their normal counterparts,[441] but there are exceptions to this rule.[424] Moreover, it is difficult to decide whether the observed changes are required for the expression of the transformed phenotype or whether they are a consequence of some of the metabolic changes associated with the expression of malignancy or even a consequence of the growth conditions of neoplastic cells.[442] The *in vitro* or *in vivo* growing conditions of cells such as mouse embryonal carcinoma cells can greatly affect DNA methylation.[443] No consistent correlation between a general hypomethylation of genomic DNA and enhanced metastatic capacity has been found in a series of murine and human melanoma cell lines, but the tumor cell populations of cell lines established from individual lung metastases exhibited marked heterogeneity for DNA methyla-tion levels.[444] Mechanisms in addition to DNA methylation are importantly involved in the control of gene expression in embryonal carcinoma cells infected with the chronic retrovirus M-MuLV.[445] Unfortunately, the molecular mechanisms related to the initiation and maintenance of DNA methylation are still poorly understood and additional basic knowledge is needed on this topic in order to assess more properly the relationship between DNA methylation and neoplasia.

2. RNA and Protein Methylation

The possibility has been discussed that, in addition to DNA methylation, the methylation of particular species of RNA, including transfer RNA (tRNA) and ribosomal RNA (rRNA), may have a role in the molecular processes related to normal or aberrant differentiation. The mammalian 5.8S rRNA contains a 2'-O-methylated uridylic acid residue which is methylated in the cytoplasm of normal tissues but is highly undermethylated in the newly synthesized RNA of rapidly growing neoplastic tissues.[446,447] In contrast, an increase in 5.8S rRNA methylation is observed in cell differentiation. It is also possible that protein methylation, which is under the control of specific enzymes, may have a role in cell differentiation and neoplastic transforma-tion.[448] However, the exact role of RNA and protein methylation in relation to cell differentiation and neoplastic transformation is unknown.

3. DNA Rearrangement, Transposition, or Amplification

In bacteria, yeast, and plants, as as well as in protozoa and invertebrates, including *Drosophila*, the shuffling of DNA modules of information, termed transposable elements or transposons, is important for genetic variation and regulation of gene expression.[449-454] Although no typical transposons have been described as yet in vertebrates, recent evidence supports the existence of transposon-like structures even in mammals, including humans.[455,456] The transpos-able elements would be produced by a process of reverse transcription to DNA of RNA molecules generated by the activity of RNA polymerase III. The segments of the genome transcribed by this enzyme would correspond to repetitive sequences interspersed in the genome.[457,458] In the human, most repetitive sequences correspond to the *Alu* family, which is composed of short-length (approximately 300 bp in length) repetitive DNA present in at least 400,000 copies per haploid genome, corresponding to 3 to 6% of the human genome. It has been suggested that *Alu*-family-like sequences may promote the transposition of other sequences of eukaryotic DNA.[459] In general, repetitive sequence transcripts may have a role in developmental processes.[460] Although most human *Alu* sequences may represent pseudogenes, the possibility exists that one or more members of the human *Alu* family may code for an as yet unidentified gene product. Interestingly, *Alu* family members are transcriptionally silent in some neoplastic cell lines, e.g., in HeLa cells.[461]

Another type of exchange of genetic information between multigene families is gene conversion, which may operate both in lower eukaryotes and in higher cells and organisms.[462] Gene conversion consists of a non-reciprocal transfer of genetic information by which a given gene acts as a sequence donor without being affected in its function and another gene, which shares extensive homology with the donor gene, receives a block of DNA sequences from the donor gene and undergoes variation. The molecular mechanisms of gene conversion as well as the possible role of gene conversion in cell differentiation and neoplastic transformation are little understood.

The precise role of DNA rearrangements and transpositions in vertebrate differentiation and development is not clear at present but, in principle, position effects may be instrumental for the regulation of gene expression. There is evidence that particular types of DNA rearrangements, including tandem duplication occurring in human cells, may result in activation of the expression of neighboring genes.[463] Vertebrate immunoglobulin genes undergo specific rearrangements of DNA segments that are instrumental for the synthesis of different immunoglobulin molecular species and, consequently, to determine an adequate immune response. These rearrangements can be used for the study and classification of human B-cell lymphomas. Similar DNA rearrangements occur in the antigen-specific T cell receptor gene and may serve as molecular markers for the diagnosis and classification of T-cell lymphoid neoplasms.[216,464,465] Moreover, in addition to DNA rearrangements, hypermutational processes which are nonrandomly distributed occur throughout sequences within the V_H region of Ig genes in both normal and tumor B-cell clones.[466] These changes result in extensive variation of nucleic acid residues among the V_H genes.

ADP-ribosyl transferase (ADPRT) activity and transient DNA breaks may be widely involved in the differentiation of eukaryotic cells, including chicken and human cells.[467-471] Since ADPRT is an enzyme required for DNA repair and efficient rejoining of DNA strand breaks, its early activation in differentiating cells suggests that transposition of DNA segments may be critically involved in certain differentiation processes occurring in eukaryotic cells. Proteins such as growth factors, involved in the induction of cell differentiation, may cause single-strand breaks in double-stranded DNA, which may be associated with changes in gene expression.[472] However, the relative importance of DNA transposition and/or rearrangement in the mechanisms of differentiation of eukaryotic cells, especially in vertebrate cells, is difficult to evaluate at present.

Whereas chromosome stability is characteristic of normal cells, chromosome instability is a general feature of tumor cells. One may then ask the question as to whether such instability is the consequence of a generalized activation of transposable elements.[473] The possibility that DNA rearrangements and transpositions as well as small deletions may be associated with the origin of neoplastic changes has been discussed.[474-482] An intriguing parallelism would exist between chromosomal changes involved in the evolutionary creation of new species of living organisms and the constitution and development of clones of cells with chromosome translocations and rearrangements that may originate new cellular clones with potential oncogenic properties.[483] At least under certain experimental conditions, the process of neoplastic transformation is too efficient to be explained only by point mutational events occurring at some specific sites of the genome. There are certain situations in which even quite low doses of mutagen are capable of initiating the process of transformation in almost every exposed cell.[484] It is difficult to explain this situation solely on the basis of point mutational events.

When early passage cultures of normal human diploid fibroblasts were exposed to various doses of X-rays and were thereafter serially pasaged and followed throughout their lifespan *in vitro*, it was observed that the irradiation produces chromosomal rearrangements which may persist throughout the lifespan of the cells.[485] Multiple chromosomal clones emerged among the progeny of cells in cultures exposed to multiple sequential radiation doses. In several cases these clones expanded to include most of the cell population before the cultures became senescent. It was hypothesized that the emergence of abnormal clones with translocations and/or rearrangements in the vicinity of critical cellular genes may be associated with the development of the transformed phenotype induced by X-irradiation.[485,486]

Cancer can be produced in animals by manipulations such as transplantation of tissues to special sites or implantation of sheets of plastic material.[487,488] Sarcomas of monoclonal origin develop in mice upon subcutaneous implantation of nonbiodegradable materials, such as millipore filters.[489,490] Unlike carcinogenic chemicals, viruses or radiation, this foreign body material is not cell invasive. Consequently, foreign body tumorigenesis may be useful for the study of "pure" initiation changes in neoplasia. Point mutations are a most unlikely mechanism for the origin of transformation in these cases but a diversity of numerical and structural chromosome changes occurs very early during foreign body tumorigenesis. Such abnormalities are unstable and variable during early preneoplasia, gaining stability during advanced stages of neoplastic progression, which leads to the presence of common structural chromosome changes in the tumor cells derived from this population.[490] It seems likely that foreign body tumorigenesis is initiated by selection of some specific chromosome changes, which may lead to expression of a transformed phenotype, as reflected by increased proliferative drive and abnormal cell behavior.

Exposure to asbestos fibers is the primary cause of human mesothelioma in industrialized countries but the mechanisms by which asbestos causes mesothelioma remain obscure. Replicative cultures of human pleural mesothelial cells exposed to asbestos fibers exhibit abnormal growth properties associated with the emergence of clones of aneuploid cells with chromosomes possessing a repetitious banding pattern but these alterations are insufficient to cause the cells to be tumorigenic.[491] Thus, although particular types of chromosome alterations may be associated with the initial changes occurring in cells exposed to asbestos, these alterations are in themselves insufficient for the expression of a malignant phenotype.

In many types of transformed cells, rearrangements and transpositions of large genomic segments can be observed by microscopical methods in form of particular types of structural chromosome aberrations, such as translocations or inversions. As mentioned before, the presence of these abnormalities is the rule, not only in neoplasia, but also in preneoplasia. In addition, amplification of specific genes, or groups of genes, can be ascertained by the presence of characteristic cytogenetic abnormalities, such as homogeneously staining regions (HSRs) and double minutes (DMs), which are also frequently observed in many different types of transformed cells.[492-497] Unregulated amplification of particular genomic segments may be considered as a pathological process, occurring readily in neoplastic cells but rarely in normal cells.[498] Gene amplification may contribute, together with other chromosome alterations, to the rapid evolution and progression of cancer.

There is clear evidence that the rearrangement of discrete cellular DNA sequences may result in the creation of sequences with oncogenic capability. A rat DNA sequence containing the 5′ half of the c-*raf* protooncogene replaced by other rat DNA sequence was produced during the procedure of DNA transfection in the NIH/3T3 assay system.[499] The newly produced recombinant sequence was transcribed in form of a fused mRNA in which the 5′ half of the sequence was replaced by an unknown rat sequence, and this mRNA coded a fused c-*raf*-related protein. The normal and recombinant c-*raf* DNAs were each connected to the long terminal repeat (LTR) of Rous sarcoma virus (RSV) and were transfected thereafter into NIH/3Ts cells.[500] Only the recombinant form of the DNA sequence exhibited transforming activity. It is thus apparent that particular types of rearrangements of cellular DNA may result in the formation of sequences with oncogenic capability.

The general role of DNA transposition, translocation, and rearrangement in the origin and/ or development of tumors is difficult to evaluate at present. In many tumors, especially in solid tumors (carcinomas, sarcomas), specific alterations of these types are not consistently observed. Transformation of some rat cell lines by tumor promoters can occur without affecting sister chromatid exchange (SCE),[501] which suggests that large-scale DNA rearrangements may not be a requisite for the origin of transformation. The results of experiments with *N*-ethyl-*N*-nitrosourea (ENU)-induced transformation in Syrian hamster embryo (SHE) cells clearly show that chromosome alterations other than SCE play a major role in the induction of morphological transformation whereas SCE and gene mutations would play only a minor role or would not be involved in the early stages of neoplastic transformation at all.[502] In addition to microscopical methods, further application of DNA hybridization studies and restriction fragment length polymorphism (RFLP) analysis are required for a better understanding of this important subject.[220,271]

C. VIRAL HYPOTHESIS

The role of viruses in the etiology of neoplastic diseases under both natural and experimental conditions is well documented for many vertebrate species, including several nonhuman primates. However, the possible role of viruses in human cancer has been for many years a subject of controversy.[503] In any case, only some particular types of human tumors would be associated with viral infection.

1. DNA Viruses

Several type of DNA viruses are ubiquituous infectious agents and some of these viruses have been postulated as possible agents in the causation of human tumors. Examples of this situation are the Epstein-Barr virus (EBV) in relation to nasopharyngeal carcinoma and African Burkitt's lymphoma, herpes simplex virus type 2 (HSV-2) and papillomaviruses in relation to carcinoma of the uterine cervix, and hepatitis B virus (HBV) in relation to hepatocellular carcinoma. The mechanisms of oncogenicity associated with infection by DNA viruses are seemingly complex and are, at present, not well understood. In any case, under natural conditions these viruses would not be capable of inducing tumors by themselves but would require the cooperation of unspecified endogenous and/or exogenous factors.

2. Retroviruses

Among RNA viruses, some retroviruses may have oncogenic potential in either natural or experimental conditions. Retroviruses are characterized by the presence of a gene encoding reverse transcriptase and may be of either exogenous or endogenous origin. Two types of exogenous retroviruses have been described, namely, acutely transforming retroviruses (acute retroviruses) and chronic retroviruses.[504] Acute retroviruses are characterized by the presence of specific transforming sequences, termed oncogenes. These sequences are not of viral but of cellular origin, and acute retroviruses act only as oncogene transducers, although they are not infectious agents transmitting malignant diseases under natural conditions. Only by means of experimental manipulations can be demonstrated the high oncogenic capability of acute retroviruses. A prototype of these viruses is the RSV, which was isolated from tumors of chickens.[505]

Under natural conditions, only chronic retroviruses would be involved in the etiology of neoplastic diseases. These viruses do not possess specific transforming sequences of cellular origin, i.e., they do not act as oncogene transducers. In contradistinction to acute retroviruses, chronic retroviruses are not capable of transforming cultured cells and would produce tumors only after a prolonged latent period. Chronic retroviruses have been implicated in the etiology of different malignant diseases, mainly leukemias and lymphomas, in numerous mammalian species, including some primates. Their possible role in the etiology of human neoplasms is not clear but, recently, certain chronic retroviruses, generically termed human T-cell lymphotropic viruses (HTLVs), have been recognized as agents probably involved in the etiology of some human malignant diseases.[506-511] HTLVs are infectious agents, being transmitted horizontally by contagion, and not through the germ line. Another class of infectious retroviruses, the human immunodeficiency viruses (HIVs) are responsible for the epidemic disease termed acquire immune deficiency syndrome (AIDS) and may be involved in the etiology of certain human tumors such as Kaposi's sarcoma through indirect mechanisms associated with a severe alteration of the immune system.[512-514]

3. Activation of Endogenous Proviruses

Endogenous proviruses are present in the mammalian genome, including the human genome, and are transmitted as cellular genes through the germ line.[515-517] Their normal functions are unknown but they could be involved in some developmental processes. The possible relation of endogenous proviruses to neoplastic diseases is not understood. In any case, factors other than viral infection or activation are of critical importance for the origin and development of tumors under natural conditions.

D. EPIGENETIC HYPOTHESIS

In contradistinction to the different kinds of genetic hypotheses discussed above, the epigenetic hypothesis of the origin of cancer postulates that structural genomic changes, either of mutational or nonmutational types, are not crucially required for the initiation of neoplastic changes and that regulatory changes alone may lead to transformation.

1. Neoplasia and Metaplasia

Abnormal cell differentiation may result in either metaplasia or neoplasia. Whereas, in metaplasia cells from an adult, fully differentiated tissue of one kind are transformed into cells from a differentiated tissue of another kind,[518] in neoplasia the proliferating cells never reach the state of terminal differentiation characteristic of the respective tissue where they arise. Metaplasia occurs by a process of transdifferentiation which consists in the switching of differentiated cells to cells with other phenotypes. Transdifferentiation processes have been observed very often in cultures of neural and ocular tissues and may occur normally between mast cell subpopulations.[519,520]

2. Blocked Ontogeny Hypothesis

Embryogenesis and carcinogenesis share striking similarities at the cellular and molecular levels. Both normal mammalian embryonic cells and and malignant cells are apparently immortal when maintained in appropriate conditions in *in vitro* culture.[139] However, the behavioral characteristics of normal and malignant cells are in clear contrast.[521] Embryogenesis represents a state of order where progressively differentiating structures are organized to build up an organism. In contrast, carcinogenesis is a pathological process which results in the production of disorganized tumor tissues which disrupt normal tissues and may lead to destruction and death of the organism.

The idea that neoplastic transformation may be considered as a consequence of some disturbance in the normal processes of differentiation (blocked ontogeny hypothesis) has been discussed during the last decades by many investigators.[189,522] Moreover, cancer has been considered in itself as a particular type of abnormal postembryonic differentiation resulting in a "caricature of the tissue of origin,"[523] or as a form of retrodifferentiation which would constitute "the only alternative against aging and death."[524] Cancer has also been considered as an "abortive attempt at differentiation by the neoplastic stem cells,"[525] or as a form of "variant differentiation."[526] Different degrees of abnormalities of differentiation are frequently seen even among different cells from a given tumor. In any case, it is apparent that normal cell differentiation almost always, with some rare exceptions (lymphoid cell differentiation), inescapably leads to cell death after the accomplishment of the differentiated function. In a particular tissue, cells undergoing differentiation are characterized by a progressive slowing of the rate of proliferation, with total arrest of proliferation when terminal differentiation is reached.

3. Lineage Infidelity and Misprogramming

Human leukemias do not represent aberrant cell types expressing new "leukemia antigens" but resemble normal hematopoietic precursor cells blocked at different stages of differentiation.[72] Although leukemic cells are not identical to normal progenitor cells, the exact differences existing between them are difficult to identify and there is a lot of controversy as to whether leukemic cells express lineage infidelity and promiscuity of marker expression due to genetic missprogramming.[527]

4. Neoplastic Transformation and the Expression of Differentiated Functions

Undoubtedly, there is a close association, and partial identity, between the mechanisms involved in the control of cell differentiation and those related to the expression of a transformed phenotype. Neoplasia occurs with increased frequency in organs and tissues affected by altered differentiation processes, e.g., in abnormal sexual differentiation.[528] Cell cycle-dependent processes involved in the control of cell differentiation and proliferation may be involved in tumor-suppressing mechanisms. Clones of BALB/c 3T3 cells expressing defects in the control of both cellular differentiation and proliferation are highly tumorigenic, whereas clones that maintain the ability to control either their differentiation or their proliferation are markedly less tumorigenic, and clones of the same cells that maintain the ability to control both their differentiation and their proliferation are nontumorigenic.[529] Preneoplastic cells may express defects in the stringency with which the integrated control of cellular differentiation and proliferation is regulated.[145] Thus, maintenance by a stem cell of its ability to efficiently regulate the control of cellular differentiation and/or proliferation can serve to suppress oncogenic transformation.

UV irradiation and other agents capable of initiating carcinogenic processes may act through a selective and stable inhibition of stem cell differentiation.[530] However, a dissociation between expression of malignant properties and expression of differentiated functions may be observed in certain experimental conditions, for example, in cultured rat thyroid cells transformed by temperature-sensitive (*ts*) mutants of Kirsten murine sarcoma virus (K-MuSV).[531] Moreover, expression of a single defect in control of the terminal phase of differentiation is not sufficient for complete carcinogenesis.[532] These results suggest that the expression of a single defect in the control of terminal differentiation may represent an early event in the multistage process of carcinogenesis but that this defect is insufficient in itself to induce complete neoplastic transformation. Additional cellular defects or changes must be expressed for a cell to be fully initiated in its neoplastic transformation.

The potential for reactivation of cell proliferation may be preserved in differentiated cells such as the hepatocytes, which may proliferate in regenerative processes when subjected to appropriate stimuli. However, it is not clear if all cells of the population can participate in these processes or if there is a specific subpopulation with preserved capacity for cell proliferation.[533] The possibility that neoplastic transformation originates in vivo in a subpopulation of cells with spontaneous or environmentally induced resistance to terminal differentiation has been suggested by the results obtained in some studies.[534,535]

5. Molecular Mechanisms of Cell Differentiation

Commitment of embryonic cells to their fate depends on both intra- and intercellular (extracellular) determinants of cell differentiation.[536] The development of specific patterns of cell differentiation in embryonic or postembryonic cells depends on both the particular genetic potential and programming of the cell and the influence of intra- and extracellular signals which include hormones, peptide growth factors, and protein products of cellular genes including protooncogenes.[86] Transcription factors that may be regulated in an either positive or negative manner are probably involved in the control of cellular gene expression during differentiation.[537] The genes involved in the expression of differentiated morphology and function are probably different in different types of cells and tissues, but these genes remain little characterized.[538]

The molecular phenomena responsible for the normal processes of cell differentiation remain poorly characterized. There is evidence that, at least in some cases, these processes may be independent of DNA synthesis.[539] The roles of DNA methylation and nonmutational genomic changes in cell differentiation phenomena were discussed in a previous section of this chapter. Interactions between sequence specific nuclear DNA binding proteins and 5′-flanking DNase I hypersensitive sites of particular genes may be instrumental for the modulation of gene transcription, and the transcriptional activation of particular genes, or set of genes, may be responsible for the expression of cell-specific differentiated functions.[540] The introduction of nicks or single-strand breaks in double-stranded DNA, which may be specifically stimulated by particular peptide growth factors, may be required for the initiation of changes involved in the regulation of gene expression.[472,541]

6. Role of Homeoboxes in Morphogenesis and Differentiation

Self-renewal and differentiation programs of multipotential stem cells are controlled by separate genes.[542] Discrete genomic protein-coding sequences, designated homeoboxes, play an important role in the regulation of morphogenesis and differentiation in *Drosophila,* and similar sequences are conserved in a variety of invertebrate and vertebrate species, including humans.[543-548] More than 11 copies of the homeobox have been characterized in flies and mutations in any of these elements can alter the normal embryonic segmentation patterns of the insect. The presence of highly conserved copies of homeobox homology in both of the great divisions of the animal kingdom, the protostomes and the deuterostomes, indicates their existence for at least 800 million years.[544] Homeobox sequences have been cloned from the genomes of *Xenopus,* mice, and humans.[545,549,550]

Homeoboxes are clustered in particular regions of the genome and are differentially expressed during prenatal and postnatal development.[546] Murine homeobox genes share with the *Drosophila* homeobox homologues several properties including sequence homology, clustering, and location on different chromosomes. They are also differentially expressed during normal embryogenesis as well as during differentiation of embryonal carcinoma cells.[551,552] Thus, in spite of the different developmental strategies adopted by *Drosophila* and mammals, functional similarities may exist with respect to the expression of homeobox genes. An important, perhaps crucial, role of homeoboxes in mammalian developmental processes is suggested by the observation that the expression of mouse homeobox genes is tissue and region specific. For example, the homeobox genes *Hox-1.2* and *Hox-1.4* are expressed in the lower myelencephalon and in the cervical central nervous system of the mouse and, in addition, the *Hox-1.2* gene is expressed in several thoracic prevertebrae.[553] The *Hox-1.4* gene is expressed not only in the mouse central nervous system but also in the germ cells of the testis, especially in meiotic prophase spermatocytes and in early (round) spermatids.[554] *Hox-1.4* gene transcripts present in the normal mouse embryo and teratocarcinoma cell cultures are larger than those present in germ cells. A homeobox sequence identified as *Hox-2.3* is strongly expressed in a tissue-specific fashion in adult mice and in a restricted region of the central nervous system during embryogenesis.[555] Treatment of pluripotent embryonal carcinoma cells with retinoic acid leads to induction of *Hox-2.3* expression. The complete nucleotide sequence of the murine *Hox-2.3* gene was determined.[556] The possible role of homeobox genes in abnormal developmental processes and neoplastic diseases is not understood at present.

A homeobox-containing gene cluster, termed m6, has been mapped to mouse chromosome 6 by somatic cell genetic analysis and a homologous locus is present on the short arm of human chromosome 7.[557] Four homeoboxes have been cloned recently from the mouse genome, and their nucleotide sequences were determined.[558] Three of these homeoboxes are linked to the *Hox-2* gene complex on mouse chromosome 11, whereas the fourth, *Hox-4*, was assigned to chromosome 12. All four homeoboxes are expressed in the mouse embryo and the expression of 4.2-kb transcripts from one of them (mh19) was found to be connected to the induced differentiation of Friend erythroleukemia cells.

Four homeobox DNA sequences have been assigned to particular regions on human chromosomes: one to 2q31-q37, other to 12q12-q13, and the other two to chromosome 17.[559] Interestingly, a collagen chain gene is located in the vicinity of each of these human homeobox genes. However, in man there are several collagen gene loci that have not been shown to be near a homeobox gene and the biological significance, if any, of the association between the two types of genes is unknown.

Unfortunately, almost nothing is known about the specific physiological role of homeobox-encoded proteins in relation to particular types of differentiation and developmental processes. The possible role of homeoboxes in oncogenic processes is supported by the observation that specific expression of homeobox-containing genes occurs during induced differentiation of embryonal carcinoma cells.[560] Induction of differentiation of embryonic carcinoma cells with retinoic acid is associated with accumulation of large amounts of homeobox transcripts. However, nonchemical treatment triggering differentiation of these cells does not lead to detectable expression of homeobox genes, which suggests that the transcriptional activation of homeobox genes is correlated with retinoic acid treatment but not with the process of differentiation as such.[561]

7. Extranuclear Cellular Factors in the Regulation of Cell Differentiation

Most probably, the processes of differentiation depend on regulatory changes occurring at the genomic level under the action of specific environmental influences acting through alterations in the plasma membrane and/or the cytoplasm. There is experimental evidence that the expression of genes in the nuclei of differentiated cells is remarkably plastic and susceptible to modulation by the cytoplasm.[562] Hormones and peptide growth factors are important environmental factors involved in the control of cell proliferation and cell differentiation in susceptible cells, and this susceptibility would depend, at least partially, on modulation of the genetic program of the particular cell.[86] Interferons are also involved in the regulation of cell proliferation and differentiation.[563] It follows that abnormalities such as those occurring in neoplastic cells, characterized by increase in the rate of cell proliferation and decrease in cell maturation and differentiation, may be a consequence of spontaneous or environmentally induced changes in the particular genetic program of the cell, responsible for the development and maintenance of normal differentiation.

Experiments with fusion of normal diploid human fibroblasts from amniotic fluid or from fetal lung with differentiated mouse muscle cells to form stable heterokaryons show an activation of at least five previously silent human muscle genes.[539] In these experiments it was clearly shown that DNA synthesis or genome structural alterations are not required for the expression of a new set of genes, such as muscle-specific genes, and that cytoplasmic factors play a critical role in regulating the expression of the differentiated state. However, the chemical nature and the mechanism of action of the latter factors are unknown. There is evidence that the expression of a transformed phenotype in RSV-transformed cultured chick embryo cells may be independent of cell division.[564] However, in mouse cultured cells at least one cell division is required for the fixation of the state of malignant transformation induced by 3-methylcholan-threne (MCA).[565]

8. Regulatory Changes Involved in Neoplastic Transformation

Alterations of cellular regulatory phenomena leading to neoplastic transformation could occur at several sites, including the nucleus and different extranuclear sites (cytoplasm, mitochondria, cytoskeleton, plasma membrane), but it is difficult to distinguish the primary from the secondary alterations. In any case, these alterations would result in a derangement of genomic functions involved in the maintenance of a normally differentiated state. Hypothetically, two types of alterations are possible: (1) the extranuclear factors involved in these regulatory phenomena would be produced in abnormal quantity or quality or (2) the response of the nucleus to normal extranuclear signals would not be adequate. The main lines of evidence that lend support to the epigenetic hypothesis of the origin of cancer are discussed next.

9. Susceptibility to Malignant Transformation

There are marked differences in the susceptibility of different animals to transformation *in vivo* and *in vitro*. As a general rule, laboratory and domestic animals are more susceptible to spontaneous or carcinogen-induced neoplasms than wild animals. Epithelial cell cultures derived from numerous rodent organs and tissues have been neoplastically transformed by chemical carcinogens, but there are only few reports of carcinogen-induced transformation of human epithelial organ or cell cultures, which indicates that transformation of human epithelial cells to immortality and malignancy is an extremely rare event.[566] The marked differences existing among different animal species in the susceptibility to transformation cannot be attributed to differences in mutation rates, which are of about the same order of magnitude in all of them. These facts suggest that nonmutational mechanisms, which may be either genetic or nongenetic, can be critically involved in the origin of neoplasia. Such mechanisms may be variable among different animals according to their respective genotypes.

Within a given population of cultured normal cells (low-passage Syrian hamster embryonic cells), there may be marked differences in the susceptibility to carcinogen-induced neoplastic transformation. These differences, however, are not due to variation in the rates of mutation among the components of the cell population, but should be attributed to subtle changes in the state of differentiation existing between apparently identical cells.[567] Again, this dissociation between mutation and neoplastic transformation indicates a fundamental difference in the nature of these two processes.

10. Environmental Influences on the Expression of the Malignant Phenotype

Factors from the microenvironment where the cells are growing may be of critical importance for the expression, or lack of expression, of a transformed phenotype. Moreover, depending on certain environmental conditions, neoplastic cells may participate in at least some normal developmental processes. Transplantation of mice teratoma cells (embryonal carcinoma cells) into mice blastulas may result in development of chimeric mice exhibiting normal adult tissues that are partially derived from the malignant cells.[568] However, the ability of embryonal carcinoma cell lines to participate in mouse embryogenesis shows great variability depending on individual clones.[569] A given clone of embryonal carcinoma cells seems to have its own intrinsic property in relation to its behavior when integrated in the developmental processes of mouse embryos; whereas some embryonal carcinoma cells differentiate completely normally into various tissues including germ cells, others cause severe morphological abnormalities at midgestational stages or produce embryonal carcinoma cell-derived tumors in the chimeric animals.

The capacity of the blastocyst to regulate the growth of embryonal carcinoma cells is limited. The blastocyst can regulate one embryonal carcinoma cell consistently and may have a slight effect on three, but it cannot regulate four or five of them.[570] Moreover, the location of the tumor cell within the blastocyst is important. Regulation occurs if the embryonal carcinoma cells is placed in the blastocoele cavity, but enhancement of tumorigenicity is obtained if it is placed between the zona pellucida and the trophoectoderm. Moreover, the blastocyst is unable to regulate the growth of other types of tumor cells. Even a single B-16 melanoma cell placed in the blastocoele cavity cannot be regulated by the blastocyst.[570] Thus, there is a degree of specificity in the regulation of tumor cell growth by the blastocyst.

Although it may be argued that teratoma cells are a very special kind of malignant cells, other types of malignant cells when injected into mice embryos can also participate in normal developmental processes. Mouse myeloma cells injected into mouse embryos *in utero* at 10 d of gestation are able to participate in normal hematopoietic differentiation, and the injected embryos may develop into normal adult mice whose granulocytes contain a marker derived from the leukemic cells.[571] Apparently, these cells are capable of responding to control mechanisms involved in the regulation of normal growth and differentiation in the embryo.[572]

Leukemic stem cells of mice, originally transformed by the Friend murine leukemia virus (F-MuLV), show malignant growth kinetics when proliferating in the spleen of the leukemic mice but revert to normal self-renewal and differentiation when grown in the spleen of irradiated syngenic hosts.[573] This behavior is independent of F-MuLV expression and the results suggests that the microenvironment to which the cells are exposed plays a fundamental role in the expression of the malignant phenotype.

Neoplastic lymphocytes from hamster leukemia induced with simian virus 40 (SV40) can retain, lose, or regain the capacity to induce leukemia or lymphoma in allogeneic animals according to the organ/tissue microenvironment in which they proliferate upon transplantation.[574] These results indicate that the malignant behavior of the neoplastic lymphocytes is not a stable, irreversible characteristic that is transmitted to the cell progeny but that, more likely, it depends on nonmutational, epigenetic events that may be modulated by the host microenvironment.

The importance of environmental factors for the expression and maintenance of the transformed phenotype is also emphasized by the changes that they may suffer under conditions of *in vitro* culture. Whereas some new phenotypic characteristics may appear when the tumor cells are cultured *in vitro*, other characteristics observed *in vivo* are not retained, and, occasionally, the cells may lose their tumorigenic properties.[575]

The human epidermoid carcinoma HEp3 exhibits highly malignant growth in chicken embryos that disappears progressively in cell culture, being essentially complete after 40 generations in culture.[576] Once lost, the malignant phenotype of the same cells reappears after exposure of the nontumorigenic cells to the *in vivo* conditions. These results suggest that the malignant phenotype of HEp3 cells is expressed in response to specific conditions existing in the physiological environment and that loss of regaining of tumorigenic properties by these cells are difficult to reconcile with mechanisms involving mutational events. Rather, humoral factors that are present, respectively, *in vivo* or *in vitro*, would contribute for modulating cell growth behavior.

11. Apparent Normal Totipotency of the Nuclei of Tumor Cells

Several investigators have demonstrated that implantation of isolated nuclei from Lucké frog adenocarcinoma cells into enucleated normal frog eggs may result in the development of apparently normal tadpoles.[577] These results suggest that Lucké adenocarcinoma cells are not malignant cells because they have mutations, since their implantation into a normal cytoplasmic environment would induce reprogramming of an essentially normal genetic information, capable of guiding normal developmental processes. However, it should be noticed that the efficiency of these experimental procedures is rather low and that the growth of the resulting embryos is always arrested at the stage of tadpole. A normal adult frog has never been created by means of such artificial procedures.

12. Suppression of Tumorigenicity in Somatic Cell Hybrids

Somatic cell hybrids can be generated *in vitro* by fusion between different types of cells, which is frequently induced by the exposure of cells to the inactivated Sendai virus. Even interspecific somatic cell hybrids, constituting heterokaryons, can be obtained by this procedure.[578] The analysis of the behavior of the malignant phenotype in somatic cell hybrids indicate that this phenotype is a recessive one because, whenever a malignant cell is fused with a cell of low tumorigenicity or with a normal diploid cell, the hybrid cells show a suppression or marked reduction of the malignant phenotype.[579-583] Suppression of the malignant phenotype can be achieved even in cells continuously expressing a transforming gene product (the protein product of a mutated human EJ c-H-*ras* protooncogene), when the transformed cells are fused to normal cells.[584-588] This suppression suggests that normal cells may contain tumor-suppressing genes, or antioncogenes, capable of inhibiting the expression of a transformed phenotype. However, the tumor-suppressive activity as demonstrated in somatic cell hybrids does not necessarily involve an antioncogene but could be due to mechanisms acting at epigenetic levels. The results obtained in hybrids of cells containing an oncogenically activated oncogene can be explained on the basis of recessivity of oncogene expression, which is in contradiction with the apparent dominant behavior of mutated oncogenes. Moreover, the lesions determining the transformed phenotype, although recessive, fail to complement each other. Only in certain virally transformed cells the transformed phenotype behaves as a dominant trait, but this behavior depends on the continuous expression of specific viral genes (oncogenes).

The expression of a transformed phenotype (anchorage independence) can be effectively suppressed by fusion of carcinogen-transformed baby hamster kidney (BHK) cells with normal human fibroblasts. Karyotype analysis of these cells indicates that only human chromosome 1 is retained in all cell hybrids in which the transformed phenotype is reexpressed.[589] These results suggest the existence of a gene, or genes, located on human chromosome 1, which have the capacity of suppressing the expression of the transformed phenotype by acting in a dominant fashion. However, human chromosome 1 is not among those chromosomes that are associated with the suppression of malignancy in other types of cells, like Chinese hamster ovary (CHO) cells or human HeLa cells. Thus, chromosome-mediated suppression of malignancy is an heterogeneous phenomenon and a chromosome, or chromosome segment, producing a general suppression of the malignant phenotype would probably not exist.

Analysis of cell hybrids between normal, early-passage Syrian hamster embryo (SHE) cells and a highly tumorigenic, chemically transformed cell line (BP6T) shows suppression of anchorage-independent growth and tumorigenicity in the hybrid cells compared with the tumorigenic BP6T cells.[590] Moreover, hybrids between BP6T cells with chemically induced immortal, but nontumorigenic, hamster cell lines showed a similar suppression. This tumor-suppressive ability was reduced in the same cells at later passages and in some cases nearly completely lost, prior to the neoplastic transformation of the immortalized cell lines. Subclones of the cell lines were heterogeneous in their ability to suppress tumorigenicity in cell hybrids. These results suggest that chemically induced neoplastic progression of SHE cells involves at least three steps: (1) induction of immortality, (2) activation of a transforming gene, and (3) loss of a tumor-suppressive function.[590] The latter would be a key step for neoplastic progression.

Although genetic models can be constructed to explain these phenomena, the results obtained with the suppression of malignancy after somatic cell hybridization are more easily explained by epigenetic processes such as regulatory circuits operating at the level of some genomic functions which would be essential for the expression of malignant cell behavior. Furthermore, the transformed and malignant (tumorigenic) phenotypes may each represent a separate phenomenon, which may often be found in association with each other but are not necessarily expressed simultaneously and may be under separate control.[580,591] Suppression of tumorigenicity in somatic cell hybrids may be associated with changes in the levels of transcriptional expression of several genes, but the biological significance of these changes is not understood.[592]

13. Suppression of Tumorigenicity and Induction of Immortalization in Cybrids

Enucleation techniques allow the separation of the nucleus from the cytoplasm, and the anucleate cytoplasms, termed cytoplasts, can be fused with whole cells, which results in the production of mononuclear cytoplasmic hybrids, termed cybrids. The construction of cybrids between tumorigenic cells and cytoplasms from nontumorigenic cells has demonstrated that the transformed phenotype is not suppressed when the tumorigenic cells are virally transformed but that a heritable suppression of the transformed phenotype occurs when spontaneously trans-formed cells are used to produce the cybrids.[593-595] These results strongly suggest that factor(s) present in the cytoplasm of nontumorigenic cells are able to induce a heritable suppression of tumorigenicity, thus supporting the hypothesis that, at least in some tumors arising spontane-ously, epigenetic factors are critically involved in the origin and maintenance of the transformed phenotype.

Fusion of normal human lymphocytes with isolated cytoplasts from transformed L929 mouse cells results in B- and T-cell lines that appear to grow indefinitely.[596] Apparently, some factor(s) present in the cytoplasm of the transformed mouse cells are capable of altering the regulation of specific nuclear functions in the human lymphocytes thus inducing their immortalization, although the fused lymphocytes do not exhibit malignant properties. The cytoplasmic factors responsible for the induction of such immortalization have not been identified, but the immortalizing activity is restricted to cytoplasts from transformed cell lines with unlimited proliferation potential.[596]

14. Suppression of Tumorigenicity Induced by Chemical Mutagens

Treatment of tumorigenic murine neoplastic cell lines *in vitro* with potent chemical mutagens followed by cloning of the surviving cells results in the selection, at extraordinary high frequencies (up to 90%), of clones unable to grow progressively in normal syngeneic mice.[597] Such clones, designated *tum⁻*, are nontumorigenic in normal hosts and are phenotypically stable in culture over a period of several weeks or months. The frequency rates of generation of *tum⁻* variants are several orders of magnitude greater than that predicted by classic genetic mutational events, which suggests that these variants are originated by epigenetic mechanisms.

15. Tumor Cells May Spontaneously Develop into Normally Differentiated Cells *In Vivo*

In some tumors of plants and animals the division of tumor cells may be associated with differentiation and consequent production of normal cells. This phenomenon has been observed in some tumors of the sunflower, in epidermoid (squamous) carcinomas of the rat, and in teratomas occurring in humans and other animal species,[598,599] but it should be considered as exceptional, not being representative of the the general behavior of tumors.

An intriguing phenomenon is the spontaneous regression of tumors, which is defined as the reduction in size or complete disappearance of a histologically identified tumor in the absence of therapy that would be considered as adequate to alter significantly the natural course of the disease.[6] Spontaneous regression of human cancer is very rare and is most frequently observed in a few types of tumors, namely, malignant melanoma, hypernephroma, choriocarcinoma, and nephroblastoma, which account together for the majority of the total cases.[600-603] Spontaneous regression of retinoblastomas has also been reported.[604,605] However, it has been suggested that the latter cases do not represent true retinoblastomas but retinomas, that is, they would correspond to more benign forms of the tumor, originated in partially differentiated cells.[606] Human retinoblastoma may originate from a primitive neuroectodermal multipotential cell.[607] The culture of human retinoblastoma cells under appropriate conditions *in vitro* may result in their differentiation into particular structures termed Flexner-Wintersteiner rosettes.[608] Sponta-neous regression of cytogenetic and hematologic anomalies was observed in a patient with Ph chromosome-positive CML followed up over 8 years.[609] The percentage of Ph-positive cells in this patient decreased from 100 to 37% and a trisomy 8 which was present initially disappeared without therapy.

Spontaneous regression has also been observed in certain experimental tumors, like the malignant lymphomas induced in Swiss and NZW mice by 1-ethyl-1-nitrosourea (ENU) and the leukemia induced in chickens with avian myeloblastosis virus (AMV).[610,611] The mechanisms involved in spontaneous regression of tumors are multiple and may be different in different cases but one mechanism may consist in the induction of terminal differentiation by unidentified endogenous and/or exogenous environmental stimuli. It is likely that only the tumors originated in partially differentiated cells can undergo spontaneous regression due to terminal differentiation. In a rare case of spontaneous regression of hepatocellular carcinoma in a Chinese patient, the evidence indicated that regression occurred by involution rather than maturation and that the tumor was replaced by surrounding tissue.[612]

Spontaneous regression of neoplasms should be distinguished from spontaneous remission, which is also a very rare event. Spontaneous remission of acute leukemia, for example, is a transient phenomenon and is frequently associated with precedent or concurrent bacterial infections.[613] The mechanisms responsible for such remissions are not known.

16. *In Vitro* Spontaneous Differentiation of Transformed Cells

Different types of neoplastic cells maintained under appropriate culture conditions *in vitro* may occasionally undergo processes of spontaneous maturation and differentiation.[608,614-618] Leukemic cells of the bone marrow from patients with acute myelocytic leukemia (AML) may be progressively and completely replaced by normal mature cells (neutrophilic granulocytes and, subsequently, macrophages) when the cells are maintained under appropriate conditions in a long-term culture system *in vitro*.[619] The cellular mechanisms associated with such reversion phenomena are not understood but mutational events are apparently not responsible for these reversions because different types of mutagenic agents, including an alkylation agent, a frameshift mutagen, and a treatment known to induce both chromosomal and point mutations, are unable to increase the frequency of revertants of hepatoma cultured cells.[620] In contrast, the same cells can be heritably induced to differentiate following a short interval of culture in the form of aggregates, which suggests that increased cell contacts may elicit differentiation *in vitro* through mechanisms evoking those operating in embryonic induction phenomena *in vivo*.[621] Obviously, such mechanisms would not be associated with mutations but would involve particular types of regulatory changes, most probably occurring at the genome level.

17. Induction of Differentiation of Transformed Cells

Reversion from a transformed to a differentiated phenotype may be induced, especially in transformed hematopoietic cells, by treatment *in vitro* with a diversity of chemical agents.[473,533,622-628] The HL-60 human promyelocytic leukemia cell line has been extensively used as a model for the induction of differentiation *in vitro*.[629,630] HL-60 cells are able to differentiate into the granulocyte or the monocytic pathway, according to the type of differentiation inducer agent. Differentiation inducers that have been applied to the study of HL-60 cells or other cellular systems *in vitro* include retinol (vitamin A) and other retinoic acid derivatives,[631-635] vitamin D_3 derivatives such as calcitriol $(1,25(OH)_2D_3)$,[636-639] dimethyl sulfoxide (DMSO),[640-642] 5-azacytidine,[643] sodium butyrate or dibutyryl cAMP,[644-646] prostaglandin E_1 and cholera toxin,[647] 5-bromodeoxyuridine,[648] naphtalene sulfonamide calmodulin,[649] 3-deaza-(±)-aristeromycin (an inhibitor of *S*-adenosylhomocysteine hydrolase),[650] adenosine dialdehyde and nitrous oxide,[651] actinomycin D,[652] and, paradoxically, tumor-promoting substances such as phorbol diesters.[653] Even natural dietary substances such as the fatty acids palmitoleic and myristoleic acids can act as differentiation inducers.[654] The wide diversity of differentiation inducers suggests that the differentiation of neoplastic cells induced by different types of agents is associated with different types of molecular mechanisms.

Differentiation induced by differentiation inducers is almost always a transient phenomenon, requiring the continuous presence of the inducer in the medium and disappearing after withdrawal of the inducer. In almost all of these cases the action of the differentiation-inducing agents is reversible and the cell returns to the expression of a transformed phenotype when cultured again in an inducer-free medium, which is accompanied by the death of the differentiated postreplicative cells. Reversion of the transformed phenotype induced by some agents, e.g., BUdr, is only partial and some of the transformation-associated changes do not revert under treatment with the inducer.[655] Moreover, the cells are usually insensitive to rechallenge with the inducers, which indicates that they are not permanently affected by these treatments. Exceptionally, the differentiated state induced in neoplastic cultured cells may be heritable, as observed in a human colonic cancer cell line (HT29) after treatment with sodium butyrate (5mM for 9 d).[644] The foci of differentiated cells induced by sodium butyrate *in vitro* are apparently of clonal origin, being originated in single cells where some permanent changes occur, allowing the creation of an heritable differentiation program. Sodium butyrate induces an irreversible differentiation of a human salivary gland adenocarcinoma cell line into myoepithelial cells.[645] Although the molecular mechanisms of sodium butyrate-induced irreversible differentiation of neoplastic cells *in vitro* have not been elucidated, it is known that this agent induces hyperacetylation of histones, mainly as a consequence of inhibition of histone deacetylase,[656] which may lead to changes in the control of gene expression.

A combined treatment of HL-60 cells with retinoic acid and aphicolidin (a specific and reversible inhibitor of DNA polymerase-α) may inhibit leukemic cell proliferation more effectively without causing severe cytotoxicity.[657] Lithium was found to inhibit the DMSO-induced commitment to differentiation of murine erythroleukemia (MEL) cells at nontoxic concentrations that have only a small effect on the rate of proliferation.[658] Mitomycin C, a drug which interacts with both single- and double-stranded DNA, also inhibits DMSO-induced differentiation of MEL cells.[659]

Transformed hamster embryo fibroblasts react to exposure to the xanthate compound D609 (tricyclodecan-9-yl-xanthogenate) with immediate reversion to the growth kinetics and flat morphology of the untransformed parental cells.[660] After six population doublings in the presence of D609, clones which display an untransformed morphology in the absence of D609 arise with a high frequency (90%) and such clones reacquire a limited *in vitro* lifetime and lose the ability to induce tumors in athymic "nude" mice. These results demonstrate the stable maintenance of the intact genetic program for a limited *in vitro* lifetime over several hundred generations in transformed cells and provide direct evidence for the complete reversibility of the property of immortality.

Growth factors produced by hematic cells, including cytokines such as IL-1, IL-3, CSF-2, IFN-γ, and TNF-α are capable of inducing differentiation of cultured leukemic cells or leukemic cell lines.[661-666] Not all leukemic cell clones respond to the same factor even though they may have the appropriate surface receptors. Combined treatments with growth factors and/or other differentiation inducers may be more effective than treatment with single factors. Combined low concentrations of TNF-α and retinoic acid are very active for inducing differentiation of HL-60 cells into both the monocyte-macrophage and the granulocyte phenotypes.[667] The differentiating capacity of retinoic acid on HL-60 cells is also enhanced by IFN-α and IFN-β, but not IFN-γ.[668]

In a few instances viruses have been used to induce differentiation of transformed cells. Highly malignant cat melanoma cells may be induced to differentiation *in vitro* into neuronal, nontumorigenic cells, when they are infected with the endogenous cat retrovirus RD114.[669] Apparently, the insertion of a promoter contained in the LTR region of the virus could alter the transcriptional control of the malignant cell, inducing its terminal differentiation.

Interestingly, differentiation can be induced in particular types of cells by oncogene products. For example, plasmid vectors encoding either the c-*fos* protooncogene or the E1A region of human adenovirus Ad5 are capable of inducing differentiation of F9 teratocarcinoma stem cells.[670,671] In experiments with transfer of the human or mouse protooncogene c-*fos* into F9 cells, a drastic alteration of the cell morphology and proliferative potential is observed in association with the onset of expression of several differentiation markers.[670] Expression of c-*fos* in certain mouse tissues is correlated with differentiation processes resulting in production of mature cells, which suggests that the normal function of this gene is tightly associated with processes involved in cell differentiation.[672] These findings provided the first evidence that the artificial transfer of a single cellular gene can promote a cellular differentiation process.

The molecular events involved in the induction of differentiation by retinoic acid, DMSO, phorbol esters, steroid hormones, and other agents are not understood but there is evidence that retinoic acid is capable of inducing acute alterations in specific gene expression in both normal and leukemic myeloid cells.[673] Retinoic acid-induced reversion of a transformed mouse embryo fibroblast cell line (AKR-MCA cells) to a nontransformed phenotype is accompanied by a greatly reduced level of phosphorylation of a 38-kDa cytosolic protein as well as by a restored ability to respond to the specific growth factor, EGF.[635] Induction of differentiation of human myeloid leukemia cells in culture by tunicamycin is associated with a decrease in the high catalase activity that is present in the leukemic cells.[674] The mechanisms involved in differentiation induced *in vitro* by different experimental procedures are not identical but different cellular metabolic pathways are activated by each type of inducer.[675] The effects of phorbol esters on various cell functions, including the induction of cell differentiation, are apparently mediated by a cell membrane alteration,[676] but the events linking the alteration at the level of the cell membrane to changes in the expression of the cellular genetic program are not understood. In general, agents that produce an increase of the intracellular level of cyclic AMP are capable of inducing differentiation in susceptible cells, such as neuroblastoma cells.[677] The possible role of protooncogene protein products in the processes of spontaneous or induced differentiation of neoplastic cells is suggested by an altered expression of specific protooncogenes in these processes. For example, a decreased expression of N-*myc* precedes retinoic acid-induced differentiation of a human neuroblastoma cell line.[678]

An important task is the characterization of cellular proteins involved in the molecular mechanisms of cell differentiation. HL-60 cells initiated to differentiation with either calcitriol or DMSO may produce an activity which is capable of inducing differentiation and loss of proliferative capacity in fresh HL-60 cells.[679] Differentiation of the U-937 human leukemia cell line by treatment with phorbol ester (TPA) is also associated with production of a factor which is present in the conditioned medium and which is capable of inducing differentiation of U-937 cells.[680] This differentiation-inducing factor (DIF) is apparently represented by a 67-kDa protein which is distinct from all factors reported to regulate the differentiation of leukemic cell lines. It is not known whether the DIFs produced by HL-60 and U-937 cells are similar or identical. A factor, called the macrophage and granulocyte inducer (MGI) is capable of inducing differentiation of normal myeloid precursors.[681-683] MGI is a protein of molecular weight 68,000 and is secreted by various types of cell, including fibroblasts and macrophages. However, at least two different molecular forms of MGI may exist. Recently, a factor, termed D-factor, inducing differentiation of mouse myeloid leukemia M1 cells into macrophages has been purified to homogeneity from serum-free conditioned medium of mouse L-929 cells.[684] The purified factor gave a single band of protein with a molecular weight of 62,000 and its half-maximal concentration for inducing differentiation was 1.7×10^{-11} *M*. A DIF that is constitutively produced in the HUT-102 malignant T-lymphocyte leukemic cell line is a protein of approximately 50,000 mol wt capable of inducing differentiation of HL-60 and U-937 leukemia cell lines.[685] This DIF is also capable of inhibiting the growth of fresh human AML cells as well as the growth of normal granulocyte-macrophage colonies. The physiological roles and the mechanisms of action of MGI and the D and DIF factors are unknown. A DIF capable of inducing the differentiation of human leukemia cells *in vitro* has been identified recently with TNF-α, a factor capable of producing tumor cell lysis.[686] Both TNF-α and IFN-γ have the ability to induce monocytic differentiation of the HL-60 cell line.[662] Combinations of TNF-α and IFN-γ act synergistically in the induction of differentiation of ML-1 human myeloblastic leukemia cells *in vitro*.[687]

The conditioned medium of a CSF-producing tumor (G2T) obtained from a patient with lung cancer contained a differentiation-inducing activity (DIA) that was capable of inducing differentiation of HL-60 cells into macrophage-like cells.[688,689] This DIA has an apparent mol wt of 36,000 and is distinct from CSFs of lower molecular weight. A well-characterized cellular growth factor, the human granulocyte colony-stimulating factor (G-CSF), which has been obtained by expression of the cloned human gene, is a 19,000-mol wt glycoprotein capable of inducing *in vitro* terminal differentiation of cultured murine and human leukemic cells into macrophages and granulocytes, including M1 cells.[690,691] However, even under optimum conditions of differentiation of M1 cells induced by G-CSF, 30 to 40% blastic cells remain.

Induction of tumor cell differentiation could represent a valuable therapeutic approach for the treatment of human cancer, including hematopoietic and solid neoplasms.[627] Unfortunately, agents that induce an efficient differentiation of transformed cells in *in vitro* systems may not cause differentiation when applied *in vivo* to animals bearing malignant diseases such as myeloblastic leukemia.[692] Growth factors involved in hematopoietic processes may induce differentiation of leukemia cells not only *in vitro*, but also *in vivo*. Myeloid regulatory proteins such as CSF-2 and IL-3 can induce differentiation of leukemic cells when injected into mice that carry myeloid leukemic cells contained in intraperitoneally implanted diffusion chambers.[693] Moreover, one type of leukemic cells that undergo differentiation in these experiments *in vivo* was resistant to differentiation induced by the same growth factors *in vitro*, which indicates that the process of differentiation was indirect and required the production of some specific DIF *in vivo*. Neuroblastoma patients treated with chemotherapy associated with maturation-inducing agents showed signs of morphological differentiation in the tumor cells, but none of them exhibited a complete disappearance or complete maturation of the tumor cells.[694]

Inhibition of malignant cell clones has been observed in patients receiving differentiation-inducing agents, e.g., in a patient with a myelodysplastic syndrome associated with refractory anemia who was treated with a retinoic acid derivative.[695] The latter phenomenon, however, should be considered as exceptional. A cautious approach should be recommended for the treatment of patients with differentiation inducers because, in addition to possible toxic effects, some of these agents are potentially dangerous. Induction of differentiation of neoplastic cells may not always be associated with a loss of their malignant behavior. For example, differentiation induced in sublines of B16 mouse melanoma cells was found to be associated with a reduction in tumorigenic capacity but, paradoxically, the differentiated cells exhibited a markedly enhanced capacity to produce metastases (pulmonary tumor nodules) after i.v. injection into syngeneic mice.[696] Moreover, in certain cases differentiation-inducing agents such as retinoic acid may act in an unpredictable manner as enhancers of carcinogenic processes.[697] Treatment of JB6 mouse epidermal cells with calcitriol can result not in differentiation but in the irreversible conversion into malignant phenotype, as reflected by the acquisition of anchorage-independent growth.[698] Thus, differentiation-inducing agents should be used with caution in clinical trials and the general use of such agents for the chemoprevention of cancer may be contraindicated.

18. Discrepancies between Mutagenicity and Carcinogenicity

Most carcinogens are also mutagens but there are some intriguing exceptions to this general rule.[363-365] For example, 2,3,7,8-tetrachlorodibenzo-*p*-dioxin is a carcinogen as potent as aflatoxin B_1 in rats but there is no evidence of its covalent binding to DNA and the evidence for its mutagenic activity is inconclusive.[699] The estrogenic compound diethylstilbestrol (DES) is as active as benzo-*a*-pyrene (BP) to induce transformation of Syrian hamster embryo fibroblasts but it is apparently not mutagenic for the same cells.[700] Although DES does not produce point mutations or chromosome structural aberrations at doses it induces cell transformation, it does induce a high degree of aneuploidy under the same conditions.[701] However, a possible relationship between numerical chromosome changes alone and malignancy is not clearly established.

An increase in the frequency of SCE is considered as an excellent parameter for demonstrating the mutagenic action of a wide number of physical, biological, and chemical agents. In cancer patients, cancer-prone families, or in patients with high risk for cancer, no significant differences in SCE frequencies have been found.[702] Many other examples of discrepancy between mutagenicity and carcinogenicity could be mentioned but there will always remain criticisms related to methodological aspects. Indeed, it is a very difficult task to exclude mutagenicity or carcinogenicity since the appropriate experimental conditions could have not been fulfilled.

19. Relationship between Exposition to X-Rays and the Yield of Transformation *In Vitro*

When C3H mouse embryo fibroblasts irradiated *in vitro* are permitted to grow to confluence, and then are resuspended and reseeded at 300 cells per dish and incubated anew for 6 weeks to allow regrowth to confluence and the development of transformed foci of cells, the yield of transformed foci per dish is independent of dilutions between 1:10 and 1:10,000, and is the same as that on dishes containing undisturbed cells.[703] In other words, in these experiments the yield of transformed foci per dish is constant, even when the confluent cells are resuspended and reseeded over a range of 25,000 to 30,000 cells per dish. These results suggest that the cell alteration that leads to the formation of a clone of transformed cells is not the immediate, direct consequence of the exposure to X-rays, and is probably not a mutational event. Rather, the exposure to X-rays would result in a cellular alteration such as a functional or metabolic change common to most or all of the surviving cells, and this change would be transmitted to the progeny during subsequent growth. Thus, the primary consequence of radiation exposure would be an unspecified epigenetic change that would determine an enhanced probability of a second event, which is rare and perhaps mutational, and is expressed as a transformed clone.[484,703] Other interpretations could also be valid for explaining the results obtained in these experiments.[130,704]

Nanomolar concentrations of a protease inhibitor (Bowman-Birk protease inhibitor) with chymotrypsin-inhibitory activity is capable of suppressing X-ray-induced transformation of C3H/10T1/2 cells, probably acting on the first, common event occurring in a large fraction of the irradiated cells.[705] A similar effect is produced by a protease inhibitor obtained from potatoes, called chymotrypsin inhibitor 1 (CI-1).[706] Oncogenic transformation of C3H/10T1/2 cells induced by either X-rays or N-methyl-N′-nitro-N-nitrosoguanidine is also inhibited if lipopoly-saccharide (LPS) is present in the culture medium.[707] The mechanisms for the LPS or protease inhibitors-induced suppression of radiation-induced transformation is unknown but epigenetic changes are more likely involved than mutational phenomena. The CI-1 inhibitor does not interact with specific receptor proteins on the surface of C3H/10T1/2 cells but may be taken up by pinocytosis, membrane turnover, or some other mechanisms leading to its internalization into the cells. However, the ultimate mechanisms of action of these inhibitors are unknown.

An assessment of the radiogenic cancer initiation frequency per clonogenic rat thyroid or mammary cell *in vivo* indicates that radiogenic initiation of thyroid and mammary cancer is a common cellular event.[708,709] The frequent, initial event proposed for the induction of transformation by ionizing radiation may consist, however, not in a purely epigenetic change but in a change affecting relatively large targets and it has been proposed that gross chromosomal lesions, including rearrangements, may be the starting point of this process.[710] This proposal is in accord with the well known clastogenic properties of radiation.

Results obtained with DNA transfection assays strongly suggest that DNAs from mammalian cells transformed into malignancy by direct exposure *in vitro* to X-radiation consistently contain genetic sequences with transforming activity in recipient cell lines.[711] Moreover, treatment of the DNAs with restriction endonucleases prior to transfection indicates that the same transforming gene (protooncogene) is present in each of the transformed cells of either mouse or hamster origin. The results of these experiments suggest that radiogenic malignant transformation is associated with genetic changes involving an oncogenic activation of discrete cellular DNA sequences.

20. Two-Dose Radiation-Induced Acute Myeloid Leukemia in the Mouse

Two-dose experiments for AML induction in mice by X- or γ-rays clearly indicate that the initiating event is not an immediate permanent change but requires to be fixed in some way.[712] A progressive reduction in observed AML frequency occurs as the time interval between two equal exposures to X-rays is increased, which shows that the first dose, which interacts with the corresponding effect produced by the second dose, decays with the passage of time. The decay in initiation effectiveness is quite rapid, the interaction disappearing, or nearly so, in less than 3 d. The results of these experiments are apparently incompatible with orthodox concepts that initiation is a stable state that must be followed by multiple events over a period of time before cells express fully malignant behavior.

21. Relationship between Exposition to UV Irradiation and Cell Transformation *In Vitro*

3T3 proadipocytes represent a nontransformed mesenchymal stem cell line that possesses the ability to regulate its proliferation at a distinct site of the G_1 phase of the cell cycle as well as the ability to regulate its proliferation at two additional G_1 states that may be induced by changes in the culture medium. A low dose of 254-nm UV irradiation selectively and stably inhibits the nonterminal and terminal differentiation of over 70% of proadipocyte stem cells *in vitro* but does not abrogate other cell cycle-dependent growth control processes.[530] Differentiation-defective proadipocyte stem cells are not completely transformed but show an increased spontaneous transformation rate, as evidenced by the formation of foci in high-density cell cultures. These results support the role of defects in the control of differentiation in the initiation of carcinogenesis. The observations also support a concept that the initiation of carcinogenesis involves multiple phases.

22. Spontaneous Generation of Highly Tumorigenic Variants in Cells Transfected with Viral Genes

Rat cells transfected with polyoma virus transforming genes may express a nontumorigenic (flat) phenotype when they carry silent copies of the polyoma virus transforming gene, *pmt*. These cells are converted spontaneously to the tumorigenic phenotype and express elevated levels of *pmt* transcripts and antigen at a rate which is much higher than would be expected for a conventional mutation in a mammalian cells.[713] The highly tumorigenic variants are probably generated from the flat cell lines by epigenetic events.

23. Effect of Thyroid Hormone on Neoplastic Transformation *In Vitro*

The results of important experimental work indicate that the presence of thyroid hormone in the medium is required for the expression of neoplastic transformation induced by X-rays, chemical carcinogens, or oncogenic viruses. When C3H mouse embryo fibroblasts are incubated in medium depleted from thyroid hormones for 1 week, the cells become completely resistant to the transforming action of an X-ray dose that yields transformation frequencies of approximately 10^{-3} in medium supplemented with triiodothyronine (T3).[714] The addition of T3 (0.1 mM) to the thyroid hormone-depleted medium reestablishes the expected frequency of transformation. Moreover, protein synthesis is required for the restoration of the transforming action of X-rays by thyroid hormone since cycloheximide abolishes the T3-dependent, X-ray-induced transformation.[714] Thyroid hormone also modulates an early stage involved in neoplastic transformation induced by type 5 adenovirus (Ad5) in rat embryo fibroblasts, and it also enhances the expression of the transformed state in cells that were previously transformed by Ad5.[715,716] Moreover, thyroid hormone plays a key role in chemically induced transformation in cultured hamster embryo cells or C3H mouse embryo fibroblasts.[717] An absolute dependence of transformation on T3 was found with the indirect carcinogen benzo(*a*)pyrene, which requires metabolic activation, and with the direct-acting carcinogen *N*-methyl-*N'*-nitro-*N*-nitrosoguanidine (MNNG). The results indicate that thyroid hormone is crucial in early phases of chemically induced neoplastic transformation and that it has no effect on the later stages of expression of the transformed state.

Thyroid hormone also modulates transformation induced by the acute transforming retrovirus K-MuSV, which contains the oncogene v-H-*ras*.[718] Moreover, in the presence of T3, transformed foci develop in C3H/10T1/2 cells following transfection with high-mol wt DNA from MCA-transformed cells (which contains an activated c-K-*ras* protooncogene), whereas no foci develop in transfected cells grown in the absence of T3.[716] The presence or absence of T3 does not alter either the level of c-K-*ras* mRNA or the quantity of c-K-*ras* p21 protein in the MCA-transformed cells.

Morphological transformation of recipient cells by transfection with DNA isolated from X-ray-transformed C3H/10T1/2 cells (XT cells) is modulated by thyroid hormone.[719] When the recipient cells are maintained in T3-deficient medium, the appearance of foci of transformed cells is greatly reduced after transfection. This reduction is due to the lack of expression of some particular function(s) in the recipient cells, since the thyroid status does not alter DNA uptake or integration.

The results of these experiments are hardly compatible with a simplistic mutational model of the origin of neoplastic transformation. Rather, they strongly suggest that at least one crucial epigenetic change is early required for the occurrence of transformation induced *in vitro* by different types of oncogenic agents. The nature of this change is unknown but there is evidence that the action of thyroid hormone, at least in certain cells, is indirect and is associated with the secretion of an autocrine growth factor.[720] A role for protooncogene expression in the modulation of neoplastic transformation by thyroid hormone is suggested by the fact that the regulation of 3-methylcholanthrene-induced transformation of C3H/10T1/2 cells by thyroid hormone correlates with the transcriptional expression of the c-K-*ras* protooncogene.[721] Interestingly, the high-affinity thyroid hormone receptor has been identified recently with the protein product of the c-*erb*-A protooncogene.[722, 723]

In conclusion, the available evidence suggests that the striking alterations occurring in the expression of a transformed phenotype under the influence of thyroid hormone are related to the regulatory effects of endogenous growth factors and/or protooncogene protein products whose synthesis depends on the presence of thyroid hormone.

E. SUMMARY

There are still many unsolved questions in relation to the origin of neoplastic transformation. Four types of hypotheses may be discussed on this subject: mutational genetic, nonmutational genetic, viral, and epigenetic.

The mutational hypothesis postulates that point mutations and/or chromosome aberrations are required for the origin and expression of neoplastic transformation. This hypothesis is supported by a host of data constituting an impressive body of evidence. Although most of this evidence is indirect, there could remain little doubt that some mutational changes are crucially involved in one or more of the multiple steps leading to neoplastic transformation. The most controversial aspect in relation to this hypothesis is the question about what kind of point mutations and/or chromosome aberrations are important, or even indispensable, for the origin of transformation. Evidence accumulated in the last years points to protooncogenes as good candidates for targets in mutational events associated with tumorigenic processes. On the other hand, recent evidence strongly suggests that the deletion of certain specific genes with tumor-suppressing properties (antioncogenes or emerogenes) may be of crucial importance in certain types of tumorigenic processes. However, it should be recognized that certain clinical and experimental observations are difficult to reconcile with a hypothesis on carcinogenesis based only on structural changes occurring at the genomic level.

According to the nonmutational genetic hypothesis, structural genomic changes that cannot be considered as true mutations would be responsible for the origin of neoplastic transformation. These changes would include either alterations in the patterns of DNA methylation or rearrangement, transposition, or amplification of individual genes or DNA segments. Such changes are heritable at the cellular level and may represent a kind of bridge between mutational and epigenetic changes. They are involved in normal processes of differentiation and control of gene expression, and they could also be involved in heritable abnormalities of differentiation such as neoplastic transformation and tumor development.

The viral hypothesis postulates that infection by some DNA and RNA viruses may be causally related to the origin of cancer. Unfortunately, most of the viruses suggested as possible agents for tumorigenic processes are ubiquitous infectious agents causing also nonmalignant diseases or may even not be associated with any disease in some individuals of the infected population. Consequently, nonviral factors of endogenous and/or exogenous origin should contribute, in addition to the putative oncogenic virus, to the transformation of susceptible cells and tumor development. Furthermore, the mechanisms that would be responsible for the oncogenic properties of these viruses remain unknown.

The RNA viruses that have been implicated as possible etiological agents of cancer under natural conditions are infectious retroviruses called chronic retroviruses, which are capable of inducing transformation in vivo in a chronic manner, after long latency periods. Chronic retroviruses do not possess specific transforming sequences (oncogenes) and are not able to induce cell transformation *in vitro*. The exact role of chronic retroviruses in the etiology of human malignant diseases is not clear, but they would act through indirect pathways and would be involved in only some relatively rare human neoplasms.

A number of retroviruses can produce the experimental transformation of cells, either *in vivo* or *in vitro*, in an acute manner. The genome of such acutely transforming retroviruses (acute retroviruses) is characterized by the presence of specific sequences, called viral oncogenes, which are responsible for the transforming potential of these viruses. These oncogenes are, however, not of viral origin but of cellular origin, and acute retroviruses act only as oncogene transducers. The cellular, original counterparts of viral oncogenes are termed protooncogenes. Acute retroviruses have been isolated most frequently from natural or experimental tumors but they do not act as infectious agents transmitting neoplastic diseases under natural conditions in any animal species.

Endogenous proviruses are contained in the mammalian genome, including the human genome, and are transmitted from one generation to another as cellular genes through the germ line. Endogenous proviruses may be involved in the control mechanisms of certain developmental processes but their possible relation to neoplastic diseases is not understood.

The epigenetic hypothesis postulates that regulatory changes alone are critically involved in the molecular events leading to neoplastic transformation. These changes may occur at either nuclear or extranuclear sites but would always be reflected in alterations of genome regulation. Moreover, according to the epigenetic hypothesis, at least in some cases regulatory changes would be sufficient not only for the appearance but also for the maintenance of the transformed phenotype.

Most probably, both genetic and epigenetic events play an important role in oncogenic processes. In the final analysis, it may be true that the transformed phenotype could result from different factors and mechanisms operating under different natural or experimental conditions but acting through a few, or perhaps only one, common pathway(s). In the last few years it has been postulated that regulatory or structural changes in specific protooncogene sequences could be at least one of the essential components of this common pathway(s). Other components may consist of different genetic and epigenetic phenomena whose complex interactions are still not understood. Although the inclusion of some particular genetic or epigenetic factors in the origin of cancer may be accepted on the ground of clinical or experimental evidence, the exclusion of any of the above-mentioned factors is probably not justified, taking into account our present state of ignorance.

REFERENCES

1. Foulds, L., *Neoplastic Development,* Vol. 1, Academic Press, London, 1969.
2. Pitot, H.C., *Fundamentals of Oncology,* 3rd ed., Marcel Dekker, New York, 1986.
3. Harada, T., Ito, K., Shimaoka, K., Hosoda, Y., and Yakumaru, K., Fatal thyroid carcinoma: anaplastic transformation of adenocarcinoma, *Cancer,* 39, 2588, 1977.
4. Kahn, S.B., Love, R.R., Sherman, C., Jr., and Chakravorty, R., Eds., *Concepts in Cancer Medicine,* Grune and Stratton, New York, 1983.
5. Manigault, P., La transformation tumorale chez les vegetaux, *Bull. Cancer,* 54, 137, 1967.
6. Dawe, C.J., Phylogeny and oncogeny, *Natl. Cancer Inst. Monogr.,* 31, 1, 1969.
7. Braun, A.C., *The Cancer Problem: A Critical Analysis and Modern Synthesis,* Columbia University Press, New York, 1969.
8. Dorn, C.R., Comparative oncology: dogs, cats, and man, *Persp. Biol. Med.,* 15, 507, 1972.
9. Madewell, B.R., Neoplasms in domestic animals: a review of experimental and spontaneous carcinogenesis, *Yale J. Biol. Med.,* 54, 111, 1981.
10. O'Gara, R.W. and Adamson, R.H., Spontaneous and induced neoplasms in nonhuman primates, in *Pathology of Simian Primates,* Fiennes, R.N.T.-W., Ed., S. Karger, Basel, 1972, 190.
11. Virchow, R., *Die krankhaften Geschwüste,* A. Hirschwald, Berlin, 1863.
12. Ben-Ze'ev, A., The cytoskeleton in cancer cells, *Biochim. Biophys. Acta,* 780, 197, 1985.
13. Goerttler, K., Haag, D., and Tasca, C., Cytophotometrische Untersuchungen an Zellkern von experimentell erzeugten Neoplasmen, *Zeitschr. Krebsforsch.,* 76, 155, 1971.
14. Harbers, E. and Sandritter, W., Gesteigerte Heterochromatisierung als pathologisches Prinzip, *Deut. Med. Wochenschr.,* 93, 269, 1968.
15. Becker, F.F., Sequential phenotypic and biochemical alterations during chemical hepatocarcinogenesis, *Cancer Res.,* 36, 2563, 1976.
16. Riggs, A.D., X-inactivation, differentiation and DNA methylation, *Cytogenet. Cell Genet.,* 14, 9, 1975.
17. Atkin, N.B., Triple sex chromatin, and other sex chromatin anomalies, in tumours of females, *Br. J. Cancer,* 21, 40, 1967.
18. Siracky, J., Sex chromatin in cancer of the uterine cervix, *Acta Cytol.,* 11, 486, 1967.
19. Straub, D.G., Lucas, L.A., McMahon, N.J., Pellett, O.L., and Teplitz, R.L., Apparent reversal of X-condensation mechanism in tumors of the female, *Cancer Res.,* 29, 1233, 1969.
20. Bertrand, S. and Cheix, F., Sex chromatin in tumors of the female breast: the problem reviewed, *Biomedicine,* 27, 82, 1977.
21. McBurney, M.W. and Adamson, E.D., Studies on the activity of the X chromosome in female teratocarcinoma cells in culture, *Cell,* 9, 57, 1976.
22. Martin, G.R., Epstein, C.J., Travis, B., Tucker, G., Yatziv, S., Martin, D.W., Jr., Clift, S., and Cohen, S., X-chromosome inactivation during differentiation of female teratocarcinoma stem cells *in vitro, Nature,* 271, 329, 1978.
23. Sandberg, A.A., *The Chromosomes in Human Cancer and Leukemia,* Elsevier/North-Holland, New York, 1981.
24. Yunis, J.J., Specific fine chromosomal defects in cancer: an overview, *Hum. Pathol.,* 12, 503, 1981.
25. Yunis, J.J., The chromosomal basis of human neoplasia, *Science,* 221, 227, 1983.
26. Chaganti, R.S.K., Significance of chromosome change to hematopoietic neoplasms, *Blood,* 62, 515, 1983.
27. Gilbert, F., Chromosomes, genes, and cancer: a classification of chromosome abnormalities in cancer, *J. Natl. Cancer Inst.,* 71, 1107, 1983.

28. Trent, J.M., Chromosomal alterations in human solid tumours: implications of the stem cell model to cancer cytogenetics, *Cancer Surv.*, 3, 395, 1984.

29. Herlyn, M., Clark, W.H., Rodeck, U., Mancianti, M.L., Jambrosic, J., and Koprowski, H., Biology of tumor progression in human melanocytes, *Lab. Invest.*, 56, 461, 1987.

30. Barlogie, B., Raber, M.N., Schumann, J., Johnson, T.S., Drewinko, B., Swartzendruber, D.E., Gohde, W., Andreeff, M., and Freireich, E.J., Flow cytometry in clinical cancer research, *Cancer Res.*, 43, 3982, 1983.

31. Friedlander, M.L., Hedley, D.W., and Taylor, I.W., Clinical and biological significance of aneuploidy in human tumours, *J. Clin. Pathol.*, 37, 961, 1984.

32. Barlogie, B., Drewinko, B., Schumann, J., Gohde, W., Dosik, G., Latreille, J., Johnston, D.A., and Freireich, E.J., Cellular DNA content as a marker of neoplasia in man, *Am. J. Med.*, 69, 195, 1980.

33. Nowell, P.C. and Hungerford, D.A., A minute chromosome in human chronic granulocytic leukemia, *Science*, 132, 1497, 1960.

34. Caspersson, T., Gahrton, G., Lindsten, J., and Zech, L., Identification of the Philadelphia chromosome as a number 22 by quinacrine mustard fluorescence, *Exp. Cell Res.*, 63, 238, 1970.

35. Rowley, J.D., A new consistent chromosomal abnormality in chronic myelogenous leukemia identified by quinacrine fluorescence and Giemsa staining, *Nature*, 243, 290, 1973.

36. Mitelman, F., Catalogue of chromosome aberrations in cancer, *Cytogenet. Cell Genet.*, 36, 1, 1983.

37. Ashman, L.K., The immunogenicity of tumour cells, *Immunol. Cell Biol.*, 65, 271, 1987.

38. Feizi, T., Demonstration by monoclonal antibodies that carbohydrate structures of glycoproteins and glycolipids are onco-developmental antigens, *Nature*, 314, 53, 1985.

39. Feizi, T., Carbohydrate antigens in human cancer, *Cancer Surv.*, 4, 245, 1985.

40. Gendler, S.J., Burchell, J.M., Duhig, T., White, R., Parker, M., and Taylor-Papadimitriou, J., Cloning and partial cDNA encoding differentiation and tumor-associated mucin glycoproteins expressed by human mammary epithelium, *Proc. Natl. Acad. Sci. U.S.A.*, 84, 6060, 1987.

41. Chakrabarty, S. and Bratain, M.G., The use of ^{125}I-lectin probes in defining plasma membrane carbohydrate moieties in 3 subpopulations of human colonic carcinoma cells, *Cancer Lett.*, 37, 99, 1987.

42. Klavins, J.V., *Tumor Markers,* Alan R. Liss, New York, 1985.

43. Neville, A.M., Tumor markers and their clinical value, *Tumour Biol.*, 7, 83, 1986.

44. Cimino, F., Birkmayer, G.D., Klavins, J.V., Pimentel, E., and Salvatore, E., *Human Tumor Markers: Biology and Clinical Applications,* Walter de Gruyter, Berlin, 1987.

45. Okada, Y., Arima, T., Togawa, K., Nagashima, H., Jinno, K., Moriwaki, S., Kunitomo, T., Thurin, J., and Koprowski, H., Neoexpression of ABH and Lewis blood group antigens in human hepatocellular carcinomas, *J. Natl. Cancer Inst.*, 78, 19, 1987.

46. Vowden, P., Lowe, A.D., Lennox, E.S., and Bleehen, N.M., Are blood group isoantigens lost from malignant prostatic epithelium? Immunohistochemical support for the preservation of the H isoantigen, *Br. J. Cancer*, 53, 307, 1986.

47. Vowden, P., Lowe, A.D., Lennox, E.S., and Bleehen, N.M., The expression of ABH and Y blood group antigens in benign and malignant breast tissue: the preservation of the H and Y antigens in malignant epithelium, *Br. J. Cancer*, 53, 313, 1986.

48. Springer, G.F., T and Tn, general carcinoma autoantigens, *Science*, 224, 1198, 1984.

49. Flavell, R.A., Allen, H., Burkly, L.C., Sherman, D.H., Waneck, G.L., and Widera, G., Molecular biology of the H-2 histocompatibility complex, *Science*, 233, 437, 1986.

50. Cunliffe, V. and Trowsdale, J., The molecular genetics of human chromosome 6, *J. Med. Genet.*, 24, 649, 1987.

51. Festenstein, H., The biological consequences of altered MHC expression on tumours, *Br. Med. Bull.*, 43, 217, 1987.

52. Goodenow, R.S., Vogel, J.M., and Linsk, R.L., Histocompatibility antigens on murine tumors, *Science*, 230, 777, 1985.

53. Hämmerling, G.J., Klar, D., Pülm, W., Momburg, F., and Moldenhauer, G., The influence of major histocompatibility complex class I antigens on tumor growth and metastasis, *Biochim. Biophys. Acta*, 907, 245, 1987.

54. Tanaka, K., Isselbacher, K.J., Khoury, G., and Jay, G., Reversal of oncogenesis by the expression of a major histocompatibility complex class I gene, *Science*, 228, 26, 1985.

55. Stauss, H.J., van Waes, C., Fink, M.A., Starr, B., and Schreiber, H., Identification of a unique tumor antigen as rejection antigen by molecular cloning and gene transfer, *J. Exp. Med.*, 164, 1516, 1986.

56. Springer, G.F., Desai, P.R., Murthy, M.S., Yang, H.J., and Scanlon, E.F., Precursors of the blood group MN antigens as human carcinoma-associated antigens, *Transfusion*, 19, 233, 1979.

57. Pollack, M.S., Heagney, S.D., Livingston, P.O., and Fogh, J., HLA-A, B, C and DR alloantigen expression on forty-six cultured human tumor cell lines, *J. Natl. Cancer Inst.*, 66, 1003, 1981.

58. Limas, C. and Lange, P., A, B, H antigen detectability in normal and neoplastic urothelium: influence of methodological factors, *Cancer*, 49, 2476, 1982.

59. Momburg, F., Degener, T., Bacchus, E., Moldenhauer, G., Hämmerling, G.J., and Möller, P., Loss of HLA-A,B,C and *de novo* expression of HLA-D in colorectal cancer, *Int. J. Cancer,* 37, 179, 1986.

60. Schoentag, R., Primus, F.J., and Kuhns, W., ABH and Lewis blood group expression in colorectal carcinoma, *Cancer Res.,* 47, 1695, 1987.

61. Van Waes, C., Urban, J.L., Rothstein, J.L., Ward, P.L., and Schreiber, H., Highly malignant tumor variants retain tumor-specific antigens recognized by T helper cells, *J. Exp. Med.,* 164, 1547, 1986.

62. Meruelo, D., Kornreich, R., Rossomando, A., Pampeno, C., Boral, A., Silver, J.L., Buxbaum, J., Weiss, E.H., Devlin, J.J., Mellor, A.L., Flavell, R.A., and Pellicer, A., Lack of class I H-2 antigens in cells transformed by radiation leukemia virus is associated with methylation and rearrangement of H-2 DNA, *Proc. Natl. Acad. Sci. U.S.A.,* 83, 4504, 1986.

63. Carraway, K.L. and Spielman, J., Structural and functional aspects of tumor cell sialomucins, *Mol. Cell. Biochem.,* 72, 109, 1986.

64. Yachnin, S., The clinical significance of human α-fetoprotein, *Ann. Clin. Lab. Sci.,* 8, 84, 1978.

65. Gold, P., Shuster, J., and Freedman, S.O., Carcinoembryonic antigen (CEA) in clinical medicine, *Cancer,* 42, 1399, 1978.

66. Wepsic, H.T., Overview of oncofetal antigens in cancer, *Ann. Clin. Lab. Sci.,* 13, 261, 1983.

67. Begent, R.H.J., The value of carcinoembryonic antigen measurement in clinical practice, *Ann. Clin. Biochem.,* 21, 231, 1984.

68. Sulitzeanu, D., Human cancer-associated antigens: present status and implications for immunodiagnosis, *Adv. Cancer Res.,* 44, 1, 1985.

69. Peiper, S.C. and Stass, S.A., Markers of cellular differentiation in acute lymphoblastic leukemia, *Arch. Pathol. Lab. Med.,* 106, 3, 1982.

70. Hyland, G.L. and Baker, M.A., Leukemia-associated antigens: recent advances in detection, characterization and diagnostic usefulness, *Med. Lab. Sci.,* 41, 55, 1984.

71. Foon, K.A. and Todd, R.F., Immunologic classification of leukemia and lymphoma, *Blood,* 68, 1, 1986.

72. Foon, K.A., Gale, R.P., and Todd, R.F., Recent advances in the immunologic classification of leukemia, *Semin. Hematol.,* 23, 257, 1986.

73. Schmidt, J.A., Marshall, J., Hayman, M.J., Doderlein, G., and Beug, H., Monoclonal antibodies to novel erythroid differentiation antigens reveal specific effects of oncogenes on the leukaemic cell phenotype, *Leukemia Res,* 10, 257, 1986.

74. Inoue, M., Sasagawa, T., Saito, J., Shimizu, H., Ueda, G., Tanizawa, O., and Nakayama, M., Expression of blood group antigens A, B, H, Lewis-a, and Lewis-b in fetal, normal, and malignant tissues of the uterine endometrium, *Cancer,* 60, 2985, 1987.

75. Oikawa, S., Nakazato, H., and Kosaki, G., Primary structure of human carcinoembryonic antigen (CEA) deduced from cDNA sequence, *Biochem. Biophys. Res. Commun.,* 142, 511, 1987.

76. Herberman, R.B., Immunogenicity of tumor antigens, *Biochim. Biophys. Acta,* 473, 93, 1977.

77. Nathrath, W.B.J., Organ and tumour antigens in malignant disease: a review, *J. R. Soc. Med.,* 71, 755, 1978.

78. Parmiani, G., Carbone, G., Invernizzi, G., Pierotti, M.A., Sensi, M.L., Rogers, M.J., and Appella, E., Alien histocompatibility antigens in tumor cells, *Immunogenetics,* 9, 1, 1979.

79. Law, L.W., Characteristics of tumour-specific antigens, *Cancer Surv.,* 4, 3, 1985.

80. Bitterman, P., Hearing, V.J., and Gersten, D.M., Melanoma antigens as modified normal gene sequences, *Life Sci.,* 40, 2207, 1987.

81. Lee, V.K., Hellström, K.E., and Nepom, G.T., Idiotypic interactions in immune responses to tumor-associated antigens, *Biochim. Biophys. Acta,* 865, 127, 1986.

82. Phillips, E.R. and Ruch, R.J., A nonviral, virus strain-specific antigen expressed on rat cells transformed by avian sarcoma virus, *Cancer Res.,* 46, 5864, 1986.

83. Fuji, H. and Iribe, H., Clonal variation in tumorigenicity of L1210 lymphoma cells: nontumorigenic variants with an enhanced expression of tumor-associated antigen and Ia antigens, *Cancer Res.,* 46, 5541, 1986.

84. Ullrich, S.J., Robinson, E.A., Law, L.W., Willingham, M., and Appella, E., A mouse tumor-specific transplantation antigen is a heat shock-related protein, *Proc. Natl. Acad. Sci. U.S.A.,* 83, 3121, 1986.

85. Yagita, H., Masuko, T., and Hashimoto, Y., Inhibition of tumor cell growth *in vitro* by murine monoclonal antibodies that recognize a proliferation-associated cell surface antigen system in rats and humans, *Cancer Res.,* 46, 1478, 1986.

86. Pimentel, E., *Hormones, Growth Factors, and Oncogenes,* CRC Press, Boca Raton, FL, 1987.

87. Ethier, S.P. and Cundiff, K.C., Importance of extended growth potential and growth factor independence on *in vivo* neoplastic potential of primary rat mammary carcinoma cells, *Cancer Res.,* 47, 5316, 1987.

88. Muraguchi, A., Nishimoto, H., Kawamura, N., Hori, A., and Kishimoto, T., B cell-derived BCGF functions as autocrine growth factor(s) in normal and transformed B lymphocytes, *J. Immunol.,* 137, 179, 1986.

89. Coffey, R.J., Jr., Derynck, R., Wilcox, J.N., Bringman, T.S., Goustin, A.S., Moses, H.L., and Pittelkow, M.R., Production and auto-induction of transforming growth factor-alpha in human keratinocytes, *Nature,* 328, 817, 1987.

90. Porter, S., Glaser, L., and Bunge, R.P., Release of autocrine growth factor by primary and immortalized Schwann cells, *Proc. Natl. Acad. Sci. U.S.A.*, 84, 7768, 1987.

91. Sjölund, M., Hedin, U., Sejersen, T., Heldin, C.-H., Thyberg, J., Arterial smooth muscle cells express platelet-derived growth factor (PDGF) A chain mRNA, secrete a PDGF-like mitogen, and bind exogenous PDGF in a phenotype- and growth state-dependent manner, *J. Cell Biol.*, 106, 403, 1988.

92. Vogt, M., Lesley, J., Bogenberger, J., Volkman, S., and Haas, M., Coinfection with viruses carrying the v-Ha-*ras* and v-*myc* oncogenes leads to growth factor independence by an indirect mechanism, *Mol. Cell. Biol.*, 6, 3545, 1986.

93. Vogt, M., Lesley, J., Bogenberger, J.M., Haggblom, C., Swift, S., and Haas, M., The induction of growth factor-independence in murine myelocytes by oncogenes results in monoclonal cell lines and is correlated with cell crisis and karyotypic instability, *Oncogene Res.*, 2, 49, 1987.

94. Straus, D.S. and Mohandas, T., Growth suppression of hybrids between transformed cells and normal fibroblasts in serum-free medium: correlation with retention of human chromosomes, *Somat. Cell Mol. Genet.*, 13, 587, 1987.

95. Paul, D., Henahan, M., and Walter, S., Changes in growth control and growth requirements associated with neoplastic transformation in vitro, *J. Natl. Cancer Inst.*, 53, 1499, 1974.

96. Pardee, A.B. and Dubrow, R.D., Control of cell proliferation, *Cancer*, 39, 2747, 1977.

97. Wille, J.J., Maercklein, P.B., and Scott, R.E., Neoplastic transformation and defective control of cell proliferation and differentiation, *Cancer Res.*, 42, 5139, 1982.

98. Marchok, A.C. and Martin, D.H., Sequential appearance of anchorage independence, uncontrolled nuclear division, and tumorigenicity in 7,12-dimethylbenz(*a*)anthracene-exposed rat tracheal epithelial cells, *Cancer Res.*, 47, 3446, 1987.

99. Andreeff, M., Cell kinetics of leukemia, *Semin. Hematol.*, 23, 300, 1986.

100. Okabe, J., Hayashi, M., Honma, Y., and Hozumi, M., Differentiation of mouse myeloid leukemia cells is inhibited by a factor from non-differentiating leukemia cells, *Int. J. Cancer*, 22, 570, 1978.

101. Bullough, W.S., The chalones: a review, *Natl. Cancer Inst. Monogr.*, 38, 5, 1972.

102. Vogler, W.R. and Winton, E.F., Humoral granulopoietic inhibitors: a review, *Exp. Hematol.*, 3, 337, 1975.

103. Bullough, W.S., Mitotic control in adult mammalian tissues, *Biol. Rev.*, 50, 99, 1975.

104. Finkler, N. and Acker, P., Chalones: a minireview, *Mount Sinai J. Med.*, 45, 258, 1978.

105. Rytömaa, T. and Toivonen, H., Chalones: concepts and results, *Mechan. Ageing Dev.*, 9, 471, 1979.

106. Patt, L.M. and Houck, J.C., The incredible shrinking chalone, *FEBS Lett.*, 120, 163, 1980.

107. Fremuth, F., Chalones and specific growth factors in normal and tumor growth, *Acta Univ. Carol. (Med. Monogr.)*, 110, 1, 1984.

108. Iversen, O.H., What is new in endogenous growth stimulators and inhibitors, *Pathol. Res. Pract.*, 180, 77, 1985.

109. Sanford, K.K. and Evans, V.J., A quest for the mechanism of "spontaneous" malignant transformation in culture with associated advances in culture technology, *J. Natl. Cancer Inst.*, 68, 895, 1982.

110. DiPaolo, J.A., Relative difficulties in transforming human and animal cells *in vitro*, *J. Natl. Cancer Inst.*, 70, 3, 1983.

111. Stanbridge, E.J. and Wilkinson, J., Analysis of malignancy in human cells: malignant and transformed phenotypes are under separate genetic control, *Proc. Natl. Acad. Sci. U.S.A.*, 75, 1466, 1978.

112. Klein, G., Lymphoma development in mice and humans: diversity of initiation is followed by convergent cytogenetic evolution, *Proc. Natl. Acad. Sci. U.S.A.*, 76, 2442, 1979.

113. Evans, C.H. and DiPaolo, J.A., Independent expression of chemical carcinogen-induced phenotypic properties frequently associated with the neoplastic state in a cultured guinea pig cell line, *J. Natl. Cancer Inst.*, 69, 1175, 1982.

114. Chakrabarty, S., Brattain, M.G., Ochs, R.L., and Varani, J., Modulation of fibronectin, laminin, and cellular adhesion in the transformation and differentiation of murine AKR fibroblasts, *J. Cell. Physiol.*, 133, 415, 1987.

115. Boreiko, C.J., Abernethy, D.J., and Stedman, B., Alterations of intercellular communication associated with the transformation of C3H/10T1/2 cells, *Carcinogenesis*, 8, 321, 1987.

116. Kanno, Y., Modulation of cell communication and carcinogenesis, *Jpn. J. Physiol.*, 35, 693, 1985.

117. Abercrombie, M., Contact inhibition: the phenomenon and its biological implications, *Natl. Cancer Inst. Monogr.*, 26, 249, 1967.

118. Martz, E. and Steinberg, M.S., The role of cell-cell contact in "contact" inhibition of cell division: a review and new evidence, *J. Cell. Physiol.*, 79, 189, 1972.

119. Martz, E. and Steinberg, M.S., Contact inhibition of what? — an analytical review, *J. Cell. Physiol.*, 81, 25, 1973.

120. Brandley, B.K. and Schnaar, R.L., Cell-surface carbohydrates in cell recognition and response, *J. Leukocyte Biol.*, 40, 97, 1986.

121. Blat, C., Chatelain, G., Desauty, G., and Harel, L., Inhibitory diffusible factor IDF45, a G1 phase inhibitor, *FEBS Lett.*, 203, 175, 1986.

122. Blat, C., Villaudy, J., Rouillard, D., Golde, A., and Harel, L., Modulation by the src oncogene of the effect of inhibitory diffusible factor IDF45, *J. Cell. Physiol.*, 130, 416, 1987.

123. Barrett, J.C. and Ts'o, P.O.P., Evidence for the progressive nature of neoplastic transformation *in vitro*, *Proc. Natl. Acad. Sci. U.S.A.*, 75, 3761, 1978.

124. Verheijen, R.H.M., Feitz, W.F.J., Beck, J.L.M., Debruyne, F.M.J., Vooys, G.P., Kenemans, P., and Herman, C.J., Cell DNA content — correlation with clonogenicity in the human tumour cloning system (HTCS), *Int. J. Cancer,* 35, 653, 1985.

125. Hamburger, A.W. and White, C.P., Autocrine growth factors for human tumor clonogenic cells, *Int. J. Cell Cloning,* 3, 399, 1985.

126. Butler, W.B., Berlinski, P.J., Hillman, R.M., Kelsey, W.H., and Toenniges, M.M., Relation of *in vitro* properties to tumorigenicity for a series of sublines of the human breast cancer cell line MCF-7, *Cancer Res.,* 46, 639, 1986.

127. Romerdahl, C.A. and Rubin, H., Variation in capacity for anchorage-independent growth among agar-derived clones of spontaneously transformed BALB/3T3 cells, *Cancer Res.,* 44, 5570, 1984.

128. Rizzino, A., Ruff, E., and Rizzino, H., Induction and modulation of anchorage-independent growth by platelet-derived growth factor, fibroblast growth factor, and transforming growth factor-beta, *Cancer Res.,* 46, 2816, 1986.

129. Hamburger, A.W., White, C.P., Lurie, K., and Kaplan, R., Monocyte-derived growth factors for human tumor clonogenic cells, *J. Leukocyte Biol.,* 40, 381, 1986.

130. Deschatrette, J. and Weiss, M.C., Characterization of differentiated and dedifferentiated clones from a rat hepatoma, *Biochimie,* 56, 1603, 1974.

131. Hayflick, L. and Moorhead, P.S., The serial cultivation of human diploid cell strains, *Exp. Cell Res.,* 25, 585, 1961.

132. Hayflick, L., The limited *in vitro* lifetime of human diploid strains, *Exp. Cell Res.,* 37, 614, 1965.

133. Holliday, R., Growth and death of diploid and transformed human fibroblasts, *Fed. Proc. Fed. Am. Soc. Exp. Biol.,* 34, 51, 1975.

134. Daniel, C.W., Aidells, B.D., Medina, D., and Faulkin, L.J., Jr., Unlimited division potential of precancerous mouse mammary cells after spontaneous or carcinogen-induced transformation, *Fed. Proc. Fed. Am. Soc. Exp. Biol.,* 34, 64, 1975.

135. Little, J.B., Characteristics of radiation-induced neoplastic transformation *in vitro*, *Leukemia Res.,* 10, 719, 1986.

136. Tevethia, M.J., Pipas, J.M., Kierstead, T., and Cole, C., Requirements for immortalization of primary mouse embryo fibroblasts probed with mutants bearing deletions in the 3′ end of SV40 gene A, *Virology,* 162, 76, 1988.

137. Smith, H.S., Wolman, S.R., Dairkee, S.H., Hancock, M.C., Lippman, M., Leff, A., and Hackett, A.J., Immortalization in culture: occurrence at a late stage in the progression of breast cancer, *J. Natl. Cancer Inst.,* 78, 611, 1987.

138. Martinez, A.O., Norwood, T.H., Prothero, J.W., and Martin, G.M., Evidence for clonal attenuation of growth potential in HeLa cells, *In Vitro,* 14, 996, 1978.

139. Suda, Y., Suzuki, M., Ikawa, Y., and Aizawa, S., Mouse embryonic stem cells exhibit indefinite proliferative potential, *J. Cell. Physiol.,* 133, 197, 1987.

140. Farber, E., Pre-cancerous types in carcinogenesis: their physiological adaptative nature, *Biochim. Biophys. Acta,* 738, 171, 1984.

141. Scherer, E., Neoplastic progression in experimental hepatocarcinogenesis, *Biochim. Biophys. Acta,* 738, 219, 1984.

142. Farber, E. and Sarma, D.S.R., Chemical carcinogenesis: the liver as a model, *Pathol. Immunopathol. Res.,* 5, 1, 1986.

143. Farber, E. and Sarma, D.S.R., Hepatocarcinogenesis: a dynamic cellular perspective, *Lab. Invest.,* 56, 4, 1987.

144. Dubreuilh, M.W., La mélanose circonscrite précancereuse, *Ann. Dermatol. Syphyl. (Paris),* 3, 129, 1912.

145. Sparks, R.L., Seibel-Ross, E.I., Wier, M.L., and Scott, R.E., Differentiation, dedifferentiation, and transdifferentiation of BALB/c 3T3 T mesenchymal stem cells: potential significance in metaplasia and neoplasia, *Cancer Res.,* 46, 5312, 1986.

146. Barbason, H., Fridman-Manduzio, A., Lelievre, P., and Betz, E.H., Variations of liver cell control during diethylnitrosamine carcinogenesis, *Eur. J. Cancer,* 13, 13, 1977.

147. Scherer, E. and Emmelot, P., Foci of altered liver cells induced by a single dose of diethylnitrosamine and partial hepatectomy: their contribution to hepatocarcinogenesis in the rat, *Eur. J. Cancer,* 11, 145, 1975.

148. Williams, G.M., Ohmori, T., and Watanabe, K., G. The persistence and phenotypic stability of transplanted rat liver neoplastic nodules, *Am. J. Pathol.,* 99, 1, 1980.

149. Baba, T.W. and Humphries, E.H., Formation of a transformed follicle is necessary but not sufficient for development of an avian leukosis virus-induced lymphoma, *Proc. Natl. Acad. Sci. U.S.A.,* 82, 213, 1985.

150. Tatematsu, M., Nagamine, Y., and Farber, E., Redifferentiation as a basis for remodeling of carcinogen-induced hepatocyte nodules to normal appearing liver, *Cancer Res.,* 43, 5049, 1983.

151. Reuber, M.D., Various degrees of susceptibility of different stocks of rats to *N*-2-fluorenyldiacetamide hepatic carcinogenesis, *J. Natl. Cancer Inst.*, 57, 111, 1976.
152. Thomassen, D.G., Role of spontaneous transformation in carcinogenesis: development of preneoplastic rat tracheal epithelial cells at a constant rate, *Cancer Res.*, 46, 2344, 1986.
153. Wolfe, H.J., Melvin, K.E.W., Cervi-Skinner, S.J., Al Saadi, A.A., Juliar, J.F., Jackson, C.E., and Tashjian, A.H., C-cell hyperplasia preceding medullary thyroid carcinoma, *N. Engl. J. Med.*, 289, 437, 1973.
154. Jordan, S.W., Smith, N.L., and Dike, L.S., The significance of cervical cytologic dysplasia, *Acta Cytol.*, 25, 237, 1981.
155. Armenian, H.K., Lilienfeld, A.M., Diamond, E.L., and Bross, I.D.J., Relation between benign prostatic hyperplasia and cancer of the prostate: a prospective and retrospective study, *Lancet*, 2, 115, 1974.
156. Greenwald, P., Kirmss, V., Polan, A.K., and Dick, V.S., Cancer of the prostate among men with benign prostatic hyperplasia, *J. Natl. Cancer Inst.*, 53, 335, 1974.
157. Williams, G.M., The pathogenesis of rat liver cancer caused by chemical carcinogens, *Biochim. Biophys. Acta*, 605, 167, 1980.
158. Goldfarb, S. and Pugh, T.D., The origin and significance of hyperplastic hepatocellular islands and nodules in hepatic carcinogenesis, *J. Am. Coll. Toxicol.*, 1, 119, 1982.
159. Rabes, H.M., Development and growth of early preneoplastic lesions induced in the liver by chemical carcinogens, *J. Cancer Res. Clin. Oncol.*, 106, 85, 1983.
160. Bannasch, P. and Zerban, H., Pathogenesis of primary liver tumors induced by chemicals, *Rec. Result. Cancer Res.*, 100, 1, 1986.
161. Bannasch, P., Preneoplastic lesions as end points in carcinogenicity testing. I. Hepatic preneoplasia, *Carcinogenesis*, 7, 689, 1986.
162. Rotstein, J., Sarma, D.S.R., and Farber, E., Sequential alterations in growth control and cell dynamics of rat hepatocytes in early precancerous steps in hepatocarcinogenesis, *Cancer Res.*, 46, 2377, 1986.
163. Iyer, A.P. and Banerjee, M.R., Sequential expression of preneoplastic and neoplastic characteristics of mouse mammary epithelial cells transformed in organ culture, *J. Natl. Cancer Inst.*, 66, 893, 1981.
164. Kunze, E., Schauer, A., Eder, M., and Seefeldt, C., Early sequential lesions during development of experimental gastric cancer with special reference to dysplasias, *J. Cancer Res. Clin. Oncol.*, 95, 247, 1979.
165. Nettesheim, P., Klein-Szanto, A.J.P., Marchok, A.C., Steele, V.E., Terzaghi, M., and Topping, D.C., Studies of neoplastic development in respiratory tract epithelium, *Arch. Pathol. Lab. Med.*, 105, 1, 1981.
166. Farber, E., The biochemistry of preneoplastic liver: a common metabolic pattern in hepatocyte nodules, *Can. J. Biochem. Cell Biol.*, 62, 486, 1984.
167. Farber E., Cellular biochemistry of the stepwise development of cancer with chemicals, *Cancer Res.*, 44, 5463, 1984.
168. Grundmann, E., Precancer histology: trends and prospects, *Zeitschr. Krebsforsch.*, 85, 1, 1976.
169. Gullino, P.M., Considerations on the preneoplastic lesions of the mammary gland, *Am. J. Pathol.*, 89, 413, 1977.
170. Christopherson, W.M., Dysplasia, carcinoma in situ, and microinvasive carcinoma of the uterine cervix, *Hum. Pathol.*, 8, 489, 1977.
171. Welch, W.R. and Scully, R.E., Precancerous lesions of the endometrium, *Hum. Pathol.*, 8, 503, 1977.
172. Cardiff, R.D., Wellings, S.R., and Faulkin, L.J., Biology of breast preneoplasia, *Cancer*, 39, 2734, 1977.
173. Koss, L.G., Dysplasia: a real concept or a misnomer?, *Obstet. Gynecol.*, 51, 374, 1978.
174. Spriggs, A.I., Natural history of cervical dysplasia, *Clin. Obstet. Gynecol.*, 8, 65, 1981.
175. Correa, P., Precursors of gastric and esophageal cancer, *Cancer*, 50, 2554, 1982.
176. Yoshida, Y., Biology of myelodysplastic syndromes, *Int. J. Cell Cloning*, 5, 356, 1987.
177. Nowell, P.C., Preleukemia: cytogenetic clues in some confusing disorders, *Am. J. Pathol.*, 89, 459, 1977.
178. Linman, J.W. and Bagby, G.C., Jr., The preleukemic syndrome (hemopoietic dysplasia), *Cancer*, 42, 854, 1978.
179. Koeffler, H.P. and Golde, D.W., Human preleukemia, *Ann. Int. Med.*, 93, 347, 1980.
180. Kleihauer, E., The preleukemic syndromes (hematopoietic dysplasia) in childhood, *Eur. J. Pediat.*, 133, 5, 1980.
181. Shively, J.A., Recognition of preleukemia, *Ann. Clin. Lab. Sci.*, 10, 95, 1980.
182. Schneider, P., Les états préleucémiques, *Schweiz. Med. Wochenschr.*, 111, 1208, 1981.
183. Nowell P.C., Preleukemias, *Hum. Pathol.*, 12, 522, 1981.
184. Koeffler, H.P., Myelodysplastic syndromes (preleukemia), *Semin. Hematol.*, 23, 284, 1986.
185. Henmi, A., Uchida, T., and Shikata, T., Karyometric analysis of liver cell dysplasia and hepatocellular carcinoma: evidence against precancerous nature of liver cell dysplasia, *Cancer*, 55, 2594, 1985.
186. Sipponen, P., Intestinal metaplasia and gastric carcinoma, *Ann. Clin. Res.*, 13, 139, 1981.
187. Sinha, D. and Dao, T.L., A direct mechanism of mammary carcinogenesis induced by 7,12-dimethylbenz(*a*)anthracene, *J. Natl. Cancer Inst.*, 53, 841, 1974.

188. Maskens, A.P. and Dujardin-Loits, R-M., Experimental adenomas and carcinomas of the large intestine behave as distinct entities: most carcinomas arise de novo in flat mucosa, *Cancer*, 47, 81, 1981.

189. Dustin, P., Jr., Cell differentiation and carcinogenesis: a critical review, *Cell Tissue Kinet.*, 5, 519, 1972.

190. Medina, D., Oborn, C.J., and Asch, B.B., Distinction between preneoplastic and neoplastic mammary cell populations *in vitro* by cytochalasin B-induced multinucleation, *Cancer Res.*, 40, 329, 1980.

191. Gullino, P.M., Natural history of breast cancer: progression from hiperplasia to neoplasia as predicted by angiogenesis, *Cancer*, 39, 2697, 1977.

192. Ivanckovic, S., Chemical and viral agents in prenatal experimental carcinogenesis, *Biol. Res. Pregnancy*, 3, 99, 1982.

193. Costa, G., Cachexia, the metabolic component of neoplastic diseases, *Cancer Res.*, 37, 2327, 1977.

194. Medline, A. and Farber, E., The multi-step theory of neoplasia, in *Recent Advances in Histopathology*, Anthony, P.F. and Macsween, R.N.M., Eds., Churchill Livingstone, Edinburgh, 1981, 19.

195. Farber, E., The multistep nature of cancer development, *Cancer Res.*, 44, 4217, 1984.

196. Weinstein, I.B., Gattoni-Celli, S., Kirschmeier, P., Lambert, M., Hsiao, W., Backer, J., and Jeffrey, A., Multistage carcinogenesis involves multiple genes and multiple mechanisms, *J. Cell. Physiol.*, Suppl. 3, 127, 1984.

197. Foulds, L., Multiple etiologic factors in neoplastic development, *Cancer Res.*, 25, 1339, 1965.

198. Berenblum, I. and Shubik, P., The role of croton oil applications associated with a single painting of a carcinogen, in tumour induction in the mouse's skin, *Br. J. Cancer*, 1, 379, 1947.

199. Pitot, H., The natural history of neoplasia: newer insights into an old problem, *Am. J. Pathol.*, 89, 401, 1977.

200. Farber, E., The sequential analysis of liver cancer induction, *Biochim. Biophys. Acta*, 605, 149, 1980.

201. Pitot, H.C., Goldsworthy, T., and Moran, S., The natural history of carcinogenesis: implications of experimental carcinogenesis in the genesis of human cancer, *J. Supramol. Struct. Cell. Biochem.*, 17, 133, 1981.

202. Farber, E., Chemical carcinogenesis: a biologic perspective, *Am. J. Pathol.*, 106, 271, 1982.

203. Pitot, H.C., The natural history of neoplastic development: the relation of experimental models to human cancer, *Cancer*, 49, 1206, 1982.

204. Pitot, H.C., Contributions to our understanding of the natural history of neoplastic development in lower animals to the cause and control of human cancer, *Cancer Surv.*, 2, 519, 1983.

205. Shubik, P., Progression and promotion, *J. Natl. Cancer Inst.*, 73, 1005, 1984.

206. Iannaccone, P.M., Weinberg, W.C., and Deamant, F.D., On the clonal origin of tumors: a review of experimental models, *Int. J. Cancer*, 39, 778, 1987.

207. Fialkow, P.J., The origin and development of human tumors studied with cell markers, *N. Engl. J. Med.*, 291, 26, 1974.

208. Gartler, S.M., Patterns of cellular proliferation in normal and tumor cell populations, *Am. J. Pathol.*, 86, 685, 1977.

209. Nowell, P., Tumors as clonal proliferation, *Virchows Arch. B Cell Pathol.*, 29, 145, 1978.

210. Fialkow, P.J., Clonal origin of human tumors, *Annu. Rev. Med.*, 30, 135, 1979.

211. Martin, P.J., Najfeld, V., and Fialkow, P.J., B-lymphoid cell involvement in chronic myelogenous leukemia: implications for the pathogenesis of the disease, *Cancer Genet. Cytogenet.*, 6, 359, 1982.

212. Waldmann, T.A., Davis, M.M., Bongiovanni, K.F., and Korsmeyer, S.J., Rearrangements of genes for the antigen receptor on T cells as markers of lineage and clonality in human lymphoid neoplasms, *N. Engl. J. Med.*, 313, 776, 1985.

213. Foa, R., Pelicci, P.-G., Migone, N., Lauria, F., Pizzolo, G., Flug, F., Knowles, D.M., II, and Dalla-Favera, R., Analysis of T-cell receptor beta chain (T_{beta}) gene rearrangements demonstrates the monoclonal nature of T-cell chronic lymphoproliferative disorders, *Blood*, 67, 247, 1986.

214. Williams, M.E., Innes, D.J., Jr., Borowitz, M.J., Lovell, M.A., Swerdlow, S.H., Hurtubise, P.E., Brynes, R.K., Chan, W.C., Byrne, G.E., Jr., Whitcomb, C.C., and Thomas, C.Y., Immunoglobulin and T cell receptor gene rearrangements in human lymphoma and leukemia. IV, *Blood*, 69, 79, 1987.

215. Foroni, L., Foldi, J., Matutes, E., Catovsky, D., O'Connor, N.J., Baer, R., Forster, A., and Rabbitts, T.H., Alpha, beta, and gamma T-cell receptor genes: rearrangements correlate with haematological phenotype in T cell leukaemias, *Br. J. Haematol.*, 67, 307, 1987.

216. Korsmeyer, S.J., Antigen receptor genes as molecular markers of lymphoid neoplasms, *J. Clin. Invest.*, 79, 1291, 1987.

217. Raffeld, M., Wright, J.J., Lipford, E., Cossman, J., Longo, D.L., Bakhshi, A., and Korsmeyer, S.J., Clonal evolution of t(14;18) follicular lymphomas demonstrated by immunoglobulin genes and the 18q21 major breakpoint region, *Cancer Res.*, 47, 2537, 1987.

218. Arnold, A., Cossman, J., Bakhshi, A., Jaffe, E., Waldmann, T.A., and Korsmeyer, S.J., Immunoglobulin-gene rearrangements as unique clonal markers in human lymphoid neoplasms, *N. Engl. J. Med.*, 309, 1593, 1983.

219. Vogelstein, B., Fearon, E.R., Hamilton, S.R., and Feinberg, A.E., Use of restriction fragment length polymorphisms to determine the clonal origin of human tumors, *Science*, 227, 642, 1985.

220. Olszewska, E., Hay, D.E., Jones, K.W., and Chetty, U., Somatic DNA variability in human breast carcinoma, *Oncogene*, 1, 403, 1987.

221. Fearon, E.R., Hamilton, S.R., and Vogelstein, B., Clonal analysis of human colorectal tumors, *Science,* 238, 193, 1987.

222. Donis-Keller, H., Green, P., Helms, C., Cartinhour, S., Weiffenbach, B., Stephens, K., Keith, T.P., Bowden, D.W., Smith, D.R., Lander, E.S., Botstein, D., Akots, G., Rediker, K.S., Gravius, T., Brown, V.A., Rising, M.B., Parker, C., Powers, J.A., Watt, D.E., Kauffman, E.R., Bricker, A., Phipps, P., Muller-Kahle, H., Braman, J.C., Knowlton, R.G., Barker, D.F., Crooks, S.M., Lincoln, S.E., Daly, M.J., and Abrahamson, J., A genetic linkage map of the human genome, *Cell,* 51, 319, 1987.

223. Vogelstein, B., Fearon, E.R., Hamilton, S.R., Preisinger, A.C., Willard, H.F., Michelson, A.M., Riggs, A.D., and Orkin, S.H., Clonal analysis using recombinant DNA probes from the X-chromosome, *Cancer Res,* 47, 4806, 1987.

224. Furth, J. and Kahn, M.C., The transmission of leukemia in mice with a single cell, *Am. J. Cancer,* 31, 276, 1937.

225. Ishibashi, K., Studies on the number of cells necessary for the transplantation of the Yoshida sarcoma, *Gann,* 41, 1, 1950.

226. Hosokawa, K., Further studies on transplantation of Yoshida sarcoma with a single cell and with cell-free tumor ascites, *Gann,* 41, 236, 1950.

227. Alexander, P., Do cancers arise from a single transformed cell or is monoclonality of tumors a late event in carcinogenesis?, *Br. J. Cancer,* 51, 453, 1985.

228. Delli Bovi, P., Donti, E., Knowles, D.M., II, Friedman-Kien, A., Luciw, P.A., Dina, D., Dalla-Favera, R., and Basilico, C., Presence of chromosomal abnormalities and lack of AIDS retrovirus DNA sequences in AIDS-associated Kaposi's sarcoma, *Cancer Res.,* 46, 6333, 1986.

229. Esumi, M., Aritaka, T., Arii, M., Suzuki, K., Tanikawa, K., Mizuo, H., Mima, T., and Shikata, T., Clonal origin of human hepatoma determined by integration of hepatitis B virus DNA, *Cancer Res.,* 46, 5767, 1986.

230. Hsiao, W.-L.W., Gattoni-Celli, S., and Weinstein, I.B., Oncogene-induced transformation of C3H 10T1/2 cells is enhanced by tumor promoters, *Science,* 226, 552, 1984.

231. Connan, G., Rassoulzadegan, M., and Cuzin, F., Focus formation in rat fibroblasts exposed to a tumour promoter after transfer of polyoma *plt* and *myc* oncogenes, *Nature,* 314, 277, 1985.

232. Hsiao, W.-L.W., Wu, T., and Weinstein, I.B., Oncogene-induced transformation of a rat embryo fibroblast cell line is enhanced by tumor promoters, *Mol. Cell. Biol.,* 6, 1943, 1986.

233. Argyris, T.S., Regeneration and the mechanism of epidermal tumor promotion, *Crit. Rev. Toxicol.,* 14, 211, 1985.

234. Berenblum, I., Challenging problems in cocarcinogenesis, *Cancer Res.,* 45, 1917, 1985.

235. Burns, F.J., Vanderlaan, M., Sivak, A., and Albert, R.E., Regression kinetics of mouse skin papillomas, *Cancer Res.,* 36, 1422, 1976.

236. Sanchez, J.H., Abernethy, D.J., and Boreiko, C.J., Reversible expression of morphological transformation in C3H/10T1/2 mouse embryo cultures exposed to 12-*O*-tetradecanoylphorbol-13-acetate, *Carcinogenesis,* 7, 1793, 1986.

237. Takahashi, K., Heine, U.I., Junker, J.L., Colburn, N.H., and Rice, J.M., Role of cytoskeleton changes and expression of the H-*ras* oncogene during promotion of neoplastic transformation in mouse epidermal JB6 cells, *Cancer Res.,* 46, 5923, 1986.

238. Colburn, N.H. and Smith, B.M., Genes that cooperate with tumor promoters in transformation, *J. Cell. Biochem.,* 34, 129, 1987.

239. Lerman, M.I., Sakai, A., Kai-Tai, Y., and Colburn, N.H., DNA sequences in human nasopharyngeal carcinoma cells that specify susceptibility to tumor promoter-induced neoplastic transformation, *Carcinogenesis,* 8, 121, 1987.

240. Kadhim, S., Burns, B.F., and Birnboim, H.C., *In vivo* induction of tumor variants by phorbol 12-myristate 13-acetate, *Cancer Lett.,* 38, 209, 1987.

241. Schmähl, D., Critical remarks on the validity of promoting effects in human carcinogenesis, *J. Cancer Res. Clin. Oncol.,* 109, 260, 1985.

242. Boswell, H.S., Srivastava, A., Burgess, J.S., Nahreini, P., Heerema, N., Inhorn, L., Padgett, F., Walker, E.B., and Geib, R.W., Cellular control of *in vitro* progression of murine myeloid leukemia: progression accompanies acquisition of independence from growth factor and stromal cells, *Leukemia,* 1, 785, 1987.

243. Kendal, W.S. and Frost, P., Genetic instability and tumor progression, *Pathol. Immunopathol. Res.,* 5, 455, 1986.

244. Goldenberg, D.M. and Pavia, R.A., Malignant potential of murine stromal cells after transplantation of human tumors into nude mice, *Science,* 212, 65, 1981.

245. Goldenberg, D.M. and Pavia, R.A., *In vivo* horizontal oncogenesis by a human tumor in nude mice, *Proc. Nat. Acad. Sci. U.S.A.,* 79, 2389, 1982.

246. Kerbel, R.S., Lagarde, A.E., Dennis, J.W., and Donaghue, T.P., Spontaneous fusion in vivo between normal host and tumor cells: possible contribution to tumor progression and metastasis studied with a lectin-resistant mutant tumor, *Mol. Cell. Biol.,* 3, 523, 1983.

247. Kompff, J., Staab, H.J., Heilbronner, H., Anderer, F.A., and Ritter, H., Cell fusion responsible for horizontal oncogenesis by human tumors in nude mice, *Biochem. Biophys. Res. Commun.,* 124, 933, 1984.

248. Sparrow, S., Jones, M., Billington, S., and Stace, B., The in vivo malignant transformation of mouse fibroblasts in the presence of human tumour xenografts, *Br. J. Cancer,* 53, 793, 1987.

249. Gupta, V., Rajaraman, S., Gadson, P., and Costanzi, J.J., Primary transfection as a mechanism for transformation of host cells by human tumor cells implanted in nude mice, *Cancer Res.,* 47, 5194, 1987.

250. Kovacs, G., Premature chromosome condensation: evidence for *in vivo* cell fusion in human malignant tumours, *Int. J. Cancer,* 36, 637, 1985.

251. Folkman, J., Tumor angiogenesis, *Adv. Cancer Res.,* 43, 175, 1985.

252. How is blood vessel growth regulated in normal and neoplastic tissue?, *Cancer Res.,* 46, 467, 1986.

253. Normann, S.J., Macrophage infiltration and tumor progression, *Cancer Metast. Rev.,* 4, 277, 1985.

254. Dexter, D.I., Neoplastic subpopulations in carcinoma, *Ann. Clin. Lab. Sci.,* 11, 98, 1981.

255. Dexter, D.L. and Calabresi, P., Intraneoplastic diversity, *Biochim. Biophys. Acta,* 695, 97, 1982.

256. Woodruff, M.F.A., Cellular heterogeneity in tumours, *Br. J. Cancer,* 47, 589, 1983.

257. Heppner, G.H., Tumor heterogeneity, *Cancer Res.,* 44, 2259, 1984.

258. Rubin, H., Early origin and pervasiveness of cellular heterogeneity in some malignant transformations, *Proc. Natl. Acad. Sci. U.S.A.,* 81, 5121, 1984.

259. Brattain, M.G., Fine, W.D., Khaled, F.M., Thompson, J., and Brattain, D.E., Heterogeneity of malignant cells from a human colonic carcinoma, *Cancer Res.,* 41, 1751, 1981.

260. Hassan, Y., Wolfson, M., and Aboud, M., Phenotypic heterogeneity in 3-methylcholanthrene-induced transformation of normal rat kidney cells infected with Moloney murine leukemia virus, *Cell Biol. Int. Rep.,* 10, 19, 1986.

261. Rubin, H., Uniqueness of each spontaneous transformant from a clone of BALB/c 3T3 cells, *Cancer Res.,* 48, 2512, 1988.

262. Fidler, I.J., Biologic heterogeneity of cancer metastases, *Breast Cancer Res. Treatm.,* 9, 17, 1987.

263. Schnipper, L.E., Clinical implications of tumor-cell heterogeneity, *N. Engl. J. Med.,* 314, 1423, 1986.

264. Heicappell, R., Naito, S., Ichinose, Y., Creasey, A.A., Lin, L.S., and Fidler, I.J., Cytostatic and cytolytic effects of human recombinant tumor necrosis factor on human renal cell carcinoma cell lines derived from a single surgical specimen, *J. Immunol.,* 138, 1634, 1987.

265. Shapiro, J.R., Yung, W.K., and Shapiro, W.R., Isolation, karyotype, and clonal growth of heterogeneous subpopulations of human malignant gliomas, *Cancer Res.,* 41, 2349, 1981.

266. Honsik, C.J., Diamant, M., and Olsson, L., Generation of stable cellular phenotypes in a human malignant cell line conditioned by alterations in the cellular microenvironment, *Cancer Res.,* 46, 940, 1986.

267. Houghton, A.N., Real, F.X., Davis, L.J., Cordon-Cardo, C., and Old, L.J., Phenotypic heterogeneity of melanoma: relation to the differentiation program of melanoma cells, *J. Exp. Med.,* 164, 812, 1987.

268. Frost, P. and Kerbel, R.S., On a possible epigenetic mechanism(s) of tumor cell heterogeneity: the role of DNA methylation, *Cancer Metastasis Rev.,* 2, 375, 1983.

269. Nicolson, G.L., Generation of phenotypic diversity and progression in metastatic tumor cells, *Cancer Metastasis Rev.,* 3, 25, 1984.

270. Kerbel, R.S., Frost, P., Liteplo, R., Carlow, D.A., and Elliot, B.E., Possible epigenetic mechanisms of tumor progression: induction of high-frequency heritable but phenotypically unstable changes in the tumorigenic and metastatic properties of tumor cell populations by 5-azacytidine treatment, *J. Cell. Physiol.,* Suppl. 3, 87, 1984.

271. Dracopoli, N.C., Houghton, A.N., and Old, L.J., Loss of polymorphic restriction fragments in malignant melanoma: implications for tumor heterogeneity, *Proc. Natl. Acad. Sci. U.S.A.,* 82, 1470, 1985.

272. Weiss, L., Orr, F.W., and Honn, K.V., Interactions of cancer cells with the microvasculature during metastasis, *FASEB J.,* 2, 12, 1988.

273. Carr, I. and Orr, F.W., Invasion and metastasis, *Can. Med. Assoc. J.,* 128, 1164, 1983.

274. Sträuli, P. and Haemmerli, G., The role of cancer cell motility in invasion, *Cancer Metastasis Rev.,* 3, 127, 1984.

275. Gabbert, H., Mechanisms of tumor invasion: evidence from in vivo observations, *Cancer Metast. Rev.,* 4, 293, 1985.

276. Grimstad, I.A., Direct evidence that cancer cell locomotion contributes importantly to invasion, *Exp. Cell. Res.,* 173, 515, 1987.

277. Tryggvason, K., Höyhtyä, M., and Salo, T., Proteolytic degradation of extracellular matrix in tumor invasion, *Biochim. Biophys. Acta,* 907, 191, 1987.

278. Liotta, L.A., Tumor invasion and metastases — role of the extracellular matrix, *Cancer Res.,* 46, 1, 1986.

279. Gerard, R.D., Chien, K.R., and Meidell, R.S., Molecular biology of tissue plasminogen activator and endogenous inhibitors, *Mol. Biol. Med.,* 3, 449, 1986.

280. Matrisian, L.M., Bowden, G.T., Krieg, P., Fürstenberger, G., Briand, J.-P., Leroy, P., and Breathnach, R., The mRNA coding for the secreted protease transin is expressed more abundantly in malignant than in benign tumors, *Proc. Natl. Acad. Sci. U.S.A.,* 83, 9413, 1986.

281. Sloane, B.F., Rozhin, J., Johnson, K., Taylor, H., Crissman, J.D., and Honn, K.V., Cathepsin B: association with plasma membrane in metastatic tumors, *Proc. Natl. Acad. Sci. U.S.A.,* 83, 2483, 1986.

282. Laiho, M., Saksela, O., and Keski-Oja, J., Transforming growth factor beta alters plasminogen activator activity in human skin fibroblasts, *Exp. Cell Res.,* 164, 399, 1986.
283. McCarthy, J.B., Basara, M.L., Palm, S.L., Sas, D.F., and Furcht, L.T., The role of cell adhesion proteins — laminin and fibronectin — in the movement of malignant and metastatic cells, *Cancer Metast. Rev.,* 4, 125, 1985.
284. Juliano, R.L., Membrane receptors for extracellular matrix macromolecules: relationship to cell adhesion and tumor metastasis, *Biochim. Biophys. Acta,* 907, 261, 1987.
285. Ouaissi, M.A. and Capron, A., Fibronectines: structures et fonctions, *Ann. Inst. Pasteur (Paris),* 136C, 169, 1985.
286. Humphries, M.J., Olden, K., and Yamada, K.M., A synthetic peptide from fibronectin inhibits experimental metastasis of murine melanoma cells, *Science,* 233, 467, 1986.
287. Leibovitch, S.A., Hillion, J., Leibovitch, M.-P., Guillier, M., Schmitz, A., and Harel, J., Expression of extracellular matrix genes in relation to myogenesis and neoplastic transformation, *Exp. Cell Res.,* 166, 526, 1986.
288. Jones, G.E., Arumugham, R.G., and Tanzer, M.L., Fibronectin glycosylation modulates fibroblast adhesion and spreading, *J. Cell Biol.,* 103, 1663, 1986.
289. Bevacqua, S.J., Greeff, C.W., and Hendrix, M.J.C., Cytogenetic evidence of gene amplification as a mechanism for tumor cell invasion, *Somat. Cell Mol. Genet.,* 14, 83, 1988.
290. Ananthaswamy, H.N., Price, J.E., Goldberg, L.H., and Bales, E.S., Simultaneous transfer of tumorigenic and metastatic phenotypes by transfection with genomic DNA from a human cutaneous squamous cell carcinoma, *J. Cell. Biochem.,* 36, 137, 1988.
291. Furcht, L.T., Critical factors controlling angiogenesis: cell products, cell matrix, and growth factors, *Lab. Invest.,* 55, 505, 1986.
292. Ingber, D.E., Madri, J.A., and Folkman, J., Endothelial growth factors and extracellular matrix regulate DNA synthesis through modulation of cell and nuclear expansion, *In Vitro Cell. Dev. Biol.,* 23, 387, 1987.
293. Folkman, J. and Klagsbrun, M., Angiogenic factors, *Science,* 235, 442, 1987.
294. Höckel, M., Sasse, J., and Wissler, J.H., Purified monocyte-derived angiogenic substance (angiotropin) stimulates migration, phenotypic changes, and "tube formation" but not proliferation of capillary endothelial cells *in vitro, J. Cell. Physiol.,* 133, 1, 1987.
295. Leibovich, S.J., Polverini, P.J., Shepard, H.M., Wiseman, D.M., Shively, V., and Nuseir, N., Macrophage-induced angiogenesis is mediated by tumour necrosis factor-alpha, *Nature,* 329, 630, 1987.
296. Coman, D.R., Mechanisms responsible for the origin and distribution of blood-borne tumor metastases: a review, *Cancer Res.,* 13, 397, 1953.
297. Pimentel, E., Metástasis: mecanismos de formación y posibilidades de control, *Acta Oncol. Venez.,* 7, 63, 1964.
298. Carter, R.L., Some aspects of the metastatic process, *J. Clin. Pathol.,* 35, 1041, 1982.
299. Tarin, D., The cell biology of metastatic tumour spread, *ICRS J. Med. Sci.,* 12, 1071, 1984.
300. Schirrmacher, V., Cancer metastasis: experimental approaches, theoretical concepts, and impacts for treatment strategies, *Adv. Cancer Res.,* 43, 1, 1985.
301. Auerbach, R., Patterns of tumor metastasis: organ selectivity in the spread of cancer cells, *Lab. Invest.,* 58, 361, 1988.
302. Mehta, P., Potential role of platelets in the pathogenesis of tumor metastasis, *Blood,* 63, 55, 1984.
303. Nelson, D.S. and Nelson, M., Evasion of host defences by tumours, *Immunol. Cell Biol.,* 65, 287, 1987.
304. Penn, I., Cancer is a complication of severe immunosuppression, *Surg. Gynecol. Obstet.,* 162, 603, 1986.
305. Penn, I., The occurrence of malignant tumors in immunosuppressed states, *Prog. Allergy,* 37, 259, 1986.
306. Ebert, E.C., Roberts, A.I., O'Connell, S.M., Robertson, F.M., and Nagase, H., Characterization of an immunosuppressive factor derived from colon cancer cells, *J. Immunol.,* 138, 2161, 1987.
307. Frost, P. and Kerbel, R.S., Immunology of metastasis: can the immune response cope with disseminated tumor?, *Cancer Metastasis Rev.,* 2, 239, 1983.
308. Prehn, R.T. and Prehn, L.M., The autoimmune nature of cancer, *Cancer Res.,* 47, 927, 1987.
309. Siegel, B.V., Immunology and oncology, *Int. Rev. Cytol.,* 96, 89, 1985.
310. Burns, G.F., Begley, C.G., Mackay, I.R., Triglia, T., and Werkmeister, J.A., "Supernatural" killer cells, *Immunol. Today,* 6, 370, 1985.
311. Herberman, R.B., Reynolds, C.W., and Ortaldo, J.R., Mechanism of cytotoxicity by natural killer (NK) cells, *Annu. Rev. Immunol.,* 4, 651, 1986.
312. Grossman, Z. and Herberman, R.B., Natural killer cells and their relationship to T-cells: hypothesis on the role of T-cell receptor gene rearrangement on the course of adaptative differentiation, *Cancer Res.,* 46, 2651, 1986.
313. Hanna, N., The role of natural killer cells in the control of tumor growth and metastasis, *Biochim. Biophys. Acta,* 780, 213, 1985.
314. Uchida, A., The cytolytic and regulatory role of natural killer cells in human neoplasia, *Biochim. Biophys. Acta,* 865, 329, 1986.

315. Fuyama, S., Yamamoto, H., Fujii, Y., and Arai, S., Mechanisms of *in vivo* generation of cytotoxic effector cells against tumor in tumor-bearing mice, *Cancer Res.*, 46, 5548, 1986.

316. Seidel, H.J., Stolz, W., Sutter, H., and Kreja, L., Natural killer cells in leukemogenesis, *Leukemia Res.*, 10, 803, 1986.

317. Patek, P.Q., Lin, Y., and Collins, J.L., Natural cytotoxic cells and tumor necrosis factor active similar lytic mechanisms, *Cancer Res.*, 138, 1641, 1987.

318. Urban, J.L., Shepard, H.M., Rothstein, J.L., Sugarman, B.J., and Schreiber, H., Tumor necrosis factor: a potent effector molecule for tumor cell killing by activated macrophages, *Proc. Natl. Acad. Sci. U.S.A.*, 83, 5233, 1986.

319. Kornbluth, R.S. and Eddington, T.S., Tumor necrosis factor production by human monocytes is a regulated event: induction of TNF-alpha-mediated cellular cytotoxicity by endotoxin, *J. Immunol.*, 137, 2585, 1986.

320. Evans, R., Macrophages and neoplasms: new insights and their implication in tumor immunobiology, *Cancer Metast. Rev.*, 1, 227, 1982.

321. Fidler, I.J., Macrophages and metastasis — a biological approach to cancer therapy, *Cancer Res.*, 45, 4714, 1985.

322. Hart, I.R. and Fidler, I.J., The implications of tumor heterogeneity for studies on the biology and therapy of cancer metastasis, *Biochim. Biophys. Acta*, 651, 37, 1981.

323. Poste, G. and Greig, R., The experimental and clinical implications of cellular heterogeneity in malignant tumors, *J. Cancer Res. Clin. Oncol.*, 106, 159, 1983.

324. Nicolson, G.L., Cell surface molecules and tumor metastasis: regulation of metastatic phenotypic diversity, *Exp. Cell Res.*, 150, 3, 1984.

325. Dennis, J.W. and Laferte, S., Tumor cell surface carbohydrate and the metastatic phenotype, *Cancer Metast. Rev.*, 5, 185, 1987.

326. Dano, K., Andreasen, P.A., Grondahl-Hansen, J., Kristensen, P., Nielsen, L.S., and Skriver, L., Plasminogen activators, tissue degradation and cancer, *Adv. Cancer Res.*, 44, 139, 1985.

327. Genton, C., Kruithof, E.K.O., and Schleuning, W.-D., Phorbol ester induces the biosynthesis of glycosylated and nonglycosylated plasminogen activator inhibitor 2 in high excess over urokinase-type plasminogen activator in human U-937 lymphoma cells, *J. Cell Biol.*, 104, 705, 1987

328. Leighton, J., Inherent malignancy of cancer cells possibly limited by genetically differing cells in the same tumor, *Acta Cytol.*, 9: 138, 1965.

329. Weiss, L., Random and nonrandom processes in metastasis, and metastatic inefficiency, *Invasion Metastasis*, 3, 193, 1983.

330. Milas, L., Peters, L.J., and Ito, H., Spontaneous metastasis: random or selective?, *Clin. Exp. Metastasis*, 1, 309, 1983.

331. Weiss, L., Holmes, J.C., and Ward, P.M., Do metastases arise from pre-existing subpopulations of cancer cells?, *Br. J. Cancer*, 47, 81, 1983.

332. Harris, J.F., Chambers, A.F., Hill, R.P., and Ling, V., Metastatic variants are generated spontaneously at a high rate in mouse KHT tumor, *Proc. Natl. Acad. Sci. U.S.A.*, 79, 5547, 1982.

333. Bernstein, S.C. and Weinberg, R.A., Expression of the metastatic phenotype in cells transfected with human metastatic tumor DNA, *Proc. Natl. Acad. Sci. U.S.A.*, 82, 1726, 1985.

334. Brodt, P., Characterization of two highly metastatic variants of Lewis lung carcinoma with different organ specificities, *Cancer Res.*, 46, 2442, 1986.

335. Mareel, M.M. and Van Roy, F.M., Are oncogenes involved in invasion and metastasis?, *Anticancer Res.*, 6, 419, 1986.

336. Van Roy, F.M., Messiaen, L., Liebaut, G., Gao, J., Dragonetti, C.H., Fiers, W.C., and Mareel, M.M., Invasiveness and metastatic capability of rat fibroblast-like cells before and after transfection with immortalizing and transforming genes, *Cancer Res.*, 46, 4787, 1986.

337. Collard, J.G., van de Poll, M., Scheffer, A., Roos, E., Hopman, A.H.M., Geurts van Kessel, A.H.M., and van Dongen, J.J.M., Location of genes involved in invasion and metastasis on human chromosome 7, *Cancer Res.*, 47, 6666, 1987.

338. Elvin, P., Kerr, I.B., McArdle, C.S., and Birnie, G.D., Isolation and preliminary characterisation of cDNA clones representing mRNAs associated with tumour progression and metastasis in colorectal cancer, *Br. J. Cancer*, 57, 36, 1988.

339. Shiosaka, T., Tanaka, Y., and Kobayashi, Y., Preferentially expressed genes in stomach adenocarcinoma cells, *Br. J. Cancer*, 56, 539, 1987.

340. Knudson, A.G., Jr., Genetics of human cancer, *Annu. Rev. Genet.*, 20, 231, 1986.

341. Hansen, M.F. and Cavenee, W.K., Genetics of cancer predisposition, *Cancer Res.*, 47, 5518, 1987.

342. Strong, L.C., Genetic etiology of cancer, *Cancer*, 40, 438, 1977.

343. Moolgavkar, S.H. and Knudson, A.G., Jr., Mutation and cancer: a model for human carcinogenesis, *J. Natl. Cancer Inst.*, 66, 1037, 1981.

344. Higginson, J., Multiplicity of factors involved in cancer patterns and trends, *J. Environ. Pathol. Toxicol.,* 3, 113, 1980.
345. Wynder, E.L., The environment and cancer prevention, *J. Environm. Pathol. Toxicol.,* 3, 171, 1980.
346. Schottenfeld, D., Genetic and environmental factors in human carcinogenesis, *J. Chron. Dis.,* 39, 1021, 1986.
347. Ibsen, K.H. and Fishman, W.H., Developmental gene expression in cancer, *Biochim. Biophys. Acta,* 560, 243, 1979.
348. Petropoulos, C.J., Lemire, J.M., Goldman, D., and Fausto, N., Homology between rat liver RNA populations during development, regeneration, and neoplasia, *Cancer Res.,* 45, 5114, 1985.
349. Rubin, H., Is somatic mutation the major mechanism of malignant transformation?, *J. Natl. Cancer Inst.,* 64, 995, 1980.
350. Straus, D.S., Somatic mutation, cellular differentiation, and cancer causation, *J. Natl. Cancer Inst.,* 67, 233, 1981.
351. Weinhouse, S., What are isozymes telling us about gene regulation and cancer?, *J. Natl. Cancer Inst.,* 68, 343, 1982.
352. Pitot, H.C., Grosso, L.E., and Goldsworthy, T., Genetics and epigenetics of neoplasia: facts and theories, *Carcinogen. Compr. Surv.,* 10, 65, 1985.
353. Bauer, K.H., Mutationstheorie der Geschwulstentstehung: Uebergang von Körperzellen, in *Geschwulstzellen durch Gen-Aenderung,* Julius Springer Verlag, Berlin, 1928.
354. Burdette, W.J., The significance of mutation in relation to the origin of tumors: a review, *Cancer Res.,* 15, 201, 1955.
355. Bauer, K.H., *Das Krebsproblem,* 2nd ed., Springer-Verlag, Berlin, 1963.
356. Quintanilla, M., Brown, K., Ramsden, M., and Balmain, A., Carcinogen-specific mutation and amplification of Ha-*ras* during mouse skin carcinogenesis, *Nature,* 322, 78, 1986.
357. Bos, J.L., Fearon, E.R., Hamilton, S.R., Verlaan-de Vries, M., van Boom, J.H., van der Eb, A.J., and Vogelstein, B., Prevalence of *ras* gene mutations in human colorectal cancers, *Nature,* 327, 293, 1987.
358. Forrester, K., Almoguera, C., Han, K., Grizzle, W.E., and Perucho, M., Detection of high incidence of K-*ras* oncogenes during human colon tumorigenesis, *Nature,* 327, 298, 1987.
359. Rodenhuis, S., van de Wetering, M.L., Mooi, W.J., Evers, S.G., van Zandwijk, N., and Bos, J.L., Mutational activation of the K-*ras* oncogene: a possible pathogenetic factor in adenocarcinoma of the lung, *N. Engl. J. Med.,* 317, 929, 1987.
360. Forrester, K., Almoguera, C., Jordano, J., Grizzle, W.E., and Perucho, M., High incidence of c-K-*ras* oncogenes in human colon cancer detected by the RNAse A mismatch cleavage method, *J. Tumor Marker Oncol.,* 2, 113, 1987.
361. Almoguera, C., Shibata, D., Forrester, K., Martin, J., Arnheim, N., and Perucho, M., Most human carcinomas of the exocrine pancreas contain mutant c-K-*ras* genes, *Cell,* 53, 549, 1988.
362. den Otter, W., Koten, J.W., and Derkideren, D.J., A new model for oncogenesis: from tumour immunology to a mathematical approach of oncogenesis, *Anticancer Res.,* 6, 509, 1986.
363. Andrews, A.W., Thibault, L.H., and Lijinsky, W., The relationship between carcinogenicity and mutagenicity of some polynuclear hydrocarbons, *Mutation Res.,* 51, 311, 1978.
364. Andrews, A.W., Thibault, L.H., and Lijinsky, W., The relationship between mutagenicity and carcinogenicity of some nitrosamines, *Mutation Res.,* 51, 319, 1978.
365. Garrett, N.E., Stack, H.F., Gross, M.R., and Waters, M.D., An analysis of the spectra of genetic activity produced by known or suspected human carcinogens, *Mutation Res.,* 134, 89, 1984.
366. Cleaver, J.E., Bootsma, D., and Friedberg, E., Human diseases with genetically altered DNA repair processes, *Genetics,* 79, 215, 1975.
367. Hanawalt, P.C. and Sarasin, A., Cancer-prone hereditary diseases with DNA processing abnormalities, *Trends Genet.,* 2, 124, 1986.
368. Hsu, T.C., Genetic predisposition to cancer with special reference to mutagen sensitivity, *In Vitro Cell. Dev. Biol.,* 23, 591, 1987.
369. Robbins, J.H., Kraemer, K.H., Lutzner, M.A., Festoff, B.W., and Coon, H.G., Xeroderma pigmentosum: an inherited disease with sun sensitivity, multiple cutaneous neoplasms, and abnormal DNA repair, *Ann. Int. Med.,* 80, 221, 1974.
370. Friedberg, E.C., Xeroderma pigmentosum: recent studies on the DNA repair defects, *Arch. Pathol. Lab. Med.,* 102, 3, 1978.
371. Robbins, J.H., Significance of repair of human DNA: evidence from studies in xeroderma pigmentosum, *J. Natl. Cancer Inst.,* 61, 645, 1978.
372. Willis, A.E., Weksberg, R., Tomlinson, S., and Lindahl, T., Structural alterations of DNA ligase I in Bloom syndrome, *Proc. Natl. Acad. Sci. U.S.A.,* 84, 8016, 1987.
373. Hansemann, D. von, Ueber asymmetrische Zellteilung in Epithelkrebsen und deren biologische Bedeutung, *Virchows Arch. Pathol. Anat. Physiol.,* 119, 299, 1890.

374. Makino, S.A., A cytological study of the Yoshida sarcoma, an ascites tumor of white rats, *Chromosoma,* 4, 649, 1952.
375. Sasaki, M., Role of chromosomal mutation in the development of cancer, *Cytogenet. Cell Genet.,* 33, 160, 1982.
376. Sasaki, M., Current statues of cytogenetic studies in animal tumors with special reference to nonrandom chromosome changes, *Cancer Genet. Cytogenet.,* 5, 153, 1982.
377. Sasaki, M.S., Chromosome abnormalities in cancer development, *Environ. Sci. Res.,* 31, 35, 1984.
378. Boveri, T., *Zur Frage der Entstehung maligner Tumoren,* Gustav Fischer, Jena, 1914.
379. Sugiyama, T., Ueda, N., Maeda, S., Shiraishi, N., Goto-Mimura, K., Murao, S., and Chattopadhyay, S.C., Chemical carcinogenesis in the rat: common mode of action of carcinogens at the chromosome level, *J. Natl. Cancer Inst.,* 67, 831, 1981.
380. Le Beau, M.M. and Rowley, J.D., Recurring chromosomal abnormalities in leukaemia and lymphoma, *Cancer Surv.,* 3, 371, 1984.
381. Fonatsch, C., Cytogenetic markers in hematoproliferative disorders, *Blut,* 51, 315, 1985.
382. Le Beau, M.M. and Rowley, J.D., Chromosomal abnormalities in leukemia and lymphoma: clinical and biological significance, *Adv. Hum. Genet.,* 15, 1, 1986.
383. Wolman, S., Cytogenetics and cancer, *Arch. Pathol. Lab. Med.,* 108, 15, 1984.
384. Schroeder, T.M., Genetically determined chromosome instability syndromes, *Cytogenet. Cell Genet.,* 33, 119, 1982.
385. Kuhn, E.M. and Therman, E., Cytogenetics of Bloom's syndrome, *Cancer Genet. Cytogenet.,* 22, 1, 1986.
386. Gustavson, K.-H., Jansson, R., and Oberg, K., Chromosomal breakage in multiple endocrine adenomatosis (types I and II), *Clin. Genet.,* 23, 143, 1983.
387. de Nuñez, M., Penchaszadeh, V., and Pimentel, E., Chromosome fragility in patients with sporadic unilateral retinoblastoma, *Cancer Genet. Cytogenet.,* 11, 139, 1984.
388. Yunis, J.J., Soreng, A.L., and Bowe, A.E., Fragile sites are targets of diverse mutagens and carcinogens, *Oncogene,* 1, 59, 1987.
389. De Braekeleer, M., Smith, B., and Lin, C.C., Fragile sites and structural rearrangements in cancer, *Hum. Genet.,* 69, 112, 1985.
390. Le Beau, M.M., Chromosomal fragile sites and cancer-specific breakpoints — a moderating viewpoint, *Cancer Genet. Cytogenet.,* 31, 55, 1988.
391. Popescu, N.C. and DiPaolo, J.A., Relationship of chromosomal alterations to gene expression in carcinogenesis, in *Carcinogenesis,* Vol. 10, Huberman, E., Ed., Raven Press, New York, 1985, 419.
392. Mitelman, F., Levan, G., and Brandt, L., Highly malignant cells with normal karyotype in G-banding, *Hereditas,* 80, 291, 1975.
393. Klein, G., Ohno, S., Rosenberg, N., Wiener, F., Spira, J., and Baltimore, D., Cytogenetic studies on Abelson-virus-induced mouse leukemias, *Int. J. Cancer,* 25, 805, 1980.
394. Muschel, R.J., Nakahara, K., Chu, E., Pozzatti, R., and Liotta, L.A., Karyotypic analysis of diploid or near diploid metastatic transformed rat embryo fibroblasts, *Cancer Res.,* 46, 4104, 1986.
395. Cerni, C., Mougneau, E., and Couzin, F., Transfer of "immortalizing" oncogenes into rat fibroblasts induces both high rates of sister chromatid exchange and appearance of abnormal karyotypes, *Exp. Cell Res.,* 168, 439, 1987.
396. DiPaolo, J.A., Karyological instability of neoplastic somatic cells, *In Vitro,* 11, 89, 1975.
397. Popescu, N.C., Amsbaugh, S.C., Milo, G., and DiPaolo, J.A., Chromosome alterations with *in vitro* exposure of human fibroblasts to chemical or physical carcinogens, *Cancer Res.,* 46, 4720, 1986.
398. Yunis, J.J., Bloomfield, C.D., and Ensrud, K., All patients with acute nonlymphocytic leukemia may have a chromosomal defect, *N. Engl. J. Med.,* 305, 135, 1981.
399. Williams, D.L., Harber, J., Murphy, S.B., Look, A.T., Kalwinsky, D.K., Rivera, G., Melvin, S.L., Stass, S., and Dahl, G.V., Chromosomal translocations play a unique role in influencing prognosis in childhood acute lymphoblastic leukemia, *Blood,* 68, 205, 1986.
400. Bloomfield, C.D. and de la Chapelle, A., Chromosome abnormalities in acute nonlymphocytic leukemia: clinical and biological significance, *Semin. Oncol.,* 14, 372, 1987.
401. Gahrton, G., Juliusson, G., Robert, K.-H., Friberg, K., and Zech, L., Pathogenetic and clinical significance of chromosomal aberrations in B-cell chronic lymphocytic leukemia, in *Molecular Biology of Tumor Cells,* Wahren, B., Ed., Raven Press, New York, 1985, 45.
402. Gahrton, G., Juliusson, G., Robèrt, K.H., and Zech, L., Specific chromosomal markers in B- and T-cell chronic lymphocytic leukemia, *Tumour Biol.,* 6, 1, 1985.
403. Wolman, S.R., Smith, H.S., Stampfer, M., and Hackett, A.J., Growth of diploid cells from breast cancers, *Cancer Genet. Cytogenet.,* 16, 49, 1985.
404. Smith, H.S., Liotta, L.A., Hancock, M.C., Wolman, S.R., and Hackett, A.J., Invasiveness and ploidy of human mammary carcinomas in short-term culture, *Proc. Natl. Acad. Sci. U.S.A.,* 82, 1805, 1985.
405. Anders, F., Scholl, E., and Schartl, M., Environmental and hereditary factors in the causation of neoplasia, based on studies of the *Xiphophorus* fish melanoma system, in *Proc. XIth Int. Pigment Cell Conference,* Seiji, M., Ed., University of Tokyo Press, 1981, 491.

406. Rowley, J.D., Biological implications of consistent chromosome rearrangements in leukemia and lymphoma, *Cancer Res.,* 44, 3159, 1984.
407. Pimentel, E., Oncogenes and human cancer, *Cancer Genet. Cytogenet.,* 14, 347, 1985.
408. Mark, J. and Dahlenfors, R., Cytogenetical observations in 100 human benign pleomorphic adenomas: specificity of the chromosomal aberrations and their relationship to sites of localized oncogenes, *Anticancer Res.,* 6, 299, 1986.
409. Bartholdi, M.F., Ray, F.A., Cram, L.S., and Kraemer, P.M., Karyotype instability of Chinese hamster cells during *in vivo* tumor progression, *Somat. Cell Mol. Genet.,* 13, 1, 1987.
410. Klein, G., The approaching era of the tumor suppressor genes, Science, 238, 1539, 1987.
411. Padmanabhan, R., Howard, T.H., and Howard, B.H., Specific growth inhibitory sequences in genomic DNA from quiescent human embryo fibroblasts, *Mol. Cell. Biol.,* 7, 1894, 1987.
412. Woodcock, D.M., Crowther, P.J., and Diver, W.P., The majority of methylated deoxycytidines in human DNA are not in the CpG dinucleotide, *Biochem. Biophys. Res. Commun.,* 145, 888, 1987.
413. Razin, A. and Riggs, A.D., DNA methylation and gene function, Science, 210, 604, 1980.
414. Doerfler, W., DNA methylation and gene activity, *Annu. Rev. Biochem.,* 52, 93, 1983.
415. Doerfler, W., DNA methylation: site-specific methylations cause gene inactivation, *Angew. Chem. (Engl. Ed.),* 23, 919, 1984.
416. Bird, A.P., CpG-rich islands and the function of DNA methylation, *Nature,* 321, 209, 1986.
417. Wigler, M., Levy, D., and Perucho, M., The somatic replication of DNA methylation, *Cell,* 24, 33, 1981.
418. Holliday, R., A new theory of carcinogenesis, *Br. J. Cancer,* 40, 513, 1979.
419. Riggs, A.D. and Jones, P.A., 5-Methylcytosine, gene regulation, and cancer, *Adv. Cancer Res.,* 40, 1, 1983.
420. Boehm, T.L.J. and Drahovsky, S., Alteration of enzymatic methylation of DNA cytosines by chemical carcinogen: a mechanism involved in the initiation of carcinogenesis, *J. Natl. Cancer Inst.,* 71, 429, 1983.
421. Nyce, J., Weinhouse, S., and Magee, P.N., 5-methylcytosine depletion during tumour development: an extension of the miscoding concept, *Br. J. Cancer,* 48, 463, 1983.
422. Holliday, R., DNA methylation and epigenetic defects in carcinogenesis, *Mutat. Res.,* 181, 215, 1987.
423. Jones, P.A., DNA methylation and cancer, *Cancer Res.,* 46, 461, 1986.
424. Chandler, L.A., DeClerck, Y.A., Bogenmann, E., and Jones, P.A., Patterns of DNA methylation and gene expression in human tumor cell lines, *Cancer Res.,* 46, 2944, 1986.
425. Cox, R. and Irving, C.C., Inhibition of DNA methylation by S-adenosylethionine with the production of methyl-deficient DNA in regenerating rat liver, *Cancer Res.,* 37, 222, 1977.
426. Pfohl-Leszkowicz, A., Salas, C., Fuchs, P.P., and Dirheimer, G., Mechanism of inhibition of enzymatic deoxyribonucleic acid methylation by 2-(acetylamino)fluorene bound to deoxyribonucleic acid, *Biochemistry,* 20, 3020, 1981.
427. Wilson, V.L., Smith, R.A., Longoria, J., Liotta, M.A., Harper, C.M., and Harris, C.C., Chemical carcinogen-induced decreases in genomic 5-methyldeoxycytidine content of normal human bronchial epithelial cells, *Proc. Natl. Acad. Sci. U.S.A.,* 84, 3298, 1987.
428. Barr, F.G., Rajagopalan, S., MacArthur, C.A., and Lieberman, M.W., Genomic hypomethylation and far-5' sequence alterations are associated with carcinogen-induced activation of the hamster thymidine kinase gene, *Mol Cell. Biol.,* 6, 3023, 1986.
429. Carr, B.I., Reilly, J.G., Smith, S.S., Winberg, C., and Riggs, A.D., The tumorigenicity of 5-azacytidine in the male Fischer rat, *Carcinogenesis,* 5, 1583, 1984.
430. Jones, P.A., Altering gene expression with 5-azacytidine, *Cell,* 40, 485, 1985.
431. Hsiao, W.-L.W., Gattoni-Celli, S., Kirschmeier, P., and Weinstein, I.B., Effects of 5-azacytidine on methylation and expression of specific DNA sequences in C3H 10T1/2 cells, *Mol. Cell Biol.,* 4, 509, 1984.
432. Hsiao, W.-L.W., Gattoni-Celli, S., and Weinstein, I.B., Effects of 5-azacytidine on the progressive nature of cell transformation, *Mol. Cell. Biol.,* 5, 1800, 1985.
433. Olsson, L., Due, C., and Diamant, M., Treatment of human cell lines with 5-azacytidine may result in profound alterations in clonogenicity and growth rate, *J. Cell Biol.,* 100, 508, 1985.
434. Babiss, L.E., Zimmer, S.G., and Fisher, P.B., Reversibility of progression of the transformed phenotype in Ad5-transformed rat embryo cells, *Science,* 228, 1099, 1985.
435. Borrello, M.G., Pierotti, M.A., Bongarzone, I., Donghi, R., Mondellini, P., and Della Porta, G., DNA methylation affecting the transforming activity of the human Ha-*ras* oncogene, *Cancer Res.,* 47, 75, 1987.
436. Mikol, Y.B., Hoover, K.L., Creasia, D., and Poirier, L.A., Hepatocarcinogenesis in rats fed methyl-deficient, amino acid-defined diets, *Carcinogenesis,* 9, 1619, 1983.
437. Hoover, K.L., Lynch, P.H., and Poirier, L.A., Profound postinitiation enhancement by short-term severe methionine, choline, vitamin B12 and folate deficiency of hepatocarcinogenesis in rats given a single low-dose diethylnitrosamine, *J. Natl. Cancer Inst.,* 73, 1327, 1984.
438. Wilson, M.J., Shivapurkar, N., and Poirier, L.A., Hypomethylation of hepatic nuclear DNA in rats fed with a carcinogenic methyl-deficient diet, *Biochem. J.,* 218, 987, 1984.
439. Bhave, M.R., Wilson, M.J., and Poirier, L.A., c-H- *ras* and c-K- *ras* gene hypomethylation in the livers and hepatomas of rats fed methyl-deficient, amino acid-defined diets, *Carcinogenesis,* 9, 343, 1988.

440. Kanduc, D., Ghoshal, A., Quagliariello, E., and Farber, E., DNA hypomethylation in ethionine-induced rat preneoplastic hepatocyte nodules, *Biochem. Biophys. Res. Commun.,* 150, 739 1988.

441. Feinberg, A.P. and Vogelstein, B., Hypomethylation distinguishes genes of some human cancers from their normal counterparts, *Nature,* 301, 89, 1983.

442. Erickson, R.P., Ferrucci, S., Rahe, B., Rosenberg, M.P., and Morello, D., Growth conditions of F9 embryonal carcinoma cells affect the degree of DNA methylation, *Mol. Biol. Rep.,* 10, 109, 1984.

443. Erickson, R.P., Ferrucci, S., Rahe, B., Rosenberg, M.P., and Morello, lD., Growth conditions of F9 embryonal carcinoma cells affect the degree of DNA methylation, *Mol. Biol. Rep.,* 10, 109, 1984.

444. Ormerod, E.J., Everett, C.A., Finch, M., and Hart, I.R., DNA methylation levels in human and murine melanoma cell lines of varying metastatic potential, *Cancer Res.,* 46, 4342, 1986.

445. Gautsch, J.W. and Wilson, M.C., Delayed *de novo* methylation in teratocarcinoma suggests additional tissue-specific mechanisms for controlling gene expression, *Nature,* 301, 32, 1983.

446. Nazar, R.N., Sitz, T.O., and Somers, K.D., Cytoplasmic methylation of mature 5.8S rRNA, *J. Mol. Biol.,* 142, 117, 1980.

447. Munholland, J.M. and Nazar, R.N., Methylation of ribosomal RNA as a possible factor in cell differentiation, *Cancer Res.,* 47, 169, 1987.

448. Paik, W.K. and Kim, S., Protein methylation, in *The Enzymology of Post-Translational Modification of Proteins,* Vol. 2, Freedman, R.B. and Hawkins, H.C., Eds., Academic Press, London, 1985, 187.

449. Nevers, P. and Saedler, H., Transposable genetic elements as agents of gene instability and chromosomal rearrangements, *Nature,* 268, 109, 1977.

450. Calos, M.P. and Jeffrey, H.M., Transposable elements, *Cell,* 20, 579, 1980.

451. Starlinger, P., IS elements and transposons, *Plasmid,* 3, 241, 1980.

452. Strobel, E., Mobile dispersed repeated DNA elements in the *Drosophila* genome, *Fed. Proc. Fed. Am. Soc. Exp. Biol.,* 41, 2656, 1982.

453. Starlinger, P., Transposable elements, *Trends Biochem. Sci.,* 9, 125, 1984.

454. Weiner, A.M., Deininger, P.L., and Efstratiadis, A., Nonviral retroposons: genes, pseudogenes, and transposable elements generated by the reverse flow of genetic information, *Annu. Rev. Biochem.,* 55, 631, 1986.

455. Jagadeeswaran, P., Forget, B.G., and Weissman, S.M., Short interspersed repetitive DNA elements in eucaryotes: transposable DNA elements generated by reverse transcription of RNA pol III transcripts?, *Cell,* 26, 141, 1981.

456. Baltimore, D., Retroviruses and transposons: the role of reverse transcription in shaping the eukaryotic genome, *Cell,* 40, 481, 1985.

457. Jelinek, W.R. and Schmid, C.W., Repetitive sequences in eukaryotic DNA and their expression, *Annu. Rev. Biochem.,* 51, 813, 1982.

458. Schmid, C.W. and Jelinek, W.R., The *alu* family of dispersed repetitive sequences, *Science,* 216, 1065, 1982.

459. Calabretta, B., Robberson, D.L., Barrera-Saldana, H.A., Lambrou, T.P., and Saunders, G.F., Genome instability in a region of human DNA enriched in *Alu* repeat sequences, *Nature,* 296, 219, 1982.

460. Davidson, E.H. and Posakony, J.W., Repetitive sequence transcripts in development, *Nature,* 297, 633, 1982.

461. Paulson, K.E. and Schmid, C.W., Transcriptional inactivity of Alu repeats in HeLa cells, *Nucleic Acids Res.,* 14, 6145, 1986.

462. Kourilsky, P., Molecular mechanisms for gene conversion in higher cells, *Trends Genet.,* 2, 60, 1986.

463. Murnane, J.P., Inducible gene expression by DNA rearrangements in human cells, *Mol. Cell. Biol.,* 6, 549, 1986.

464. Knowles, D.M. II, Pelicci, P.-G., and Dalla-Favera, R., Immunoglobulin and T cell receptor beta chain gene DNA probes in the diagnosis and classification of human lymphoid neoplasia, *Mol. Cell. Probes,* 1, 15, 1987.

465. Toyonaga, B. and Mak, T.W., Genes of the T-cell antigen receptor in normal and malignant T cells, *Annu. Rev. Immunol.,* 5, 585, 1987.

466. Levy, R., Levy, S., Cleary, M.L., Carroll, W., Kon, S., Bird, J., and Sklar, J., Somatic mutations in human B-cell tumors, *Annu. Rev. Immunol.,* 96, 43, 1987.

467. Farzaneh, F., Zalin, R., Brill, D., and Shall, S., DNA strand breaks and ADP-ribosyl transferase activation during cell differentiation, *Nature,* 300, 362, 1982.

468. Johnstone, A.P. and Williams, G.T., Role of DNA breaks and ADP-ribosyl transferase activity in eukaryotic differentiation demonstrated in human lymphocytes, *Nature,* 300, 368, 1982.

469. Francis, G.E., Ho, A.D., Gray, D.A., Berney, J.J., Wing, M.A., Yaxley, J.J., Ma, D.D.F., and Hoffbrand, A.V., DNA strand breakage and ADP-ribosyl transferase mediated DNA ligation during stimulation of human bone marrow cells by granulocyte-macrophage colony stimulating activity, *Leukemia Res.,* 8, 407, 1984.

470. Farzaneh, F., Meldrum, R., and Shall, S., Transient formation of DNA strand breaks during the induced differentiation of a human promyelocytic leukaemic cell line, HL-60, *Nucleic Acids Res.,* 15, 3493, 1987.

471. Farzaneh, F., Feon, S., Lebby, R.A., Brill, D., and Shall, S., DNA repair in human promyelocytic cell line, HL-60, *Nucleic Acids Res.,* 15, 3503, 1987.

472. Weisinger, G., Korn, A.P., and Sachs, L., Protein that induces cell differentiation causes nicks in double-stranded DNA, *FEBS Lett.,* 200, 107, 1986.

473. Sager, R., Genetic instability, suppression and human cancer, *Cancer Surv.,* 3, 321, 1984.

474. de Grouchy, J. and de Nava, C., A chromosomal theory of carcinogenesis, *Ann. Int. Med.,* 69, 381, 1968.

475. Sager, R., Transposable elements and chromosomal rearrangements in cancer — a possible link, *Nature,* 282, 447, 1979.

476. Cairns, J., The origin of human cancers, *Nature,* 289, 353, 1981.

477. Klein, G., The role of gene dosage and genetic transpositions in carcinogenesis, *Nature,* 294, 313, 1981.

478. Radman, M., Jeggo, P., and Wagner, R., Chromosomal rearrangement and carcinogenesis, *Mutation Res.,* 98, 249, 1982.

479. Klein, G., Specific chromosomal translocations and the genesis of B-cell-derived tumors in mice and men, *Cell,* 32, 311, 1983.

480. Sandberg, A.A., A chromosomal hypothesis of oncogenesis, *Cancer Genet. Cytogenet.,* 8, 277, 1983.

481. Chorazy, M., Sequence rearrangements and genome instability, *J. Cancer Res. Clin. Oncol.,* 109, 159, 1985.

482. Turner, D.R., Morley, A.A., Haliandros, M., Kutlaca, R., and Sanderson, B.J., *In vivo* somatic mutations in human lymphocytes frequently result from major gene alterations, *Nature,* 315, 343, 1985.

483. de Grouchy, J., Cancer and the evolution of species: a ransom, *Biomedicine,* 18, 6, 1973.

484. Kennedy, A.R., Cairns, J., and Little, J.B., Timing of the steps in transformation of C3H 10T1/2 cells by X-irradiation, *Nature,* 307, 85, 1984.

485. Kano, Y. and Little, J.B., Mechanisms of human cell neoplastic transformation: X-ray-induced abnormal clone formation in long-term cultures of human diploid fibroblasts, *Cancer Res.,* 45, 2550, 1985.

486. Little, J.B., Mutagenic and chromosomal events in radiation transformation, *Biochimie,* 67, 405, 1985.

487. Brand, K.G., Buoen, L.C., Johnson, K.H., and Brand, I., Etiological factors, stages, and the role of the foreign body in foreign body tumorigenesis: a review, *Cancer Res.,* 35, 279, 1975.

488. Brand, K.G., Diversity and complexity of carcinogenic processes: conceptual inferences from foreign-body tumorigenesis, *J. Natl. Cancer Inst.,* 57, 973, 1976.

489. Karp, R.D., Johnson, K.H., Buoen, L.C., Ghobrial, H.K.G., Brand, I., and Brand, K.G., Tumorigenesis by milliopore filters in mice: histology and ultrastructure of tissue reactions as related to pore size, *J. Natl. Cancer Inst.,* 51, 1275, 1973.

490. Rachko, D. and Brand, K.G., Chromosomal aberrations in foreign body tumorigenesis in mice, *Proc. Soc. Exp. Biol. Med.,* 172, 382, 1983.

491. Lechner, J.F., Tokiwa, T., LaVeck, M., Benedict, W.F., Banks-Schlegel, S., Yeager, H., Jr., Banerjee, A., and Harris, C.C., Asbestos-associated chromosomal changes in human mesothelial cells, *Proc. Natl. Acad. Sci. U.S.A.,* 82, 3884, 1985.

492. Levan, A., Levan, G., and Mitelman, F., *Chromosomes Cancer,* 86, 15, 1977.

493. Barker, P.E., Double minutes in human tumor cells, *Cancer Genet. Cytogenet.,* 5, 81, 1982.

494. Casartelli, C., Cancer and chromosomes: a review, *Rev. Brasil. Genet.,* 3, 595, 1982.

495. Gebhart, E., Tulusan, A.H., Maillot, K.V., and Mulz, D., Double minutes: new markers in cells of human solid tumors, *J. Genet. Hum.,* 31, 45, 1983.

496. Arrighi, F.E., Gene amplification in human tumor cells, in *Proc. 13th Int. Cancer Congress,* Part C, Alan R. Liss, New York, 1983, 259.

497. Sakai, K., Kanda, N., Shiloh, Y., Donlon, T., Schreck, R., Shipley, J., Dryja, T., Chaum, E., Chaganti, R.S.K., and Latt, S., Molecular and cytogenetic analysis of DNA amplification in retinoblastoma, *Cancer Genet. Cytogenet.,* 17, 95, 1985.

498. Sager, R., Gadi, I.K., Stephens, L., and Grabowy, C.T., Gene amplification: an example of accelerated evolution in tumorigenic cells, *Proc. Natl. Acad. Sci. U.S.A.,* 82, 7015, 1985.

499. Ishikawa, F., Takaku, F., Hayashi, K., Nagao, M., and Sugimura, T., Activation of rat c-*raf* during transfection of hepatocellular carcinoma DNA, *Proc. Natl. Acad. Sci. U.S.A.,* 83, 3209, 1986.

500. Ishikawa, F., Takaku, F., Nagao, M., and Sugimura, T., Rat c-*raf* oncogene activation by a rearrangement that produces a fused protein, *Mol. Cell. Biol.,* 7, 1226, 1987.

501. Cerni, C., The transformation of a rat cell line induced by a tumor promoter occurs without affecting sister chromatid exchange, *Oncology,* 41, 357, 1984.

502. de Kok, A.J., Tates, A.D., Den Engelse, L., and Simons, J.W.I.M., Genetic and molecular mechanisms of the *in vitro* transformation of Syrian hamster embryo cells by the carcinogen *N*-ethyl-*N*-nitrosourea. I. Correlation of morphological transformation and enhanced fibrinolytic activity to gene mutation, chromosomal alterations and lethality, Carcinogenesis, 6, 1565, 1985.

503. Pimentel, E., Human oncovirology, *Biochim. Biophys. Acta,* 560, 169, 1979.

504. Robinson, H.L., Retroviruses and cancer, *Rev. Infect. Dis.,* 4, 1015, 1982.

505. Rous, P., A sarcoma of the fowl transmissible by an agent separable from the tumor cells, *J. Exp. Med.,* 13, 397, 1911.

506. Gallo, R.C. and Wong-Staal, F., Current thoughs on the viral etiology of certain human cancers, *Cancer Res.*, 44, 2743, 1984.

507. Hinuma, Y., Retrovirus in adult T-cell leukemia, *Progr. Med. Virol.*, 30, 156, 1984.

508. Sugamura, K. and Hinuma, Y., Human retrovirus in adult T-cell leukemia/lymphoma, *Immunol. Today*, 6, 83, 1985.

509. Gallo, R.C., The human T-cell leukemia/lymphotropic retroviruses (HTLV) family: past, present, and future, *Cancer Res.*, 45 (Suppl.), 4524s, 1985.

510. Hunsmann, G. and Hinuma, Y., Human adult T-cell leukemia virus and its association with disease, *Adv. Viral Oncol.*, 5, 147, 1985.

511. Gallo, R.C., Human tumor and immunodeficiency viruses, *AIDS Res. Hum. Retrovir.*, 3 (Suppl. 1), 187, 1987.

512. Gallo, R.C., Sarngadharan, M.G., Popovic, M., Shaw, G.M., Hahn, B., Wong-Staal, F., Robert-Guroff, M., Salahuddin, S.Z., and Markham, P.D., HTLV-III and the etiology of AIDS, *Progr. Allergy*, 37, 1, 1986.

513. Montagnier, L., Lymphadenopathy associated virus: its role in the pathogenesis of AIDS and related diseases, *Progr. Allergy*, 37, 46, 1986.

514. Ho, D.D., Pomeranz, R.J., and Kaplan, J.C., Pathogenesis of infection with human immunodeficiency virus, *N. Engl. J. Med.*, 317, 278, 1987.

515. Jaenisch, R., Endogenous retroviruses, *Cell*, 32, 5, 1983.

516. Risser, R., Horowitz, J.M., and McCubrey, J., Endogenous mouse leukemia viruses, *Annu. Rev. Genet.*, 17, 85, 1983.

517. Kozak, C.A., Retroviruses as chromosomal genes in the mouse, *Adv. Cancer Res.*, 44, 295, 1985.

518. Lugo, M., Metaplasia: an overview, *Arch. Pathol. Lab. Med.*, 108, 185, 1984.

519. Okada, T.S., Recent progress in studies of the transdifferentiation of eye tissue *in vitro, Cell Differ.*, 13, 177, 1983.

520. Kitamura, Y., Nakano, T., and Kanakura, Y., Transdifferentiation between mast cell subpopulations, *Dev Growth Differ.*, 28, 321, 1986.

521. Tsonis, P.A., Embryogenesis and carcinogenesis: order and disorder, *Anticancer Res.*, 7, 617, 1987.

522. Potter, V.R., The present status of the blocked ontogeny hypothesis of neoplasia: the thalassemia connection, *Oncodev. Biol. Med.*, 2, 243, 1981.

523. Pierce, G.B., Relationship between differentiation and carcinogenesis, *J. Toxicol. Environ. Health*, 2, 1335, 1977.

524. Uriel, J., Cancer, retrodifferentiation, and the myth of Faust, *Cancer Res.*, 36, 4269, 1976.

525. Pierce, G.B., Differentiation of normal and malignant cells, *Fed. Proc.Fed. Am. Soc. Exp. Biol.*, 29, 1248, 1970.

526. Finckh, E.S., Aberrant, variant and deviant differentiation in pathology, *Pathology*, 14, 443, 1982.

527. Greaves, M.F., Chan, L.C., Furley, A.J.W., Watt, S.M., and Molgaard, H.V., Lineage promiscuity in hemopoietic differentiation and leukemia, *Blood*, 67, 1, 1986.

528. Verp, M.S. and Simpson, J.L., Abnormal sexual differentiation and neoplasia, *Cancer Genet. Cytogenet.*, 25, 191, 1987.

529. Wille, J.J., Jr. and Scott, R.E., Suppression of tumorigenicity by the cell-cycle-dependent control of cellular differentiation and proliferation, *Int. J. Cancer*, 37, 875, 1986.

530. Scott, R.E. and Maercklein, P.B., An initiator of carcinogenesis selectively and stably inhibits stem cell differentiation: a concept that initiation of carcinogenesis involves multiple phases, *Proc. Natl. Acad. Sci. U.S.A.*, 82, 1995, 1985.

531. Colletta, G., Pinto, A., Di Fiore, P.P., Fusco, A., Ferrentino, M., Avvedimento, V.E., Tsuchida, N., and Vecchio, G., Dissociation between transformed and differentiated phenotype in rat thyroid epithelial cells after transformation with a temperature-sensitive mutant of the Kirsten murine sarcoma virus, *Mol. Cell. Biol.*, 3, 2099, 1983.

532. Wier, M.L. and Scott, R.E., Defective control of terminal differentiation and its role in carcinogenesis in the 3T3 T proadipocyte stem cell line, *Cancer Res.*, 45, 3339, 1985.

533. Freshney, R.I., Induction of differentiation in neoplastic cells, *Anticancer Res.*, 5, 111, 1985.

534. Yuspa, S.H. and Morgan, D.L., Mouse skin cells resistant to terminal differentiation associated with initiation of carcinogenesis, *Nature*, 293, 72, 1981.

535. Kilkenny, A.E., Morgan, D., Spangler, E.F., and Yuspa, S.H., Correlation of initiating potency of skin carcinogens with potency to induce resistance to terminal differentiation in cultured mouse keratinocytes, *Cancer Res.*, 45, 2219, 1985.

536. Stent, G.S., Cell lineage in development, *FEBS Lett.*, 1, 1, 1987.

537. La Thangue, N.B. and Rigby, P.W.J., An adenovirus E1A-like transcription factor is regulated during the differentiation of murine embryonal carcinoma stem cells, *Cell*, 49, 507, 1987.

538. The nucleotide sequence of three genes participating in the adipose differentiation of 3T3 cells, *J. Biol. Chem.*, 261, 10821, 1986.

539. Chiu, C-P. and Blau, H.M., Reprogramming cell differentiation in the absence of DNA synthesis, *Cell*, 37, 879, 1984.

540. Plumb, M.A., Lobanenkov, V.V., Nicolas, R.H., Wright, C.A., Zavou, S., and Goodwin, G.H., Characterisation of chicken erythroid nuclear proteins which bind to the nuclease hypersensitive regions of the beta^A- and beta^B-globin genes, *Nucleic Acids Res.*, 14, 7675, 1986.

541. Basu, M., Frick, K., Sen-Majumdar, A., Scher, C.D., and Das, M., EGF receptor-associated DNA-nicking activity is due to a M_r-100,000 dissociable protein, *Nature*, 316, 640, 1985.

542. von Melchner, H. and Höffken, K., Disconnection of genes coding for self-renewal and differentiation: a possible mechanism of diversity in acute myeloid leukemias, *Blut*, 50, 257, 1985.

543. Nusslein-Volhard, C. and Wieschaus, E., Mutations affecting segment number and polarity in *Drosophila*, *Nature*, 287, 795, 1980.

544. McGinnis, W., Garber, R.L., Kuroiwa, A., and Gehring, W.J., A homologous protein-coding sequence in *Drosophila* homeotic genes and its conservation in other metazoans, *Cell*, 37, 403, 1984.

545. Hart, C.P., Awgulewitsch, A., Fainsod, A., McGinnis, W., and Ruddle, F.H., Homeo box gene complex on mouse chromosome 11: molecular cloning, expression in embryogenesis, and homology to a human homeo box locus, *Cell*, 43, 9, 1985.

546. Colberg-Poley, A.M., Voss, S.D., Chowdhury, K., Stewart, C.L., Wagner, E.F., and Gruss, P., Clustered homeo boxes are differentially expressed during murine development, *Cell*, 43, 39, 1985.

547. Ruddle, F.H., Hart, C.P., and McGinnis, W., Structural and functional aspects of the mammalian homeo-box sequences, *Trends Genet.*, 1, 48, 1985.

548. Scott, M.P. and Carroll, S.B., The segmentation and homeotic gene network in early *Drosophila* development, *Cell*, 51, 689, 1987.

549. Carrasco, A.E., McGinnis, W., Gehring, W.J., and De Robertis, E.M., Cloning of an *X. laevis* gene expressed during early embryogenesis coding for a peptide region homologous to *Drosophila* homeotic genes, *Cell*, 37, 49, 1984.

550. Levine, M., Rubin, G.M., and Tjian, R., Human DNA sequences homologous to a protein coding region conserved between homeotic genes of *Drosophila*, *Cell*, 38, 667, 1984.

551. Breier, G., Bucan, M., Francke, U., Colberg-Poley, A.M., and Gruss, P., Sequential expression of murine homeo box genes during F9 EC cell differentiation, *EMBO J.*, 5, 2209, 1986.

552. Utset, M.F., Awgulewitsch, A., Ruddle, F.H., and McGinnis, W., Region-specific expression of two mouse homeo box genes, *Science*, 235, 1379, 1987.

553. Toth, L.E., Slawin, K.L., Pintar, J.E., and Nguyen-Huu, M.C., Region-specific expression of mouse homeobox genes in the embryonic mesoderm and central nervous system, *Proc. Natl. Acad. Sci. U.S.A.*, 84, 6790, 1987.

554. Wolgemuth, D.J., Viviano, C.M., Gizang-Ginsberg, E., Frohman, M.A., Joyner, A.L., and Martin G.R., Differential expression of the mouse homeobox-containing gene *Hox-1.4* during male germ cell differentiation and embryonic development, *Proc. Natl. Acad. Sci. U.S.A.*, 84, 5813, 1987.

555. Meijlink, F., de Laaf, R., Verrijzer, O., Kroezen, V., Hilkens, J., and Deschamps, J., A mouse homeobox containing gene on chromosome 11: sequence and tissue-specific expression, *Nucleic Acids Res.*, 15, 6773, 1987.

556. Verrijzer, P., de Graaff, W., Deschamps, J., and Meijlink, F., Nucleotide sequence of the Hox2.3 gene region, *Nucleic Acids Res.*, 16, 2729, 1988.

557. Bucan, M., Yang-Feng, T., Colberg-Poley, A.M., Wolgemuth, D.J., Guenet, J.L., Francke, U., and Lehrach, H., Genetic and cytogenetic localisation of the homeo box containing genes on mouse chromosome 6 and human chromosome 7, *EMBO J.*, 5, 2899, 1986.

558. Lonai, P., Arman, E., Czosnek, H., Ruddle, F.H., and Blatt, C., New murine homeoboxes: structure, chromosomal assignment, and differential expression in adult erythropoiesis, *DNA*, 6, 409, 1987.

559. Cannizzaro, L.A., Croce, C.M., Griffin, C.A., Simeone, A., Boncinelli, E., and Huebner, K., Human homeo box-containing genes located at chromosome regions 2q31-2q37 and 12q12-12q13, *Am. J. Hum. Genet.*, 41, 1, 1987.

560. Tsonis, P.A. and Adamson, E.D., Specific expression of homeobox-containing genes during induced differentiation of embryonal carcinoma cells, *Biochem. Biophys. Res. Commun.*, 137, 520, 1986.

561. Deschamps, J., de Laaf, R., Joosen, L., Meijlink, F., and Destrée, O., Abundant expression of homeobox genes in mouse embryonal carcinoma cells correlates with chemically induced differentiation, *Proc. Natl. Acad. Sci. U.S.A.*, 84, 1304, 1987.

562. Blau, H.M., Pavlath, G.K., Hardeman, E.C., Chiu, C-P., Silberstein, L., Webster, S. G., Miller, S.C., and Webster, C., Plasticity of the differentiated state, *Science*, 230, 758, 1985.

563. Clemens, M.J. and McNurlan, M.A., Regulation of cell proliferation and differentiation by interferon, *Biochem. J.*, 226, 345, 1985.

564. Bader, J.P., Virus-induced transformation without cell division, *Science*, 180, 1069, 1973.

565. Kasunaga, T., The role of cell division in the malignant transformation of mouse cells treated with 3-methylcholanthrene, *Cancer Res.*, 35, 1637, 1975.

566. Stampfer, M.R. and Bartley, J.C., Induction of transformation and continuous cell lines from normal human mammary epithelial cells after exposure to benzo(*a*)pyrene, *Proc. Natl. Acad. Sci. U.S.A.*, 82, 2394, 1985.

567. Nakano, S., Ueo, H., Bruce, S.A., and Ts'o, P.O.P., A contact-insensitive subpopulation in Syrian hamster cell cultures with a greater susceptibility to chemically induced neoplastic transformation, *Proc. Natl. Acad. Sci. U.S.A.,* 82, 5005, 1985.

568. Illmensee, K. and Mintz, B., Totipotency and normal differentiation of single teratocarcinoma cells cloned by injection into blastocysts, *Proc. Natl. Acad. Sci. U.S.A.,* 73, 549, 1976.

569. Hanaoka, K., Hayasaka, M., Noguchi, T., and Kato, Y., Viable chimeras between embryonal carcinoma cells and mouse embryos: comparison of aggregation and injection methods, *Dev. Growth Differ.,* 29, 263, 1987.

570. Pierce, G.B., Lewis, S.H., Miller, G.J., Moritz, E., and Miller, P., Tumorigenicity of embryonal carcinoma as an assay to study control of malignancy by the murine blastocyst, *Proc. Natl. Acad. Sci. U.S.A.,* 76, 6649, 1979.

571. Gootwine, E., Webb, C.G., and Sachs, L., Participation of myeloid leukaemic cells injected into embryos in haematopoietic differentiation in adult mice, *Nature,* 299, 63, 1982.

572. DiBerardino, M.A. and Hoffner, N.J., Gene reactivation in erythrocytes: nuclear transplantation in oocytes and eggs of *Rana, Science,* 219, 862, 1983.

573. Matioli, G., Friend leukemic mouse stem cell reversion to normal growth in irradiated hosts, *J. Reticuloendo-thel. Soc.,* 14, 380, 1973.

574. Diamandopoulos, G.T., Microenvironmental influences on the *in vivo* behavior of neoplastic lymphocytes. *Proc. Natl. Acad. Sci. U.S.A.,* 76, 6456, 1979.

575. Tveit, K.M. and Pihl, A., Do cell lines *in vitro* reflect the properties of the tumours of origin? — a study of lines derived from human melanoma xenografts, *Br. J. Cancer,* 44, 775, 1981.

576. Ossowski, L. and Reich, E., Changes in malignant phenotype of a human carcinoma conditioned by growth environment, *Cell,* 33, 323, 1983.

577. McKinnell, R.G., Deggins, B.A., and Labat, D.D., Transplantation of pluripotential nuclei from triploid frog tumors, *Science,* 16, 394, 1969.

578. Harris, H. and Watkins, J.F., Hybrid cells derived from mouse and man: artificial heterokaryons of mammalian cells from different species, *Nature,* 205, 640, 1965.

579. Harris, H., Cell fusion and the analysis of malignancy, *Proc. R. Soc. London,* B179, 1, 1971.

580. Stanbridge, E.J., Genetic analysis of tumorigenicity in human cell hybrids. *Cancer Surv.,* 3, 336, 1984.

581. Sager, R., Genetic suppression of tumor formation, Adv. *Cancer Res.,* 44, 43, 1985.

582. Sager, R., Genetic suppression of tumor formation: a new frontier in cancer research, *Cancer Res.,* 46, 1573, 1986.

583. Harris, H. and Bramwell, M.E., The suppression of malignancy by terminal differentiation: evidence from hybrids between tumour cells and keratinocytes, *J. Cell Sci.,* 87, 383, 1987.

584. Craig, R.W. and Sager, R., Suppression of tumorigenicity in hybrids of normal and oncogene-transformed CHEF cells, *Proc. Natl. Acad. Sci. U.S.A.,* 82, 2062, 1985.

585. Geiser, A.G., Der, C.J., Marshall, C.J., and Stanbridge, E.J., Suppression of tumorigenicity with continued expression of the c-Ha-*ras* oncogene in EJ bladder carcinoma-human fibroblast hybrid cells, *Proc. Natl. Acad. Sci. U.S.A.,* 83, 5209, 1986.

586. Griegel, S., Traub, O., Willecke, K., and Schäfer, R., Suppression and re-expression of transformed phenotype in hybrids of Ha-*ras*-1-transformed Rat-1 cells and early-passage rat embryonic fibroblasts, *Int. J. Cancer,* 38, 697, 1986.

587. Willecke, K., Griegel, S., Martin, W., Traub, O., and Schäfer, R., The Ha-*ras*-induced transformed phenotype of Rat-1 cells can be suppressed in hybrids with rat embryonic fibroblasts, *J. Cell. Biochem.,* 34, 23, 1987.

588. Schäfer, R., Suppression of the neoplastic phenotype and "anti-oncogenes", *Blut,* 54, 257, 1987.

589. Stoler, A. and Bouck, N., Identification of a single chromosome in the normal human genome essential for suppression of hamster cell transformation, *Proc. Natl. Acad. Sci. U.S.A.,* 82, 570, 1985.

590. Koi, M. and Barrett, J.C., Loss of tumor-suppressive function during chemically induced neoplastic progression of Syrian hamster embryo cells, *Proc. Natl. Acad. Sci. U.S.A.,* 83, 5992, 1986.

591. Chopan, M. and Kopelovich, L., The suppression of tumorigenicity in human x mouse cell hybrids. II. The relationship between tumorigenicity and parameters of transformation *in vitro, Exp. Cell Biol.,* 49, 132, 1981.

592. O'Hara, B.M., Klinger, H.P., Curran, T., Zhang, Y-D., and Blair, D.G., Levels of *fos, ets2,* and *myb* proto-oncogene RNAs correlate with segregation of chromosome 11 of normal cells and with suppression of tumorigenicity in human cell hybrids, *Mol. Cell. Biol.,* 7, 2941, 1987.

593. Howell, A.N. and Sager, R., Tumorigenicity and its suppression in cybrids of mouse and Chinese hamster cell lines, *Proc. Natl. Acad. Sci. U.S.A.,* 75, 2358, 1978.

594. Shay, J.W., Lorkowski, G., and Clark, M.A., Suppression of tumorigenicity in cybrids, *J. Supramol. Struct. Cell. Biochem.,* 16, 75, 1981.

595. Israel, B.A. and Schaeffer, W.I., Cytoplasmic suppression of malignancy, *In Vitro Cell. Dev. Biol.,* 23, 627, 1987.

596. Abken, H., Jungfer, H., Albert, W.H.W., and Willecke, K., Immortalization of human lymphocytes by fusion with cytoplasts of transformed mouse L cells, *J. Cell Biol.,* 103, 795, 1986.

597. Frost, P., Kerbel, R.S., Bauer, E., Tartamella-Biondo, R., and Cefalu, W., Mutagen treatment as a means for selecting immunogenic variants from otherwise poorly immunogenic malignant murine tumors, *Cancer Res.,* 43, 125, 1983.

598. Braun, A.C., *The Biology of Cancer,* Addison-Wesley, Reading, MA, 1974.
599. O'Hare, M.J., Teratomas, neoplasia and differentiation: a biological overview. I. The natural history of teratomas, *Invest. Cell Pathol.,* 1: 39, 1978.
600. Pierce, G.B., Neoplasms, differentiation and mutations, *Am. J. Pathol.,* 77, 103, 1974.
601. McGovern, V.J., Spontaneous regression of melanoma, *Pathology,* 7, 91, 1975.
602. Woodruff, M., Interaction of cancer and host, *Br. J. Cancer,* 46, 313, 1982.
603. Bolande, R.P., Spontaneous regression and cytodifferentiation of cancer in early life: the oncogenic grace period, *Surv. Synth. Pathol. Res.,* 4, 296, 1985.
604. Sanborn, G.E., Augsburger, J.J., and Shields, J.A., Spontaneous regression of bilateral retinoblastoma, *Br. J. Ophthalmol.,* 66, 685, 1982.
605. Migdal, C., Spontaneous regression of retinoblastoma in identical twins, *Br. J. Ophthalmol.,* 66, 691, 1982.
606. Gallie, B.L., Ellsworth, R.M., Abramson, D.H., and Phillips, R.A., Retinoma: spontaneous regression of retinoblastoma or benign manifestation of the mutation?, *Br. J. Cancer,* 45, 513, 1982.
607. Tsokos, M., Kyritsis, A.P., Chader, G.J., and Triche, T.J., Differentiation of human retinoblastoma *in vitro* into cell types with characteristics observed in embryonal or mature retina, *Am. J. Pathol.,* 123, 542, 1986.
608. Bogenmann, E., Retinoblastoma cell differentiation in culture, *Int. J. Cancer,* 38, 883, 1986.
609. Smadja, N., Krulik, M., Audebert, A.A., de Gramont, A., and Debray, J., Spontaneous regression of cytogenetic and haematologic anomalies in Ph[1]-positive chronic myelogenous leukaemia, *Br. J. Haematol.,* 63, 257, 1986.
610. Rice, J.M., Spontaneous regression of autochtonous malignant lymphomas induced in Swiss and NZW mice by 1-ethyl-1-nitrosourea, *Natl. Cancer Inst. Monogr.,* 35, 197, 1972.
611. Silva, R.F. and Moscovici, C., Spontaneous regression of leukemia in chickens infected with avian myeloblastosis virus, *Proc. Soc. Exp. Biol. Med.,* 143, 604, 1973.
612. Lam, K.C., Ho, J.C.I., and Yeung, R.T.T., Spontaneous regression of hepatocellular carcinoma: a case study, *Cancer,* 50, 332, 1982.
613. Jehn, U.W. and Mempel, M.A., Spontaneous remission of acute myeloid leukemia: a report of a case and brief review of the literature, *Blut,* 52, 165, 1986.
614. Rabinowitz, Z. and Sachs, L., Reversion of properties in cells transformed by polyoma virus, *Nature,* 220, 1203, 1968.
615. Aubert, C., Cultures de melanomes malins primitifs humains: mise en evidence d'un controle de la differenciation cellulaire *in vitro, C.R. Acad. Sci. Paris,* 280, 1641, 1975.
616. Kreider, J.W. and Schmoyer, M.E., Spontaneous maturation and differentiation of B16 melanoma cells in culture, *J. Natl. Cancer Inst.,* 55, 641, 1975.
617. Jakob, H., Buckingham, M.E., Cohen, A., Dupont L., Fiszman, M., and Jacob, F., A skeletal muscle cell line isolated from a mouse teratocarcinoma undergoes apparently normal terminal differentiation *in vitro, Exp. Cell Res.,* 114, 403, 1978.
618. Bogenmann, E. and Mark, C., Routine growth and differentiation of primary retinoblastoma cells in culture, *J. Natl. Cancer Inst.,* 70, 95, 1983.
619. Iland, H.J., Croaker, G.M., Repka, E., Radloff, T.J., and Vincent, P.C., Long-term bone marrow culture induces terminal differentiation of human myeloid leukemic cells, *Exp. Hematol.,* 15, 1109, 1987.
620. Deschatrette, J., Moore, E.E., Dubois, M., and Weiss, M.C., Dedifferentiated variants of a rat hepatoma: reversion analysis, *Cell,* 19, 1043, 1980.
621. Deschatrette, J., Dedifferentiated variants of a rat hepatoma: partial reversion induced by cell aggregation, *Cell,* 22, 501, 1980.
622. Koeffler, H.P., Induction of differentiation of human acute myelogenous leukemia cells: therapeutic implications, *Blood,* 62, 709, 1983.
623. Ross, D.W., Leukemic cell maturation, *Arch. Pathol. Lab. Med.,* 109, 309, 1985.
624. Sartorelli, A.C., Malignant cell differentiation as a potential therapeutic approach, *Br. J. Cancer,* 52, 293, 1985.
625. Tsiftsoglou, A.S. and Robinson, S.H., Differentiation of leukemic cell lines: a review focusing on murine erythroleukemia and human HL-60 cells, *Int. J. Cell Cloning,* 3, 349, 1985.
626. Niles, R.M., Chemical induction of tumor cell differentiation, *Surv. Synth. Pathol. Res.,* 4, 282, 1985.
627. Reiss, M., Gamba-Vitalo, C., and Sartorelli, A.C., Induction of tumor cell differentiation as a therapeutic approach: preclinical models for hematopoietic and solid neoplasms, *Cancer Treat. Rep.,* 70, 201, 1986.
628. Sachs, L., Cell differentiation and bypassing of genetic defects in the suppression of malignancy, *Cancer Res.,* 47, 1981, 1987.
629. Collins, S.J., The HL-60 promyelocytic leukemia cell line: proliferation, differentiation, and cellular oncogene expression, *Blood,* 70, 1233, 1987.
630. Leukemic cell maturation: phenotypic variability and oncogene expression in HL60 cells: a review, *Blood Cells,* 13, 319, 1988.
631. Sporn, M.B. and Roberts, A.B., Role of retinoids in differentiation and carcinogenesis, *Cancer Res.,* 43, 3034, 1983.
632. Pahlman, S., Ruusala, A.-I., Abrahamsson, L., Mattson, M.E.K., and Esscher, T., Retinoic acid-induced differentiation of cultured neuroblastoma cells: a comparison with phorbolester-induced differentiation, *Cell Different.,* 14, 135, 1984.

633. Kyritsis, A., Joseph, G., and Chader, G.J., Effects of butyrate, retinol, and retinoic acid on human Y-79 retinoblastoma cells growing in monolayer cultures, *J. Natl. Cancer Inst.,* 73, 649, 1984.

634. Williams, J.B. and Napoli, J.L., Metabolism of retinoic acid and retinol during differentiation of F9 embryonal carcinoma cells, *Proc. Natl. Acad. Sci. U.S.A.,* 82, 4658, 1985.

635. Levine, A.E., Crandall, C.A., Brattain, D., Chakrabarty, S., and Brattain, M.G., Retinoic acid restores normal growth control to a transformed mouse embryo fibroblastic cell line, *Cancer Lett.,* 33, 33, 1986.

636. Tanaka, H., Abe, E., Miyaura, C., Shiina, Y., and Suda, T., 1-α,25-Dihydroxyvitamin D_3 induces differentiation of human promyelocytic leukemia cells (HL-60) into monocyte-macrophages, but not into granulocytes, *Biochem. Biophys. Res. Commun.,* 117, 86, 1983.

637. Miyaura, C., Abe, E., Honma, Y., Hozumi, M., Nishii, Y., and Suda, T., Cooperative effect of 1-α,25-dihydroxyvitamin D_3 and dexamethasone in inducing differentiation of mouse myeloid leukemia cells, *Arch Biochem. Biophys.,* 227, 379, 1983.

638. Koeffler, H.P., Amatruda, T., Ikekawa, N., Kobayashi, Y., and DeLuca, H.F., Induction of macrophage differentiation of human normal and leukemic myeloid stem cells by 1,25-dihydroxyvitamin D_3 and its fluorinated analogues, *Cancer Res.,* 44, 5624, 1984.

639. Abe, J., Moriya, Y., Saito, M., Sugawara, Y., Suda, T., and Nishii, Y., Modulation of cell growth, differentiation, and production of interleukin-3 by 1a,25-dihydroxyvitamin D_3 in the murine myelomonocytic leukemia cell line WEHI-3, *Cancer Res.,* 46, 6316, 1986.

640. Preisler, H.D. and Giladi, M., Differentiation of erythroleukemic cells *in vitro* irreversible induction by dimethyl sulfoxide (DMSO), *J. Cell. Physiol.,* 85, 537, 1975.

641. Kimhi, Y., Palfrey, C., Spector, I., Barak, Y., and Littauer, U.Z., Maturation of neuroblastoma cells in the presence of dimethylsulfoxide, *Proc. Natl. Acad. Sci. U.S.A.,* 73, 462, 1976.

642. Collins, S.J., Ruscetti, F.W., Gallagher, R.E., and Gallo, R.C., Terminal differentiation of human promyelocytic leukemia cells induced by dimethyl sulfoxide and other polar compounds, *Proc. Natl. Acad. Sci. U.S.A.,* 75, 2458, 1978.

643. Darmon, M., Nicolas, J.-F., and Lamblin, D., 5-Azacytidine is able to induce the conversion of teratocarcinoma-derived mesenchymal cells into epithelial cells, *EMBO J.,* 3, 961, 1984.

644. Augeron, C. and Laboisse, C.L., Emergence of permanently differentiated cell clones in a human colonic cancer cell line in culture after treatment with sodium butyrate, *Cancer Res.,* 44, 3961, 1984.

645. Azuma, M., Hayashi, Y., Yoshida, H., Yanagawa, T., Yura, Y., Ueno, A., and Sato, M., Emergence of differentiated subclones from a human salivary adenocarcinoma cell clone in culture after treatment with sodium butyrate, *Cancer Res.,* 46, 770, 1986.

646. Giuffré, L., Schreyer, M., Mach, J.-P., and Carrel, S., Cyclic AMP induces differentiation *in vitro* of human melanoma cells, *Cancer,* 61, 1132, 1988.

647. Somers, K.D., Increased cyclic AMP content directly correlated with morphological transformation of cells infected with a temperature-sensitive mutant of mouse sarcoma virus, *In Vitro,* 16, 851, 1980.

648. Silagi, S., Reversible suppression of malignancy and differentiation of melanoma cells, *Am. J. Pathol.,* 89, 671, 1977.

649. Veigl, M.L., Sedwick, W.D., Niedel, J., and Branch, M.E., Induction of myeloid differentiation of HL-60 cells with naphthalene sulfonamide calmodulin antagonists, *Cancer Res.,* 46, 2300, 1986.

650. Aarbakke, J., Miura, G.A., Prytz, P.S., Bessesen, A., Slordal, L., Gordon, R.K., and Chiang, P.K., Induction of HL-60 cell differentiation by 3-deaza-($\pm$)-aristeromycin, an inhibitor of S-adenosylhomocysteine hydrolase, *Cancer Res.,* 46, 5469, 1986.

651. Pilz, R.B., Van den Berghe, G., and Boss, G.R., Adenosine dialdehyde and nitrous oxyde induce HL-60 differentiation, *Blood,* 70, 1161, 1987.

652. Fischkoff, S.A., Kishi, K., Benjamin, W.R., Rossi, R.M., Hoessly, M.C., Hoxie, J.A., Seals, C., Anderson, L., Ishizaka, T., and Hakimi, J., Induction of differentiation of the human leukemia cell line, KU812, *Leukemia Res.,* 11, 1105, 1987.

653. Vandenbark, G.R. and Niedel, J.E., Phorbol diesters and cellular differentiation, *J. Natl. Cancer Inst.,* 73, 1013, 1984.

654. Jenis, D.M., Keyes, S.R., and Sartorelli, A.C., Induction of the differentiation of HL-60 promyelocytic leukemia cells by palmitoleic and myristoleic acids, *Leukemia Res.,* 11, 935, 1987.

655. Lage-Davila, A., Krust, B., Hoffmann-Clercq, F., Torpier, G., and Montagnier, L., Bromodeoxyuridine-induced reversion of transformed characteristics in BHK21 cells: changes at the plasma membrane level, *J. Cell. Physiol.,* 100, 95, 1979.

656. Boffa, L.C., Vidali, G., Mann, R.S., and Allfrey, V.G., Suppression of histone deacetylation *in vivo* and *in vitro* by sodium butyrate, *J. Biol. Chem.,* 253, 3364, 1978.

657. Chou, R.H. and Chervenick, P.A., Combined effects of aphidicolin and retinoic acid on proliferation and differentiation of human leukaemic (HL-60) cells, *Cell Tissue Kinet.,* 18, 387, 1985.

658. Zaricznyj, C. and Macara, I.G., Lithium inhibits terminal differentiation of erythroleukemia cells: evidence for a pre-commitment "priming" event, *Exp. Cell Res.,* 168, 402, 1987.

659. Foresti, M., Gaudio, L., Geraci, G., and Manduca, P., Inhibition of dimethyl sulfoxide induced erythropoietic differentiation of murine erythroleukemia cells in culture, *Cancer Res.,* 46, 6260, 1986.

660. Amtmann, E., Müller, K., Knapp, A., and Sauer, G., Reversion of bovine papillomavirus-induced transformation and immortalization by a xanthate compound, *Exp. Cell Res.,* 161, 541, 1985.

661. Resch, K., Martin, M., Lovett, D.H., Kyas, U., and Gemsa, D., The receptor for interleukin 1 in plasma membranes of the human leukemia cell K562: biological and biochemical characterization, *Immunobiology,* 172, 336, 1986.

662. Glazer, R.I., Chapekar, M.S., Hartman, K.D., and Knode, M.C., Appearance of membrane-bound tyrosine kinase during differentiation of HL-60 leukemia cells by immune interferon and tumor necrosis factor, *Biochem. Biophys. Res. Commun.,* 140, 908, 1986.

663. Michalevicz, R. and Revel, M., Interferons regulate the *in vitro* differentiation of multilineage lympho-myeloid stem cells in hairy cell leukemia, *Proc. Natl. Acad. Sci. U.S.A.,* 84, 2307, 1987.

664. Trinchieri, G., Rosen, M., and Perussia, B., Induction of differentiation of human myeloid cell lines by tumor necrosis factor in cooperation with 1 α,25-dihydroxyvitamin D_3, *Cancer Res.,* 47, 2236, 1987.

665. Lyons, A.B. and Ashman, L.K., Studies on the differentiation of the human myelomonocytic cell line RC-2A in response to lymphocyte-derived factors, *Leukemia Res.,* 11, 797, 1987.

666. Lotem, J., Shabo, Y., and Sachs, L., Role of different normal hematopoietic regulatory proteins in the differentiation of myeloid leukemic cells, *Int. J. Cancer,* 41, 101, 1988.

667. Trinchieri, G., Rosen, M., and Perussia, B., Retinoic acid cooperates with tumor necrosis factor and immune interferon in inducing differentiation and growth inhibition of the human promyelocytic leukemic cell line HL-60, *Blood,* 69, 1218, 1987.

668. Lin, J. and Sartorelli, A.C., Stimulation by interferon of the differentiation of human promyelocytic leukemia (HL-60) cells produced by retinoic acid and actinomycin D, *J. Interferon Res.,* 7, 379, 1987.

669. Rasheed, S., Role of endogenous cat retrovirus in cell differentiation, *Proc. Natl. Acad. Sci. U.S.A.,* 79, 7371, 1982.

670. Müller, R. and Wagner, E.F., Differentiation of F9 teratocarcinoma stem cells after transfer of c-*fos* proto-oncogenes, *Nature,* 311, 438, 1984.

671. Montano, X. and Lane, D.P., The adenovirus E1a gene induces differentiation of F9 teratocarcinoma cells, *Mol. Cell. Biol.,* 7, 1782, 1987.

672. Müller, R., Müller, D., and Guilbert, L., Differential expression of c-*fos* in hematopoietic cells: correlation with differentiation of monomyelocytic cells *in vitro*, *EMBO J.,* 3, 1887, 1984.

673. Murtaugh, M.P., Dennison, O., Stein, J.P., and Davies, P.J.A., Retinoic acid-induced gene expression in normal and leukemic myeloid cells, *J. Exp. Med.,* 163, 1325, 1986.

674. Kos, Z., Pavelic, L., Pekic, B., and Pavelic, K., Reversal of human myeloid leukemia cells into normal granulocytes and macrophages: activity and intracellular distribution of catalase, *Oncology,* 44, 245, 1987.

675. Mita, S., Nakaki, T., Yamamoto, S., and Kato, R., Phosphorylation and dephosphorylation of human promyelocytic leukemia cell (HL-60) proteins by tumor promoter, *Exp. Cell Res.,* 154, 492, 1984.

676. Cooper, R.A., Braunwald, A.D., and Kuo, A.L., Phorbol ester induction of leukemic cell differentiation is a membrane-mediated process, *Proc. Natl. Acad. Sci. U.S.A.,* 79, 2865, 1982.

677. Prasad, K.N., Sahu, S.K., and Sinha, P.K., Cyclic nucleotides in the regulation of expression of differentiated functions in neuroblastoma cells, *J. Natl. Cancer Inst.,* 57, 619, 1976.

678. Thiele, C.J., Reynolds, C.P., and Israel, M.A., Decreased expression of N-*myc* precedes retinoic acid-induced morphological differentiation of human neuroblastoma, *Nature,* 313, 404, 1985.

679. Djulbegovic, B., Christmas, S.E., and Moore, M., Differentiated HL-60 promyelocytic leukaemia cells produce a factor inducing differentiation, *Leukemia Res.,* 11, 259, 1987.

680. Kurata, N., Sawada, M., Ito, Y., and Marunouchi, T., A factor inducing differentiation of the human monocytic cell line U-937 produced by 12-*O*-tetradecanoylphorbol 13-acetate-treated U-937, *Jpn. J. Cancer Res.,* 78, 219, 1987.

681. Sachs, L., Control of growth and normal differentiation in leukemic cells: regulation of the developmental program and restoration of the normal phenotype in myeloid leukemia, *J. Cell. Physiol.,* Suppl. 1, 151, 1982.

682. Sachs, L., The molecular regulators of normal and leukaemic blood cells, *Proc. R. Soc. London,* B231, 289, 1987.

683. Sachs, L., The molecular control of blood cell development, *Science,* 238, 1374, 1987.

684. Tomida, M., Yamamoto-Yamaguchi, Y., and Hozumi, M., Purification of a factor inducing differentiation of mouse myeloid leukemic M1 cells from conditioned medium of mouse fibroblast L929 cells, *J. Biol. Chem.,* 259, 10978, 1984.

685. Gullberg, U., Nilsson, E., Sarngadharan, M.G., and Olsson, I., T lymphocyte-derived differentiation-inducing factor inhibits proliferation of leukemic and normal hemopoietic cells, *Blood,* 68, 1333, 1986.

686. Takeda, K., Iwamoto, S., Sugimoto, H., Takuma, T., Kawatani, N., Noda, M., Masaki, A., Morise, H., Arimura, H., and Konno, K., Identity of differentiation inducing factor and tumour necrosis factor, *Nature,* 323, 338, 1986.

687. Takuma, T., Takeda, K., and Konno, K., Synergism of tumor necrosis factor and interferon-gamma in induction of differentiation of human myeloblastic leukemic ML-1 cells, *Biochem. Biophys. Res. Commun.*, 145, 514, 1987.

688. Ikeda, K., Motoyoshi, K., Ishizaka, Y., Hatake, K., Kajigaya, S., Saito, M., and Miura, Y., Human colony-stimulating activity-producing tumor: production of very low mouse-active colony-stimulating activity and induction of marked granulocytosis in mice, *Cancer Res.*, 45, 4144, 1985.

689. Hanamura, T., Motoyoshi, K., Hatake, K., Miura, Y., and Saito, M., Human colony-stimulating factor-producing lung cancer tissue releases a differentiation-inducing factor for human leukemic cells, *Leukemia*, 1, 497, 1987.

690. Souza, M., Boone, T.C., Gabrilove, J., Lai, P.H., Zsebo, K.M., Murdock, D.C., Chazin, V.R., Bruszewski, J., Lu, H., Chen, K.K., Barendt, J., Platzer, E., Moore, M.A.S., Mertelsmann, R., and Welte, K., Recombinant human granulocyte colony-stimulating factor: effects on normal and leukemic myeloid cells, *Science*, 232, 61, 1986.

691. Tomida, M., Yamamoto-Yamaguchi, Y., Hozumi, M., Okabe, T., and Takaku, F., Induction by recombinant human granulocyte colony-stimulating factor of differentiation of mouse myeloid leukemic M1 cells, *FEBS Lett.*, 207, 271, 1986.

692. Weinberg, J.B. and Misukonis, M.A., Comparison of *in vitro* and *in vivo* differentiation of myeloblastic leukemia of the RFM/Un mouse, *Cancer Res.*, 44, 5594, 1984.

693. Lotem, J. and Sachs, L., *In vivo* control of differentiation of myeloid leukemic cells by recombinant granulocyte-macrophage colony-stimulating factor and interleukin 3, *Blood*, 71, 375, 1988.

694. Ogita, S., Tokiwa, K., Arizono, N., and Takahashi, T., Neuroblastoma: incomplete differentiation of the way to maturation or morphological alteration resembling maturity?, *Oncology*, 45, 148, 1988.

695. Abrahm, J., Besa, E.C., Hyzinski, M., Finan, J., and Nowell, P., Disappearance of cytogenetic abnormalities and clinical remission during therapy with 13-*cis*-retinoic acid in a patient with myelodysplastic syndrome: inhibition of growth of the patient's malignant monocytoid clone, *Blood*, 67, 1323, 1986.

696. Bennett, D.C., Dexter, T.J., Ormerod, E.J., and Hart, I.R., Increased experimental metastatic capacity of a murine melanoma following induction of differentiation, *Cancer Res.*, 46, 3239, 1986.

697. Kulesz-Martin, M., Blumenson, L., and Lisafeld, B., Retinoic acid enhancement of an early step in the transformation of mouse epidermal cells *in vitro*, *Carcinogenesis*, 7, 1425, 1986.

698. Hosoi, J., Abe, E., Suda, T., Colburn, N.H., and Kuroki, T., Induction of anchorage-independent growth of JB6 mouse epidermal cells by 1 α,25-dihydroxyvitamin D_3, Cancer Res., 46, 5582, 1986.

699. Poland, A. and Glover, E., An estimate of the maximum *in vivo* covalent binding of 2,3,7,8,tetrachlorodibenzo-*p*-dioxin to rat liver protein, ribosomal RNA, and DNA, *Cancer Res.*, 39, 3341, 1979.

700. Barrett, J.C., Wong, A., and McLachlan, J.A., Diethylstilbestrol induces neoplastic transformation without measurable gene mutation at two loci, *Science*, 212, 1402, 1981.

701. Tsutsui, T., Maizumi, H., McLachlan, J.A., and Barrett, J.C., Aneuploidy induction and cell transformation by diethylstilbestrol: a possible chromosomal mechanism in carcinogenesis, *Cancer Res.*, 43, 3814, 1983.

702. Sandberg, A.A., Some comments on sister chromatid exchange (SCE) in human neoplasia, *Cancer Genet. Cytogenet.*, 1, 197, 1980.

703. Kennedy, A.R., Fox, M., Murphy, G., and Little, J.B., Relationship between x-ray exposure and malignant transformation in C3H 10T1/2 cells, *Proc. Natl. Acad. Sci. U.S.A.*, 77, 7262, 1980.

704. Little, J.B., Cellular mechanisms of oncogenic transformation *in vitro*, in *Transformation Assay of Established Cell Lines*, Kakunaga, T. and Yamasaki, H., Eds., International Agency for Research on Cancer, Lyon, France, 1985, 9.

705. Yavelow, J., Collins, M., Birk, Y., Troll, W., and Kennedy, A.R., Nanomolar concentrations of Bowman-Birk soybean protease inhibitor suppress x-ray-induced transformation *in vitro*, *Proc. Natl. Acad. Sci. U.S.A.*, 82, 5395, 1985.

706. Billings, P.C., Clair, W.S., Ryan, C.A., and Kennedy, A.R., Inhibition of radition-induced transformation of C3H/10T1/2 cells by chymotrypsin inhibitor 1 from potatoes, *Carcinogenesis*, 8, 809, 1987.

707. Sakiyama, H., Yasukawa, M., Terasima, T., and Kanegasaki, S., Inhibition of X-ray or chemical carcinogen-induced neoplastic transformation of C3H10T1/2 fibroblasts by lipopolysaccharides, *Cancer Res.*, 46, 3862, 1986.

708. Mulcahy, R.T., Gould, M.N., and Clifton, K.H., Radiation initiation of thyroid cancer: a common cellular event, *Int. J. Radiat. Biol.*, 45, 417, 1984.

709. Clifton, K.H., Tanner, M.A., and Gould, M.N., Assessment of radiogenic cancer initiation frequency per clonogenic rat mammary cell *in vivo*, *Cancer Res.*, 46, 2390, 1986.

710. Elkind, M.M., Hill, C.K., and Han, A., Repair and misrepair in radiation-induced neoplastic transformation, in *Carcinogenesis*, Vol. 10, Huberman, E. and Barr, S.H., Eds., Raven Press, New York, 1985, 317.

711. Borek, C., Ong, A., and Mason, H., Distinctive transforming genes in x-ray-transformed mammalian cells, *Proc. Natl. Acad. Sci. U.S.A.*, 84, 794, 1987.

712. Mole, R.H., Radiation-induced acute myeloid leukemia in the mouse: experimental observations *in vivo* with implications for hypothesis about the basis of carcinogenesis, *Leukemia Res.,* 10, 859, 1986.

713. Bouchard, L., Vass-Marengo, J., and Bastin, M., Expression of the malignant phenotype in rat fibroblasts transfected with the polyomavirus transforming genes, *Virology,* 155, 1986.

714. Guernsey, D.L., Borek, C., and Edelman, I.S., Crucial role of thyroid hormone in x-ray-induced neoplastic transformation in cell culture, *Proc. Natl. Acad. Sci. U.S.A.,* 78, 5708, 1981.

715. Fisher, P.B., Guernsey, D.L., Weinstein, I.B., and Edelman, I.S., Modulation of adenovirus transformation by thyroid hormone, *Proc. Natl. Acad. Sci. U.S.A.,* 80, 196, 1983.

716. Babiss, L.E., Guernsey, D.L., and Fisher, P.B., Regulation of anchorage-independent growth by thyroid hormone in type 5 adenovirus-transformed rat embryo cells, *Cancer Res.,* 45, 6017, 1985.

717. Borek, C., Guernsey, D.L., Ong, A., and Edelman, I.S., Critical role played by thyroid hormone in induction of neoplastic transformation by chemical carcinogens in tissue culture, *Proc. Natl. Acad. Sci. U.S.A.,* 80, 5749, 1983.

718. Borek, C., Ong, A., and Rhim, J.S., Thyroid hormone modulation of transformation induced by Kirsten murine sarcoma virus, *Cancer Res.,* 45, 1985.

719. Leuthauser, S.W.C. and Guernsey, D.L., Thyroid hormone affects the expression of neoplastic transformation induced by DNA-transfection, *Cancer Lett.,* 35, 321, 1987.

720. Hinkle, P.M. and Kinsella, P.A., Thyroid hormone induction of an autocrine growth factor secreted by pituitary tumor cells, *Science,* 234, 1549, 1986.

721. Guernsey, D.L. and Leuthauser, S.W.C., Correlation of thyroid hormone dose-dependent regulation of K-*ras* proto-oncogene expression with oncogene activation by 3-methylcholanthrene: loss of thyroidal regulation in the transformed mouse cell, *Cancer Res.,* 47, 3052, 1987.

722. Sap, J., Muñoz, A., Damm, K., Goldberg, Y., Ghysdael, J., Leutz, A., Beug, H., and Vennström, B., The c-*erb*-A protein is a high-affinity receptor for thyroid hormone, *Nature,* 324, 635, 1986.

723. Weinberger, C., Thompson, C.C., Ong, E.S., Lebo, R., Gruol, D.J., and Evans, R.M., The c-*erb*-A gene encodes a thyroid hormone receptor, *Nature,* 324, 641, 1986.

Chapter 2

ACUTE RETROVIRUSES

I. INTRODUCTION

The possible role of viruses in the etiology of malignant diseases is currently a subject of high controversy. Both RNA and DNA viruses have been suspected as possible causal factors of cancer in different animal species, including humans.[1-4] Exogenous viruses with oncogenic potential are retroviruses, which are characterized by an RNA genome and the presence of a gene encoding the RNA-dependent DNA polymerase, reverse transcriptase. Retroviruses may be associated with a diversity of diseases in human and nonhuman vertebrate species, including immunologic, inflammatory, and neoplastic diseases.[5] However, most frequently retroviruses are nonpathogenic and may rather be involved in certain normal developmental processes. In the last years, retroviral vectors have become extremely useful in biotechnology as instruments for mediating gene transfer into higher eukaryotic cells.[6]

Retroviruses have been classified into three families: oncovirinae, spumavirinae, and lentivirinae. The viruses from the first of these families, also called oncoviruses, have been subgrouped, mainly on the basis of morphological criteria according to electron microscopic studies, into A-, B-, C-, and D-type oncoviruses.[7-9] According to their biological properties, exogenous retroviruses with oncogenic potential are classified in two groups: acutely transforming retroviruses (acute retroviruses), which are highly and directly oncogenic viruses, and nonacute, slow, or chronic retroviruses, which have a weaker oncogenic potential and would transform cells only through indirect mechanisms (Table 1). In addition, since the genome of most, if not all, vertebrate species contains endogenous retroviruses, the possible role of these integrated viruses (endogenous proviruses) in the origin and/or development of malignant diseases should also be considered.

II. GENERAL CHARACTERISTICS OF ACUTE RETROVIRUSES

The possible role of viruses in the etiology of cancer was suggested for the first time at the beginning of this century by work on avian leukemia.[10] A few years later it was observed that sarcomas in chickens can be transmitted by injection of cell-free extracts of these tumors.[11] The agent responsible for this experimental transmission of a tumor was recognized to be a virus, the Rous sarcoma virus (RSV), which is capable of inducing the acute neoplastic transformation of susceptible cells either *in vivo* or *in vitro*.[12,13] RSV represents a prototype of retroviruses with defined potential for inducing the rapid malignant transformation of susceptible cells.

Acutely transforming, highly oncogenic retroviruses, also called in an abbreviated manner "acute retroviruses", are defective, replication-incompetent viruses resulting from recombinational events that occurred between nondefective, replication-competent type C retroviruses and cellular DNA sequences called protooncogenes. Acute retroviruses have been isolated from tumors occurring in different animal species but they are not infectious agents involved in the natural transmission of diseases from one animal to another. Since viruses are generally considered as agents with an infectious potential under natural conditions, the use of the term virus for designating these isolates is not totally appropriate but has become common. One of these viruses, the Harvey murine sarcoma virus (H-MuSV), was isolated from solid tumors that developed in rats previously injected with a chronic transforming mouse ecotropic retrovirus, the Moloney murine leukemia virus (M-MuLV).[14] Presumably, this virus picked up genetic information from the rat cells in which M-MuLV had been propagated. A closely related acute retrovirus isolated thereafter by a similar procedure was called Kirsten murine sarcoma virus (K-

TABLE 1
Characteristics of Chronic and Acute Retroviruses

	Chronic	Acute
Latency period for disease induction	Long	Short
Transformation of cells *in vitro*	No	Yes
Structure of the genome	Complete	Defective
Presence of oncogenes	No	Yes

MuSV).[15] An acute retrovirus, the Rasheed rat sarcoma virus, was isolated by *in vitro* cocultivation of rat cultured cells producing an endogenous rat retrovirus with chemically transformed rat tumor cells.[16] Another acute retrovirus, the Abelson murine leukemia virus (A-MuLV), arose in a steroid-treated mouse infected with M-MuLV,[17] probably as a consequence of recombination of MuLV with cellular sequences.

In contrast to chronic retroviruses, the genome of acute retroviruses is characterized by the presence of different structural defects and, with few exceptions (some strains of RSV), these viruses cannot replicate without the aid of "helper viruses" that supply the defective functions. A-MuLV, for example, is replication-defective but contains in its genome all the information required for transformation of susceptible cells such as bone marrow cells *in vitro* or for tumor induction *in vivo* in susceptible animals such as weanling BALB/c mice.[18] Helper M-MuLV is not necessary for A-MuLV-induced transformation. In general, acute retroviruses do not require replication for expressing their transformation capabilities.

The ability of acute retroviruses to induce in a relatively rapid manner the malignant transformation of cells is not due to intrinsic viral sequences. The structural defects occurring in the genomes of acute retroviruses are related to the acquisition of specific cellular sequences called cellular oncogenes, c-*onc* genes, or protooncogenes. Upon their acquisition by retroviral genomes, these sequences are called viral oncogenes, v-*onc* genes, or true oncogenes. The acquired viral sequences code for proteins (oncoproteins) that are responsible for the initiation and/or maintenance of malignant transformation induced by the transducing virus in susceptible cells.[19-28] Cloned viral oncogenes are capable of inducing foci of transformed cells *in vitro* and their injection into susceptible animals *in vivo* may result in the formation of malignant tumors. Transfection of mouse fibroblasts *in vitro* with cloned oncogenes may result in their conversion into cells with metastatic capability.[29] After deletion of the oncogene sequences, acute retroviruses are not able to acutely transform cultured cells *in vitro* or to induce the rapid appearance of malignant tumors *in vivo*. Thus, all the available evidence indicates that nucleotide sequences derived from the cellular counterparts of viral oncogenes, i.e., from the protooncogenes, are responsible for the neoplastic transformation induced by acute retroviruses. A list of some of the best characterized acute retroviruses with their species of origin and the respective oncogenes, which are indicated by symbols usually composed of three letters, appears in Table 2.

A. STRUCTURE OF ACUTE RETROVIRUSES

Acute retroviruses are replication defective, noninfectious viruses due to the presence of different types of genomic deletions in the structural genes (*gag*, *pol*, and *env*) of the chronic retrovirus from which they are derived. Viral oncogene sequences substitute for the deleted parts of the viral genome and are fused in different combinations to the 3' side of the remaining portion of the viral genome. Long terminal repeats (LTRs) are situated at both ends of the integrated proviral genome, flanked by cellular DNA sequences corresponding to the site of viral integration in a host cell chromosome. The general structure of acute and chronic retroviruses is indicated in Figure 1.

TABLE 2
Acute Transforming Retroviruses and Their
Respective Oncogenes

Oncogene	Isolate origin	Prototype virus strain
abl	Rodent (mouse)	Abelson murine leukemia virus
crk	Avian (chicken)	Avian sarcoma virus CT10
erb-A	Avian (chicken)	Avian erythroblastosis virus
erb-B	Avian (chicken)	Avian erythroblastosis virus
ets	Avian (chicken)	Avian leukemia virus E26
fes/fps	Feline (cat)	Snyder-Theilen feline sarcoma virus
fgr	Feline (cat)	Gardner-Rasheed feline sarcoma virus
fms	Feline (cat)	McDonough feline sarcoma virus
fos	Rodent (mouse)	FBJ murine osteosarcoma virus
jun	Avian (chicken)	ASV-17 avian sarcoma virus
Kit	Feline (cat)	Hardy-Zuckerman 4 feline sarcoma virus
mht/mil	Avian (chicken)	Mill Hill 2 avian carcinoma virus
mos	Rodent (mouse)	Moloney murine sarcoma virus
myb	Avian (chicken)	Avian myeloblastosis virus
myc	Avian (chicken)	MC29 avian myelocytomatosis virus
raf	Rodent (mouse)	3611 murine sarcoma virus
H-*ras*	Rodent (rat)	Harvey murine sarcoma virus
K-*ras*	Rodent (rat)	Kirsten murine sarcoma virus
rel	Avian (turkey)	Avian reticuloendotheliosis virus
ros	Avian (turkey)	Rochester URII avian sarcoma virus
sis	Primate (monkey)	Simian sarcoma virus
ski	Avian (chicken)	SKV 770 avian virus
src	Avian (chicken)	Rous sarcoma virus
yes	Avian (chicken)	Y73 Avian sarcoma virus

1. Origin of Viral Oncogenes

Viral oncogenes are derived by genetic recombination between retroviruses and specific cellular DNA sequences, the protooncogenes. Two different recombinational events may be required for the transduction of protooncogene sequences by an acute retrovirus.[30] The first event would occur between the genome of an integrated provirus and specific cellular protooncogene sequences, and the second event would take place between a hybrid RNA molecule transcribed from the product of the first recombination and the RNA genome of a chronic retrovirus. It can be assumed that such a combination of events occur with a very low frequency. Moreover, since acute retroviruses are not integrated as proviruses into the germ line, but are found only in rare natural or experimental tumors, and, since acute retroviruses are not infectious agents under natural conditions and the acquisition of protooncogene-derived sequences does not represent any advantage for the survival of the retrovirus, it can be deduced that the survival of acute retroviruses depends only on their maintenance in laboratories.[31]

2. Structure of Viral Oncogenes

The genome organization and complete nucleotide sequences of several acute retroviral genomes, or the sequences of their transforming genes, have been determined, including the sequences of M-MuSV,[32-34] simian sarcoma virus (SSV),[35,36] avian sarcoma virus (ASV) Y73,[37] avian myeloblastosis virus (AMV),[38] H-MuSV and K-MuSV,[39,40] RSV,[41,42] avian myelocytomatosis virus (AMCV) MC29,[43] avian reticuloendotheliosis virus (REV),[44] Rasheed rat sarcoma virus,[45] avian erythroblastosis virus (AEV),[46,47] m1 MuSV,[48] ASV PRCII,[49] MuSV 3611,[50] avian carcinoma virus MH2,[51-53] ASV UR2,[54] and BALB/c MuSV.[55]

Almost all of the protooncogene sequences transduced by acute retroviruses have undergone

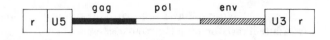

GENOME OF A CHRONIC RETROVIRUS

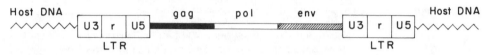

PROVIRUS OF A CHRONIC RETROVIRUS

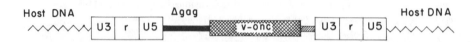

ACUTE TRANSFORMING RETROVIRAL PROVIRUS

FIGURE 1. Schematic representation of the general structure of chronic and acute retroviral genomes.

extensive deletions in their amino- and/or carboxy-terminal regions during recombination with the helper virus.[55] For example, in M-MuSV and SSV the amino-terminal regions of c-*mos* and c-*sis* protooncogene sequences, respectively, have been replaced by *env*-derived sequences. In MC29 AMCV and A-MuLV genomes, 5′ terminal sequences of the c-*myc* and c-*abl* protooncogenes, respectively, have been replaced by *gag* gene sequences. With AMV and the Finkel-Biskis-Jenkins strain of MuSV (FBJ MuSV), the carboxy-terminal regions of the c-*myb* and c-*fos* protooncogenes, respectively, have been replaced by sequences derived from the helper virus. The v-*mil* oncogene transduced by the MH2 acute avian retrovirus is a truncated version of the c-*mil* protooncogene contained in the chicken genome, lacking the 5′ coding region that specifies the amino-terminal portion of the cellular protein.[56] One exception to general rule is represented by the *ras* oncogene family, in which the entire coding region of the respective protooncogenes can be incorporated in the transducing retroviruses.

The oncogenic potential of some acute retroviruses may depend not exclusively on v-*onc* sequences of cellular origin contained within the respective oncogene but also on oncogenic determinants from the parental chronic retrovirus genome. For example, sequence analysis of K-MuSV reveals recombinational regions representing potential leukemogenic determinants on the parental MuLV genome.[57] Moreover, chronic retroviruses that are replication-defective as a consequence of structural changes that occurred during passage *in vivo* may display acute transforming capability without the acquisition of v-*onc* sequences of cellular origin. For example, the myeloproliferative leukemia virus (MPLV) is an acute leukemogenic virus that was generated during *in vivo* passage of F-MuLV.[58] Comparison of the physical maps of MPLV and F-MuLV indicates that MPLV derived from F-MuLV with conservation of the *gag* and *pol* regions but that the *env* region was deleted and rearranged.

Acute retroviruses inserted in the host cell genome contain at both the 5′ and 3′ ends LTRs that enable the proviruses to exploit the transcriptional apparatus of the host cells in a *cis*-acting fashion. The transcriptional control signals within the LTRs of acute retroviruses such as M-MuSV are composed of several physically separated elements containing distinct nucleotide sequences.[59] Such elements may display promoter or enhancer activities and may exhibit different functions in different types of cells.

B. TRANSDUCTION OF ONCOGENE SEQUENCES

The molecular mechanisms by which protooncogene sequences are captured by nonacute retroviruses, giving origin to acute, highly oncogenic retroviruses, are largely unknown. It has been suggested that nucleotide sequence homologies between limited regions of the protoonco-gene and structural genes of chronic transforming retroviruses may facilitate the events required for transduction or that, alternatively, recombination could proceed via RNA splicing proc-esses.[60] A multistep model for oncogene transduction that has received general acceptance include the following sequential steps: (1) proviral integration within or upstream of a protooncogene in the same transcriptional orientation; (2) deletion of the 3' proviral DNA including the 3' LTR, thereby fusing the protooncogene to the viral transcriptional unit; (3) transcription from the 5' LTR promoter to generate a fusion transcript encompassing both proviral and protooncogene sequences; (4) packaging of the chimeric (hybrid) transcripts and wild-type viral genomes as heterodimers into virus particles; and (5) template switching by reverse transcriptase between the heterodimers during viral DNA synthesis, thereby restoring 3' viral sequences to the chimeric molecule.[61] The overall consequences of this process are the incorporation of the protooncogene sequences into the internal portion or the retrovirus genome and the retention of the terminal *cis*-acting viral elements essential for replication. The second recombination event in the generation of an acute retrovirus appears to occur at the RNA level and would be facilitated by homologous sequences.

1. Dual Transduction of Oncogenes

Usually, only one oncogene is contained in the genome of each acute retrovirus but some of these viruses may contain two oncogenes. For example, AEV contains the oncogenes *erb*-A and *erb*-B,[62-66] E26 AMCV contains the oncogenes *myb* and *ets*,[67] and the avian retrovirus MH2 contains the oncogenes *mht/mil* and *myc*.[68-71] The oncogene v-*mht* of the MH2 virus contains at the 3' end sequences related to the v-*raf* oncogene of MuSV 3611 but the v-*mht*-specific sequences are derived from the same protooncogene as the v-*raf* sequences, i.e., they are derived from a c-*mht/raf* protooncogene contained in the chicken genome.[72]

Although AEV and MH2 are generally considered as viruses transducing two oncogenes, both viruses can transform fibroblasts with only one of two potential transforming genes, namely, *gag-erb*-B and *gag-myc*, respectively.[73] It has thus been postulated that these retro-viruses cannot be considered as a model for two-gene oncogenesis, in which two oncogenes must cooperate for transforming function. A spontaneous deletion mutant of MH2, the PA200-MH2 virus, transduces only the v-*mil* oncogene.[74] The PA220-MH2 virus is capable of inducing morphological transformation of CEF cells in culture but, in contrast to MH2, it is inefficient in inducing colonies in semisolid medium and is totally unable to induce wing tumors by inoculation into young birds. Mutant MH2 viruses carrying only the v-*mil* oncogene are able to induce proliferation in cultures of chicken embryo neuroretina cells, but do not induce neoplastic transformation of these cells.[75]

Mutants of the MH2 virus may lack either the v-*mil* or the v-*myc* oncogene.[76,77] MH2 retroviruses lacking a functional v-*mil* oncogene have a reduced oncogenic potential, being unable to induce myeloid neoplasms *in vivo*, although they are capable of inducing kidney tumors.[78] Whereas v-*myc* induces chick macrophages to proliferate in the presence of an appropriate growth factor (the chicken myelomonocytic growth factor) and is necessary for maintenance of a transformed phenotype in macrophages, v-*mil* induces autocrine growth by triggering the production of the growth factor.[79] Thus, v-*mil* may cooperate with v-*myc* at the functional level and may contribute to the specific development of myelomonocytic neoplasms induced by the MH2 virus. MH2 viruses expressing only the v-*myc* oncogene fail to induce any detectable change in neuroretina cells. The results of these studies indicate that expression of v-*myc* in addition to v-*mil* is necessary to induce complete transformation of MH2-infected chicken neuroretina cells.[80] The mechanisms involved in the cooperation between the two oncogenes, v-*myc* and v-*mil*, are unknown.

The mechanisms involved in dual transduction of nonlinked protooncogenes are not understood. The protooncogene sequences transduced in a dual form by a single acute retrovirus are dispersed among different chromosomes in almost every animal species examined.[81,82] The protooncogenes c-*erb*-A and c-*erb*-B are located on different human and chicken chromosomes but in the mouse these oncogenes are syntenic, being located on chromosome 11.[83] However, although linked, the physical distance between c-*erb*-A and c-*erb*-B in mouse is apparently significant since two somatic hybrid cell lines carrying a portion of mouse chromosome 11 that were positive of c-*erb*-A were negative for c-*erb*-B.[83] At least three different mechanisms should be considered as possible in relation to dual oncogene transduction by retroviruses: (1) chromosome translocation in the original tumor cells prior to transduction by the retroviral vector, (2) existence of a precursor virus containing only one of the two oncogenes and recombination for a second time with the cellular genome, and (3) recombination of two retroviruses transducing each one a single oncogene.

Oncogenes transduced in a dual form by some retroviruses may be contained in single form by variants of the same viruses. For example, the oncogenes v-*erb*-A and v-*erb*-B are not always carried together by acute retroviruses. The AEV-H variant has the genomic structure 5′-*gag-pol-erb*-B-3′, not containing v-*erb*-A sequences.[84] In spite of transducing a single oncogene, AEV-H is capable of inducing both erythroblastosis and sarcomas in susceptible recipient animals. Another virus, the RSV-associated virus type 1 (RAV-1), transduces only the v-*erb*-B oncogene.[85] The three viruses, AEV, AEV-H, and RAV-1, are capable of inducing rapid-onset erythroblastosis when inoculated into 1-week-old chickens.

The four carboxy-terminal amino acids of v-*erb*-A are encoded by a c-*erb*-B intron-derived sequence, thus demonstrating that AEV acquired a truncated c-*erb*-A gene.[86] The v-*erb*-B gene is a truncated version of c-*erb*-B and the observations suggest that the recombination events involved in the generation of v-*erb*-B occurred at the DNA level. The v-*erb*-A oncogene is also a truncated version of its cellular homologue and c-*erb*-A is 42 nucleotides longer than v-*erb*-A at its 5′ coding extremity.[87] In contrast to v-*erb*-B, the v-*erb*-A oncogene is unable by itself to induce neoplastic transformation of cells but is capable of inducing a strong enhancement of cellular growth *in vitro* and *in vivo*.[88] The v-*erb*-A and v-*erb*-B oncogenes can cooperate in the induction of a fully transformed phenotype in chicken embryo erythroblasts and fibroblasts.[89]

2. Transduction of Homologous Protooncogene Sequences from Different Animal Species

The number of cellular oncogenes, as defined by transduction by acute, highly oncogenic retroviruses, is probably limited to no more than two or three dozens, and retroviruses of different taxonomic groups may act as transducers of the same protooncogene sequences from different species. For example, common c-*onc* sequences are transduced by the avian retrovirus MH2, which transduces two oncogenes, v-*mht* and v-*myc*, and MuSV 3611, which transduces the oncogene v-*raf*. The oncogenes v-*mht* and v-*raf* have sequences showing about 95% of homology in relation to the corresponding amino acids.[52,71] Thus, v-*mht*, v-*mil*, and v-*raf* represent different isolates derived from cognate cellular genes of avian and mammalian species and may be considered as variants of one and the same oncogene. Murine retroviruses carrying recombinant *raf*/*myc* oncogenes rapidly induce hematopoietic neoplasms in newborn mice.[90]

The oncogenes v-H-*ras* and v-K-*ras* are present in the acute retroviruses H-MuLV and K-MuLV, respectively. These viruses were isolated from solid tumors of rats that had been inoculated with the chronic ecotropic mouse retrovirus M-MuLV.[14,15] Other v-*ras* genes, including one designated v-*bas*, were detected in acute retroviruses from mouse tumors.[91,92] The rat- and mouse-derived v-*ras* genes exhibit extensive nucleotide homology and display similar or identical transforming capabilities. Acute retroviruses carrying v-*ras* oncogenes contain deletions in the viral genome sequences and are replication-defective viruses.

3. Structural and Functional Differences between Different Viral Oncogene Isolates

Qualitative differences are frequently observed among different isolates of a given oncogene. For example, the oncogene v-*myc* is present in the avian acute retroviruses MH2 and MC29, but both the 5′ and 3′ borders of these oncogene isolates are not identical, which suggests that transduction of c-*myc*-related sequences involved different sequence elements in the generation of MH2 and MC29 viruses, respectively.[93] The structural differences existing among different acute retroviruses carrying the v-*myc* oncogene can be studied by using specific proteases including the p15 viral protease.[94] A DNA segment of approximately 345 bp corresponding to the third exon of the chicken c-*myc* gene is not present in the sequence of the MC29 AMCV v-*myc* oncogene.[95] However, a comparison of all mutations present in four v-*myc* alleles from different acute retroviruses carrying this oncogene (MC29, CMII, OK10, and MH2) indicates that there is no common specific mutation in all of the alleles.[96]

Specific sequences responsible for transformation may be recognized by studying mutations or deletions that produce specific changes in the oncogene protein product. The study of variants of A-MuLV indicates that most of the sequences corresponding to the 3′-coding region of the v-*abl* oncogene are not required for cell transformation.[97] The v-*abl* oncogene is transduced by the acute retrovirus A-MuLV, isolated from the mouse, as well as by the Hardy-Zuckerman-2 FeSV (HZ2-FeSV), isolated from a fibrosarcoma of a cat infected with the chronic retrovirus FeLV.[98] The organization of the genomes of A-MuLV derived from mouse and HZ2 FeSV derived from cat are similar, with genetic sequences arranged in the order 5′-*gag*-*abl*-*env*-3′. However, there are differences in some genetic elements of these two viruses as well as in their respective translational products.[99] Some A-MuLV variants may have an increased oncogenic potential which depends on particular recombination that may occur between viral and cellular sequences.[100] The molecular analysis of two strains of A-MuLV (P120 and P160) that have been cloned, and their comparison with murine c-*abl* clones, indicates that both strains have deleted 114 codons at the 5′ end and replaced these sequences with 240 codons derived from the *gag* gene of M-MuLV.[101] In addition, the two strains of A-MuLV contain deletions or alterations in the middle coding sequences of the oncogene. The v-*abl* oncogene contained in the feline isolate HZ2 FeSV has eliminated 51 codons from the 5′ end and all the sequences downstream to the 490th codon of the c-*abl* sequences.[102] In addition to the 3′ and 5′ deletions, acute retroviruses transducing the v-*abl* oncogene may have frame-shift and point mutations within the oncogene sequences, as compared with the c-*abl* protooncogene.

Structural and functional differences exist among different retroviral isolates from avian and feline origin containing the *fps*/*fes* oncogene.[103-105] An ASV containing the v-*fps* oncogene was isolated independently in Japan (Fujinami sarcoma virus or FSV) and Scotland (PRCII ASV), and other ASV isolates, including the variant PRCIIp, were described later. The different isolates of ASV probably correspond to independent transductional events. The most striking differences between these isolates are their respective oncogenic potentials. Injection of FSV or PRCIIp ASV into chicks under 2-weeks old nearly always causes fibromyxosarcomas, with an average latent period of 1 week. On the other hand, PRCII ASV is much less oncogenic, causing tumors in only 15% of chicks, after a latent period of 3 to 4 weeks.[106] Also, in cultured chick embryo fibroblasts, PRCII ASV causes only a partially transformed phenotype. The diminished oncogenicity of PRCII ASV may be attributed to a 1020-nucleotide deletion in the 5′ half of the genome.[103,104] The deletion does not include the 3′ end of the v-*fps* gene, which is directly related to the tyrosine-specific kinase activity of the oncogene protein product, but may produce changes in the subcellular location and solubility of this product, which could be responsible for its diminished oncogenic properties. PRCIIp ASV is a highly oncogenic variant which encodes a *gag-fps* transforming protein of about 170 kDa and has a genome at least 1 kbp larger than that of PRCII ASV.[107] Probably, PRCII ASV is a deletion mutant of PRCIIp ASV.

The v-*fps* oncogene of PRCII ASV and the c-*fps* protooncogene contained in the chicken genome have been cloned.[108] The c-*fps* sequences span approximately kbp, including a number of introns not represented in v-*fps*. The v-*fps* oncogene is highly homologous to the feline v-*fes* oncogene contained in the Gardner-Arnstein and Snyder-Theilen strains of FeSV. Each of these FeSV strains has a large deletion in the 5' half of v-*fes*, partially overlapping the deletion in PRCII AVS.[109] All of the protein products of the *fps/fes* viral oncogenes possess tyrosine-specific protein kinase activity but the precise role of this type of activity in oncogenicity is not understood. The less oncogenic PRCII variant of ASV induces a level of tyrosine phosphorylation in total cell proteins which is as high or higher than that found in cells transformed by the more tumorigenic FSV.[110] A recombinant gene in which 3' human c-*fps/fes* sequences replaced over 80% of the v-*fes* sequences was able to induce transformation in NIH/3T3 mouse fibroblasts and encoded tyrosine-specific protein kinase activity.[111] Whereas the normal human c-*fps/fes* protooncogene lacks transforming capacity, its oncogenic potential can be activated by fusion of the *gag* gene from Gardner-Arnstein ASV, which results in a fourfold increase in the specific kinase activity of the gene product.[112]

Some AEV isolates contain v-*erb*-B oncogenes that lack codons for the immediate carboxyl terminus of the EGF receptor, and the biological properties (tumor-inducing ability and specificity) of these variant viruses are different from those of the prototype virus.[113,114] Thus, differences in the transforming potential of v-*erb*-B-carrying acute retroviruses correlate with differences in *erb*-B sequences encoding the carboxy-terminal domain of the EGF receptor protein.

III. ONCOGENIC POTENTIAL OF VIRAL ONCOGENES

All retroviral oncogenes so far examined are mutant or structurally altered, frequently truncated versions of the respective protooncogenes contained in the normal cellular genome. Several types of structural differences between v- and c-*onc* genes are probably responsible for the acute transforming ability of v-*onc* genes as compared to c-*onc* genes, which would not possess such an ability.

A. STRUCTURAL AND FUNCTIONAL PROPERTIES OF VIRAL ONCOGENES

Specific structural alterations occurring in protooncogene-derived sequences, including deletion and linkage as well as point mutations, are responsible for the oncogenic potential of the resulting acute retroviruses. Virus-specific sequences contained in viral oncogenes may also provide functions required for transformation. Viral oncogene sequences may not be species specific. For example, a murine retrovirus encoding an avian v-*myc* oncogene may induce transformation of mammalian fibroblasts and macrophages *in vitro*.[115] Recombinant murine retroviruses containing the avian v-*myc* oncogene induce a wide spectrum of neoplasms in mammals, including newborn mice.[116,117] A murine retrovirus containing the avian v-*erb*-B oncogene can induce transformation of mammalian cells.[118]

In general, the rates of evolutionary changes (nucleotide substitutions per site per year) in viral oncogenes (or other RNA viral genes) are several orders of magnitude higher than those of cellular oncogenes, which are comparable to that of many functional DNA genes.[119] As a consequence of qualitative differences generated by such mutational events, as well as differences generated during the recombinational events that occurred between the parental infectious retrovirus and the cellular genome, the transforming ability of the protein products of cellular oncogenes may be markedly reduced, or may be absent, when it is compared with their viral counterparts. For example, RSV variants that carry the cellular *src* gene instead of the viral *src* gene are not able to transform chicken embryo fibroblasts.[120] Plasmids carrying the c-*src* gene are also not able to induce focus formation in NIH/3T3 cells in spite of the presence of high levels of the c-*onc* protein product, whereas plasmids carrying the v-*src* gene, either alone or associated with c-*src*, are very efficient for the induction of oncogenic transformation in the same cell system.[121]

The transforming activity of acute retroviruses may depend on the state of DNA methylation at cytosine residues in the provirus sequences. The transforming activity of cloned M-MuSV proviral DNA containing the v-*mos* oncogene can be inhibited by *in vitro* methylation of the DNA at cytosine residues.[122] This inhibition can be reversed by treatment of the transfected cells with the demethylating agent, 5-azacytidine. Inhibition of MuSV-induced transformation by DNA methylation needs not to have site specificity but may have region specificity within the provirus genome. The transformed phenotype of NIH/3T3 cells transfected with a retroviral vector carrying the v-*mos* oncogene can be reversibly suppressed by treatment with interferon (IFN-γ), which downregulates the expression of v-*mos* transcripts.[123] These results indicate that the v-*mos* product plays a direct role in the expression of a transformed phenotype by cells carrying the v-*mos* oncogene.

The relevance of particular point mutations in relation to the transforming ability of oncogene protein products may be difficult to evaluate even in the case of mutations conditioning temperature sensitivity *ts* alteration of the protein. A single amino acid change (from histidine to aspartic acid) located in the center of the tyrosine-specific protein kinase domain of the v-*erb*-B oncogene product confers a thermolabile phenotype to *ts* 167 AEV-transformed HD6 erythroid precursor cells.[124] However, the precise relationship between the structural and functional change could not be ascertained.

The presence of altered AMV proviral sequences integrated into the genome of chicken embryo fibroblasts is responsible for the expression of a transformed phenotype in the cells transfected with the virus, but it is not known whether this transformation results from the production of a high level of an intact v-*myb* product, from the expression of an abnormal v-*myb*-related polypeptide, or from other mechanisms.[125] AMV *ts* mutants for production of p45^{v-myb} are defective for inducing cellular transformation at the nonpermissive temperature.[126] However, expression of the v-*myb* product may not be sufficient for the induction of neoplastic transformation in particular cells. Expression of molecular vectors carrying the v-*myb* oncogene in avian and mammalian cells may be independent of transformation.[127]

Site-directed mutagenesis procedures can be conveniently used for the evaluation of the intracellular localization of oncogene products and the biological activity of these products.[128] However, the sole presence of point mutational differences between a viral oncogene and the respective cellular protooncogene does not necessarily indicate that the transforming potential of the viral oncogene is due to the presence of such differences. The v-*myc* domains of several different acute transforming retroviruses carrying the v-*myc* oncogene (MC29, OK10, MH2, CMII) differ from proto-*myc* in private point mutations and each one of these could be necessary to convert the c-*myc* protooncogene into a true oncogene, but since a common mutation is not found in all v-*myc* genes it is unlikely that such mutations are essential for oncogenicity.[96,129] At least in this case, it is more likely that particular types of deletions and conjugations of c-*myc* sequences with viral sequences, rather than specific point mutations, would be responsible for converting a normal cellular gene into a true oncogene. The apparent conservation of carboxyl-terminal sequences in all v-*myc* gene products of four different ALVs indicate their functional significance but no mutants of v-*myc*-containing oncogene retroviruses have been isolated that direct the synthesis of smaller v-*myc* gene products terminating at positions internal to the gene.[130] Several spontaneous non-conditional mutants of the MC29 retrovirus contain internal deletions and generate altered *gag-myc* products of 90 to 100 kDa which have strongly reduced potential to transform hematopoietic cells *in vitro* or to induce tumors in animals but which are capable of transforming cultured fibroblasts.[131] Comparison of tryptic phosphopeptide mapping of wild-type and mutant *gag-myc* hybrid proteins showed that a large peptide sequence extensively phosphorylated at serine and threonine residues is present in the wild-type protein but is absent in the mutant viral proteins.

Deletion of sequences present in the parental protooncogene may be critically relevant for the acquisition of oncogenic potential by retroviral oncogenes. The v-*ros* oncogene contained in the UR2 ASV is truncated at both 5′ and 3′ ends, compared to the normal chicken c-*ros* protooncogene.[132,133] The v-*ets* oncogene of E26 ALV is also characterized by truncation of sequences present at both the 5′ and 3′ ends of the normal chicken c-*ets* protooncogene as well as by the acquisition of noncoding sequences of c-*ets* into the virus.[134]

The v-*rel* oncogene is contained in reticuloendotheliosis virus strain T (REV-T).[135,136] The minimal events required to generate v-*rel* from its cellular counterpart, the c-*rel* protooncogene contained in the turkey's genome, involves recombination between helper virus (REV-A) and c-*rel*, splicing of large introns, point mutations, and deletion of at least part of a 3′ c-*rel* exon which is not present in v-*rel*.[137-139] Changes in relatively small regions of the virus genome are sufficient to convert REV-T into a strongly transforming virus.[140] The v-*rel* oncogene is transcribed into 3.0-kb subgenomic, polyadenylated RNA in REV-T-transformed cells, while the c-*rel* protooncogene is expressed in form of a 4.0-kb transcript in avian cells of hematopoietic origin. The protein product of the v-*rel* oncogene represents a truncated and mutated version of the normal c-*rel* protooncogene product and contains 12 amino acids at its 5′ terminus derived from REV-A *env* sequences. Activation of the c-*rel* protooncogene into a fully transforming gene in REV-T requires at least the following changes: deletion of the c-*rel* 3′ noncoding sequences, deletion of most of the helper virus-related *env* gene, and alterations of the amino-terminal and central regions of the c-*rel* protein.[141] It is thus apparent that the generation of highly oncogenic retroviruses such as REV-T requires a series of complex events with multiple genetic rearrangements that affect both the protooncogene and the replication-competent parental retrovirus. Tumorigenicity induced by the p57^{v-rel} product of the REV-T virus may be associated with the production of an autogenous growth factor.[142]

The v-*erb*-B oncogene was derived from the avian EGF receptor gene by truncation as a consequence of the recombination event involved in the genesis of AEV. Both the v-*erb*-B protein and the EGF receptor are transmembrane tyrosine-specific protein kinases but they have important structural differences; when aligned with the human EGF receptor sequences, the v-*erb*-B protein lacks the signal peptide for membrane translocation (24 amino acids), most of the extracellular ligand-binding domain (amino acids 1 to 555), and 32 carboxy-terminal amino acids.[143] A chimeric gene encoding the extracellular and the transmembrane domains of the human EGF receptor joined to sequences coding for the cytoplasmic domain of the AEV v-*erb*-B oncogene was constructed in order to test the possibility that replacement of the receptor domain may be sufficient to restore a normal ligand-responsive receptor from a transforming protein.[144] When expressed in rodent cells (Rat 1) fibroblasts, this reconstituted gene product was transported to the cell surface and bound EGF, and its autophosphorylation activity was stimulated by interaction with the ligand. Expression of the chimeric EGF receptor/v-*erb*-B gene led to neoplastic transformation in the transfected Rat 1 cells (anchorage-independent cell growth in soft agar). Moreover, exposure of the cells to EGF led to focus formation in monolayers, which suggests that the transforming potential of the chimeric gene resides in intracellular features unique to v-*erb*-B oncogene sequences. The carboxy-terminal deletion in the chimeric gene (and v-*erb*-B) is likely to be predominantly responsible for the transforming action of this protein by altering the regulation of its phosphorylation activity or its substrate specificity.[144] The transforming capacity of v-*erb*-B is gradually diminished and finally lost in proportion to the extension of deletions introduced in the 3′-terminal region of the oncogene sequences.[39] The capacity to transform erythroblasts is lost before fibroblast transformation is severely affected, suggesting that a large part of the carboxy-terminal domain of the v-*erb*-B protein is required for mitogenic signaling in erythroid cells than in fibroblasts.

Deletion of DNA sequences encoding the amino-terminal region of the c-*raf* protooncogene protein product, with partial replacement by *gag*-derived sequences, characterizes the v-*raf* oncogene of the acute murine retrovirus MuSV 3611.[145] This deletion is sufficient to confer transforming capability to c-*raf*-derived proteins.[146]

Deletions at both the 5' and 3' ends distinguish the v-*myb* oncogene of AMV from its normal c-*myb* chicken counterpart and these deletions would be responsible for the acquisition of an oncogenic capability by the truncated viral protein product.[147] In addition to these deletions which determine that the protein encoded by v-*myb* represents a truncated version at both its ends of the chicken c-*myb* product, there are 11 amino acid substitutions distinguishing these two products, and the AMV allele of v-*myb* is fused to a small portion of viral *gag* sequences by the splice that generates mRNA for v-*myb*.[148] The amino acid substitutions present in the v-*myb* product do not appear to be responsible for its transforming potential, since a constructed v-*myb* oncogene which lacks all 11 of the specific amino acid substitutions present in p48^{v-myb} of AMV retains, although with lowered efficiency, the transformation capability.[149] A constructed recombinant clone (KXA 3457) in which the v-*myb* sequences are flanked by the two AMV LTRs generate abnormal *myb*-specific RNA species and *myb*-related polypeptides and is capable of inducing transformation when expressed in CEF cells.[150] These results suggest that transformation of cells by v-*myb* might require qualitative alterations related to amino- and/or carboxy-terminal deletions, but not substitutions in the amino acid sequences of the oncogene protein product. However, the structural origins of tumorigenicity induced by the products of *myb* DNA sequences remain enigmatic.

The protooncogene c-*fps* contained in the avian genome would have acquired oncogenic potential upon transduction as v-*fps* in the ASV genome due to several structural alterations, including the following possibilities: (1) the proteins encoded by the various forms of v-*fps* may be truncated versions of the protein encoded by c-*fps*, (2) the polypeptides encoded by v-*fps* are fused to a portion of viral protein encoded by the structural gene *gag*, (3) several amino acid substitutions distinguish the v-*fps* protein from the c-*fps* protein, and (4) in some ASV strains the v-*fps* gene has suffered deletions that remove amino acid sequences from the encoded protein.[105] Rodent cells (Rat-2 cells) transfected with a constructed vector carrying the human c-*fes*/*fps* protooncogene express approximately 50-fold more human p92^{c-fes} protein than is found in human myeloid leukemic cells but remain morphologically normal and failed to grow in soft agar.[151] Despite this elevated level of expression, human p92^{c-fes} does not induce substantial increase of phosphotyrosine in the transfected cells and the p92^{c-fes} protein is not phosphorylated itself on tyrosine. Thus, even cells ectopically expressing high levels of a normal protooncogene product may control the specific kinase activity of this product but are not able to restrain the activity of the respective viral oncogene product.

While the intact c-*fps* gene product lacks transformation ability by itself even when overexpressed by means of molecular vectors, its transformation potential can be activated by either mutation in the *fps* coding region or by fusion with viral *gag* gene sequences.[112,152] It has been suggested that the oncogenic potential of v-*fps*, in contradistinction to the lack of such a potential in the c-*fps* protooncogene, is more probably associated with the substitution of the 5' c-*fps* specific suppressor domain by δ-*gag* viral sequences than with the possible existence of point mutational differences between the respective coding sequences.[153] The avian v-*fps* gene is closely related to the v-*fes* gene of FeSV and the respective protooncogenes, c-*fps* and c-*fes*, would represent the avian and feline copies of the same gene. Another FeSV isolate, the Theilen-Pedersen strain of FeSV, encodes for a *gag-onc* fusion protein of 83,000 mol wt whose v-*onc* nucleotide sequences are related, but not identical, to the v-*fps* and v-*fes* oncogenes.[154]

A novel FeSV isolate, the Hardy-Zuckerman 4 strain of FeSV (HZ4-FeSV) carries an oncogene, termed v-*kit*, which is a member of the tyrosine-protein kinase oncogene family.[155,156] The oncogene v-*kit* is closely related in its structure to the v-*fms* oncogene which is present in the Susan McDonough strain of FeSV (SM-FeSV).[157,158] The v-*fms* oncogene product has all the structural features of the receptor for the mononuclear phagocyte colony-stimulating factor, CSF-1, except that at its distal carboxyl terminus the last 40 amino acids of the CSF-1 receptor have been substituted for 11 unrelated v-*fms*-coded amino acids.[159] In membrane preparations, the tyrosine-specific protein kinase activity of the normal CSF-1 receptor is stimulated by CSF-1, whereas the v-*fms* kinase activity appears to act constitutively and is refractory to the ligand. Treatment of SM-FeSV-transformed REF cells with the glycosylation processing inhibitor, castanospermine, decreases the association of the gp14^{v-fms} product with the plasma membrane without affecting its tyrosine kinase activity, and a reversion to the nontransformed phenotype is observed in the castanospermine-treated cells.[160]

Quantitative alterations in the expression of oncogene sequences may be responsible, at least in some cases, for the transforming capability of these sequences. Neither major structural changes, such as in-frame fusion with virion genes or internal deletions, nor specific, if any, missense mutations of the c-*myc* coding region are necessary for oncogenic activation of transduced *myc* alleles.[96,161] However, some mutations can affect the transforming activity of *myc* sequences. Substitution of threonine-61 for a methionine (as in the v-*myc* product of the MC29 virus) significantly enhances the fibroblast-transforming capacity of the recombinant oncogene.[162] Such a hybrid v-*myc*/c-*myc* gene is still severalfold less active in transformation than the authentic v-*myc* oncogene of the MC29 retrovirus.

The protein product of M-MuSV strain 124 is the protein p37^{v-mos}, which contains the sequences corresponding to the viral oncogene v-*mos*.[163] The variant M-MuSV virus *ts* 110 is a temperature-sensitive (*ts*) mutant which produces at the permissive temperature (33°C) an 85,000-Da *gag-mos* hybrid protein, termed p85$^{gag-mos}$, but at the restricted temperature (39°C) expresses a 58,000-Da *gag* protein, termed p58^{gag}, which does not contain a viral oncogene product.[164-166] This phenomenon is due to a *ts* RNA splicing event in which the message at the permissive temperature contains *gag* and *mos* sequences fused in an ORF whose translation results in the synthesis of p85$^{gag-mos}$. This protein possesses kinase activity and induces transformation of susceptible cells. Thus, temperature manipulations allow for examination of phenotypic changes associated with the synthesis of the hybrid protein containing the transforming viral sequences.[165] Another transforming protein produced by a *ts* mutant of M-MuSV is termed p100$^{gag-mos}$ and results from the translation of a continuous ORF from the *gag* to the *mos* gene due to a 5-base deletion at intron-exon border of the 3′ splice site.[166] The p100$^{gag-mos}$ protein is translated from the ORF at any growth temperature.

Molecular vector constructs can be used to demonstrate that, depending on the amount of intracellular v-*mos* product, different stages of morphological transformation can be observed.[167] A strong correlation exists between the cell transformation activity of various mutant v-*mos* gene constructs and the serine/threonine-specific protein kinase activity of the products of these constructs.[168] Deletion mutants assayed with retroviral vectors may also contribute to define the biological properties of the v-*mos* oncogene.[169] The results of all of these studies support the concept that the transforming properties of the v-*mos* oncogene protein product crucially depend on its specific kinase activity. However, the exact biochemical mechanisms by which the v-*mos* protein-associated kinase induce neoplastic transformation remain unknown.

Different intracellular levels of the v-*onc* protein p37^{v-mos} can be obtained by regulation of recombinant vectors containing MMTV LTR fused to the entire coding region of v-*mos*.[167,170] The results obtained in experiments performed with these vectors demonstrate that a critical intracellular level of p37^{v-mos} is required for both the initiation and maintenance of the transformed phenotype in transfected NIH/3T3 cells. Moreover, there is a direct correlation between the amounts of cytoplasmic v-*mos*-specific RNA and p37^{v-mos} protein in these cells and their stage of transformation as defined by several transformation-characteristic parameters.[167] LTR sequences may have a critical role in determining the target cell specificities of different v-*mos*-carrying acute transforming retroviruses as well as in imparting oncogenic properties to molecular vectors carrying a c-*mos* gene.[171] However, the oncogenic potential of c-*mos* appears to be rather low. Transgenic mice expressing high levels of c-*mos* as a consequence of embryo injection of a murine c-*mos* gene linked to M-MuSV LTR are characterized only by changes in secondary lens fiber differentiation.[172] No neoplastic changes were detected in the transgenic mice in spite of the fact that c-*mos* transcripts are widely expressed in the tissues of the animals.

B. ONCOGENIC POTENTIAL OF PROTOONCOGENES

Although the term "oncogene" may be appropriate for the transforming genes contained in acute retroviruses, the same may not be true when applied to the original cellular counterparts, whose functions are essentially normal and, probably, indispensable ones. The term protooncogene should be more conveniently used when reference is made to the cellular counterpart of viral oncogenes. A most important issue is to know whether altered protooncogenes can acquire oncogenic potential and can thus play an essential role in carcinogenic processes. At least under the conditions of strict experimental protocols, structurally or functionally altered protooncogenes (or the products of these genes) are capable of inducing neoplastic transformation of susceptible cells.

Quantitative changes in *myc* gene expression rather than qualitative changes in the structure of the gene product may be essential for the function of *myc* as an efficient transforming gene. A retroviral vector containing the complete chicken c-*myc* gene in which the native promoter has been replaced by a retroviral LTR is sufficient to convert the c-*myc* protooncogene into a transforming gene, without requiring truncation of the first exon of the gene as it occurs in c-*myc*-transducing acute retroviruses.[173] A mouse retrovirus that contains the protein-coding exons from the mouse c-*myc* gene expresses high levels of LTR-c-*myc* RNA and induces transformation and tumorigenic properties in established lines of mouse fibroblasts.[174] The mouse fibroblast cell lines infected with this constructed retrovirus express high levels of LTR-c-*myc* RNA and are tumorigenic in nude mice. Cotransfection of rat 3Y1 cells, established from a Fisher rat embryo, with a transcriptionally activated c-*myc* gene and PSV2 *neo* DNA results in the appearance of colonies of transformed cells which are capable of inducing tumors in syngeneic rats.[175] Both c-*myc* and N-*myc* genes can induce morphological transformation, anchorage independence, and tumorigenicity in established rat fibroblasts (Rat-1 cells) when they are expressed at high levels from a transfected constructed vector.[176] The number of passages in culture is apparently important for the expression of the transforming potential of the c-*myc* gene. Late passage (60 generation) FR3T3 rat fibroblasts are transformed to a tumorigenic phenotype after transfection with a retroviral vector carrying an activated c-*myc* gene, whereas cells from early passage are resistant to the acquisition of a fully transformed phenotype.[177] In contrast to the diploid early passage cells, the late passage FR3T3 cells contain karyotypic abnormalities which may be important for the expression of neoplastic transformation.

The oncogenic potential of a c-*myc* protooncogene altered by replacement of the 5′ regulatory region by those of another gene and by deletion of the first c-*myc* exon has been demonstrated in transgenic mice.[178] Up to 80% of female transgenic mice expressing the c-*myc* transgene specifically in the mammary gland during late pregnancy and lactation develop mammary adenocarcinomas. The tumors appear as early as 2 months after the onset of c-*myc* transgene expression and their appearance is associated with deregulated milk protein gene expression and acquisition of hormone- and growth factor-independent growth. Since only a fraction of the mammary gland cells expressing the deregulated c-*myc* transgene become neoplastically transformed, it follows that additional genetic and/or epigenetic alterations are required in order to malignant transformation to occur.

The transformation efficiency of constructs carrying qualitatively unaltered c-*myc* sequences is usually significantly lower than that of constructs carrying v-*myc*-derived sequences, which suggests that mutations and other structural changes may play an important role for the evolution of fully tumorigenic v-*myc* oncogenes.[96,161] Only slight morphological changes are observed in mouse or rat cells transfected with c-*myc* genes linked to viral promoters.[179] Primary REF cells are moderately stimulated to growth but are not transformed and do not acquire tumorigenic properties after transfection with a plasmid carrying the normal human c-*myc* gene.[180,181] An established rat fibroblast cell line (F2408), expressing high level of human c-*myc* transcripts as a consequence of transfection with a constructed plasmid containing the c-*myc* gene under the control of polyoma virus regulatory elements, may acquire anchorage-independent growth and may become tumorigenic upon inoculation into young syngeneic rats.[182] However, the transformed cells appeared with a low frequency among the population of transfected cells, which suggests that additional mutational or epigenetic events may be required for the development of clones expressing high levels of c-*myc* transcripts and anchorage independency. Constructed plasmids in which the human c-*myc* gene is linked to the BPV-1 genome can induce immortalization in primary rat embryo cells but cell lines derived from the transfected cells do not usually display a transformed phenotype although some of them express a high level of c-*myc* and/or BPV-1 mRNAs.[183] It may be concluded that the normal c-*myc* protooncogene may confer immortal properties when expressed at high levels in some types of cells *in vitro* but the genetic and/or epigenetic changes in addition to high levels of c-*myc* gene expression are required for the malignant transformation of cells.

Transgenic mice bearing a c-*myc* protooncogene subjected to the lymphoid-specific Ig heavy chain enhancer develop primarily benign polyclonal overproliferation of pre-B cells and a second genetic accident is apparently required for progression of these cells to malignancy.[184] Even the complete *gag-myc* sequences of the acute MC29 retrovirus cloned in a plasmid vector may not be sufficient to induce neoplastic transformation in cells such as C3H/10T1/2 mouse embryo fibroblasts, which require cotransfection of the v-*myc* oncogene with a mutated T24 c-H-*ras* gene to become morphologically transformed and to exhibit anchorage-independent growth in soft agar.[185] These results lend support to the multistep hypothesis of malignant transformation.

The product of the osteosarcoma-associated FBJ strain of MuSV, p55[v-fos], shows an altered carboxy-terminal region compared to the c-*fos* product.[186] Both v- and c-*fos* may be capable of inducing experimental transformation.[187] Activation of the transforming potential of c-*fos* requires two experimental manipulations: (1) linkage of transcriptional enhancer elements to the gene and (2) disruption of interacting sequences at the 3′ end of the gene. The c-*fos* gene is expressed in certain normal cells (amnion cells) at levels comparable to that of v-*fos* in FBJ MuSV-transformed cells and it has been suggested that expression of the normal c-*fos* gene at high levels in an inappropriate cell type can lead to transformation.[188,189] Removal of a 67-bp sequence located in the noncoding region of c-*fos*, 123-189 nucleotides downstream from the polyadenylation signal, in the 3′ untranslated part of the gene, is sufficient to activate its transforming potential.[190] These results suggest that posttranscriptional regulation of c-*fos* expression may be important in preventing the normal gene to become an oncogene with transforming capability.

The v-*fos* oncogene is also contained in an avian transforming retrovirus, NK24, which was isolated from a chicken with nephroblastoma.[191] The NK24 virus transforms CEF cells *in vitro* and is capable of inducing fibrosarcomas, osteosarcomas, and nephroblastomas after injection *in vivo*. Unlike the v-*fos* oncogene products of FBJ and FBR murine osteosarcoma viruses, which suffer a structural alteration at their carboxyl termini, the NK24 v-*fos* oncogene product seems to have the same carboxyl-terminal structure as the chicken c-*fos* gene product.

The c-*mos* protooncogene from all species tested can be activated by an LTR to transform NIH/3T3 cells in culture or to produce tumors in nude mice.[192-194] However, there are species-specific differences in the transforming efficiency of c-*mos* genes. The transforming activity of human c-*mos* is 100-fold lower than that of mouse c-*mos*. Chicken c-*mos* can transform mouse cells as efficiently as mouse c-*mos* and is also able to transform chicken cells, although with lower efficiency. Human cells are resistant to transformation induced by retroviral constructions containing the human c-*mos* gene.

Protooncogenes altered by apparently spontaneous mutations may also acquire oncogenic potential. For example, c-*ras* genes isolated from human tumors or tumor cell lines are capable of inducing oncogenic transformation of NIH/3T3 cells. These genes are characterized by the presence of mutations consisting in nucleotide substitutions at particular sites of the protoonco-gene exonic sequences (codons 12 and 61), which determine changes in the functional properties of the p21$^{c\text{-}ras}$ protein products. In addition to point mutations, c-*ras* genes can acquire oncogenic potential as a consequence of other structural alterations, especially by truncation of a 5′ exon of the gene.[195] Interestingly, a point mutation in the last intron of the c-H-*ras* protooncogene has been characterized as responsible for the increased expression of the gene and the acquisition of transforming activity.[196]

IV. VIRAL ONCOGENE PRODUCTS AND NEOPLASTIC TRANSFORMATION

The protein products of the oncogenes contained in acute retroviruses are oncoproteins responsible for the high oncogenic potentialities of these viruses. Expression of constructed vectors carrying cloned v-*onc* genes can induce malignant transformation of susceptible cells. For example, molecular chimeras containing the LTR of MMTV fused to the v-H-*ras* oncogene are able to induce transformation of NIH/3T3 cells.[197] However, the expression of viral oncogene products such as the products of v-*mos* and v-*fes* is not always associated with the expression of a transformed phenotype.[198-200] Moreover, at least certain cells may be able to differentiate along a normal pathway in spite of the persistent expression of a viral oncogene.[201]

A. PHENOTYPIC CHANGES IN ONCOGENE-TRANSFECTED CELLS

Transfection of an oncogene into susceptible cells can bypass the specific requirements for growth control or can alter the behavioral properties of the cell. The MCF7 human breast carcinoma cell line possesses estrogen receptors and responds to estrogen by increasing invasiveness properties. After transfection with an v-H-*ras* oncogene these cells acquire higher malignant characteristics, with increased invasion of reconstituted basement membranes, and estrogen has no discernible effect in the oncogene-transfected cells.[202] Thus, although the malignant phenotype of MCF7 cells is under hormonal control, this control is bypassed after v-H-*ras* transfection. However, v-*ras* oncogenes may not produce a malignant phenotype when expressed in other types of cells. Infection of mature murine splenic B lymphocytes by K-MuSV pseudotyped with an amphotropic MuLV helper virus results in the production of immortalized B-cell lines which retain the same mature phenotype as the starting cell population, including hapten-specific binding.[203]

B. HOST FACTORS IN RELATION TO THE ONCOGENIC POTENTIAL OF VIRAL ONCOGENE PROTEINS

The type of cell and its physiological condition, including the stage of maturation, may be critical for the induction or lack of induction of neoplastic transformation by viral oncogene protein products. There may be marked differences in the susceptibilities of cells from different animal species for v-*onc*-induced transformation. While rodent cells are frequently susceptible to transformation induced by viral oncogene products, human cells are generally resistant to such transformation. The oncogene v-*src* readily transforms and establishes embryonic rodent fibroblasts, but not diploid human fibroblasts.[204] The p21 protein products of v-*ras* oncogenes can easily transform mouse fibroblasts, as demonstrated with the NIH/3T3 DNA transfection assay, but normal human cells (fibroblasts or lymphocytes) are resistant to v-*ras*-induced transformation.[205] Normal quiescent human lymphocytes are not induced to cell growth and are not immortalized by either v-H-*ras* of v-*myc* oncogenes in spite of their efficient expression by means of molecular constructs. Some types of mouse cells may also exhibit resistance to v-*ras*-induced tumorigenicity. Skin grafts constructed with mouse epidermal cells carrying a v-H-*ras* oncogene produce only benign tumors (papillomas) on athymic nude mouse recipients.[206,207] Expression of the exogenous oncogene seems to be regulated at the transcriptional level in the differentiated portions of the benign tumor. Murine macrophage-like cell lines immortalized *in vitro* with a recombinant retrovirus carrying two oncogenes, v-*raf* and v-*myc*, can proliferate *in vitro* in the absence of exogenous growth factors but exhibit many of the constitutional and/or inducible phenotypic properties characteristic of normal peritoneal exudate macrophages.[208]

Human cells may be rendered susceptible to v-*onc*-induced transformation when they are treated with certain genetic constructs. Human FS-2 fibroblasts can acquire tumorigenic capacity when they express SV40 T antigen and are infected with K-MuSV pseudotyped with BaEV.[207] The relevance of such complex artificial manipulations in relation to the natural tumorigenic processes occurring in humans and other animal species is dubious.

The direct injection of mouse pups or rat fetuses during the second half of pregnancy with acute retroviruses (M-MuSV and K-MuSV) results in the induction of different and multiple tumors.[209,210] A variety of neoplasms characteristic of early life, including mixed mesenchymal sarcomas and epithelial tumors of the brain, appear in the injected newborns within the first 5 weeks of life. Unexpectedly, many tumors induced in these experiments appeared at targets distant from the site of virus inoculation, e.g., in the brain, which suggests a virus-cell interaction event likely to depend on particular stages of cellular maturation and organization.[210]

Rat thyroid epithelial cell lines are transformed by K-MuSV and the transformed cells are blocked in the expression of differentiated functions, including iodide uptake and thyroglobulin synthesis.[211] However, $p21^{v-ras}$ expression does not seem to be continuously required in order to cause this block in the differentiation properties of the transformed cell lines since the block is not reversed when cells infected with a *ts* mutant of K-MuSV are shifted to the temperature nonpermissive for transformation.[212]

The susceptibility of cells to be transformed by oncogene products may depend on their efficiency to synthesize these products. Transfection of a recombinant plasmid containing the human c-*myc* gene into quail embryo fibroblast cells results in phenotypic transformation, whereas an established rat embryo fibroblastic cell line (208F) is resistant to such transformation.[213] This difference is apparently related to differences in the capacity of the cells to synthesize the c-*myc* protein product. Although c-*myc* mRNAs are expressed in the two cell types (quail embryo cells and rat embryo fibroblasts), the p64/p67 human c-*myc* proteins are only detected in quail embryo fibroblasts. The molecular mechanisms responsible for this specific blocking of the translational machinery of 208F cells for reading the human c-*myc* message is unknown.

Transfected v-*myc* oncogenes can induce morphological changes and anchorage independence in immortal mouse fibroblasts and epithelial cell lines but these cells require further events to become tumorigenic.[214] A constructed transgenic mouse strain in which an MMTV LTR/c-*myc* fusion gene is anomalously expressed by induction with glucocorticoid show an increased incidence of a variety of tumors including those of testicular, mammary, lymphocytic (B-cell and T-cell), and mast cell origin.[215] However, transformation was not seen in all tissues in which the fusion gene was expressed. Expression of molecular vectors carrying the v-*myb* oncogene in avian and mammalian cells may be independent of transformation.[127] It is thus evident that host factors are of critical importance in the expression of neoplastic transformation induced by the oncogene protein products of acute retroviruses.

C. REGRESSION OR SUPPRESSION OF A V-*ONC*-INDUCED MALIGNANT PHENOTYPE

Spontaneous regression of tumors induced by acute retroviruses has been observed occasionally, for example, in chickens infected with AMV carrying the v-*myb* oncogene.[216] Moreover, AMV-transformed cultured chicken cells may be chemically induced to differentiate without a decrease in the synthesis or obvious alteration of the $p45^{v-myb}$ protein product.[217] This result reinforces the concept that a transformed phenotype can be suppressed by a mechanism not involving the switching off of the synthesis or obvious alteration of a viral protein with high oncogenic potential. Unfortunately, the mechanisms involved in the regression of oncogene-induced tumors *in vivo* and in the reversion of oncogene-transformed cells *in vitro* are unknown.

V. PROTEIN PRODUCTS OF VIRAL ONCOGENES

The polypeptide products of viral oncogenes are frequently represented not only by amino acid sequences specifically derived from the respective cellular sequences, the protooncogenes, but may also also contain sequences derived from the viral genes and may be expressed in form of hybrid proteins (polyproteins).

A. HYBRID PROTEINS

The transforming proteins of many acute retroviruses, including ASVs, MuSVs, FeSV, and SSV, are hybrid or fused proteins (polyproteins) in which *gag* or *env* viral genes initiate their translation.[130,218-223] The possible role of the nononcogenic components of these hybrid proteins in the processes of viral-induced malignant transformation remains to be defined. *gag* sequences are not required for transformation of cultured chicken cells by the *fps* oncogene contained in FSV.[224] Although FSV encodes a 130,000-Da *gag-fps* fusion protein (p130[gag-fps]), molecularly cloned DNA expressing only *fps* sequences can induce transformation of chicken embryo fibroblasts. Constructed in-phase insertion mutations throughout the FSV genome suggest that both the amino- and carboxyl-terminal v-*fps*-specific regions of p130[gag-fps] may function in concert to bring about some of the cellular changes associated with fibroblast transformation.[225]

The *gag* gene of FeLV encodes from 5′ to 3′ proteins of different molecular weights designated as p15, p12, p27, and p10.[226] Deletion of different lengths of the 3′ end of the *gag* gene during the generation of FeSV usually involves p27 and/or p10 and results in the formation of different strains of FeSV with fused *gag-onc* sequences. The collection of strains of FeSV may thus represent a resource of *onc* genes and of different segments of the p27[gag] gene that can be used for the preparation of monoclonal antibodies capable of recognizing different epitopes of the p27[gag] and v-*fes* proteins.[227] The following gene polyprotein products of different FeSV strains have been described: p85[gag-fes] of the Snyder Theilen (ST) strain, p95[gag-fes] of the Gardner-Arnstein (GA) strain, gp180[gag-fms] of the Susan McDonough (SM) strain, p70[gag-fgr] of the Gardner-Rasheed (GR) strain, p98[gag-abl] of the Hardy-Zuckerman 2 (HZ2) strain, p80[gag-kit] of the Hardy-Zuckerman 4 (HZ4) strain, and p83[gag-fgr] of the TP1 strain.[227]

The construction and analysis of AMV which produced a truncated form of the p48[v-myb] protein served to demonstrate that the *env*-encoded carboxyl terminus of p48[v-myb] is not required for transformation.[228] The influence of nononcogene polypeptide sequences encoded by acute retroviruses on the induction of neoplastic transformation varies according to the virus. Sequences derived from the *gag* gene are present in the p75[gag-fos] protein of FBR MuSV but are absent in the product of a related acute retrovirus, the FBJ MuSV, and it is interesting to observe that the v-*fos* gene could have similar oncogenic potential whether expressed as p75[gag-fos] or as p55[fos].[222] The oncogenic capacity of p75[gag-fos] was found to be greater than that of p55[fos] in another study using nonestablished cultures of mouse connective tissue cells, but the enhanced oncogenic activity of p75[gag-fos] is apparently due to structural differences other than the presence of *gag* sequences.[229] Removal of all *gag*-related sequences from FBR MuSV does not affect the transformation potential of the virus.[230] On the other hand, *gag* sequences seem to be indispensable for the induction of B-cell lymphomas in mice by A-MuLV, which contains the oncogene *abl*.[97] A-MuLV has the unique capability of transforming early B-lineage hematopoietic cells in culture, which has provided a useful model for studying B cell development.[231] Determinants derived from *gag*, but not from *abl*, are exposed on the surface of A-MuLV-transformed cells.[232] In contrast to RSV, A-MuLV does not induce sarcoma when injected into newborn mice, but recombinant virus constructs in which the *gag* sequence of A-MuLV is replaced with the 5′ end of the v-*src* oncogene can transform both fibroblasts and lymphoid cells *in vitro*.[233] The mentioned examples indicate that, although the production of hybrid proteins composed of viral structural gene products (*gag* and/or *env* products) fused to the respective v-*onc* product are not a general requisite for the oncogenic potential of acute retroviruses, they may be important in certain cases for determining the transforming capabilities of acute retroviruses in different types of cells. Nononcogene sequences from acute retroviruses may influence the expression of oncogenes in inserted proviruses. For example, sequences from the *gag-pol* region of the RSV provirus are apparently involved in regulating the level of expression of the v-*src* oncogene in RSV-infected cells.[234] The protein encoded by the v-*sis* oncogene contains a signal sequence, derived from the *env* gene of the parental SSV retrovirus, and removal of this sequence correlates with loss of biological activity.[235] Hypothetically, the signal sequence would be required for localization of the v-*sis* protein product at the cell membrane and for the interaction with the PDGF receptor.

B. MECHANISMS OF GENERATION OF HYBRID RETROVIRAL PROTEINS

In addition to controls operating at the level of transcription, RNA splicing processes may be critically involved in the generation of hybrid protein products from acute retroviruses. Rodent cells (NRK 6m2 cell line) infected with a *ts* mutant of M-MuSV display a transformed phenotype at 28 to 33°C and a normal phenotype at 39°C. At temperatures permissive for transformation, 6m2 cells contain both p58^{gag} and p85$^{gag-mos}$ proteins, whereas at 39°C only the p50^{gag} product is detected.[236] This difference is due to a structural defect in the 4.0-kb *ts* M-MuSV genomic RNA which prevents its splicing at restrictive temperatures.

C. POSTTRANSLATIONAL MODIFICATION OF V-*ONC* PROTEIN PRODUCTS

The protein products of acute retroviruses may be subjected to different co- or posttranslational modifications, including acylation, phosphorylation, and glycosylation.

Myristyl acylation of retrovirus protein products is an unusual type of posttranslational modification consisting in addition of myristic acid (a rare fatty acid) in amide linkage to the amino-terminal portion of the protein.[237] Myristylation occurs in *gag-onc* fusion proteins of retroviruses containing different oncogenes (v-*fes*, v-*abl*, v-*ras*, and v-*raf*).[238] Myristic acid is attached to the RSV protein product, pp60^{v-src}, during or immediately after synthesis and is present in both the soluble and membrane-bound forms of the protein.[239,240] Amino-terminal myristylation may contribute to the membrane localization of proteins.[241] The same posttranslational modification has been detected in cellular proteins involved in intracellular growth control mechanisms, for example, in cAMP-dependent protein kinase, which is involved in regulatory phenomena induced by insulin and several growth factors, and in calcineurin, which binds calmodulin in a Ca^{2+}-dependent fashion.[242]

Phosphorylation of acute retrovirus protein products, especially at tyrosine residues, may also have important influences on their respective biological activities. This influence is demonstrated by experiments of site-directed mutagenesis where specific phosphotyrosyl residues are substituted by nonphosphorylated amino acids. For example, substitution of phosphotyrosine at position 416 of RSV pp60^{src} and substitution of phosphotyrosine at position 1073 of FSV p130$^{gag-fps}$ results in diminished tyrosine-specific protein kinase activity and decreased oncogenic potential of the respective oncogene products.[242-244]

D. INTRACELLULAR LOCALIZATION OF VIRAL ONCOGENE PROTEIN PRODUCTS

The products of some viral oncogenes (v-*myc*, v-*myb*, v-*fos*, v-*ski*, v-*jun*, and v-*erb*-A) are located mainly in the nucleus of the host cell. The product of the MC29 AMCV oncogene, v-*myc*, is a hybrid protein or polyprotein of 110,000 Da, p110$^{gag-myc}$, resulting from the fusion of viral *gag* and *onc* genes. In MC29 AMCV-transformed cells this protein is located mainly in the nucleus, and the purified protein binds to double-stranded DNA.[245] Another strain of AMCV, OK10, encodes a nonhybrid protein, $p55^{v\text{-}myc}$, which would correspond to the viral oncogene sequences alone.[246] Both v-*myc*- and c-*myc*-encoded proteins are associated with the nuclear matrix.[247] The product of the AMV oncogene v-*myb* is a 45,000- or 48,000-Da protein, termed $p45^{v\text{-}myb}$ or $p48^{v\text{-}myb}$, respectively.[248,249] E26 ALV is an acute transforming virus whose genome contains two oncogenes, v-*myb* and v-*ets*.[67,250] The protein product of E26 ALV is a 135,000-Da tripartite protein, $p135^{gag\text{-}myb\text{-}ets}$ encoded by three genetic domains of the virus fused in the order *gag-myb-ets*.[47,25] Although the oncogenic properties of AMV and E26 ALV differ considerably, the protein products of both viruses are located in the nucleus of the transformed cells.[248] The product of FBR MuSV is a 55,000-Da protein, $p55^{v\text{-}fos}$, which is also predominantly located in the nucleus of the virus-transformed cells.[188]

The protein products of other acute viruses are located in the cytoplasm or other extranuclear cellular structures. The protein product of M-MuSV is a 37,000-Da phosphoprotein, $p37^{v\text{-}mos}$, which is predominantly a soluble cytoplasmic protein.[251] ASV PRCII and FSV share the oncogene v-*fps* and encode hybrid *gag-fps*-transforming proteins associated with different cytoplasmic fractions.[104] Virus mutants carrying insertions or large deletions in the 5′ portion of v-*fps* have reduced or absent transforming potential.[252,253] Tyrosine-specific protein kinase activity seems to be intact in these mutants, which suggests that sequences required for association of the oncogene protein product with cellular components are essential for preservation of the transforming capacity of acute retroviruses.

Other oncogene products are localized in the cell membrane and its associated structures, including adhesion plaques and cell-cell junctions. The protein products of the v-*ras* oncogene family, $p21^{v\text{-}ras}$, are located mainly on the plasma membrane.[254] The RSV oncogene protein product, $pp60^{v\text{-}src}$, the A-MuLV oncogene protein product, $p120^{gag\text{-}abl}$, and the protein product of the AEV oncogene, v-*erb*-B, are also associated with the plasma membrane.[255-257] The significance of these associations in relation to the mechanisms of cell transformation remains unclear. Many membrane-associated proteins produced by acute retroviruses, especially those of the tyrosine kinase family, are characterized by the presence of a bound fatty acid (myristate or palmitate) but there is no strict and general correlation between the presence of bound fatty acid and the membrane association of the viral products.[258]

VI. MECHANISMS OF TRANSFORMATION BY V-*ONC* PROTEIN PRODUCTS

Transformation induced by acute retroviruses may depend on derangement of particular cellular functions due to the continued presence within the cell of altered proteins corresponding to the products of retroviral oncogenes. Different acute retroviruses may employ different schemes for expressing their oncogenic potentiality.[259] Many cellular functions might be disturbed by the presence of products of acute viruses. The cellular localization of oncogene protein products may give clues in relation to their cellular mechanisms of action.

A. CONTINUED PRESENCE OF THE ONCOGENE PRODUCTS

The continued presence of a v-*onc* protein product with clear transforming ability may not be sufficient for the maintenance of the transformed phenotype in cells infected with acute retroviruses. A-MuLV-transformed mouse cells are able to differentiate without a decrease in the amount expressed or the specific kinase activity of the $p21^{gag\text{-}abl}$ product.[260] Persistent expression of the v-*mos* oncogene in M-MuSV-transformed mouse fibroblasts is compatible with their reversion to apparent nonmalignancy after prolonged treatment with α/β IFN.[199] Moreover, the reverted nonmalignant phenotype remains stable even after 60 to 100 passages in the absence of IFN. This reversion occurs in spite of the continued presence and expression of the v-*mos* oncogene from the integrated M-MuSV genome. The mechanism of such reversion is unknown but these observations clearly demonstrate that persistent integration of an acute retrovirus and persistent expression of its oncogene product is compatible with reversion to a nonmalignant phenotype.

The continued presence of a viral oncogene may not always be required for the maintenance of a malignant phenotype in oncogene-transformed cells. DNA sequences representing the v-*src* oncogene may be lost during successive passages of RSV-infected marmoset cells either *in vivo* or *in vitro*, but the transformed phenotype may persist in these cells, whose altered behavior does not depend any more on the presence of the v-*src* gene.[261] The mechanism of loss of the integrated viral oncogene may be associated with destabilization of the host cell genome. In turn, this destabilization may contribute to the continued expression of a transformed phenotype.

Perturbed hematopoiesis and the generation of multipotential stem cell clones in v-*src*-infected bone marrow cultures may be an indirect or transient effect of the oncogene.[262] Multipotential stem cell lines derived from long-term bone marrow cells infected with a recombinant M-MuLV carrying the v-*src* oncogene may lack the v-*src* gene. Thus, stable consequences of the infection must result from either direct, transient actions on the altered cells, by a sort of "hit-and-run" mechanism, or from indirect effects of v-*src* on other cells. The latter possibility is favored by the finding of a mosaic pattern of v-*src* expression in the marrow cultures.[262] However, other studies indicate that inactivation of the oncogene product in RSV-infected cells may result in reversion from the transformed phenotype to the normal phenotype. Inactivation of the pp60[v-*src*] by benzoquinoid ansamycin antibiotics (herbimycin, macbecin, and geldanamycin) in RSV-infected NRK cells results in morphological reversion of the transformed phenotype to normalcy.[263] Removal of the antibiotics results in the reappearance of the transformed morphology. Thus, at least in some cases the continued presence of the active oncogene product is required for the maintenance of the transformed phenotype in cells transformed by acute retroviruses.

B. CELL DIFFERENTIATION PROCESSES

Interference with the molecular processes involved in cell differentiation may be a common mechanism leading to neoplastic transformation induced by the oncogene products of acute retroviruses. Oncogene products may induce the neoplastic transformation of cells by blocking the normal mechanisms associated with cell differentiation. Immature cells can be more readily transformed by acute retroviruses and infection with these viruses may result in a block in the normal differentiation pathway. The target cells for AEV-induced neoplastic transformation are early erythroid precursors,[264] which may explain the induction of erythroblastosis by AEV *in vivo*.

Acute retroviruses whose oncogenes have different functional properties (v-*fes*, v-*ras*, v-*abl*, and v-*src*) can all induce transformation of early B-lineage cells *in vitro*, which results in cell lines that possess rearrangements at the Ig heavy chain locus.[265] A-MuLV-transformed cell lines have been used for the characterization of the molecular mechanisms responsible for the sequential rearrangements of Ig genes associated with the early stages of B-cell differentiation.[231,266] The v-*myc* oncogene from HB1 AMCV can induce expansion of stem cell population and preneoplastic transformation of lymphoid B cells in a bursal transplantation assay.[267,268] The preneoplastically transformed lymphoid cells fail to differentiate but are not malignant and no active protooncogenes are detected in these cells by means of the NIH/3T3 DNA transfection assay. It is difficult to distinguish between a direct effect of the oncogene products on the expression of the cellular developmental program and an indirect effect resulting from disruption of the control of cell proliferation that would prevent the necessary withdrawal from the cell cycle.[269]

Expression of viral oncogenes may be compatible with normal cellular differentiation processes. Progeny cells from pluripotent multilineage hematopoietic colonies may show no obvious alteration after infection of the blast cells with H-MuSV in spite of the fact that they express the p21[v-*ras*] product.[270] Thus, expression of the v-*ras* oncogene does not preclude maturation of the hematopoietic progenitors. Viral oncogene products may not always transform target cells by simply blocking differentiation processes.[271] Moreover, a block of cell differentiation is apparently not an indispensable requisite for the immortalizing action of viral oncogene products.[272,273] The relationship between oncogene-induced neoplastic transformation and alteration of the cell differentiation program may not be a simple one. Uncontrolled growth of hematopoietic precursors induced by acute retroviruses or their oncogene products needs not be accompanied by a block of differentiation.[274] AEV-infected cells pursue their differentiation and then become transformed.[275] Whereas chick myelomonocytic cells transformed by the v-*myb* oncogene exhibit an immature phenotype, those transformed by the v-*myc* oncogene resemble mature macrophages.[276] Thus, retroviruses that cause hematopoietic malignancies can transform cells and produce an apparently uncontrolled cell growth through mechanisms that do not necessarily involve a complete blockade in the processes of cell differentiation. Even when interrupted by the action of the transforming gene, the epigenetic program of the transformed cells may not be irreversibly canceled but can be reassumed when the action of the transforming virus is suppressed.[277]

In certain types of cells the oncogene products of acute retroviruses may not suppress but enhance the expression of differentiated functions. For example, expression of a v-*myc* oncogene in cultured mouse mammary epithelial cells (HC14 cells) results in an estimated 50-fold increased induction of β-casein protein and at least a 60-fold increase in β-casein mRNA.[278] Production of β-casein is stimulated in HC14 cells by lactogenic hormones (cortisol, insulin, and prolactin). However, expression of v-*myc* in HC14 cells does not totally abrogate the requirement for the lactogenic hormones, since they are still required for a maximal synergistic response. Introduction of the v-H-*ras* oncogene into cultured human medullary thyroid carcinoma cells results in the acquisition of increased endocrine differentiation properties by these cells, with decreased cell proliferation and DNA synthesis.[279]

C. PLASMA MEMBRANE AND CYTOSKELETON

The plasma membrane of cells transformed by acute retroviruses may exhibit important structural and functional alterations. As in other types of neoplastically transformed cells, the cells transformed by acute retroviruses show an increased glucose uptake. Malignant transformation of cells by RSV results in a marked increase in the rate of hexose transport across the plasma membrane. Interestingly, the mechanism of this increase appears to be different in different types of cells. Whereas in chicken cells (CEF cells) RSV-induced transformation affects predominantly the rate at which the glucose transporter is turned over, in rodent cells (Rat-1 cells) the v-*src* oncogene affects primarily the rate of transporter biosynthesis.[280] REF cells expressing the v-*fms* oncogene as a consequence of FeSV infection exhibit a marked increase in the uptake of (^{3}H)-deoxyglucose and reversion of these cells to the normal phenotype by treatment with the glycosylation processing inhibitor, castanospermine, is associated with a severalfold decrease in (^{3}H)-deoxyglucose uptake.[160] The inhibitor decreases the association of the gp140[v-*fms*] product with the plasma membrane.

Particular components of the plasma membrane may be altered upon expression of oncogene protein products. Acidic glycosphingolipids, which are characterized by a higher degree of sialylation, are markedly altered in mouse fibroblasts (BALB/c 3T3 cells) after transfection with a plasmid carrying the v-H-*ras* oncogene.[281] Transformation of the hamster fibroblast cell line Nil-8 with the hamster sarcoma virus (a derivative of H-MuSV) is associated with changes in N-linked glycan processing of different glycoproteins and can exert selective effects at different glycosylation sites on particular polypeptide chains.[282] Transfection into the rat fibroblastic cell line 3Y1 of several viral oncogenes (v-*ras*, v-*src*, v-*fes*, and v-*fps*), whose products are located at extranuclear sites, results in induction of synthesis of sialosylparagloboside, which is a very rare ganglioside in normal rat cells.[283] In contrast, transfection of 3Y1 cells with oncogenes coding for products with intranuclear localization results in neosynthesis of GD3 ganglioside.[284] These results suggest that oncogenes may activate sialyltransferases and that this alteration may lead to structural and functional disturbances at the level of the plasma membrane. Such changes may contribute to the expression of a transformed phenotype and/or to the escape from immunosurveillance mechanisms by the tumor cells.

Transformed cells exhibit important alterations in the cytoskeletal system. One of the early cellular changes in M-MuSV-induced malignant transformation of NRK cells is an alteration in cell morphology and cytoplasmic microtubule complex, followed by diminution of F-actin cables.[285] It is generally recognized that the microtubule-microfilament system is crucially involved in the transformation process.

D. ADENYLATE CYCLASE SYSTEM

Regulation of the adenylate cyclase system may be disturbed by the presence of viral oncogene products such as v-*ras* p21 proteins.[286,287] However, the role of this alteration in the expression of a transformed phenotype is unclear and it may be secondary to other cellular changes induced by oncogene functions. Studies with site-selective cAMP analogs tested for their growth regulatory effects on H-MuSV-transformed NIH/3T3 clone 13-3B-4 cells grown in a serum-free defined medium have yielded interesting results.[288] The analogs are capable of exerting a major regulatory effect on the growth of the v-H-*ras*-transformed cells. However, a mere decrease or increase in the intracellular level of cAMP does not appear to determine neoplastic transformation or reverse transformation, respectively, but the cellular cAMP effectors, cAMP-dependent protein kinases, play an important role in these processes.

E. PROTEIN PHOSPHORYLATION

Tyrosine-specific protein kinase activity is present in the protein products of most members of the v-*src* oncogene family, including the products of v-*src*, v-*yes*, v-*abl*, v-*fes/fps*, v-*fgr*, v-*fms*, v-*ros*, v-*kit*, and v-*erb*-B.[289-293] A similar activity is involved in the normal cellular mechanisms of action of several hormones and growth factors, including insulin, IGF-I, EGF, TGFs, PDGF, and acidic FGF.[294-298] Moreover, tyrosine protein kinase activity is present in normal, terminally differentiated cells.[299] The exact role of this activity in the malignant transformation of cells is not understood, but there is evidence that tyrosine phosphorylation of specific cellular substrates may be of critical importance for transformation induced by the oncogene protein products possessing this type of kinase activity. For example, the product of ASV UR2 is the fusion protein p68$^{gag-ros}$, and the characterization of *ts* mutants of UR2 virus indicates that p68$^{gag-ros}$ is associated with the membrane of UR2-infected cells at both the permissive and nonpermissive temperatures, but tyrosine protein kinase activity is greatly reduced at the nonpermissive temperature.[300] These results suggest that p68$^{gag-ros}$ is a membrane-associated protein whose specific kinase activity plays a crucial role in UR2-mediated cell transformation. Similar results have been obtained with other acute retroviruses whose oncogene products possess tyrosine-specific protein kinase activity. The study of mutants of the v-*abl* oncogene which are temperature-sensitive for transformation indicates that the specific tyrosine protein kinase activity of the hybrid p210$^{gag-abl}$ product is crucial to its transforming function.[301,302] Moreover, the v-*abl*-associated tyrosine kinase activity is required to maintain the transformed phenotype because cells transformed with the *ts* kinase mutants revert back to normal morphology shortly after a shift to the nonpermissive temperature. The thermolabile phosphorylation, kinase activity, and transforming ability of p140$^{gag-fps}$ encoded by a *ts* FeSV variant are restored at the nonpermissive temperature for transformation by incubation of the infected cells with sodium orthovanadate.[303] This compound is an efficient inhibitor of phosphotyrosyl phosphatases and augments the content of phosphotyrosine in the treated cells, which may result in the reversible expression of a transformed phenotype.[304]

In addition to their intrinsic tyrosine-specific protein kinase, acute retroviruses whose oncogenes possess this activity can secondarily induce an increase in the activity of cellular kinases with specificity for serine and threonine residues. For example, infection of mouse thymocytes with A-MuLV results in the induction of a remarkable increment of protein kinase C activity in both soluble and particulate cellular functions.[305] A similar increment is observed in casein kinase-2 activity in the A-MuLV-transformed cells, while cAMP-dependent protein kinase and casein kinase-1 do not undergo significant changes. In contrast, thymocytes infected with the chronic retrovirus M-MuLV, which do not possess oncogene sequences, do not exhibit increased protein kinase C activity, although the activity of casein kinase-2 is augmented in the M-MuLV-infected cells. The results suggest that the rise of protein kinase C activity in A-MuLV-transformed cells is directly or indirectly augmented by the tyrosine protein kinase associated with the v-*abl* oncogene product.[305] The role of protein kinases in A-MuLV-induced transformation is not understood, however.

In cells transformed by acute retroviruses whose oncogene products possess tyrosine-specific protein kinase activity, at least some of the transformation parameters may depend on biochemical lesions residing at sites downstream of substrate phosphorylation by the specific tyrosine kinase. Revertants of mink cells transformed by the Gardner-Arnstein strain of FeSV expressed high levels of the v-*fes* oncogene product and its associated tyrosine protein kinase activity, but were contact inhibited and unable to grow in semisolid medium in spite of expressing wild-type levels of the kinase and cellular phosphotyrosine-containing proteins at levels indistinguishable from those of the fully transformed parental cell line.[200] However, the revertant cells had tumorigenic potential.

Tyrosine protein kinase activity is absent in the oncogene products of other members of the v-*src* oncogene family, including the products of v-*raf/ mil* and v-*mos*, as well as in the protein products of other oncogenes. The protein products of oncogenes with tyrosine-specific protein kinase activity may also have kinase activity with specificity for the phosphorylation of serine and threonine residues, and a similar type of activity may be present in the protein products of oncogenes with no tyrosine protein kinase activity.[306] Kinase activity is possibly also associated with the product of the REV-T virus, the protein p59$^{v\text{-}rel}$.[307] This protein contains the first 12 amino acid residues of the *env* polyprotein signal sequence of the REV-T genome. The translation product of the MH2 acute retrovirus is the hybrid protein of 100 kDa, p100$^{gag\text{-}mil}$. The biological effects of this product, including its ability for inducing the production of myelomonocytic growth factor by v-*myc*-transformed chicken macrophages and the sustained proliferation of chicken neuroretinal cells, are mediated by the phosphorylation at serine/threonine residues of key cellular substrates.[308] Substitution of lysine 622 for methionine in the ATP-binding domain of p100$^{gag\text{-}mil}$ by site-directed mutagenesis results in the inactivation of serine/threonine-specific autophosphorylation of p100$^{gag\text{-}mil}$ and suppression of the biological characteristics of the oncogene product.

F. MONOVALENT AND DIVALENT CATIONS

In addition to protein phosphorylation, many other different types of biochemical changes may occur in cells infected by acute retroviruses, including changes in calcium compartments and fluxes.[309] A serum growth factor-independent intracellular alkalinization produced by activation of the Na$^+$/H$^+$ antiporter is observed in cells transformed with oncogenes such as v-*mos* or the activated form of c-H-*ras*.[310] This may lead to cytoplasmic alkalinization, alteration of the mitogenic signal response, and initiation of DNA synthesis. The normal c-H-*ras* protooncogene does not induce intracellular alkalinization and has only a weak mitogenic effect. The possible role of these changes in the origin and expression of the transformed phenotype are not understood.

G. PHOSPHOINOSITIDE METABOLISM

Metabolic breakdown of phosphoinositol by activation of phospholipase C results in the generation, via inositol mono- and bisphosphate intermediators, of inositol-1,4,5 trisphosphate, which induces intracellular mobilization of Ca^{2+}, and 1,2-diacylglycerol, which activates protein kinase C. These biochemical changes may be associated with important physiological effects, including the activation of particular mitogenic signals.[311-313]

The products of certain oncogene products may induce an activation of phosphoinositide metabolism. An example of this activation is represented by the cellular action of the v-*fms* oncogene that is contained in the acute retrovirus SM-FeSV, which was isolated from a spontaneously arising fibrosarcoma of a domestic cat.[314] The v-*fms* oncogene is able to transform fibroblast cell lines of several mammalian species.[157,315] SM-FeSV is also capable of inducing clonal proliferation of bone marrow progenitors *in vivo*, which may ultimately result in malignancies of different hematopoietic lineages.[316] The primary translation product of the SM-FeSV genome is a *gag-fms* fusion protein consisting of 536 amino-terminal *gag*-encoded residues and 975 carboxy-terminal v-*fms*-encoded amino acids. Addition of carbohydrate to this polypeptide chain yields a 180-kDa glycoprotein, gp180$^{gag\text{-}fms}$, and the subsequent cellular processing of this glycoprotein leads to a 140-kDa oncogene product, gp140$^{v\text{-}fms}$, which is expressed in a receptor-like manner at the level of the cell membrane.[317] The protein product of the respective protooncogene, c-*fms*, is identical to the receptor for an important hematopoietic growth factor, the macrophage colony-stimulating factor (M-CSF), also named colony-stimulating factor 1 (CSF-1).[318] The protein products of v-*fms* and c-*fms* genes differ at the extreme carboxyl terminus but are apparently identical at the extracellular amino-terminal, ligand-binding domain expressed at the cell surface. Transformation induced by the v-*fms* oncogene does not depend, however, on an exogenous source of CSF-1, and neutralizing antibodies to CSF-1 do not affect the transformed phenotype. The v-*fms* product is apparently capable of functioning as an unregulated enzyme in the absence of the growth factor ligand.[319] The altered structure at the carboxyl terminus of the v-*fms* protein may affect the tyrosine kinase activity of the v-*fms*-coded receptor-like protein. The v-*fms* products in membranes of SM-FeSV-infected cells exhibit tyrosine phosphorylation in the absence of CSF-1 and this phosphorylation is not enhanced by addition of CSF-1.[317] Moreover, cells transformed by v-*fms* have a constitutively elevated specific activity of a guanine nucleotide-dependent phospholipase C that activates phosphoinositide turnover.

The cellular effects of v-*ras* oncogene products may be intimately associated with alterations of phosphoinositide metabolism. In particular, the v-*ras* protein products may alter the effects of growth factors in the activation of phospholipase C-mediated phosphoinositide hydrolysis.[320] A revertant cell line (C11), derived from K-MuSV-transformed NIH/3T3 cells (DT cells), expresses high levels of the v-K-*ras* p21 product and rescuable transforming virus but is morphologically untransformed and is resistant to the transforming effects of the viral oncogene protein.[321] C11 cells have reduced levels of protein kinase C when compared to v-*ras*-sensitive NIH/3T3 cells and do not have the ability to phosphorylate an 80-kDa substrate of protein kinase C.[322] In addition, in C11 cells phosphoinositide levels return from elevated as in the transformed DT cells to those observed in parental NIH/3T3 cells. These results suggest the existence of a correlation between a protein kinase C-dependent cellular metabolic pathway and the expression of a K-MuSV-induced transformed phenotype.

H. HOST CELL GENOME FUNCTIONS

The predominant localization of certain oncogene products within the nucleus suggests a possible role for these products in regulation of the host cell genome functions. An alteration of genomic functions has been detected in cells infected by different acute retroviruses, with activation of some previously inactive cellular genes,[269,323,324] possibly including protooncogenes. Expression of a viral oncogene such as v-*myb* does not necessarily prevent the expression of the respective endogenous protooncogene.[325] Some oncogene products may not activate, but may inactivate specific genes, especially those whose function is related to cell differentiation processes. For example, the product of the v-*erb*-A oncogene from AEV specifically suppresses transcription of the cellular erythrocyte anion transporter (band 3) gene which is involved in erythroid differentiation.[326] Not only can the products of viral oncogenes that are primarily or predominantly localized within the nucleus induce alterations in cell genome regulation, but also the products of oncogenes with a membrane or cytoplasmic localization such as the v-H-*ras* protein, which is associated with the plasma membrane.[327] One possible mechanism by which viral oncogenes induce neoplastic transformation is by disruption of the activity of the respective protooncogene through a kind of dominant negative effect.[328] However, it is not known if alterations in host cell genome functions are a necessary prerequisite or rather a consequence of the process of malignant transformation.

I. REQUIREMENT FOR EXOGENOUS GROWTH FACTORS AND AUTOCRINE STIMULATION

Infection of cells by acute retroviruses may result in the partial or complete abolishment of the requirement for the exogenous supply of specific hormones and growth factors.[298] For example, infection of differentiated, TSH-responsive rat thyroid cell lines with acute retroviruses carrying the oncogenes v-H-*ras*, v-K-*ras*, v-*mos*, v-*raf*, or v-*src* results in the suppression of the requirement for six exogenous growth factors, and the cells become independent of TSH for their growth.[329] These observations, and the fact that the products of several oncogenes have been shown to be structurally and functionally similar to growth factors or their receptors, led to the suggestion that the relatively autonomous growth of oncogene-transformed cells may be due to the endogenous production of growth factors which would act, via specific receptors, on the same cells that produce them.[330] However, such an autocrine mechanism is apparently not universally involved in the neoplastic transformation of cells induced by acute retroviruses or cloned oncogenes. Neither the autonomous proliferation nor the spontaneous differentiation of A-MuLV-induced leukemic cell transformation seems to involve autocrine secretion of growth factors.[331]

Cells expressing a viral oncogene may initially require the presence of specific growth factors to become oncogenically transformed. For example, primary mammary gland epithelial cells transfected with a molecular vector containing the v-H-*ras* oncogene require the presence of EGF and insulin in the medium to grow in soft agar and to display tumorigenic properties.[332] However, these cells progress to growth factor-independent growth at higher passage numbers. In any case, the effects of v-H-*ras* on diploid normal mammary epithelial cells are dependent on the concentration of the oncogene product and high levels of v-H-*ras* expression are required to overcome density arrest of cell division, to cause morphological change, and to induce growth in semisolid medium and tumorigenicity.

Cells infected with acute retroviruses or transfected with cloned viral oncogenes may exhibit altered responses to exogenous growth factors. For example, Chinese hamster lung fibroblast cells (CC239 cell line) transfected with a plasmid vector expressing the v-*fps* oncogene exhibit a high level of tyrosine-specific protein kinase activity and a reduced requirement for exogenous growth factors.[337] Moreover, these cells are hypersensitive to growth factor stimulation and acquire metastatic potential even when their growth factor requirements are not abrogated, but simply reduced.

Oncogene-transformed cells may produce endogenous growth factors and may utilize them in an autocrine fashion or may become independent of the exogenous supply of growth factors by other mechanisms.[298] The autocrine hypothesis of oncogene action is supported by the findings that oncogenes may encode proteins that are structurally and functionally similar to growth factors or growth factor receptors. The products of viral oncogenes such as the v-*sis* protein, which is functionally equivalent to PDGF, can interact not only with the specific receptors located on the cell surface but also with receptors located on intracellular compartments, which may result in functional activation of the receptors.[334]

TGFs are frequently produced by cells transformed with acute retroviruses.[335-340] High amounts of both TGF-α and TGF-β are produced and secreted by SSV-transformed NRK cells.[341] As a result of this secretion, SSV-transformed NRK cells have greatly reduced ability to bind external growth factors such as PDGF and EGF and can be cultured in the absence of externally added growth factors. Since TGF-α and TGF-β in combination are sufficient to induce phenotypic transformation of NRK cells, it may be concluded that the expression of TGF cellular genes might well be essential for transformation induced by SSV. TGFs, especially TGF-α, are also produced by rodent cells transfected with activated c-*ras* oncogenes,[342,343] The oncogene-induced activation of TGF-α expression may occur at the transcriptional level. PDGF or PDGF-like mitogenic factors can also be produced by cells expressing a v-*ras* oncogene, but not by cells expressing the pp60[v-*src*] oncoprotein.[344] Endogenous growth factors produced by cells infected with acute retroviruses may play an important role in the process of their neoplastic transformation as well as in the continued expression of a transformed phenotype.

Endogenous production and secretion of growth factors may contribute in either an autocrine or paracrine manner to the expression of a transformed phenotype in cells expressing viral oncogenes. AEV-transformed chicken erythroleukemia cells secrete into the medium several different factors that are both mitogenic and enable normal CEF cells and NIH/3T3 cells to form colonies in soft agar.[345] Secretion of these factors depends on the expression of the v-*erb*-B oncogene contained in the AEV genome, as demonstrated with *ts* mutants of the virus. In addition, the AEV-transformed cells secrete a 40-kDa nonmitogenic factor which indirectly promotes the proliferation of hematopoietic cells by preventing their differentiation into proliferating inactive erythroid cells.

Abrogation of the requirement for exogenous supply of specific growth factors may be observed in cells that constitutively express a receptor corresponding to the altered version of the normal growth factor receptor. The v-*erb*-B oncogene represents an amino-terminal truncated form of the EGF receptor with constitutive tyrosine-specific protein kinase activity. Transfection of an expression vector containing the v-*erb*-B oncogene into the 32D myeloid cell line, which is devoid of EGF receptors and absolutely dependent on IL-3 for its proliferation and survival, results not only in abrogation of the requirement of exogenous supply of IL-3 but also the cells become tumorigenic when transplanted into nude mice.[346]

Cooperation between growth factors and oncogene protein products may be instrumental for the expression of a transformed phenotype. The results obtained with *ts* mutants of MH2 virus, which transduces two oncogenes (v-*mil* and v-*myc*), indicate that the gene products of both oncogenes may function independently of each other and that, whereas v-*mil* is necessary for the maintenance of cell proliferation by inducing the production of a growth factor (the chicken myelomonocytic growth factor), v-*myc* is required to maintain a transformed phenotype in the infected macrophages.[74] Mouse fibroblasts (BALB/c 3T3 cells) transformed by the v-*myc* oncogene require only insulin and PDGF or EGF for anchorage-dependent growth, but only PDGF or coexpression of a v-*ras* oncogene can induce sustained anchorage-independent growth in these cells.[347]

Infection of multilineage hematopoietic colonies with A-MuLV results in the production of an hematopoietic growth factor, CSF-2.[348] Infection of Friend cells, mast cells, myeloid cells, or lymphoid cells with A-MuLV results in abrogation of the requirement for exogenous supply of IL-3.[349-354] A-MuLV has a similar effect on IL-2-dependent T lymphocytes, relieving these cells from the exogenous supply of IL-2.[355] Expression of a cloned v-*src* oncogene in the IL-3-dependent murine cell line FD.C/1 results in IL-3 independence.[356] In contrast, the requirement of the IL-2-dependent murine cell line CTLL-2 for the specific factor is not abrogated by v-*src* oncogene expression. The mechanisms of the oncogene-induced abrogations of growth factor requirement are little understood but do not seem to necessarily involve an autocrine phenomenon with endogenous production of the growth factor and expression of its receptor.[331] Moreover, growth factor abrogation occurs in only a small fraction of the cells expressing the oncogene, suggesting that its expression is not sufficient for the acquisition of growth factor independence and that secondary progression events are crucially involved in the acquisition of growth factor-independent growth. Oncogene-transformed cells may remain dependent on the supply of exogenous growth factors. Infection of a murine helper/inducer T cell clone (D10.G4) with K-MuSV results in altered mitogenic response to certain cytokines (IL-1, IL-2, and BSF-1), but the infected cells remain dependent on exogenous factors for continued growth.[357]

The MCF-7 human breast cancer cell line responds to estrogen stimulation by increased secretion of growth factors and proliferation *in vitro* and by tumor formation in nude mice *in vivo*. Transfection of a v-H-*ras* oncogene into these cells results in tumorigenicity in the absence of estrogens as well as in elevated levels of secreted growth factors which include TGF-α, TGF-β, and IGF-I.[358] Furthermore, conditioned medium from the MCF-7 cells transfected with the v-H-*ras* oncogene can replace estrogen in stimulating MCF-7 colony formation *in vitro*. These results strongly suggest that v-*onc*-induced transformation may be mediated, at least in part, by the production and secretion of particular growth factors which may function as mitogens in an autocrine manner.[359] However, the abrogation of growth factor requirement in v-*onc*-transformed cells could occur by pathways different from the endogenous production of growth factors.

Production of specific endogenous growth factors by certain types of cells may alter their susceptibility to transformation by acute retroviruses. For example, mutants of the MC29 AMCV whose v-*myc* protein product contains amino acid deletions in the central part of the protein are not able to transform chicken bone marrow cells but can induce transformation in quail macrophages.[360] These results suggest that quail macrophages produce endogenous growth factors which act like chicken macrophage growth factor to complement v-*myc* functions, resulting in stably transformed macrophage cell lines which grow in the absence of exogenously added growth factors.

Expression of receptors for specific growth factors may be required for the malignant behavior of cells transformed by acute retroviruses. A-MuLV-transformed fibroblasts lacking the EGF receptor are not tumorigenic in nude mice.[361] In addition, cells infected with acute retroviruses may express high levels of receptors for specific growth factors. For example, myeloid cell lines infected by the malignant histiocytosis virus (MHSV), formerly called AF-1,[362] which contains v-H-*ras*-related oncogene sequences, express unusually high levels of receptors for various CSFs.[363] Such expression of growth factor receptors may be causally related to the transformed state through mechanisms of a nonautocrine nature.

Known growth factors such as TGFs and PDGF, or molecules similar to these factors, are produced by many cells transformed by acute retroviruses.[364-367] Some growth factors produced by cells transformed by acute retroviruses remain poorly characterized.[368,369] These factors are probably not specific of transformation induced by acute retroviruses but may be also produced by cells transformed by other agents and may be even produced by a variety of normal cells. A correlation may exist between the ability of a cell to respond to growth factors and its susceptibility to transformation by acute retroviruses such as K-MuSV and A-MuLV.[370] The expression of a viral oncogene and the production of growth factors may be necessary, but not sufficient, to maintain the transformed phenotype in cells infected by acute retroviruses. Flat revertants of cell lines derived from K-MuSV-transformed cells do not exhibit all the properties associated with transformation in spite of the fact that they express the v-K-*ras* oncogene and produce TGFs.[371] These results indicate that the expression of a transformed phenotype may be blocked at a point distal to the expression of oncogene products and growth factors such as TGFs.

J. NUCLEOCYTOPLASMIC TRANSPORT AND EXPRESSION OF NUCLEAR PROTEINS

Nucleocytoplasmic transport of ions and macromolecules may have great influence on essential nuclear functions such as DNA synthesis and gene expression. Hormones and growth factors are involved in the normal regulation of diffusion-mediated nuclear transport of macromolecules. K-MuSV-induced transformation of mouse 3T3 fibroblasts results in maximally stimulated nuclear transport rates which are not further enhanced by the addition of growth factors.[372]

Certain nuclear proteins are crucially involved in the regulation of genomic functions. Transformation of cells by different acute retroviruses (ASV, K-Mu-SV, H-MuSV, M-MuSV), as well as by polyoma virus, results enhanced expression of nuclear phosphoproteins of the high mobility group, designated HMG proteins.[373] While some of these proteins (HMG14 and HMG17) are normally present in all terminally differentiated mammalian and avian cells examined so far, appearance of high levels of other particular types, described as HMGI-like proteins, show a strong correlation to acute retrovirus-independent neoplastic transformation. The function of HMGI-like proteins is unknown but at least one of these proteins binds preferentially to DNA containing stretches of adenine and thymine and may be associated with satellite chromatin.

K. EXPRESSION OF CELLULAR ANTIGENS

Changes in the expression of particular cellular antigens are observed in cells infected with acute retroviruses or transfected with cloned viral oncogenes. For example, human melanocytes transformed by H-MuSV of K-MuSV express class II MHC antigens that are not present in normal melanocytes.[374] Mouse fibroblasts infected with the chronic retrovirus M-MuLV express increased levels of H-2 antigens on the cell surface, but this increase is not evident when the cells are coinfected with the acute retrovirus M-MuSV.[375] However, the possible role of these changes in v-*onc*-induced transformation is not understood. Pre-B cell lymphomas induced by retroviruses whose oncogene products are expressed at extranuclear sites, but not those expressing the intranuclear v-*myc* product, are positive for the presence of a cell surface antigen, which is a glycoprotein of 160 kDa.[376] This glycoprotein is detected by the monoclonal antigen 6C3 and is named gp160[6C3]. Although expression of gp160[6C3] is associated with acquisition of a fully transformed phenotype in early B lymphocytes, it is not known whether its expression is directly involved in the origin of B cell neoplasms. The same antigen is expressed at low levels in normal thymocytes and bone marrow cells.

Cells infected with acute retroviruses may not express MHC antigens on the cell surface. Since cytotoxic T lymphocytes recognize foreign antigen in the context of self MHC antigens, lack of expression of these antigens induced by viral products in cells transformed by acute retroviruses or other viruses may contribute to elude the immune mechanisms of the host. Infection of murine embryo fibroblasts with K-MuSV results in abolishment of the inducibility of IFN-γ expression of class II MHC antigens, and this effect is probably due to the v-K-*ras* oncogene.[377]

L. COOPERATION BETWEEN ACUTE RETROVIRUSES AND OTHER VIRUSES

Cells infected with chronic retroviruses may acquire tumorigenic properties when they are superinfected with an acute retrovirus. Murine myeloid cells immortalized by the chronic retrovirus, F-MuLV, are converted into tumorigenic cells lines upon superinfection with the acute retrovirus, A-MuLV, which transduces the v-*abl* oncogene.[349] The v-*abl* oncogene is not able *per se* to convert myeloid cells obtained from normal mouse bone marrow into growth factor-independent cell lines and at least another previous genetic change is required for such a conversion. However, another viral oncogene, v-H-*ras*, is unable to induce the malignant conversion of F-MuLV-infected cells.[349]

Expression of acute retroviruses may be altered when the cells are infected by a DNA virus. The M-MuSV LTR harbors two distinct positive activators of transcription, namely, a distal signal and an enhancer, and infection by HSV can markedly affect the utilization of these two transcription signals.[378]

VII. MULTISTAGE PROCESSES IN TRANSFORMATION INDUCED BY ACUTE RETROVIRUSES

The speed which would characterize acute retroviruses for the completion of a transformed phenotype in infected cells has been considered as exceptional. It has been taken as a proof that at least some oncogenic agents can transform cells by a kind of one-step process leading directly from a normal condition to malignancy and autonomy. A single component of the virus genome, the oncogene, would be responsible through its specific oncoprotein product of conferring to the infected cells the rapid appearance of a transformed phenotype. However, several lines of evidence suggest that the oncogenic transformation induced by acute retroviruses is a multistep process and that this process is at least partially subjected to environmental influences acting through epigenetic regulatory phenomena.[379-381]

A. CLONALITY OF TUMORS INDUCED BY ACUTE RETROVIRUSES

Tumors induced *in vivo* by acute retroviruses such as A-MuLV are usually clonal, which would not be expected if many cells are transformed by the potent oncogenic properties of the virus.[382] The simplest interpretation to these results is that very few cells are initially transformed *in vivo* by the acute retrovirus and that this very early event constitutes the rate-limiting step in the disease. Within clones of initially transformed cells, subsequent events should occur to increase the tumorigenic efficiencies of the transformed cells. The exact role of the viral oncogene or endogenous protooncogenes in promoting these secondary events is not known. Malignant progression of K-MuSV-transformed mouse fibroblasts (BALB/c 3T3 cells) is associated with amplification, rearrangement, and overexpression of the v-K-*ras* oncogene, in relation to the originally infected and transformed cell population.[383] These subsequent changes may give a selective advantage to a subpopulation of cells for invasion and metastasization after inoculation into athymic mice.

B. SUSCEPTIBILITY OF DIFFERENT CELLS TO TRANSFORMATION INDUCED BY RETROVIRAL ONCOGENES

Transformation by acute retroviruses may be rapid, lasting for only a few weeks, when either established cell lines or embryo cultures are used as a test system. However, established cell lines have probably undergone some initial changes in the progression to malignancy, i.e., they are already premalignant cells, and infection by an acute virus may represent only the last step.[384] Chicken and rodent embryo cultures, although usually considered to be "normal", have many characteristics in common with malignant cells. Transformation induced by K-MuSV can remain latent for several months through suppression of the transformed phenotype by epigenetic factors.[379] Physiologically occurring environmental factors, including factors contained in serum, regulate the progression of v-K-*ras*-induced transformation in populations of freshly explanted adult rat adrenal cells, in the continued presence of elevated levels of p21^{v-ras}.[381] Furthermore, the transformed phenotype induced by K-MuSV in the cultured cells (explants from adult rat adrenal cortex) can be reversed to epithelial-like morphology and the growth rate can be reduced by changes in the culture medium. The full transformation of K-MuSV-infected adrenal cortex cultures after many passages in 25% fetal bovine serum is not accompanied by increased expression of p21^{v-ras} since both early- and late-passage cells synthesize similar amounts of the K-MuSV oncogene product, which suggests that additional genetic and/or epigenetic alterations would be required for the progression of the cells to an overtly transformed phenotype.[385]

In cultured rat thyroid cells the infection with a *ts* mutant of K-MuSV demonstrates the interesting fact that the expression of malignant properties may be dissociated from an alteration in the expression of differentiated functions.[212] Whereas a reversion of the transformed phenotype is observed at the nonpermissive temperature, a persistent blockade of differentiated thyroid cell functions (iodide uptake and thyroglobulin synthesis) occurs at the same temperature. Apparently, the previous action of the p21^{v-ras} product irreversibly altered some transcriptional processes required for the expression of normal differentiated functions but the expression of a malignant phenotype would require the continued expression of the v-K-*ras* protein product. Revertants of H-MuSV-transformed MDCK cells express reduced levels of p21^{v-ras} and possess a more normal phenotype.[386]

Normal Syrian hamster embryo (SHE) cells in culture, which are stable nontumorigenic cells when injected in nude mice, remained nontumorigenic after transfection with the v-H-*ras* oncogene cloned in a plasmid vector.[380] In contrast, a preneoplastic cell line (DES-4), isolated after treatment of SHE cells with the human carcinogen diethylstilbestrol (DES), was highly susceptible to transformation following transfection with the same cloned v-H-*ras* oncogene. There was a good correlation between tumorigenicity and expression of v-H-*ras* in the latter cells but the cell clones were highly variable in terms of their latency periods for tumorigenicity *in vivo* and anchorage-independent growth *in vitro* and neither of these two parameters correlated with the level of expression of v-H-*ras* RNA. These results suggest that v-H-*ras* expression is necessary, but not sufficient, for the tumorigenicity of DES-4 cells.[380] The results may be compared with those obtained in transfection of a cloned v-*src* gene.[387] Transfection of v-*src* into early passage SHE cells resulted in a low but significant number of tumors when the treated cells are injected into nude mice. The tumors were formed only after long latency periods (14 weeks). In contrast, several different carcinogen-induced preneoplastic immortal SHE cell lines were highly susceptible to transformation by the v-*src* oncogene and tumors were formed with high efficiency and a short latency period. The mechanisms responsible for the relative resistance of normal, diploid SHE cells to the transforming action of the v-*src* oncogene were not characterized but the results are consistent with a multistep model involving initial suppression of the transfected v-*src* oncogene and subsequent loss of the cellular factors responsible for this suppression.[387]

The v-*myc* oncogene may confer to rat embryo fibroblasts (REF cells) in primary culture a series of new properties, including immortality and reduced requirement for serum, but do not induce the appearance of transformed foci. However, a constructed murine retrovirus, termed MMCV, carrying a v-*myc* oncogene from OK10 ALV, was able to transform fibroblasts of established cell lines (mouse NIH/3T3 and rat 208F cells) to anchorage-independent growth in agarose.[115] MMCV also induced transformation of mouse macrophages to increased proliferative capacity.

C. COOPERATION BETWEEN DIFFERENT VIRAL ONCOGENES

Different viral oncogenes may have complementary effects on cell proliferation and the expression of differentiated properties. Moreover, it has been suggested that cooperation between different oncogenes, including v-*myc*, may result in the induction of neoplastic transformation.[388-391] Cultured chicken embryo chondroblasts are induced to proliferate by expression of the v-*myc* protein product but the cells continue to express the chondroblast-specific products (type II collagen and cartilage-type sulfated proteoglycan).[392] In contrast to v-*myc*, expression of v-*src* appears to have an effect on the synthesis of the differentiated cell products which is independent on its effects of cell proliferation. The combined effect of v-*myc* and v-*mil* oncogenes in the MH2 retrovirus provides a stronger suppression of the chondroblast phenotype than can be produced by expression of v-*src*.[393] No chondroblast products can be detected in the MH2-infected cells and their morphology is completely distinct from that of normal chondroblasts.

Multiple examples may be given in which it is demonstrated that cooperation between two different oncogene functions can determine the malignant transformation of susceptible cells under specific experimental conditions. The v-*erb*-A oncogene cooperates with sarcoma virus oncogenes in the leukemic transformation of cells.[393] Synergistic action of v-*myc* and v-H-*ras* is observed in the *in vitro* neoplastic progression of murine lymphoid cells.[394] The oncogene v-*mil* induces autocrine growth and enhances tumorigenicity in v-*myc*-transformed avian macrophages.[79] Rapid induction of hematopoietic neoplasms occurs in newborn mice by the action of a recombinant murine retrovirus containing both v-*raf*/*mil* and v-*myc* oncogenes.[90,395] The recombinant virus accelerates tumor induction relative to v-*raf*- or v-*myc*-transducing viruses by a factor of about 3 and, in addition to the lymphomas and erythroblastosis which generally are the cause of death of inoculated mice, fibrosarcomas and pancreatic dysplasia also develop. Viruses expressing only the v-*myc* oncogene fail to induce any detectable changes in chicken embryo neuroretina cells and viruses expressing v-*mil* can only induce cell proliferation without transformation, but constructed recombinant viruses expressing both v-*myc* and v-*mil* are able to induce transformation in the same cells.[75] Monocytic cells from fresh murine bone marrow are immortalized by action of recombinant retrovirus carrying the combination of v-*raf* and v-*myc* oncogenes, and the proliferating cells do not require any more the addition of a specific growth factor supplement.[396] Both v-*myc* and v-*raf* oncogenes have to be expressed to induce proliferation of the bone marrow cells in standard medium, since viruses carrying either oncogene alone do not promote cell growth. The results suggest that the expression of both oncogenes may overrun the need for specific exogenous growth factor.[396] Moreover, these results could be interpreted on the basis of a model in which a competence signal is originated by v-*myc* expression and a progression signal by v-*raf*/*mil* expression.[90,395]

Epistatic phenomena (interaction between the products of two non allelic genes) can be seen in cells expressing two different viral oncogene products. Hematopoietic cells of the myelomonocytic lineage expressing either the v-*myb* or v-*myc* oncogene exhibit characteristic and different phenotypes. Cells expressing both v-*myb* and v-*myc* oncogenes as a consequence of dual retroviral infection also exhibit an abnormal phenotype but some of the phenotypic characteristics elicited by v-*myb* are interfered by v-*myc* and vice versa.[271] The molecular mechanisms involved in this interference are not understood.

The v-*erb*-A and v-*erb*-B oncogenes transduced by AEV can cooperate for the induction of neoplastic transformation in chicken fibroblasts and erythroblasts.[89] The v-*erb*-A oncogene induces a fully transformed phenotype in CEF cells partially transformed by a v-*erb*-B oncogene containing a deletion in its 3′ terminus.

D. COOPERATION BETWEEN VIRAL AND CELLULAR ONCOGENES FOR THE INDUCTION OF NEOPLASTIC TRANSFORMATION

Some retroviral oncogenes may depend on the cooperation of the protein products of specific protooncogenes for the induction and maintenance of a transformed phenotype. For example, v-*src*, v-*fms*, and v-*fes*, which code for membrane-associated growth factor receptor-like proteins, depend on the function of c-*ras* proteins for the expression of a transformed phenotype.[397] Microinjection of a monoclonal antibody that neutralizes c-*ras* proteins results in the morphological reversion of the transformed phenotype induced by the mentioned viral oncogenes. On the other hand, transformation induced by other viral oncogenes, such as v-*mos* and v-*raf*, whose products are localized mainly in the cytoplasm, is apparently independent of the c-*ras* protooncogene protein products.[397]

E. COOPERATION BETWEEN DIFFERENT PROTOONCOGENES FOR THE NEOPLASTIC TRANSFORMATION OF CELLS

Cotransfection not of v-*onc* genes but of c-*onc* genes may result in the malignant conversion of cells. Cotransfection of an expression vector carrying a human N-*myc* gene and a mutant c-H-*ras*-1 gene (derived from the EJ human bladder carcinoma cell line) may result in conversion of secondary rat embryo cells into transformed cells that can elicit tumors in athymic mice and isogeneic rats.[398] However, there is no definite evidence that cooperation between two or more protooncogenes is involved in the origin of natural, nonexperimental tumors.

F. COOPERATION BETWEEN DIFFERENT TYPES OF CELLS

Cooperation between different types of cells is probably important for the development of tumors *in vivo*. The ability of A-MuLV to transform cells derived *in vitro* from pluripotent hematopoietic progenitors of high proliferative potential and to allow progression to a tumorigenic state depends on the presence of soluble growth factors.[399] Autonomous cell lines developed only when their precursors were cocultivated for at least two or three months after infection with irradiated NIH/3T3 feeder cells. No cell lines were obtained if the cell feeders were not initially present. Thus, factors of mesenchymal origin, produced and secreted by the feeder fibroblasts, may play an essential role in the acquisition of autonomy by the acute retrovirus-infected cells. The role of A-MuLV products at this later stage is not clear, although all the lines examined in these studies contained an integrated v-*abl* oncogene.[399]

G. INTERACTION WITH CHEMICAL CARCINOGENS AND TUMOR PROMOTERS

Treatment of animals with chemical carcinogens may affect the induction of tumors by acute retroviruses. Inoculation into chickens of MCA of DMBA at times before the injection of ASV results in a stimulatory effect on the growth of tumors induced by the acute retrovirus.[400] However, this effect is dependent on both the source of the animals and the type of chemical carcinogen. There is no simple correlation between prior treatment with carcinogen and subsequent susceptibility to neoplasia. While stimulation of tumor growth is clearly observed in many occasions, such an outcome is probably governed by a wide range of genetic and environmental factors.

Tumor promoters can act in concert with viral oncogenes or activated protooncogenes during the multistage development of carcinogenic processes. Potent tumor promoters such as phorbol esters and teleocidin can enhance the transformation of cultured rodent fibroblast cell lines that have been transfected with the activated (mutated) human gene T24 c-H-*ras*.[401,402] An unidentified endogenous factor present in serum has similar enhancing effect in the T24 gene-induced neoplastic transformation of mouse and rat fibroblasts.[403] In cultured REF cells, formation of foci of transformed cells is not observed after either v-*myc* of *plt* transfer but focus formation can be induced when the oncogene transfer is followed by treatment with TPA.[404] Mouse basal keratinocytes are blocked in their differentiation processes by infection with MuSV expressing either v-H-*ras* or v-K-*ras* oncogenes and these cells respond to phorbol ester tumor promoters by undergoing phenotypic reversion to a less mature stage.[405] These results suggest that conditionally initiated cells are produced by v-*ras* oncogenes but the full expression of tumorigenicity may depend on the exposure to additional factors like tumor promoters.

A v-H-*ras* oncogene can replace chemical carcinogens and can act as an initiator of carcinogenesis in the mouse skin *in vivo*.[406] However, the introduction into epidermal cells of an activated v-H-*ras* gene, even in the form of a virus with transcriptional enhancer elements intact, is not sufficient to complete the carcinogenic process. Mice that are initiated with H-MuSV or chemical carcinogens but receive no further treatment can survive for almost 1 year without developing skin tumor of any kind. The initiated cells can survive in the epidermis for at least 4 months, since commencement of promoter treatment at this stage results in the rapid appearance of papillomas.[406] The complete dependence on promoter treatment indicates that a critical interaction must take place between the H-MuSV-initiated cell and the tumor promoter.

Phorbol esters can paradoxically act as differentiation inducers in some, but not all, cells transformed by acute retroviruses. Hematopoietic cells of the myelomonocytic lineage transformed with AMV, which carries the v-*myb* oncogene, can be induced to differentiate to fully mature macrophages by the tumor promoter TPA. In contrast, cells transformed by retroviruses expressing both v-*myb* and v-*myc* oncogenes cannot be induced to differentiate beyond the immature phenotype caused by the v-*myc* oncogene alone.[271] The reason for this difference is unknown.

H. EXPRESSION OF DIFFERENTIATED FUNCTIONS IN CELLS TRANSFORMED BY VIRAL ONCOGENES

Transformation induced by acute retroviruses is probably not a simple and direct phenomenon but may represent a particular step of the complex, multistage processes leading to oncogenesis.[407,408] Expression of a viral oncogene may not be sufficient for interrupting the normal process of differentiation or for inducing the expression of a fully malignant, tumorigenic phenotype in susceptible cells. Embryonic chick erythroid cells infected *in vitro* with AEV regularly show spontaneous differentiation in spite of the continuous expression of the v-*erb*-B oncogene.[409] Spontaneous or chemically induced differentiation of AEV-transformed erythroid cells is associated with changes at the level of the plasma membrane including expression of the anion transporter and assembly of membrane cytoskeleton components.[410] Differentiation of A-MuLV-infected immature B cells can proceed in spite of the presence of v-*abl* functions.[201] A-MuLV-induced leukemic monocytic-lineage cells can undergo extensive differentiation to cells that acquire characteristics of mature monocytes and macrophages.[411] Expression of the v-*ras* oncoprotein in pluripotent hematopoietic cells infected with H-MuSV is compatible with their normal maturation.[270]

Oncogene protein products may be capable of inducing the expression of differentiated functions. Adrenal fibroblasts from adult rats share a common embryonic origin with adrenocortical parenchymal cells and they can acquire some differentiated characteristics, including steroidogenic properties, as a consequence of transformation in early passage with K-MuSV.[412,413] Microinjection of *ras* oncogene protein into PC12 cells results in induction of morphological differentiation.[414] Differentiation can occur in cells infected with acute retroviruses, such as AEV-transformed embryonic erythroid cells,[409] especially when the cells are submitted to certain environmental changes. For example, a selective inhibition of the anchorage-independent growth induced in fibroblasts transfected with v-*myc* is produced by the differentiation-inducing agent, retinoic acid.[415] When NIH/3T3 cells adapted to grow in a medium containing 5 mM butyrate are infected with H-MuSV, addition of butyrate to the medium does not prevent the expression of the p21$^{v\text{-}ras}$ oncogene product on the inner aspect of the plasma membrane, but the appearance of foci of transformed cells is reversibly inhibited by butyrate.[416] K-MuSV-induced transformation of human skin fibroblasts is associated with their neodifferentiation into preadipocytes and addition of hydrocortisone promotes the differentiation of these preadipocytes into mature fat cells.[417] AMV-transformed cells express the oncogene protein product p45$^{v\text{-}myb}$, but may be induced to differentiate by treatment with lipopolysaccharide (LPS) without altered expression of the viral oncogene.[217] These examples indicate that the effects of viral oncogene products on transformation may be blocked at points distal to their expression.

VIII. HOST FACTORS IN TRANSFORMATION INDUCED BY ACUTE RETROVIRUSES

Many different factors depending on the host may have a critical role for the expression, or lack of expression, of a transformed phenotype induced by the products of acute retroviruses. Some acute retroviruses, albeit integrated, are not efficiently expressed in particular cells. Normal early chicken embryonic cells can be infected at high efficiency with RSV but, in spite of the fact that RSV DNA is integrated into the host cell genome, the levels of viral mRNA produced by the infected cells are very low and are not sufficient to generate fully competent viral particles. The chicken embryo is capable of regulating the malignant potential of RSV.[419] The embryo can regulate the susceptibility of tissues to RSV infection and/or expression and can modulate the spread of the virus through tissues that may or may not be transformation competent. RSV infection and expression are compatible with differentiation and expression of differentiated characteristics *in ovo*. It is thus apparent that not all cells are susceptible to the effects of infection with acute retrovirus or to the effects of transfection with cloned oncogenes. The details of the complex interactions occurring between viral and cellular functions in cells infected by acute retroviruses are little understood.

A. EXPRESSION OF FUNCTIONS DEPENDING ON CELLULAR GENES

In addition to retroviral oncogene expression, cellular functions, which may depend on the expression of protooncogenes or other cellular genes, may be required for the expression of the transformed phenotype induced by infection with acute retroviruses.[324,420] The isolation of revertants of acute retrovirus-transformed cells which contain wild-type virus genomes clearly indicates the involvement of cellular functions in the expression, or lack of expression, of a transformed phenotype.[421-426] Particular types of DNA methylation patterns may contribute to the regulation of transcriptional expression of both cellular genes and proviral DNA in cells transformed by acute transforming retroviruses.[427]

The transformation-associated factors encoded by cellular genes after infection by acute retroviruses are little characterized but may be represented, at least in part, by several types of growth factors, including TGFs and IGFs.[358] Transformation induced by M-MuSV in NRK cells is associated with the appearance of at least three different types of cellular proteins, called transformation associated proteins (TAPs).[428] TAPs differ from the known products of M-MuSV, including the fusion protein p85$^{gag-mos}$, in terms of MW, antigenic determinants, and associated protein kinase activity, which indicates that TAPs may be cellular factors activated specifically by the M-MuSV genome.

B. EXPRESSION OF PROTOONCOGENES

The possibility should be considered that acute retroviruses or their cloned oncogenes induce cell transformation through an altered expression of protooncogenes in the host cells. However, little evidence exists in favor of this possibility. Expression of a viral oncogene does not necessarily prevent the expression of the normal endogenous protooncogene counterpart. The AEV-transformed chicken erythroblastoid cell line 6C2 expresses the endogenous protein p75^{c-myb} in spite of the presence of high levels of the viral product, p48^{v-myb}.[325]

Transformation of lymphoid cells with reticuloendotheliosis virus strain t (REV-T), which carries the v-*rel* oncogene, does not result in significantly enhanced transcription of protooncogenes in the infected cells (compared with the herpesvirus-transformed cell line MSB-1), including the protooncogenes c-*rel*, c-*myc*, c-*myb*, c-*abl*, c-*src*, c-H-*ras*, c-K-*ras*, c-*sis*, c-*yes*, c-*fms*, and c-*mos*.[429] Moreover, the level of expression of the viral oncogene v-*rel* itself was only moderately increased, which suggests that transformation of lymphoid cells by the REV-T virus depends on qualitative, more than quantitative, differences between the v-*rel* and c-*rel* proteins. The REV-T-transformed cells express 2.9- to 3.0-kb v-*rel* transcripts, while MSB-1 cells express 4.0-kb c-*rel* transcripts. These cells exhibit lymphoblastoid morphology, acquire infinite growth potential, and are tumorigenic.[430]

Protooncogenes may cooperate with viral oncogenes in the expression of a fully transformed phenotype. However, the exact role of endogenous protooncogenes in the oncogenic transformation induced by viral oncogenes is not clear. Mouse NIH/3T3 fibroblasts transformed by the v-*sis* oncogene are known to be stimulated in an autocrine fashion by a PDGF-like molecule (PDGF-2 homodimer), and these cells have elevated levels of c-*fos* protooncogene expression in relation to nontransformed controls. The transfection and integration of a plasmid vector directing the synthesis of an antisense RNA to the c-*fos* protooncogene leads to restoration of density-dependent growth arrest in monolayer cultures of the v-*sis*-transformed fibroblasts, although colony formation in soft agar is not inhibited.[431] Transfer of the v-*fos* oncogene into an RSV-transformed rat cell line resulted in increased metastasization capacity of the cells expressing the viral oncogene, but the levels of expression of the endogenous c-*src*, c-*myc*, and c-*ras* genes were not clearly altered.[432] The mechanism by which the v-*fos* oncogene induces progression of the malignant phenotype remains to be elucidated.

C. CHROMOSOMAL CHANGES AND POINT MUTATIONS

Nonrandom chromosomal changes may contribute to the expression of a transformed phenotype in cells transformed by viral oncogenes. Tumors induced in nude mice by SHE cells cotransfected with v-H-*ras* and v-*myc* oncogenes have a nonrandom chromosome change which consists in a monosomy of chromosome 15.[433] It is not known whether the loss of one chromosome 15 is an early event necessary for the genesis of tumors or whether this change represents a cellular progression that occurs with high frequency and is strongly selected.

Coinfection of growth factor-dependent human hematopoietic cells with the acute retroviruses H-MuSV (which carries the oncogene v-H-*ras*) and AMCV (which carries the oncogene v-*myc*) resulted in acquisition of growth factor independency only after a lag of 2 to 3 months, and all growth factor-independent cells exhibited great variability in their karyotypes.[434] Similar results were obtained when the growth factor-dependent cells were coinfected with the acute retroviruses AMCV and A-MuLV (which carries the oncogene v-*abl*).[354] The acquisition of growth factor-independent growth by these cells is a rare event observed only after crisis of the culture and is apparently not due to the occurrence of chromosomal changes including near-triploidy or -tetraploidy. Interestingly, studies with somatic cell hybrids formed by crossing mouse melanoma cells with mouse embryo fibroblasts or neoplastic mouse L cells with human fibroblasts indicate that the hybrid cells have a reduced ability to proliferate in growth factor-unsupplemented serum-free medium relative to the parental neoplastic cells and that this reduction is associated with the presence of specific chromosome combinations in the mouse x human hybrid cells.[435] These results suggest a role for chromosomal genes in the suppression of growth in serum-free medium. However, it is rather unlikely that acute retroviruses induce the neoplastic transformation of cells via specific chromosome aberrations.

Some common pathways of oncogene-induced transformation may include as a component specific point mutation(s) in the host cell genome. Two classes of morphologic revertants of FBJ MuSV-transformed Rat-1 fibroblasts were isolated and one of these classes contained sustained point mutations in cellular genes.[436] The latter class of revertants was resistant to retransformation not only by v-*fos* but also by v-H-*ras*, v-*abl*, and v-*mos*, although it could be retransformed by polyoma virus middle T antigen or the *trk* gene. This result suggest that polyoma virus and *trk* may use for transformation a biochemical pathway which is distinct from that used by oncogenes from acute retroviruses.

D. STAGE OF DEVELOPMENT

Some characteristics of the target cells, including specificity, age, and environment, may be of critical importance to determine the response to the oncogenic potential of acute retroviruses or oncogenic viruses in general. A dividing target cell is an essential prerequisite for retroviral integration into the host cell genome and subsequent neoplastic transformation. Inhibitors of ornithine decarboxylase (ODC) activity block polyamine synthesis and reduce the number of erythroid colonies transformed by retroviruses such as F-MuLV, H-MuSV, and RSV.[437] Putrescine, a product of ODC activity, is able to overcome the effect of ODC inhibitors. Expression of certain protooncogenes (c-*myc*, c-*myb*, and p53) is markedly reduced in the cells treated with ODC inhibitors.

Susceptible cells may become completely insensitive to the transforming action of viral oncogene products after they reach a certain stage of differentiation.[438] RSV is unable to cause sarcomas in the chicken embryo *in ovo*, in spite of high levels of expression of pp60^{v-src}-associated tyrosine protein kinase activity, but the ability to display a transformed phenotype is rapidly acquired after the infected cells are placed in culture.[439,440] The effects of the injection of the v-*myc*-carrying AMCV MC29 virus strain into avian embryos shows a striking tissue specificity and time restriction.[441] The injection of MC29 at embryonic day 2 or 3 caused, about 10 days later, rhabdomyosarcomas of the heart and, in some cases, skin muscle hypertrophy. When injection was performed at day 4 or 5, the number of heart tumors declined, whereas the number of skin muscle tumors increased significantly. The protein p110$^{gag-myc}$ was found in all tumors analyzed.[441] When the MC29 virus was injected intravenously into embryos at day 10, no tumors appeared during the embryonic life.

E. GENETIC CONSTITUTION OF THE HOST

The genetic constitution of the host is of paramount importance for determining the susceptibility to infection by different viruses, including acute retroviruses, as well as for determining the possible consequences of such infection. The phenomenon is more conveniently studied in experiments performed *in vitro*. Cultured skin fibroblasts from patients with familial bilateral retinoblastoma, but not from sporadic unilateral retinoblastoma or from patients with the 13q- chromosome deletion form of the tumor, show an extremely high sensitivity to transformation by M-MuSV.[442] Fibroblasts from patients with certain inherited diseases associated with high cancer risk (Gardner syndrome, familial polyposis coli) are highly susceptible to transformation by K-MuSV but not susceptible to RSV.[443-445] Dermal fibroblasts from patients with the autosomal dominant cancer-prone disease basal cell nevus syndrome show an extended lifespan *in vitro* after transfection with either the v-*myc* oncogene of the *pro*-1 gene (a gene which specifies sensitivity to promotion of neoplastic transformation in JB6 mouse epidermal cells), as compared to normal matched fibroblasts transfected with the same genes.[446] However, the transfected fibroblasts from patients with basal cell nevus syndrome are not morphologically transformed or anchorage independent, even after treatment with tumor promoters, suggesting that they require additional genetic changes for further neoplastic progression. In general, normal human cells are resistant to transformation induced *in vitro* by acute retroviruses, although positive results have been obtained in some instances with retroviruses of murine, feline, and avian origin.[447] The oncogene v-*src* transforms and establishes rodent fibroblasts but not diploid human fibroblasts.[204]

F. IMMUNE STATUS OF THE HOST

Growth of tumors induced by acute retroviruses is influenced by the immune status of the host. The immune competence of the host may determine not only susceptibility to the induction of tumor by acute retroviruses but also the fate of the tumor once it is induced and clinically detectable.[448] Sarcomas induced in chickens by inoculation of RSV into the wing web usually regress within a few weeks after the initial growth, due to an immune response directed against viral and/or tumor antigens.[499,450]

Natural killer (NK) cells may have an active role in the lysis of oncogene-transformed cells, but their effects are probably not directed to the oncoprotein itself. Although it has been reported that NK cells can recognize preferentially murine fibroblast cell lines transformed *in vitro* by v-*ras* oncogenes,[451,452] NK sensitivity in cells transfected with v-*ras* oncogenes or oncogenically activated c-*ras* protooncogenes may depend on the induction of specific cellular characteristics in the recipient fibroblast lines and is apparently not related to the transformation event.[453] Moreover, *ras*-transformed cells expressing high levels of the gene may be able to break through the immune control of the host and proliferate rapidly.[454] Thus, oncogene-induced neoplastic transformation may alter the cell in some way that eventually allows escape from immune attack. Immunosupressive or immunodepressive conditions usually enhance or accelerate the growth of tumors induced by acute retroviruses. For example, generalized immune suppression of chickens induced by cyclophosphamide enhances the growth of ASV-induced sarcomas.[455]

IX. CONCLUSION

Acute retroviruses are noninfectious, defective retroviruses that are formed by occasional recombination events occurring between retroviral genomic sequences and DNA sequences derived from specific cellular genes, the protooncogenes. The modified protooncogene-derived sequences contained in the genome of acute retroviruses are termed viral oncogenes or v-*onc* genes. These genes possess defined potential for inducing in a relatively rapid and direct fashion the malignant transformation of susceptible cells *in vitro* as well as the formation of tumors in susceptible animals *in vivo*. The neoplastic transformation of cells induced by acute retroviruses essentially depends on the cellular actions of the protein products of the viral oncogenes but, in spite of numerous studies, the mechanisms by which these products induce the malignant phenotype are little known. Many cellular structures and functions may be altered in cells transformed by acute retroviruses but the precise importance and sequence of these alterations remain to be determined. Cells transformed by acute retroviruses may be able to differentiate without a decrease in the amount of the specific activity of the viral oncogene product. Thus, viral oncogene products are necessary for the induction of a transformed phenotype by acute retroviruses, but expression of the oncogene product may be insufficient by itself for maintaining transformation. In any case, the study of malignant transformation induced by viral oncogenes may contribute to elucidate the general molecular mechanisms involved in carcinogenic processes.

REFERENCES

1. Pimentel, E., Human oncovirology, *Biochim. Biophys. Acta*, 560, 169, 1979.
2. Rapp, F., Viral carcinogenesis, *Int. Rev. Cytol.,* Suppl. 15, 203, 1983.
3. Mackowiak, P.A., Microbial oncogenesis, *Am. J. Med.,* 82, 79, 1987.
4. Onions, D.E. and Jarett, O., Viral oncogenesis: lessons from naturally occurring animal viruses, *Cancer Surv.,* 6, 161, 1987.
5. Levy, J.A., The multifaceted retrovirus, *Cancer Res.,* 46, 5457, 1986.
6. Gilboa, E., Eglitis, M.A., Kantoff, P.W., and Anderson, W.F., Transfer and expression of cloned genes using retroviral vectors, *BioTechniques,* 4, 504, 1986.
7. Bernhard, W., The detection and study of tumor viruses with the electron microscope, *Cancer Res.,* 20, 712, 1960.
8. Dalton, A.J., RNA tumor viruses — terminology and ultrastructural aspects of virion morphology and replication, *J. Natl. Cancer Inst.,* 49, 323, 1972.
9. Fine, D. and Schochetman, G., Type D primate retroviruses: a review, *Cancer Res.,* 38, 3123, 1978.
10. Ellermann, V. and Bang, O., Experimentelle Leukämie bei Hühnern, *Zentralbl. Bakteriol.,* 46, 595, 1908.
11. Rous, P., A sarcoma of the fowl transmissible by an agent separable from the tumor cells, *J. Exp. Med.,* 13, 397, 1911.
12. Makowski, D.R., Rothberg, P.G., and Astrin, S.M., Cellular transformation by avian viruses, *Pharmacol. Ther.,* 27, 63, 1985.
13. Hayman, M.J., Oncogenes of avian leukemia viruses, *Life Sci. Res. Rep.,* 30, 163, 1985.
14. Harvey, T.T., An unidentified virus which causes the rapid production of tumors in mice, *Nature,* 204, 1104, 1964.
15. Kirsten, W.H. and Mayer, L.A., Morphologic responses to a murine erythroblastosis virus, *J. Natl. Cancer Inst.,* 39, 311, 1967.
16. Rasheed, S., Retroviruses and oncogenes in rats, in *Retroviruses and Human Pathology,* Gallo, R.C., Stehelin, D., and Varnier, O.E., Eds., Humana Press, Clifton, NJ, 1985, 153.

17. Abelson, H.T. and Rabstein, L.S., Influence of prednisolone on Moloney leukemogenic virus in BALB/c mice, *Cancer Res.*, 30, 2208, 1970.

18. Green, P.L., Kaehler, D.A., and Risser, R., Cell transformation and tumor induction by Abelson murine leukemia virus in the absence of helper virus, *Proc. Natl. Acad. Sci. U.S.A.*, 84, 5932, 1987.

19. Bishop, J.M., Retroviruses and cancer genes, *Adv. Cancer Res.*, 37, 1, 1982.

20. Gallo, R.C. and Wong-Staal, F., Retroviruses as etiologic agents of some animal and human leukemias and lymphomas and as tools for elucidating the molecular mechanism of leukemogenesis, *Blood,* 60, 545, 1982.

21. Bishop, J.M., Cellular oncogenes and retroviruses, *Annu. Rev. Biochem.*, 52, 301, 1983.

22. Bishop, J.M., Viruses, genes, and cancer, *Harvey Lect.*, 78, 137, 1984.

23. Hunter, T., Oncogenes and proto-oncogenes: how do they differ?, *J. Natl. Cancer Inst.*, 73, 773, 1984.

24. Bishop, J.M., Viral oncogenes, *Cell,* 42, 23, 1985.

25. Bishop, J.M., Viruses, genes, and cancer. II. Retroviruses and cancer genes, *Cancer,* 55, 2329, 1985.

26. Bishop, J.M., Oncogenes and proto-oncogenes, *J. Cell. Physiol.*, Suppl. 4, 1, 1986.

27. Garrett, C.T., Oncogenes, *Clin. Chim. Acta,* 156, 1, 1986.

28. Temin, H.M., Evolution of cancer genes as a mutation-driven process, *Cancer Res.*, 48, 1697, 1988.

29. Egan, S.E., Wright, J.A., Jarolim, L., Yanagihara, K., Bassin, R.H., and Greenberg, A.H., Transformation by oncogenes encoding protein kinases induces the metastatic phenotype, *Science,* 238, 202, 1987.

30. Huang, C.-C., Hay, N., and Bishop, J.M., The role of RNA molecules in transduction of the proto-oncogene c-*fps, Cell,* 44, 935, 1986.

31. Duesberg, P.H., Nunn, M., Kan, N., Watson, D., Seeburg, P.H., and Papas, T., Are activated proto-*onc* genes cancer genes?, *Haematol. Blood Transfus.*, 29, 9, 1985.

32. Van Beveren, C., Galleshaw, J.A., Jonas, V., Berns, A.J.M., Doolittle, R.F., Donoghue, D.J., and Verma, I.M., Nucleotide sequence and formation of the transforming gene of a mouse sarcoma virus, *Nature,* 289, 258, 1981.

33. Reddy, E.P., Smith, M.J., and Aaronson, S.A., Complete nucleotide sequence of the Moloney murine sarcoma virus genome, *Science,* 214, 445, 1981.

34. Van Beveren, C., van Straaten, F., Galleshaw, J.A., and Verma, I.M., Nucleotide sequence of the genome of a murine sarcoma virus, *Cell,* 27, 97, 1981.

35. Gelmann, E.P., Wong-Staal, F., Kramer, R.A., and Gallo, R.C., Molecular cloning and comparative analyses of the genome of simian sarcoma virus and its associated helper virus, *Proc. Natl. Acad. Sci. U.S.A.*, 78, 3373, 1981.

36. Devare, S.G., Reddy, E.P., Robbins, K.C., Andersen, P.R., Tronick, S.R., and Aaronson, S.A., Nucleotide sequence of the transforming gene of simian sarcoma virus, *Proc. Natl. Acad. Sci. U.S.A.*, 79, 3179, 1982.

37. Kitamura, N., Kitamura, A., Toyoshima, K., Hirayama, Y., and Yoshida, M., Avian sarcoma virus Y73 genome sequence and structural similarity of its transforming gene product to that of Rous sarcoma virus, *Nature,* 297, 205, 1982.

38. Rushlow, K.E., Lautenberger, J.A., Papas, T.S., Baluda, M.A., Perbal, B., Chirikjian, J.G., and Reddy, E.P., Nucleotide sequence of the transforming gene of avian myeloblastosis virus, *Science,* 216, 1421, 1982.

39. Dhar, R., Ellis, R.W., Shih, T.Y., Oroszlan, S., Shapiro, B., Maizel, J., Lowy, D., and Scolnick, E., Nucleotide sequence of the p21 transforming protein of Harvey murine sarcoma virus, *Science,* 217, 934, 1982.

40. Tsuchida, N., Ryder, T., and Ohtsubo, E., Nucleotide sequence of the oncogene encoding the p21 transforming protein of Kirsten murine sarcoma virus, *Science,* 217, 937, 1982.

41. Takeya, T., Feldman, R.A., and Hanafusa, H., DNA sequence of the viral and cellular *src* gene of chickens. I. Complete nucleotide sequence of an *Eco*RI fragment of recovered avian sarcoma virus which codes for gp37 and pp60^{src}, *J. Virol.*, 44, 1, 1982.

42. Schwartz, D.E., Tizard, R., and Gilbert, W., Nucleotide sequence of Rous sarcoma virus, *Cell,* 32, 853, 1983.

43. Watson, D.K., Reddy, E.P., Duesberg, P.H., and Papas, T.S., Nucleotide sequence analysis of the chicken c-*myc* gene reveals homologous and unique coding regions by comparison with the transforming gene of avian myelocytomatosis virus MC29, delta*gag-myc*, *Proc. Natl. Acad. Sci. U.S.A.*, 80, 2146, 1983.

44. Stephens, R.M., Rice, N.R., Hiebsch, R.R., Rose, H.R., Jr., and Gilden, R.V., Nucleotide sequence of v-*rel*: the oncogene of reticuloendotheliosis virus, *Proc. Natl. Acad. Sci. U.S.A.*, 80, 6229, 1983.

45. Rasheed, S., Norman, G.L., and Heidecker, G., Nucleotide sequence of the Rasheed rat sarcoma virus oncogene: new mutations, *Science,* 221, 155, 1983.

46. Yamamoto, T., Nishida, T., Miyajima, N., Kawai, S., Ooi, T., and Toyoshima, K., The *erbB* gene of avian erythroblastosis virus is a member of the *src* gene family, *Cell,* 35, 71, 1983.

47. Nunn, M.F., Seeburg, P.H., Moscovici, C., and Duesberg, P.H., Tripartite structure of the avian erythroblastosis virus E26 transforming gene, *Nature,* 306, 391, 1983.

48. Brow, M.A.D., Sen, A., and Sutcliffe, J.G., Nucleotide sequence of the transforming gene of m1 murine sarcoma virus, *J. Virol.*, 49, 579, 1984.

49. Huang, C.-C., Hammond, C., and Bishop, J.M., Nucleotide sequence of v-*fps* in the PRCII strain of avian sarcoma virus, *J. Virol.*, 50, 125, 1984.

50. Mark, G.E. and Rapp, U.R., Primary structure of v-*raf*: relatedness to the *src* family of oncogenes, *Science*, 224, 285, 1984.

51. Sutrave, P., Bonner, T.L., Rapp, U.R., Jansen, H.W., Patschinsky, T., and Bister, K., Nucleotide sequence of avian retroviral oncogene v-*mil*: homologue of murine retroviral oncogene v-*raf*, *Nature*, 309, 85, 1984.

52. Kan, N.C., Flordellis, C.S., Mark, C.E., Duesberg, P.H., and Papas, T.S., Nucleotide sequence of avian carcinoma virus MH2: two potential *onc* genes, one related to avian virus MC29 and the other related to murine sarcoma virus 3611, *Proc. Natl. Acad. Sci. U.S.A.*, 81, 3000, 1984.

53. Jansen, H.W. and Bister, K., Nucleotide sequence analysis of the chicken gene c-*mil*, the progenitor of the retroviral oncogene v-*mil*, *Virology*, 143, 359, 1985.

54. Neckameyer, W.S. and Wang, L.-H., Nucleotide sequence of avian sarcoma virus UR2 and comparison of its transforming gene with other members of the tyrosine protein kinase oncogene family, *J. Virol.*, 53, 879, 1985.

55. Reddy, P., Lipman, D., Andersen, P.R., Tronick, S.R., and Aaronson, S.A., Nucleotide sequence analysis of the BALB/c murine sarcoma virus transforming gene, *J. Virol.*, 53, 984, 1985.

56. Koenen, M., Sippel, A.E., Trachmann, C., and Bister, K., Primary structure of the chicken c-*mil* protein: identification of domains shared with or absent from the retroviral v-*mil* protein, *Oncogene*, 2, 179, 1988.

57. Norton, J.D., Connor, J., and Avery, R.J., Genesis of Kirsten murine sarcoma virus: sequence analysis reveals recombination points and potential leukaemogenic determinant on parental leukaemia virus genome, *Nucleic Acids Res.*, 12, 6839, 1984.

58. Wendling, F., Varlet, P., Charon, M., and Tambourin, P., MPLV: a retrovirus complex inducing an acute myeloproliferative leukemia disorder in adult mice, *Virology*, 149, 242, 1986.

59. Graves, B.J., Eisenman, R.N., and McKnight, S.L., Delineation of transcriptional control signals within the Moloney murine sarcoma virus long terminal repeat, *Mol. Cell. Biol.*, 5, 1948, 1985.

60. Walther, N., Lurz, R., Patschinsky, T., Jansen, H.W., and Bister, K., Molecular cloning of proviral DNA and structural analysis of the transduced *myc* oncogene of avian oncovirus CMII, *J. Virol.*, 54, 576, 1985.

61. Raines, M.A., Maihle, N.J., Moscovici, C., Crittenden, L., and Kung, H.-J., Mechanism of c-*erbB* transduction: newly released transducing viruses retain poly(A) tracts of *erbB* transcripts and encode C-terminally intact *erbB* proteins, *J. Virol.*, 62, 2437, 1988.

62. Roussel, M., Saule, S., Lagrou, C., Rommens, C., Beug, H., Graf, T., and Stehelin, D., Three new types of viral oncogene of cellular origin specific for hematopoietic cell transformation, *Nature*, 281, 452, 1979.

63. Bister, K. and Duesberg, P.H., Structure and specific sequences of avian erythroblastosis virus RNA: evidence for multiple classes of transforming genes among avian tumor viruses, *Proc. Natl. Acad. Sci. U.S.A.*, 76, 5023, 1979.

64. Vennstrom, B. and Bishop, J.M., Isolation and characterization of chicken DNA homologous to the two putative oncogenes of avian erythroblastosis virus, *Cell*, 28, 135, 1982.

65. Graf, T. and Beug, H., Role of the v-*erbA* and v-*erbB* oncogenes of avian erythroblastosis virus in erythroid cell transformation, *Cell*, 34, 7, 1983.

66. Saule, S., Dozier, C., Denhez, F., Martin, P., and Stehelin, D., Retroviruses with two oncogenes, *Nucl. Med. Biol.*, 14, 441, 1987.

67. Leprince, D., Gegonne, A., Coll, J., de Taisne, C., Schneeberger, A., Lagrou, C., and Stehelin, D., A putative second cell-derived oncogene in the avian leukaemia retrovirus E26, *Nature*, 306, 395, 1983.

68. Kan, N.C., Flordellis, C.S., Garon, C.F., Duesberg, P.H., and Papas, T.S., Avian carcinoma virus MH2 contains a transformation-specific sequence, *mht*, and shares the *myc* sequence with MC29, CMII, and OK10 viruses, *Proc. Natl. Acad. Sci. U.S.A.*, 80, 6566, 1983.

69. Coll, J., Righi, M., de Taisne, C., Dissous, C., Gegonne, A., and Stehelin, D., Molecular cloning of the avian acute transforming retrovirus MH2 reveals a novel cell-derived sequence (v-*mil*) in addition to the c-*myc* oncogene, *EMBO J.*, 2, 2189, 1983.

70. Jansen, H.W., Lurz, R., Bister, K., Bonner, T.I., Mark, G.E., and Rapp, U.R., Homologous cell-derived oncogenes in avian carcinoma virus MH2 and murine sarcoma virus 3611, *Nature*, 307, 281, 1984.

71. Kan, N.C., Flordellis, C.S., Mark, G.E., Duesberg, P.H., and Papas, T.S., A common *onc* gene sequence transduced by avian carcinoma virus MH2 and by murine sarcoma virus 3611, *Science*, 223, 813, 1984.

72. Flordellis, C.S., Kan, N.C., Lautenberger, J.A., Samuel, K.P., Garon, C.F., and Papas, T.S., Analysis of the cellular proto-oncogene *mht/raf*: relationship to the 5′ sequences of v-*mht* in avian carcinoma virus MH2 and v-*raf* in murine sarcoma virus 3611, Virology, 141, 267, 1985.

73. Zhou R.-P., Kan, N., Papas, T., and Duesberg, P., Mutagenesis of avian carcinoma virus MH2: only one of two potential transforming genes (d-*gag-myc*) transforms fibroblasts, *Proc. Natl. Acad. Sci. U.S.A.*, 82, 6389, 1985.

74. Palmieri, S. and Vogel, M.L., Fibroblast transformation parameters induced by the avian v-*mil* oncogene, *J. Virol.*, 61, 1717, 1987.

75. Bechade, C., Calothy, G., Pessac, B., Martin, P., Coll, J., Denhez, F., Saule, S., Ghysdael, J., and Stéhelin, D., Induction of proliferation or transformation of neuroretina cells by the *mil* and *myc* viral oncogenes, *Nature*, 316, 559, 1985.

76. Martin, P., Henry, C., Ferre, F., Bechade, C., Begue, A., Calothy, C., Debuire, B., Stehelin, D., and Saule, S., Characterization of a *myc*-containing retrovirus generated by propagation of an MH2 viral subgenomic RNA, *J. Virol.,* 57, 1191, 1986.

77. Martin, P., Henry, C., Denhez, F., Amouyel, P., Bechade, C., Calothy, G., Debuire, B., Stehelin, D., and Saule, S., Characterization of a MH2 mutant lacking the v-*myc* oncogene, *Virology,* 153, 272, 1986.

78. Graf, T., Weizsäcker, F.V., Grieser, S., Coll, J., Stehelin, D., Patschinsky, T., Bister, K., Bechade, C., Calothy, G., and Leutz, A., v-*mil* induces autocrine growth and enhanced tumorigenicity in v-*myc*-transformed avian macrophages, *Cell,* 45, 357, 1986.

79. von Weizsäcker, F., Beug, H., and Graf, T., Temperature-sensitive mutatants of MH2 avian leukemia virus that map in the v-*mil* and the v-*myc* oncogene, respectively, *EMBO J.,* 5, 1521, 1986.

80. Béchade, C., Dambrine, G., David-Pfeuty, T., Esnault, E., and Calothy, G., Transformed and tumorigenic phenotypes induced by avian retroviruses containing the v-*mil* oncogene, *J. Virol.,* 62, 1211, 1988.

81. Symonds, G., Stubblefield, E., Guyaux, M., and Bishop, J.M., Cellular oncogenes (c-*erb*-A and c-*erb*-B) located on different chicken chromosomes can be transduced into the same viral genome, *Mol. Cell. Biol.,* 4, 1627, 1984.

82. Symonds, G., Quintrell, N., Subblefield, E., and Bishop, J.M., Dispersed chromosomal localization of the proto-oncogenes transduced into the genome of Mill Hill 2 or E26 leukemia virus, *J. Virol.,* 59, 172, 1986.

83. Zabel, B.U., Fournier, R.E.K., Lalley, P.A., Naylor, S.A., and Sakaguchi, A.Y., Cellular homologs of the avian erythroblastosis virus *erb*-A and *erb*-B genes are syntenic in mouse but asyntenic in man, *Proc. Natl. Acad. Sci. U.S.A.,* 81, 4874, 1984.

84. Yamamoto, T., Hihara, H., Nishida, T., Kawai, S., and Toyoshima, K., A new avian erythroblastosis virus, AEV-H, carries *erbB* gene responsible for the induction of both erythroblastosis and sarcomas, *Cell,* 34, 225, 1983.

85. Miles, B.D. and Robinson, H.L., High-frequency transduction of c-*erb*B in avian leukosis virus-induced erythroblastosis, *J. Virol.,* 54, 295, 1985.

86. Henry, C., Coquillaud, M., Saule, S., Stehelin, D., and Debuire, B., The four C-terminal amino acids of the v-*erbA* polypeptide are encoded by an intronic sequence on the v-*erbB* oncogene, *Virology,* 140, 179, 1985.

87. Zahraoui, A. and Cuny, G., Nucleotide sequence of the chicken proto-oncogene c-*erbA* corresponding to domain 1 of v-*erbA*, *Eur J. Biochem.,* 166, 63, 1987.

88. Gandrillon, O., Jurdic, P., Benchaibi, M., Xiao, J.-H., Ghysdael, J., and Samarut, J., Expression of the v-*erbA* oncogene in chicken embryo fibroblasts stimulates their proliferation *in vitro* and enhances tumor growth *in vivo, Cell,* 49, 687, 1987.

89. Jansson, M., Beug, H., Gray, C., Graf, T., and Vennström, B., Defective v-*erbB* genes can be complemented by v-*erbA* in erythroblast and fibroblast transformation, *Oncogene,* 1, 167, 1987.

90. Rapp, U.R., Cleveland, J.L., Fredrickson, T.N., Holmes, K.L., Morse, H.C., III, Jansen, H.W., Patschinsky, T., and Bister, K., Rapid induction of hemopoietic neoplasms in newborn mice by a *raf(mil)/myc* recombinant murine retrovirus, *J. Virol.,* 55, 23, 1985.

91. Andersen, P.R., Tronick, S.R., and Aaronson, S.A., Structural organization and biological activity of molecular clones of the integrated genome of BALB/c mouse sarcoma virus, *J. Virol.,* 40, 431, 1981.

92. Fredrickson, T.N., O'Neill, R.R., Rutledge, R.A., Theodore, T.S., Martin, M.A., Ruscetti, S.K., Austin, J.B., and Hartley, J.W., Biologic and molecular characterization of two newly isolated *ras*-containing murine leukemia viruses, *J. Virol.,* 6, 2109, 1987.

93. Jansen, H.W., Trachmann, C., and Bister, K., Structural relationship between the chicken protooncogene c-*mil* and the retroviral oncogene c-*mil*, *Virology,* 137, 217, 1984.

94. Sovová, V., Trávnicek, M., Hlozánek, I., Cerna, H., Alitalo, K., and Vaheri, A., Evidence for p15 cleavage site in myc-specific proteins of avian MC29 and OK10 viruses, *J. Cell. Biochem.,* 28, 165, 1985.

95. Linial, M. and Groudine, M., Transcription of three c-*myc* exons is enhanced in chicken bursal and lymphoma cell lines, *Proc. Natl. Acad. Sci. U.S.A.,* 82, 53, 1985.

96. Walther, N., Jansen, H.W., Trachmann, C., and Bister, K., Nucleotide sequence of the CMII v-*myc* allele, *Virology,* 154, 219, 1986.

97. Prywes, R., Foulkes, J.G., Rosenberg, N., and Baltimore, D., Sequences of the A-MuLV protein needed for fibroblast and lymphoid cell transformation, *Cell,* 34, 569, 1983.

98. Besmer, P., Hardy, W.D., Jr., Zuckerman, E.E., Bergold, P., Lederman, L., and Snyder, H.W., Jr., The Hardy-Zuckerman 2-FeSV, a new feline retrovirus with oncogene homology to Abelson-MuLV, *Nature,* 303, 825, 1983.

99. Schalken, J.A., van den Ouweland, A.M.W., Bloemers, H.P.J., and van de Ven, W.J.M., Characterization of the feline c-*abl* proto-oncogene, *Biochim. Biophys. Acta,* 824, 104, 1985.

100. Murtagh, K., Skladany, G., Hoag, J., and Rosenberg, N., Abelson murine leukemia virus variants with increased oncogenic potential, *J. Virol.,* 60, 599, 1986.

101. Oppi, C., Shore, S.K., and Reddy, E.P., Nucleotide sequence of testis-derived c-*abl* cDNAs: implications for testis-specific transcription and *abl* oncogene activation, *Proc. Natl. Acad. Sci. U.S.A.,* 84, 8200, 1987.

102. Bergold, P.J., Blumentahl, J.A., D'Andrea, E., Snyder, H.W., Lederman, L., Silverstone, A., Nguyen, H., and Besmer, P., Nucleic acid sequence and oncogenic properties of the HZ2 feline sarcoma virus v-*abl* insert, *J. Virol.,* 61, 1193, 1987.

103. Carlberg, K., Chamberlin, M.E., and Beemon, K., The avian sarcoma virus PRCII lacks 1020 nucleotides of the *fps* transforming gene, *Virology,* 135, 157, 1984.

104. Woolford, J. and Beemon, K., Transforming proteins of Fujinami and PRCII avian sarcoma viruses have different subcellular locations, *Virology,* 135, 168, 1984.

105. Huang, C.-C., Hammond, C., and Bishop, J.M., Nucleotide sequence and topography of chicken c-*fps*: genesis of retroviral oncogene encoding a tyrosine-specific protein kinase, *J. Mol. Biol.,* 181, 175, 1985.

106. Breitman, M.L., Neil, J.C., Moscovici, C., and Vogt, P.K., The pathogenicity and defectiveness of PRCII: a new type of avian sarcoma virus, *Virology,* 108, 1, 1981.

107. Duesberg, P.H., Phares, W., and Lee, W.H., The low tumorigenic potential of PRCII, among viruses of the Fujinami sarcoma virus subgroup, corresponds to an internal (*fps*) deletion of the transforming gene, *Virology,* 131, 144, 1983.

108. Hammond, C.I., Vogt, P.K., and Bishop, J.M., Molecular cloning of the PRCII sarcoma viral genome and the chicken proto-oncogene c-*fps*, *Virology,* 143, 300, 1985.

109. Hampe, A., Laprevotte, I., and Galibert, F., Nucleotide sequences of feline retroviral oncogenes (v-*fes*) provide evidence for a family of tyrosine-specific protein kinase genes, *Cell,* 30, 775, 1982.

110. Beemon, K., Transforming proteins of some feline and avian sarcoma viruses are related structurally and functionally, *Cell,* 24, 145, 1981.

111. Sodroski, J.G., Goh, W.C., and Haseltine, W.A., Transforming potential of a human proto-oncogene (c-*fps*/*fes*) locus, *Proc. Natl. Acad. Sci. U.S.A.,* 81, 3039, 1984.

112. Feldman, R.A., Vass, W.C., and Tambourin, P.E., Human cellular *fps*/*fes* cDNA rescued via retroviral shuttle vector encodes myeloid cell NCP92 and has transforming potential, *Oncogene Res.,* 1, 441, 1987.

113. Tracy, S.E., Woda, B.A., and Robinson, H.L., Induction of angiosarcoma by a c-*erb*B transducing virus, *J. Virol.,* 54, 304, 1985.

114. Gamett, D.C., Tracy, S.E., and Robinson, H.L., Differences in sequences encoding the carboxyl-terminal domain of the epidermal growth factor receptor correlate with differences in the disease potential of viral *erb*B genes, *Proc. Natl. Acad. Sci. U.S.A.,* 83, 6053, 1986.

115. Vennström, B., Kahn, P., Adkins, B., Enrietto, P., Hayman, M.J., Graf, T., and Luciw, P., Transformation of mammalian fibroblasts and macrophages *in vitro* by a murine retrovirus encoding an avian v-*myc* oncogene, *EMBO J.,* 3, 3223, 1984.

116. Morse, H.C., III, Hartley, J.W., Fredrickson, T.N., Yetter, R.A., Majumdar, C., Cleveland, J.L., and Rapp, U.R., Recombinant murine retroviruses containing avian v-*myc* induce a wide spectrum of neoplasms in newborn mice, *Proc. Natl. Acad. Sci. U.S.A.,* 83, 6868, 1986.

117. Brigthman, B.K., Pattengale, P.K., and Fan, H., Generation and characterization of a recombinant Moloney murine leukemia virus containing the v-*myc* oncogene of avian MC29 virus: *in vitro* transformation and *in vivo* pathogenesis, *J. Virol.,* 60, 68, 1986.

118. Gazint, A., Pierce, J.H., Kraus, M.H., DiFiore, P.P., Pennington, C.Y., and Aaronson, S.A., Mammalian cell transformation by a murine retrovirus vector containing the avian erythroblastosis virus *erb*B gene, *J. Virol.,* 60, 19, 1986.

119. Gojobori, T. and Yokoyama, S., Rates of evolution of the retroviral oncogene of Moloney murine sarcoma virus and of its cellular homologues, Proc. Natl. Acad. Sci. U.S.A., 82, 4198, 1985.

120. Iba, H., Takeya, T., Cross, F.R., Hanafusa, T., and Hanafusa, H., Rous sarcoma virus variants that carry the cellular *src* gene instead of the viral *src* gene cannot transform chicken embryo fibroblasts, *Proc. Natl. Acad. Sci. U.S.A.,* 81, 4424, 1984.

121. Shalloway, D., Coussens, P.M., and Yaciuk, P., Overexpression of the c-*src* protein does not induce transformation of NIH 3T3 cells, *Proc. Natl. Acad. Sci. U.S.A.,* 81, 7071, 1984.

122. McGeady, M.L., Jhappan, C., Ascione, R., and Vande Woude, G.F., *In vitro* methylation of specific regions of the cloned Moloney sarcoma virus genome inhibits its transforming activity, *Mol. Cell. Biol.,* 3, 305, 1983.

123. Seliger, B., Kruppa, G., and Pfizenmaier, K., Murine gamma interferon inhibits v-*mos*-induced fibroblast transformation via down regulation of retroviral gene expression, *J. Virol.,* 61, 2567, 1987.

124. Choi, O.-R., Trainor, C., Graf, T., Beug, H., and Engel, J.D., A single amino acid subsitution in v-*erb*B confers a thermolabile phenotype to *ts*167 avian erythroblastosis virus-transformed erythroid cells, *Mol. Cell. Biol.,* 6, 1751, 1986.

125. Soret, J., Kryceve-Martinerie, C., Crochet, J., and Perbal, B., Transformation of Brown Leghorn chicken embryo fibroblasts by avian myeloblastosis virus proviral DNA, *J. Virol.,* 55, 193, 1985.

126. Moscovici, M.G., Klempnauer, K.-H., Symonds, G., Bishop, J.M., and Moscovici, C., Transformation-defective mutant of avian myeloblastosis virus that is temperature sensitive for production of transforming protein p45^{v-myb}, *Mol. Cell. Biol.*, 5, 3301, 1985.

127. Lipsick, J.S., Ibanez, C.E., and Baluda, M.A., Expression of molecular clones of v-*myb* in avian and mammalian cells independently of transformation, *J. Virol.*, 59, 267, 1986.

128. Heaney, M.L., Pierce, J., and Parsons, J.T., Site-directed mutagenesis of the *gag-myc* gene of avian myelocytomatosis virus 29: biological activity and intracellular localization of structurally altered proteins, *J. Virol.*, 60, 167, 1986.

129. Hayflick, J., Seeburg, P.H., Ohlsson, R., Pfeiffer-Ohlsson, S., Watson, D., Papas, T., and Duesberg, P.H., Nucleotide sequence of two overlapping *myc*-related genes in avian carcinoma virus OK10 and their relation to the *myc* genes of other viruses and the cell, *Proc. Natl. Acad. Sci. U.S.A.*, 82, 2718, 1985.

130. Patchinsky, T., Walter, G., and Bister, K., Immunologic analysis of v-*myc* gene products using antibodies against a *myc*-specific synthetic peptide, *Virology*, 136, 348, 1984.

131. Bister, K., Trachmann, C., Jansen, H.W., Schroeer, B., and Patschinsky, T., Structure of mutant and wild-type MC29 v-*myc* alleles and biochemical properties of their protein products, *Oncogene*, 1, 97, 1987.

132. Neckameyer, W.S., Shibuya, M., Hsu, M.-T., and Wang, L.-H., Proto-oncogene c-*ros* codes for a molecule with structural features common to those of growth factor receptors and displays tissue-specific and developmentally regulated expression, *Mol. Cell. Biol.*, 6, 1478, 1986.

133. Podell, S.B. and Sefton, B.M., Chicken proto-oncogene c-*ros* cDNA clones: identification of a c-*ros* RNA transcript and deduction of the amino acid sequence of the carboxyl terminus of the c-*ros* product, *Oncogene*, 2, 9, 1987.

134. Watson, D.K., McWilliams, M.J., and Papas, T.S., Molecular organization of the chicken *ets* locus, *Virology*, 164, 99, 1988.

135. Theilen, G.H., Zeigel, R.F., and Twiehaus, M.J., Biological studies with RE virus (strain T) that induces reticuloendotheliosis in turkeys, chickens, and Japanese quails, *J. Natl. Cancer Inst.*, 37, 731, 1966.

136. Moore, B.E. and Bose, H.R., Jr., Transformation of avian lymphoid cells by reticuloendotheliosis virus, *Mutat. Res.*, 195, 79, 1988.

137. Chen, I.S.Y. and Temin, H.M., Substitution of 5′ helper virus sequences into non-*rel* portion of reticuloendotheliosis virus strain T suppresses transformation of chicken spleen cells, *Cell*, 31, 111, 1982.

138. Chen, I.S.Y., Wilhelmsen, K.C., and Temin, H.M., Structure and expression of c-*rel*, the cellular homolog to 1 oncogene of reticuloendotheliosis virus strain T, *J. Virol.*, 45, 104, 1983.

139. Wilhelmsen, K.C. and Temin, H.M., Structure and dimorphism of c-*rel* (turkey), the cellular homolog to the oncogene of reticuloendotheliosis virus strain T, *J. Virol.*, 49, 521, 1984.

140. Miller, C.K., Embretson, J.E., and Temin, H.M., Transforming viruses spontaneously arise from nontransforming reticuloendotheliosis virus strain T-derived viruses as a result of increased accumulation of spliced viral RNA, *J. Virol.*, 62, 1219, 1988.

141. Sylla, B.S. and Temin, H.M., Activation of oncogenicity of the c-*rel* proto-oncogene, *Mol. Cell. Biol.*, 6, 4709, 1986.

142. Garry, R.F. and Bose, H.R., Jr., Autogenous growth factor production by reticuloendotheliosis virus-transformed hematopoietic cells, *J. Cell. Biochem.*, 37, 327, 1988.

143. Ullrich, A., Coussens, L., Hayflick, J.S., Dull, T.J., Gray, A., Tam, A.W., Lee, J., Yarden, Y., Libermann, T.A., Schlessinger, J., Downward, J., Mayes, E.L.V., Whittle, N., Waterfield, M.D., and Seeburg, P.H., Human epidermal growth factor receptor cDNA sequence and aberrant expression of the amplified gene in A431 epidermoic carcinoma cells, *Nature*, 309, 418, 1984.

144. Riedel, H., Schlessinger, J., and Ullrich, A., A chimeric, ligand-binding v*erb*B/EGF receptor retains transforming potential, Science, 236, 197, 1987.

145. Rapp, U.R., Reynolds, F.H., Jr., and Stephenson, J.R., New mammalian transforming retrovirus: demonstration of a polyprotein gene product, *J. Virol.*, 45, 914, 1983.

146. Schultz, A.M., Copeland, T., Oroszlan, S., and Rapp, U.R., Identification and characterization of c-*raf* phosphoproteins in transformed murine cells, *Oncogene*, 2, 187, 1988.

147. Rosson, D. and Reddy, E.P., Nucleotide sequence of chicken c-*myb* complementary DNA and implications for *myb* oncogene activation, *Nature*, 319, 604, 1986.

148. Gerondakis, S. and Bishop, J.M., Structure of the protein encoded by the chicken proto-oncogene c-*myb*, *Mol. Cell. Biol.*, 6, 3677, 1986.

149. Stober-Grässer, U. and Lipsick, J.S., Specific amino acid substitutions are not required for transformation by v-*myb* of avian myeloblastosis virus, *J. Virol.*, 62, 1093, 1988.

150. Kryceve-Martinerie, C., Soret, J., Crochet, J., Baluda, M., and Perbal, B., Expression of a truncated v-*myb* product in transformed chicken embryo fibroblasts, *FEBS Lett.*, 214, 81, 1987.

151. Greer, P.A., Meckling-Hansen, K., and Pawwon, T., The human c-*fps/fes* gene product expressed ectopically in rat fibroblasts is nontransforming and has restrained protein-tyrosine kinase activity, *Mol. Cell. Biol.*, 8, 578, 1988.

152. Foster, D.A., Shibuya, M., and Hanafusa, H., Activation of the transformation potential of the cellular *fps* gene, *Cell,* 42, 105, 1985.

153. Pfaff, S.L., Zhou, R.-P., Young, J.C., Hayflick, J., and Duesberg, P.H., Defining the borders of the chicken proto-*fps* gene, a precursor of Fujinami sarcoma virus, *Virology,* 146, 307, 1985.

154. Ziemicki, A., Hennig, D., Gardner, L., Ferdinand, F.-J., Friis, R.R., Bauer, H., Pedersen, N.C., Johnson, L., and Theilen, G.H., Biological and biochemical characterization of a new isolate of feline sarcoma virus: Theilen-Pedersen (TP1-FeSV), *Virology,* 138, 324, 1984.

155. Besmer, P., Murphy, J.E., George, P.C., Qiu, F., Bergold, P.J., Lederman, L., Snyder, H.W., Jr., Brodeur, D., Zuckerman, E.E., and Hardy, W.D., A new acute transforming feline retrovirus and relation of its oncogene v-*kit* with the protein kinase gene family, *Nature,* 320, 415, 1986.

156. Besmer, P., Lader, E., George, P.C., Bergold, P.J., Qiu, F.H., Zuckerman, E.E., and Hardy, W.D., A new acute transforming feline retrovirus with *fms* homology specifies a C-terminally truncated version of the c-*fms* protein that is different from SM-feline sarcoma virus v-*fms* protein, *J. Virol.,* 60, 194, 1986.

157. Donner, L., Fedele, L.A., Garon, C.F., Anderson, S.J., and Sherr, C.J., McDonough feline sarcoma virus: characterization of the molecularly cloned provirus and its feline oncogene (v-*fms*), *J. Virol.,* 41, 489, 1982.

158. Heisterkamp, N., Groffen, J., and Stephenson, J.R., Isolation of v-*fms* and its human cellular homolog, *Virology,* 126, 248, 1983.

159. Sherr, C.J., Fibroblast and hematopoietic cell transformation by the *fms* oncogene (CSF-1 receptor), *J. Cell. Physiol.,* Suppl. 5, 83, 1987.

160. Nichols, E.J., Manger, R., Hakomori, S.-I., and Rohrschneider, L.R., Transformation by the oncogene v-*fms*: the effects of castanospermine on transformation-related parameters, *Exp. Cell Res.,* 173, 486, 1987.

161. Patschinsky, T., Jansen, H.W., Blöcker, H., Frank, R., and Bister, K., Structure and transforming function of transduced mutant alleles of the chicken c-*myc* gene, *J. Virol.,* 59, 341, 1986.

162. Frykberg, L., Graf, T., and Vennström, B., The transforming activity of the chicken c-*myc* gene can be potentiated by mutations, *Oncogene,* 1, 415, 1987.

163. Papkoff, J., Verman, I.M., and Hunter, T., Detection of a transforming gene product in cells transformed by Moloney murine sarcoma virus, *Cell,* 29, 417, 1982.

164. Nash, M., Brown, N.V., Wong, J.L., Arlinghaus, R.B., and Murphy, E.C., Jr., S1 nuclease mapping of viral RNAs from a temperature-sensitive transformation mutant of murine sarcoma virus, *J. Virol.,* 50, 478, 1984.

165. Gallick, G.E., Hamelin, R., Maxwell, S., Duyka, D., and Arlinghaus, R.B., The *gag-mos* hybrid protein of ts110 Moloney murine sarcoma virus: variation of gene expression with temperature, *Virology,* 139, 366, 1984.

166. Cizdziel, P.E., Nash, M.A., Blair, D.G., and Murphy, E.C. Jr., Molecular basis underlying phenotypic revertants of Moloney murine sarcoma virus MuSV*ts*110, *J. Virol.,* 57, 310, 1986.

167. van der Hoorn, F.A. and Müller, V., Differential transformation of C3H10T1/2 cells by v-*mos*: sequential expression of transformation parameters, *Mol. Cell. Biol.,* 5, 2204, 1985.

168. Singh, B., Hannink, M., Donoghue, D.J., and Arlinghaus, R.B., p37^{mos}-associated serine/threonine protein kinase activity correlates with the cellular transformation function of v-*mos*, *J. Virol.,* 60, 1148, 1986.

169. Bold, R.J. and Donoghue, D.J., Biologically active mutants, with deletions in the v-*mos* oncogene assayed with retroviral vectors, *Mol. Cell. Biol.,* 5, 3131, 1985.

170. Papkoff, J. and Ringold, G.M., Use of the mouse mammary tumor virus long terminal repeat to promote steroid-inducible expression of v-*mos*, *J. Virol.,* 52, 420, 1984.

171. Stocking, C., Kollek, R., Bergholz, U., and Ostertag, W., Long terminal repeat sequences impart hematopoietic transformation properties to the myeloproliferative sarcoma virus, *Proc. Natl. Acad. Sci. U.S.A.,* 82, 5746, 1985.

172. Khillan, J.S., Oskarsson, M.K., Propst, F., Kuwabara, T., Vande Woude, G.F., and Westphal, H., Defects in lens fiber differentiation are linked to c-*mos* overexpression in transgenic mice, *Genes Dev.,* 1, 1327, 1987.

173. Zhou, R.-P. and Duesberg, P.H., *myc* protooncogene linked to retroviral promoter, but not to enhancer, transforms embryo cells, *Proc. Natl. Acad. Sci. U.S.A.,* 85, 2924, 1988.

174. Baumbach, W.R., Keath, E.J., and Cole, M.D., A mouse c-*myc* retrovirus transforms established fibroblast lines *in vitro* and induces monocyte-macrophage tumors *in vivo,* *J. Virol.,* 59, 276, 1986.

175. Shiroki, K., Segawa, K., Koita, Y., and Shibuya, M., Neoplastic transformation of rat 3Y1 cells by a transcriptionally activated c-*myc* gene and stabilization of p53 cellular tumor antigen in the transformed cells, *Mol. Cell. Biol.,* 6, 4379, 1986.

176. Small, M.B., Hay, N., Schwab, M., and Bishop, J.M., Neoplastic transformation by the human gene N-*myc*, *Mol. Cell. Biol.,* 7, 1638, 1987.

177. Zerlin, M., Julius, M.A., Cerni, C., and Marcu, K.B., Elevated expression of an exogenous c-*myc* gene is insufficient for transformation and tumorigenic conversion of established fibroblasts, *Oncogene,* 1, 19, 1987.

178. Schoenenberger, C.-A., Andres, A.-C., Groner, B., van der Valk, M., LeMeur, M., and Gerlinger, P., Targeted c-*myc* gene expression in mammary glands of transgenic mice induces mammary tumours with constitutive milk protein gene transcription, *EMBO J.,* 7, 169, 1988.

179. Keath, E.J., Caimi, P.G., and Cole, M.D., Fibroblast lines expressing activated c-*myc* oncogenes are tumorigenic in nude mice and syngeneic animals, *Cell*, 39, 339, 1984.

180. Nicolaiew, N. and Dautry, F., Growth stimulation of rat primary embryo fibroblasts by the human *myc* gene, *Exp. Cell Res.*, 166, 357, 1986.

181. Storer, R.D., Allen, H.L., Kraynak, A.R., and Bradley, M.O., Rapid induction of an experimental metastatic phenotype in first passage rat embryo cells by cotransfection of EJ c-Ha-*ras* and c-*myc* oncogenes, *Oncogene*, 2, 141, 1988.

182. Pellegrini, S. and Basilico, C., Rat fibroblasts expressing high levels of human c-myc transcripts are anchorage-independent and tumorigenic, *J. Cell. Physiol.*, 126, 107, 1986.

183. Modjtahedi, N., Feunteun, J., and Brison, O., *cis* activation of the c-*myc* gene in bovine papilloma virus type 1/human c-*myc* hybrid plasmis, *Exp. Cell Res.*, 174, 58, 1988.

184. Langdon, W.Y., Harris, A.W., Cory, S., and Adams, J.M., The c-*myc* oncogene perturbs B lymphocyte development in E$_{mu}$-*myc* transgenic mice, *Cell*, 47, 11, 1986.

185. Taparowsky, E.J., Heaney, M.L., and Parsons, J.T., Oncogene-mediated multistep transformation of C3H10T1/2 cells, *Cancer Res.*, 47, 4125, 1987.

186. van Beveren, C., Enami, S., Curran, and Verma, I.M., FBR murine osteosarcoma virus. II. Nucleotide sequence of the provirus reveals that the genome contains sequences acquired from two cellular genes, *Virology*, 135, 229, 1984.

187. Miller, A.D., Curran, T., and Verma, I.M., c-*fos* protein can induce cellular transformation: a novel mechanism of activation of a cellular oncogene, *Cell*, 36, 51, 1984.

188. Curran, T., Miller, A.D., Zokas, L., and Verma, I.M., Viral and cellular *fos* proteins: a comparative analysis, *Cell*, 36, 259, 1984.

189. Müller, R., Müller, D., and Guilbert, L., Differential expression of c-*fos* in hematopoietic cells: correlation with differentiation of monomyelocytic cells *in vitro*, *EMBO J.*, 3, 1887, 1984.

190. Meijlink, F., Curran, T., Miller, A.D., and Verma, I.M., Removal of a 67-base-pair sequence in the noncoding region of protooncogene *fos* converts it to a transforming gene, *Proc. Natl. Acad. Sci. U.S.A.*, 82, 4987, 1985.

191. Nishizawa, M., Goto, N., and Kawai, S., An avian transforming retrovirus isolated from a nephroblastoma that carries the *fos* gene as the oncogene, *J. Virol.*, 61, 3733, 1987.

192. Blair, D.G., Oskarsson, M., Wood, T.G., McClements, W.L., Fischinger, P.J., and Vande Woude, G.G., Activation of the transforming potential of a normal cell sequence: a molecular model for oncogenesis, *Science*, 212, 941, 1981.

193. Blair, D.G., Oskarsson, M.K., Seth, A., Dunn, K.J., Dean, M., Zweig, M., Tainsky, M.A., and Vande Woude, G.F., Analysis of the transforming potential of the human homolog of *mos*, *Cell*, 46, 785, 1986.

194. Schmidt, M., Oskarsson, M.K., Dunn, J.K., Blair, D.G., Hughes, S., Propst,F., and Vande Woude, G.F., Chicken homolog of the *mos* proto-oncogene, *Mol. Cell. Biol.*, 8, 923, 1988.

195. Cichutek, K. and Duesberg, P.H., Harvey *ras* genes transform without mutant codons, apparently activated by truncation of a 5' exon (exon-1), *Proc. Natl. Acad. Sci. U.S.A.*, 83, 2340, 1986.

196. Cohen, J.B. and Levinson, A.D., A point mutation in the last intron responsible for increased expression and transforming activity of the c-Ha-*ras* oncogene, *Nature*, 334, 119, 1988.

197. Huang, A.L., Ostrowski, M.C., Berard, D., and Hager, G.L., Glucocorticoid regulation of the Ha-MuSV p21 gene conferred by sequences from mouse mammary tumor virus, *Cell*, 27, 245, 1981.

198. Seliger, B., Kollek, R., Stocking, C., Franz, T., and Ostertag, W., Viral transfer, transcription, and rescue of a selectable myeloproliferative sarcoma virus in embryonal cell lines: expression of the *mos* oncogene, *Mol. Cell. Biol.*, 6, 286, 1986.

199. Sergiescu, D., Gerfaux, J., Joret, A.-M., and Chany, C., Persistent expression of v-*mos* oncogene in transformed cells that revert to nonmalignancy after prolonged treatment with interferon, *Proc. Natl. Acad. Sci. U.S.A.*, 83, 5764, 1986.

200. Haynes, J.R. and Downing, J.R., A recessive cellular mutation in v-*fes*-transformed mink cells restores contact inhibition and anchorage-dependent growth, *Mol. Cell. Biol.*, 8, 2419, 1988.

201. Maeda, T., Owada, M.K., Sugiyama, H., Miyake, S., Tani, Y., Ogawa, H., Oka, Y., Komori, T., Soma, T., Kishimoto, S., Seki, J., Sakato, N., and Hakura, A., Differentiation of an Abelson virus-transformed immature B precursor cell line under the expression of tyrosine kinase activity of v-abl oncogene product, *Cell Differ.*, 20, 263, 1987.

202. Albini, A., Graf, J., Kitten, G.T., Kleinman, H.K., Martin, G.R., Veillette, A., and Lippman, M.E., 17 beta-estradiol regulates and v-Ha-*ras* transfection constitutively enhances MCF7 breast cancer cell interactions with basement membrane, *Proc. Natl. Acad. Sci. U.S.A.*, 8182, 1986.

203. Lichtman, A.H., Reynolds, D.S., Faller, D.V., and Abbas, A.K., Mature murine B lymphocytes immortalized by Kirsten sarcoma virus, *Nature*, 324, 489, 1986.

204. Hjelle, B., Liu, E., and Bishop, J.M., Oncogene v-*src* transforms and establishes embryonic rodent fibroblasts but not diploid human fibroblasts, *Proc. Natl. Acad. Sci. U.S.A.*, 85, 4355, 1988.

205. Stevenson, M. and Volsky, D.J., Activated v-*myc* and v-*ras* oncogenes do not transform normal human lymphocytes, *Mol. Cell. Biol.*, 6, 3410, 1986.

206. Roop, D.R., Lowy, D.R., Tambourin, P.E., Strickland, J., Harper, J.R., Balaschak, M., Spangler, E.F., and Yuspa, S.H., An activated Harvey *ras* oncogene produces benign tumours on mouse epidermal tissue, *Nature,* 323, 822, 1986.

207. O'Brien, W., Stenman, G., and Sager, R., Suppression of tumor growth by senescence in virally transformed human fibroblasts, *Proc. Natl. Acad. Sci. U.S.A.,* 83, 8659, 1986.

208. Blasi, E., Radzioch, D., Durum, S.K., and Varesio, L., A murine macrophage cell line, immortalized by v-*raf* and v-*myc* oncogenes, exhibits normal macrophage functions, *Eur. J. Immunol.,* 17, 1491, 1987.

209. Hirano, T., Miyajima, H., Watanabe, T., Tsukudo, R., and Shimamoto, K., Enhancement of tumor induction in rats with Moloney murine sarcoma viruses by a new method based on direct injection into fetuses, *J. Natl. Cancer Inst.,* 58, 73, 1977.

210. Rossi, L., Barbieri, O., Astigiano, S., Ugolini, D., and Varnier, O.E., Stage-dependent induction of prenatal tumors in mice by the Kirsten and Moloney strains of murine sarcoma viruses, *Cancer Res.,* 45, 6107, 1985.

211. Ferrentino, M., Di Fiore, P.P., Fusco, A., Colletta, G., Pinto, A., and Vecchio, G., Expression of the *onc* gene of the Kirsten murine sarcoma virus in differentiated rat thyroid epithelial cell lines, *J. Gen. Virol.,* 65, 1955, 1984.

212. Colletta, G., Pinto, A., Di Fiore, P.P., Fusco, A., Ferrentino, M., Avvedimento, V.E., Tsuchida, N., and Vecchio, G., Dissociation between transformed and differentiated phenotype in rat thyroid epithelial cells after transformation with a temperature-sensitive mutant of the Kirsten murine sarcoma virus, *Mol. Cell. Biol.,* 3, 2099, 1983.

213. Ferré, F., Martin, P., Begue, A., Ghysdael, J., Saule, S., and Stéhelin, D., Préparation et caractérisation d'antisera spécifiques dirigés contre différents domaines polypeptidiques codés par l'oncogène c-*myc* humain pour étudier l'expression de ce gène introduit dans des cellules de caille ou de rat, *C.R. Acad. Sci. (Paris),* 303, 633, 1986.

214. Falcone, G., Summerhayes, I.C., Paterson, H., Marshall, C.J., and Hall, A., Partial transformation of mouse fibroblastic and epithelial cell lines with the v-*myc* oncogene, *Exp. Cell Res.,* 168, 273, 1987.

215. Leder, A., Pattengale, P.K., Kuo, A., Stewart, T.A., and Leder, P., Consequences of widespread deregulation of the c-*myc* gene in transgenic mice: multiple neoplasms and normal development, *Cell,* 45, 485, 1986.

216. Silva, R.F. and Moscovici, C., Spontaneous regression of leukemia in chickens infected with avian myeloblastosis virus, *Proc. Soc. Exp. Biol. Med.,* 143, 604, 1973.

217. Symonds, G., Klempnauer, K.-H., Evan, G.I., and Bishop, J.M., Induced differentiation of avian myeloblastosis virus-transformed myeloblasts: phenotypic alteration without altered expression of the viral oncogene, *Mol. Cell. Biol.,* 4, 2587, 1984.

218. Khan, A.S., Deobagkar, D.N., and Stephenson, J.R., Isolation and characterization of a feline sarcoma virus-coded precursor polyprotein: competition immunoassay for the nonstructural component(s), *J. Biol. Chem.,* 253, 8894, 1978.

219. Chen, A.P., Essex, M., Kelliher, M., de Noronha, F., Shadduck, J.A., Niederkorn, J.Y., and Albert, D., Feline sarcoma virus-specific transformation-related proteins and protein kinase activity in tumor cells, *Virology,* 124, 274, 1983.

220. Devare, S.G., Reddy, E.P., Law, J.D., Robbins, K.C., and Aaronson, S.A., Nucleotide sequence of the simian sarcoma virus genome: demonstration that its acquired cellular sequences encode the transforming gene product p28^{sis}, *Proc. Natl. Acad. Sci. U.S.A.,* 80, 731, 1983.

221. Stanker, L.H., Horn, J.P., Gallick, G.E., Kloetzer, W.S., Murphy, E.C., Jr., Blair, D.G., and Arlinghaus, R.B., *gag-mos* polyproteins encoded by variants of the Moloney strain of mouse sarcoma virus, *Virology,* 126, 336, 1983.

222. Curran, T. and Verma, I.M., FBR murine osteosarcoma virus. I. Molecular analysis and characterization of a 75,000-Da *gag-fos* fusion product, *Virology,* 135, 218, 1984.

223. Hayman, M.J., Kitchener, G., Vogt, P.K., and Beug, H., The putative transforming protein of S13 avian erythroblastosis virus is a transmembrane glycoprotein with an associated protein kinase activity, *Proc. Natl. Acad. Sci. U.S.A.,* 82, 8237, 1985.

224. Foster, D.A. and Hanafusa, H., A *fps* gene without *gag* gene sequences transforms cells in culture and induces tumors in chickens, *J. Virol.,* 48, 744, 1983.

225. Stone, J.C., Atkinson, T., Smith, M., and Pawson, T., Identification of functional regions in the transforming protein of Fujinami sarcoma virus by in-phase insertion mutagenesis, *Cell,* 37, 549, 1984.

226. Eisenman, R.N. and Vogt, V.M., The biosynthesis of oncovirus proteins, *Biochim. Biophys. Acta,* 473, 187, 1978.

227. Ishida, T., Pedersen, N.C., and Theilen, G.H., Monoclonal antibodies to the v-*fes* product and to feline leukemia: virus p27 interspecies-specific determinants encoded by feline sarcoma viruses, *Virology,* 155, 678, 1986.

228. Lipsick, J.S. and Ibanez, C.E., *env*-encoded residues are not required for transformation by p48$^{v\text{-}myb}$, *J. Virol.,* 61, 933, 1987.

229. Jenuwein, T., Müller, D., Curran, T., and Müller, R., Extended life span and tumorigenicity of nonestablished mouse connective tissue cells transformed by the *fos* oncogene of FBR-MuSV, *Cell,* 41, 629, 1985.

230. Miller, A.D., Verma, I.M., and Curran, T., Deletion of the *gag* region from FBR murine osteosarcoma virus does not affect its enhanced transforming activity, *J. Virol.,* 55, 521, 1985.

231. Alt, F.W., Blackwell, T.K., DePinho, R.A., Reth, M.G., and Yancopoulos, G.D., Regulation of genome rearragement event during lymphocyte differentiation, *Immunol. Rev.,* 89, 5, 1986.

232. Schiffmaker, L. and Rosenberg, N., *gag*-derived but not *abl*-derived determinants are exposed on the surface of Abelson virus-transformed cells, *Virology,* 154, 286, 1986.

233. Mathey-Prevot, B. and Baltimore, D., Specific transforming potential of oncogenes encoding protein-tyrosine kinases, *EMBO J.,* 4, 1769, 1985.

234. Levantis, P., Gillespie, D.A.F., Hart, K., Bissell, M.J., and Wyke, J.A., Control of expression of an integrated Rous sarcoma provirus in rat cells: role of 5′ genomic duplications reveals unexpected patterns of gene transcription and its regulation, *J. Virol.,* 57, 907, 1986.

235. Hannink, M. and Donoghue, D.J., Requirement for a signal sequence in biological expression of the v-*sis* oncogene, *Science,* 226, 1197, 1984.

236. Hamelin, R., Kabat, K., Blair, D., and Arlinghaus, R.B., Temperature-sensitive splicing defect of *ts*110 Moloney murine sarcoma virus is virus encoded, *J. Virol.,* 57, 301, 1986.

237. Schultz, A. and Oroszlan, S., Myristylation of *gag-onc* fusion proteins in mammalian transforming retroviruses, *Virology,* 133, 431, 1984.

238. Schultz, A.M., Henderson, L.E., Oroszlan, S., Garber, E.A., and Hanafusa, H., Amino terminal myristylation of the protein kinase p60*src*, a retroviral transforming protein, *Science,* 227, 427, 1985.

239. Buss, J.E., Kamps, M.P., and Sefton, B.M., Myristic acid is attached to the transforming protein of Rous sarcoma virus during or immediately after synthesis and is present in both soluble and membrane-bound forms of the protein, *Mol. Cell. Biol.,* 4, 2697, 1984.

240. Buss, J.E. and Sefton, B.M., Myristic acid, a rare fatty acid, is the lipid attached to the transforming protein of Rous sarcoma virus and its cellular homolog, *J. Virol.,* 53, 7, 1985.

241. Cross, F.R., Garber, E.A., Pellman, D., and Hanafusa, H., A short sequence in the p60*src* N terminus is required for p60*src* myristylation and membrane association and for cell transformation, *Mol. Cell. Biol.,* 4, 1834, 1984.

242. Snyder, M.A. and Bishop, J.M., A mutation at the major phosphotyrosine in pp60*v-src* alters oncogenic potential, *Virology,* 136, 375, 1984.

243. Weinmaster, G., Zoller, M.J., Smith, M., Hinze, E., and Pawson, T., Mutagenesis of Fujinami sarcoma virus: evidence that tyrosine phosphorylation of p130*gag-fps* modulates its biological activity, *Cell,* 37, 559, 1984.

244. Auersperg, N., Pawson, T., Worth, A., and Weinmaster, G., Modifications of tumor histology by point mutations in the v-*fps* oncogene: possible role of extracellular matrix, *Cancer Res.,* 47, 6341, 1987.

245. Donner, P., Greiser-Wilke, I., and Moelling, K., Nuclear localization and DNA binding of the transforming gene product of avian myelocytomatosis virus, *Nature,* 296, 262, 1982.

246. Bunte, T., Donner, P., Pfaff, E., Reis, B., Greiser-Wilke, I., Schaller, H., and Moelling, K., Inhibition of DNA binding of purified p55*v-myc* *in vitro* by antibodies against bacterially expressed *myc* protein and a synthetic peptide, *EMBO J.,* 3, 1919, 1984.

247. Eisenman, R.N., Tachibana, C.Y., Abrams, H.D., and Hann, S.R., v-*myc* and c-*myc*-encoded proteins are associated with the nuclear matrix, *Mol. Cell. Biol.,* 5, 114, 1985.

248. Klempnauer, K.-H., Symonds, G., Evan, G.I., and Bishop, J.M., Subcellular localization of proteins encoded by the oncogenes of avian myeloblastosis virus and avian leukemia virus E26 and by the chicken c-*myb* gene, *Cell,* 37, 537, 1984.

249. Boyle, W.J., Lampert, M.A., Lipsick, J.S., and Baluda, M.A., Avian myeloblastosis virus and E26 virus oncogene products are nuclear proteins, *Proc. Natl. Acad. Sci. U.S.A.,* 81, 4265, 1984.

250. Nunn, M., Weiher, H., Bullock, P., and Duesberg, P., Avian erythroblastosis virus E26: nucleotide sequence of the tripartite *onc* gene and the LTR, and analysis of the cellular prototype of the viral *ets* sequence, *Virology,* 139, 330, 1984.

251. Papkoff, J., Nigg, E.A., and Hunter, T., The transforming protein of Moloney murine sarcoma virus is a soluble cytoplasmic protein, *Cell,* 33, 161, 1983.

252. Ariizumi, K. and Shibuya, M., Construction and biological analysis of deletion mutants of Fujinami sarcoma virus: 5′-*fps* sequence has a role in the transforming activity, *J. Virol.,* 55, 660, 1985.

253. Stone, J.C. and Pawson, T., Correspondence between immunological and functional domains in the transforming protein of Fujinami sarcoma virus, *J. Virol.,* 55, 721, 1985.

254. Willingham, M.C., Pastan, I., Shih, T.Y., and Scolnick, E.M., Localization of the *src* gene product of the Harvey strain of MSV to plasma membrane of transformed cells by electron immunocytochemistry, *Cell,* 19, 1005, 1980.

255. Courtneidge, S.A., Levinson, A.D., and Bishop, J.M., The protein encoded by the transforming gene of avian sarcoma virus (pp60*src*) and a homologous protein in normal cells (pp60*proto-src*) are associated with the plasma membrane, *Proc. Natl. Acad. Sci. U.S.A.,* 77, 3783, 1980.

256. Rohrschneider, L.R. and Najita, L.M., Detection of the v-*abl* gene product at cell-substratum contact sites in Abelson murine leukemia virus-transformed fibroblasts, *J. Virol.,* 51, 547, 1984.

257. Privalsky, M.L. and Bishop, J.M., Subcellular localization of the v-*erb*-B protein, the product of a transforming gene of avian erythroblastosis virus, *Virology,* 135, 356, 1984.

258. Beemon, K. and Mattingly, B., Avian sarcoma virus *gag-fps* and *gag-yes* transforming proteins are not myristylated or palmitylated, *Virology,* 2, 716, 1986.

259. Sheiness, D., Vennstrom, B., and Bishop, J.M., Virus-specific RNAs in cells infected by avian myelocytomatosis virus and avian erythroblastosis virus: modes of oncogene expression, *Cell,* 23, 291, 1981.

260. Hines, D.L., Viral oncogene expression during differentiation of Abelson virus-infected murine promonocytic leukemia cells, *Cancer Res.,* 48, 1702, 1988.

261. Marczynska, B., Gilles, P.N., and Ogston, C.W., Instability of v-*src* sequences in nonhuman primate tumors cultured *in vitro, Virology,* 159, 154, 1987.

262. Wyke, J.A., Stocker, A.W., Searle, S., Spooncer, E., Simmons, P., and Dexter, T.M., Perturbed hemopoiesis and the generation of multipotential stem cell clones in *src*-infected bone marrow cultures is an indirect or transient effect of the oncogene, *Mol. Cell. Biol.,* 6, 959, 1986.

263. Uehara, Y., Hori, M., Takeuchi, T., and Umezawa, H., Phenotypic change from transformed to normal induced by benzoquinonoid ansamycins accompanies inactivation of p60^{src} in rat kidney cells infected with Rous sarcoma virus, *Mol. Cell. Biol.,* 6, 2198, 1986.

264. Gazzolo, L., Samarut, J., Bouabdelli, M., and Blanchet, J.P., Early precursors in the erythroid lineage are the specific target cells of avian erythroblastosis virus *in vitro, Cell,* 22, 683, 1980.

265. Holmwa, K.L., Pierce, J.H., Davidson, W.F., and Morse, H.C., III, Murine hematopoietic cells with pre-B or pre-B/myeloid characteristics are generated by in vitro transformation with retroviruses containing *fes, ras, abl,* and *src* oncogenes, *J. Exp. Med.,* 164, 443, 1986.

266. Hagiya, M., Davis, D.D., Takahashi, T., Okuda, K., Raschke, W.C., and Sakano, H., Two types of immunoglobulin-negative Abelson murine leukemia virus-transformed cells: implications for B-lymphocyte differentiation, *Proc. Natl. Acad. Sci. U.S.A.,* 83, 145, 1986.

267. Neiman, P., Wolf, C., Enrietto, P.J., and Cooper, G.M., A retroviral *myc* gene induces preneoplastic transformation of lymphocytes in a bursal transplantation assay, *Proc. Natl. Acad. Sci. U.S.A.,* 82, 222, 1985.

268. Thompson, C.B., Humphries, E.H., Carlson, L.M., Chen, C.-L. H., and Neiman, P.E., The effect of alterations in *myc* gene expression on B cell differentiation in the bursa of Fabricius, *Cell,* 51, 371, 1987.

269. Falcone, G., Tato, F., and Alema, S., Distinctive effects of the viral oncogenes *myc, erb, fps,* and *src* on the differentiation program of quail myogenic cells, *Proc. Natl. Acad. Sci. U.S.A.,* 82, 426, 1985.

270. Pharr, P.N., Ogawa, M., and Hankins, W.D., *In vitro* retroviral transfer of ras genes to single hemopoietic progenitors, *Exp. Hematol.,* 15, 323, 1987.

271. Symonds, G., Klempnauer, K.-H., Snyder, M., Moscovici, G., Moscovici, C., and Bishop, J.M., Coordinate regulation of myelomonocytic phenotype by v-*myb* and v-*myc, Mol. Cell. Biol.,* 6, 1796, 1986.

272. Hankins, W.D. and Scolnick, E.M., Harvey and Kirsten sarcoma viruses promote the growth and differentiation of erythroid precursor cells *in vitro, Cell,* 26, 91, 1981.

273. Rein, A., Keller, J., Schultz, A.M., Holmes, K.L., Medicus, R., and Ihle, J.N., Infection of immune mast cells by Harvey sarcoma virus: immortalization without loss of requirement for interleukin-3, *Mol. Cell. Biol.,* 5, 2257, 1985.

274. Scolnick, E.M., Hyperplastic and neoplastic erythroproliferative diseases induced by oncogenic murine retroviruses, *Biochim. Biophys. Acta,* 651, 273, 1982.

275. Samarut, J. and Gazzolo, L., Target cells infected by avian erythroblastosis virus differentiate and become transformed, *Cell,* 28, 921, 1982.

276. Ness, S.A., Beug, H., and Graf, T., v-*myb* dominance over v-*myc* in doubly transformed chick myelomonocytic cells, *Cell,* 51, 41, 1987.

277. Holtzer, H., Biehl, J., Yeoh, G., Meganathan, R., and Kaji, A., Effect of oncogenic virus on muscle differentiation, *Proc. Natl. Acad. Sci. U.S.A.,* 72, 4051, 1975.

278. Ball, R.K., Ziemicki, A., Schönenberger, C.A., Reichmann, E., Redmond, S.M.S., and Groner, B., v-*myc* alters the response of a cloned mouse mammary epithelial cell line to lactogenic hormones, *Mol. Endocrinol.,* 2, 133, 1988.

279. Nakagawa, T., Mabry, M., de Bustros, A., Ihle, J.N., Nelkin, B.D., and Baylin, S.B., Introduction of v-Ha-*ras* oncogene induces differentiation of cultured human medullary thyroid carcinoma cells, *Proc. Natl. Acad. Sci. U.S.A.,* 84, 5923, 1987.

280. White, M.K. and Weber, M.J., Transformation by the *src* oncogene alters glucose transport into rat and chicken cells by different mechanisms, *Mol. Cell. Biol.,* 8, 138, 1988.

281. Takimoto, M., Hirakawa, T., Oikawa, T., Naiki, M., Miyoshi, I., and Kobayashi, H., Synergistic effects of the myc and ras oncogenes on ganglioside synthesis by BALB/c 3T3 fibroblasts, *J. Biochem.,* 100, 813, 1986.

282. Hubbard, S.C., Differential effects of oncogenic transformation on *N*-linked oligosaccharide processing at individual glycosylation sites of viral glycoproteins, *J. Biol. Chem.,* 262, 16403, 1987.

283. Nakaishi, H., Sanai, Y., Shibuya, M., and Nagai, Y., Analysis of cellular expression of gangliosides by gene transfection II: rat 3Y1 cells transformed with several DNAs containing oncogenes (*fes, fps, ras* & *src*) invariably express sialosylparagloboside, *Biochem. Biophys. Res. Commun.,* 150, 766, 1988.

284. Nakaishi, H., Sanai, Y., Shiroki, K., and Nagai, Y., Analysis of cellular expression of gangliosides by gene transfection I: GD3 expression in *myc*-transfected and transformed 3Y1 correlates with anchorage-independent growth activity, *Biochem. Biophys. Res. Commun.,* 150, 760, 1988.

285. Brown, R.L., Horn, J.P., Wible, L., Arlinghaus, R.B., and Brinkley, B.R., Sequence of events in the transformation process in cells infected with a temperature-sensitive transformation mutant of Moloney murine sarcoma virus, *Proc. Natl. Acad. Sci. U.S.A.,* 78, 5593, 1981.

286. Saltarelli, D., Fischer, S., and Gacon, G., Modulation of adenylate cyclase by guanine nucleotides and Kirsten sarcoma virus mediated transformation, *Biochem. Biophys. Res. Commun.,* 127, 318, 1985.

287. Franks, D.J., Whitfield, J.F., and Durkin, J.P., Viral *p21* Ki-RAS protein: a potent intracellular mitogen that stimulates adenylate cyclase activity in early G_1 phase of cultured rat cells, *J. Cell. Biochem.,* 33, 87, 1987.

288. Tagliaferri, P., Katsaros, D., Clair, T., Neckers, L., Robins, R.K., and Cho-Chung, Y.S., Reverse transformation of Harvey murine sarcoma virus-transformed NIH/3T3 cells by site-selective cyclic AMP analogs, *J. Biol. Chem.,* 263, 409, 1988.

289. Cooper, J.A. and Hunter, T., Regulation of cell growth and transformation by tyrosine-specific protein kinases: the search for important cellular substrates, *Curr. Top. Microbiol. Immunol.,* 107, 125, 1983.

290. Hunter, T. and Cooper, J.A., Protein-tyrosine kinases, *Annu. Rev. Biochem.,* 54, 897, 1985.

291. Sefton, B.M., Oncogenes encoding protein kinases, *Trends Genet.,* 1, 306, 1985.

292. Sefton, B.M., The viral tyrosine protein kinases, *Curr. Top. Microbiol. Immunol.,* 123, 39, 1986.

293. Mäkelä, T.P. and Alitalo, K., Tyrosine kinases in control of cell growth and transformation, *Med. Biol.,* 64, 325, 1986.

294. Heldin, C.-H. and Westermark, B., Growth factors: mechanism of action and relation to oncogenes, *Cell,* 37, 9, 1984.

295. James, R. and Bradshaw, R.A., Polypeptide growth factors, *Annu. Rev. Biochem.,* 53, 259, 1984.

296. Feige, J.-J. and Chambaz, E.M., Membrane receptors with protein-tyrosine kinase activity, *Biochimie,* 69, 379, 1987.

297. Goustin, A.S., Leof, E.B., Shipley, G.D., and Moses, H.L., Growth factors and cancer, *Cancer Res.,* 46, 1015, 1986.

298. Pimentel, E., *Hormones, Growth Factors, and Oncogenes,* CRC Press, Boca Raton, FL, 1987.

299. Tuy, F.P.H., Henry, J., Rosenfeld, C., and Kahn, A., High tyrosine kinase activity in normal nonproliferating cells, *Nature,* 305, 435, 1983.

300. Garber, E.A., Hanafusa, T., and Hanafusa, H., Membrane association of the transforming protein of avian sarcoma virus UR2 and mutants temperature sensitive for cellular transformation and protein kinase activity, *J. Virol.,* 56, 790, 1985.

301. Kipreos, E.T., Lee, G.J., and Wang, J.Y.J., Isolation of temperature-sensitive tyrosine kinase mutants of v-*abl* oncogene by screening with antibodies for phosphotyrosine, *Proc. Natl. Acad. Sci. U.S.A.,* 84, 1345, 1987.

302. Takemori, T., Miyazoe, I., Shirasawa, T., Taniguchi, M., and Graf, T., A temperature-sensitive mutant of Abelson murine leukemia virus confers inducibility of IgM expression to transformed lymphoid cells, *EMBO J.,* 6, 951, 1987.

303. Meckling-Hansen, K., Nelson, R., Branton, P., and Pawson, T., Enzymatic activation of Fujinami sarcoma virus *gag-fps* transforming proteins by autophosphorylation at tyrosine, *EMBO J.,* 6, 659, 1987.

304. Klarlund, J.K., Transformation of cells by an inhibitor of phosphatases acting on phosphotyrosine in proteins, *Cell,* 41, 707, 1985.

305. Brunati, A.M., Saggioro, D., Chieco-Bianchi, L., and Pinna, L.A., Altered protein kinase activities of lymphoid cells transformed by Abelson and Moloney leukemia viruses, *FEBS Lett.,* 206, 59, 1986.

306. Edelman, A.M., Blumenthal, D.K., and Krebs, E.G., Protein serine/threonine kinases, *Annu. Rev. Biochem.,* 56, 567, 1987.

307. Rice, N.R., Copeland, T.D., Simek, S., Oroszlan, S., and Gilden, R.V., Detection and characterization of the protein encoded by the v-*rel* oncogene, *Virology,* 149, 217, 1986.

308. Denhez, F., Heimann, B., d'Auriol, L., Graf, T., Coquillaud, M., Coll, J., Galibert, F., Moelling, K., Stehelin, D., and Ghysdael, J., Replacement of lys 622 in the ATP binding domain of P10[gag-mil] abolishes the *in vitro* autophosphorylation of the protein and the biological properties of the v-*mil* oncogene of MH2 virus, *EMBO J.,* 7, 541, 1988.

309. Seuwen, K. and Adam, G., Calcium compartments and fluxes are affected by ths *src* gene product of Rat-1 cells transformed by temperature-sensitive Rous sarcoma virus, *Biochem. Biophys. Res. Commun.,* 125, 337, 1984.

310. Doppler, W., Jaggi, R., and Groner, B., Induction of v-*mos* and activated Ha-*ras* oncogene expression in quiescent NIH 3T3 cells causes intracellular alkalinisation and cell-cycle progression, *Gene,* 54, 147, 1987.

311. Berridge, M.J., Growth factors, oncogenes and inositol lipids, *Cancer Surv.,* 5, 413, 1986.
312. Whitfield, J.F., Durkin, J.P., Franks, D.J., Kleine, L.P., Raptis, L., Rixon, R.H., Sikorska, M., and Walker, P.R., Calcium, cyclic AMP and protein kinase C — partners in mitogenesis, *Cancer Metast. Rev.,* 5, 205, 1987.
313. Berridge, M.J., Inositol lipids and cell proliferation, *Biochim. Biophys. Acta,* 907, 33, 1987.
314. McDonough, S.K., Larsen, S., Brodey, R.S., Stock, N.D., and Hardy, W.D., Jr., A transmissible feline fibrosarcoma of viral origin, *Cancer Res.,* 31, 953, 1971.
315. Sarma, P.S., Sharar, A., and McDonough, S., The SM strain of feline sarcoma virus. Biologic and antigenic characterization of the virus, *Proc. Soc. Exp. Biol. Med.,* 140, 1365, 1972.
316. Heard, J.M., Roussel, M.F., Rettenmier, C.W., and Sherr, C.J., Multilineage hematopoietic disorders induced by transplantation of bone marrow cells expressing the v-*fms* oncogene, *Cell,* 51, 663, 1987.
317. Rettenmier, C.W., Jackowski, S., Rock, C.O., Roussel, M.F., and Sherr, C.J., Transformation by the v-*fms* oncogene product: an analog of the CSF-1 receptor, *J. Cell. Biochem.,* 33, 109, 1987.
318. Sherr, C.J., Rettenmier, C.W., Sacca, R., Roussel, M.F., Look, A.T., and Stanley, E.R., The c-*fms* proto-oncogene product is related to the receptor for the mononuclear phagocyte growth factor, CSF-1, *Cell,* 41, 665, 1985.
319. Wheeler, E.F., Rettenmier, C.W., Look, A.T., and Sherr, C.J., The v-*fms* oncogene induces factor independence and tumorigenicity in CSF-1 dependent macrophage cell line, *Nature,* 324, 377, 1986.
320. Parries, G., Hoebel, R., and Racker, E., Opposing effects of a *ras* oncogene on growth factor-stimulated phosphoinositide hydrolysis: desensitization to platelet-derived growth factor and enhanced sensitivity to bradykinin, *Proc. Natl. Acad. Sci. U.S.A.,* 84, 2648, 1987.
321. Noda, M., Selinger, Z., Scolnick, E.M., and Bassin, R.H., Flat revertants isolated from Kirsten sarcoma virus-transformed cells are resistant to the action of specific oncogenes, *Proc. Natl. Acad. Sci. U.S.A.,* 80, 5602, 1983.
322. Kamata, T., Sullivan, N.F., and Wooten, M.W., Reduced protein kinase C activity in a *ras*-resistant cell line derived from Ki-MSV transformed cells, *Oncogene,* 1, 37, 1987.
323. Groudine, M. and Weintraub, H., Activation of cellular genes by avian RNA tumor viruses, *Proc. Natl. Acad. Sci. U.S.A.,* 77, 5351, 1980.
324. Lane, M.-A., Neary, D., and Cooper, G.M., Activation of a cellular transforming gene in tumours induced by Abelson murine leukaemia virus, *Nature,* 300, 659, 1982.
325. Lipsick, J.S., v-*myb* does not prevent the expression of c-*myb* in avian erythroblastosis, *J. Virol.,* 61, 3284, 1987.
326. Zenke, M., Kahn, P., Disela, C., Vennström, B., Leutz, A., Keegan, K., Hayman, M.J., Choi, H.-R., Yew, N., Engel, J.D., and Beug, H., v-*erbA* specifically suppresses transcription of the avian erythrocyte anion transporter (band 3) gene, *Cell,* 52, 107, 1988.
327. Owen, R.D. and Ostrowski, M.C., Rapid and selective alterations in the expression of cellular genes accompany conditional transcription of Ha-v-*ras* in NIH 3T3 cell, *Mol. Cell. Biol.,* 7, 2512, 1987.
328. Herskowitz, I., Functional inactivation of genes by dominant negative mutations, *Nature,* 329, 219, 1987.
329. Fusco, A., Berlingieri, M.T., Di Fiore, P.P., Portella, G., Grieco, M., and Vecchio, G., One- and two-step transformations of rat thyroid epithelial cells by retroviral oncogenes, *Mol. Cell. Biol.,* 7, 3365, 1987.
330. Sporn, M.B. and Roberts, A.B., Autocrine growth factors and cancer, *Nature,* 313, 745, 1985.
331. Hines, D.L., Proliferation and differentiation of Abelson virus-infected murine myeloid leukemia cell lines does not involve an autocrine mechanism, *J. Cell. Physiol.,* 135, 108, 1988.
332. Redmond, S.M.S., Reichmann, E., Müller, R.G., Friis, R.R., Groner, B., and Hynes, N.E., The transformation of primary and established mouse mammary epithelial cells by p21-*ras* is concentration dependent, *Oncogene,* 2, 259, 1988.
333. Sadowski, I., Pawson, T., and Lagarde, A., v-*fps* protein-tyrosine kinase coordinately enhances the malignancy and growth factor responsiveness of pre-neoplastic lung fibroblasts, *Oncogene,* 2, 241, 1988.
334. Keating, M.T. and Williams, L.T., Autocrine stimulation of intracellular PDGF receptors in v-*sis*-transformed cells, *Science,* 239, 914, 1988.
335. Todaro, G.J., De Larco, J.E., and Cohen, S., Transformation by murine and feline sarcoma viruses specifically blocks binding of epidermal growth factor to cells, *Nature,* 264, 26, 1976.
336. De Larco, J.E. and Todaro, G.F., Growth factors from murine sarcoma virus-transformed cells, *Proc. Natl. Acad. Sci. U.S.A.,* 75, 4001, 1978.
337. Roberts, A.B., Lamb, L.C., Newton, D.L., Sporn, M.B., De Larco, J.E., and Todaro, G.J., Transforming growth factors: isolation of polypeptides from virally and chemically transformed cells by acid/ethanol extraction, *Proc. Natl. Acad. Sci. U.S.A.,* 77, 3494, 1980.
338. Todaro, G.J., De Larco, J.E., Fryling, C., Johnson, P.A., and Sporn, M.B., Transforming growth factors' properties and possible mechanisms of action, *J. Supramol. Struct. Cell. Biochem.,* 15, 287, 1981.
339. Roberts, A.B., Frolik, C.A., Anzano, M.A., and Sporn, M.B., Transforming growth factors from neoplastic and nonneoplastic tissues, *Fed. Proc. Fed. Am. Soc. Exp. Biol.,* 42, 2621, 1983.
340. Roberts, A.B. and Sporn, M.B., Transforming growth factors, *Cancer Surv.,* 4, 683, 1985.
341. van Zoelen, E.J.J., van Rooijen, M.A., van Oostwaard, T.M.J., and de Laat, S.W., Production of transforming growth factors by simian sarcoma virus-transformed cells, *Cancer Res.,* 47, 1582, 1987.

342. Perucho, M. and Massague, J., Reversible induction of transforming growth factor-alpha by human *ras* oncogenes, *J. Tumor Marker Oncol.*, 1, 81, 1986.

343. Buick, R.N., Filmus, J., and Quaroni, A., Activated H-*ras* transforms rat intestinal epithelial cells with expression of TGF-alpha, *Exp. Cell Res.*, 170, 300, 1987.

344. Durkin, J.P. and Whitfield, J.F., Evidence that the viral Ki-RAS protein, but not the pp60^{v-src} protein of ASV, stimulates proliferation through the PDGF receptor, *Biochem. Biophys. Res. Commun.*, 148, 376, 1987.

345. Fasciotto, B., Kanazir, D., Durkin, J.P., Whitfield, J.F., and Krsmanovic, V., AEV-transformed chicken erythroid cells secrete autocrine factors which promote soft agar growth and block erythroleukemia cell differentiation, *Biochem. Biophys. Res. Commun.*, 143, 775, 1987.

346. Pierce, J.H., Ruggiero, M., Fleming, T.P., Di Fiore, P.P., Greenberger, J.S., Varticovski, L., Schlessinger, J., Rovera, G., and Aaronson, S.A., Signal transduction through the EGF receptor transfected in IL-3-dependent hematopoietic cells, *Science*, 239, 628, 1988.

347. Vennström, B. and Bravo, R., Anchorage-independent growth of v-*myc*-transformed Balb/c 3T3 cells is promoted by platelet-derived growth factor or co-transformation by other oncogenes, *Oncogene*, 1, 271, 1987.

348. Chung, S.W., Wong, P.M.C., Shen-Ong, G., Ruscetti, S., Ishizaka, T., and Eaves, C.J., Production of granulocyte-macrophage colony-stimulating factor by Abelson virus-induced tumorigenic mast cell lines, *Blood*, 68, 1074, 1986.

349. Oliff, A., Agranovsky, O., McKinney, M.D., Murty, V.V.V.S., and Bauchwitz, R., Friend murine leukemia virus-immortalized myeloid cells are converted into tumorigenic cell lines by Abelson leukemia virus, *Proc. Natl. Acad. Sci. U.S.A.*, 82, 3306, 1985.

350. Cook, W.D., Metcalf, D., Nicola, N.A., Burgess, A.W., and Walker, F., Malignant transformation of a growth factor-dependent myeloid cell line by Abelson virus without evidence of an autocrine mechanism, *Cell*, 41, 677, 1985.

351. Pierce, J.H., Di Fiore, P.P., Aaronson, S.A., Potter, M., Pumphrey, J., Scott, A., and Ihle, J.N., Neoplastic transformation of mast cells by Abelson-MuLV: abrogation of IL-3 dependence by a nonautocrine mechanism, *Cell*, 41, 685, 1985.

352. Mathey-Prevot, B., Nabel, G., Palacios, R., and Baltimore, D., Abelson murine leukemia virus abrogation of interleukin 3 dependence in a lymphoid cell line, *Mol. Cell. Biol.*, 6, 4133, 1986.

353. Rovera, G., Valtieri, M., Mavilio, F., and Reddy, E.P., Effect of Abelson murine leukemia virus on granulocytic differentiation and interleukin-3 dependence of a murine progenitor cell line, *Oncogene*, 1, 29, 1987.

354. Vogt, M., Lesley, J., Bogenberger, J.M., Haggblom, C., Swift, S., and Haas, M., The induction of growth factor-independence in murine myelocytes by oncogenes results in monoclonal cell lines and is correlated with cell crisis and karyotypic instability, *Oncogene Res.*, 2, 49, 1987.

355. Cook, W.D., Fazekas de St. Groth, B., Miller, J.F.A.P., MacDonald, H.R., and Gabathuler, R., Abelson virus transformation of an interleukin 2-dependent antigen-specific T-cell line, *Mol. Cell. Biol.*, 7, 2631, 1987.

356. Overell, R.W., Watson, J.D., Gallis, B., Weisser, K.E., Cosman, D., and Widmer, M.B., Nature and specificity of lymphokine independence induced by a selectable retroviral vector expressing v-*src*, *Mol. Cell. Biol.*, 7, 3394, 1987.

357. Lichtman, A.H., Williams, M.E., Ohara, J., Paul, W.E., Faller, D.V., and Abbas, A.K., Retrovirus infection alters growth factor responses of T lymphocytes, *J. Immunol.*, 138, 3276, 1987.

358. Dickson, R.B., Kasid, A., Huff, K.K., Bates, S.E., Knabbe, C., Bronzert, D., Gelmann, E.P., and Lippman, M.E., Activation of growth factor secretion in tumorigenic states of breast cancer induced by 17 b-estradiol of v-Ha-*ras* oncogene, *Proc. Natl. Acad. Sci. U.S.A.*, 84, 837, 1987.

359. Kasid, A., Knabbe, C., and Lippman, M.E., Effects of v-*ras*^{H} oncogene transfection on estrogen-independent tumorigenicity of estrogen-dependent human breast cancer cells, *Cancer Res.*, 47, 5733, 1987.

360. Biegalke, B.J., Heaney, M.L., Bouton, A., Parsons, J.T., and Linial, M., MC29 deletion mutants which fail to transform chicken macrophages are competent for transformation of quail macrophages, *J. Virol.*, 61, 2138, 1987.

361. Gebhardt, A., Bell, J.C., and Foulkes, J.G., Abelson transformed fibroblasts lacking the EGF receptor are not tumorigenic in nude mice, *EMBO J.*, 5, 2191, 1986.

362. Franz, T., Löhler, J., Fusco, A., Pragnell, I, Nobis, P., Padua, R., and Ostertag, W., Transformation of mononuclear phagocytes in vivo and malignant histiocytes caused by a novel murine spleen focus-forming virus, *Nature*, 315, 149, 1985.

363. Klingler, K., Johnson, G.R., Walker, F., Nicola, N.A., Decker, T., and Ostertag, W., Macrophage cell lines transformed by the malignant histocytosis sarcoma virus: increase of CSF receptors suggests a model for transformation, *J. Cell. Physiol.*, 132, 22, 1987.

364. Anzano, M.A., Roberts, A.B., De Larco, J.E., Wakefield, L.M., Assoian, R.K., Roche, N.S., Smith, J.M., Lazarus, J.E., and Sporn, M.B., Increased secretion of type beta transforming growth factor accompanies viral transformation of cells, *Mol. Cell. Biol.*, 5, 242, 1985.

365. Ozanne, B., Fulton, R.J., and Kaplan, P.L., Kirsten murine sarcoma virus transformed cell lines and a spontaneously transformed rat cells line produce transforming factors, *J. Cell. Physiol.*, 105, 163, 1980.

366. Twardzick, D.R., Todaro, G.J., Marquardt, H., Reynolds, F.H., and Stephenson, J.R., Transformation induced by Abelson murine leukemia virus involves production of polypeptide growth factor, *Science,* 216, 894, 1982.

367. Bowen-Pope, D.F., Vogel, A., and Ross, R., Production of platelet-derived growth factor-like molecules and reduced expression of platelet-derived growth factor receptors accompany transformation by a wide spectrum of agents, *Proc. Natl. Acad. Sci. U.S.A.,* 81, 2396, 1984.

368. Hirai, R., Yamaoka, K., and Mitsui, H., Isolation and partial purification of a new class of transforming growth factors from an avian sarcoma virus-transformed rat cell line, *Cancer Res.,* 43, 5742, 1983.

369. Yamaoka, K., Hirai, R., Tsugita, A., and Mitsui, H., The purification of an acid- and heat-labile transforming growth factor from an avian sarcoma virus-transformed rat cell line, *J. Cell. Physiol.,* 119, 307, 1984.

370. Kaplan, P.L. and Ozanne, B., Cellular responsiveness to growth factors correlates with a cell's ability to express the transformed phenotype, *Cell,* 33, 931, 1983.

371. Salomon, D.S., Zwiebel, J.A., Noda, M., and Bassin, R.H., Flat revertants derived from Kirsten murine sarcoma virus-transformed cells produce transforming growth factors, *J. Cell. Physiol.,* 121, 22, 1984.

372. Jiang, L.-W., and Schindler, M., Nuclear transport in 3T3 fibroblasts: effects of growth factors, transformation, and cell shape, *J. Cell Biol.,* 106, 13, 1988.

373. Giancotti, V., Pani, B., D'Andrea, P., Berlingieri, M.T., Di Fiore, P.P., Fusco, A., Vecchio, G., Philp, R., Crane-Robinson, C., Nicolas, R.H., Wright, C.A., and Goodwin, G.H., Elevated levels of a specific class of nuclear phosphoproteins in cells transformed with v-*ras* and v-*mos* oncogenes and by cotransfection with c-*myc* and polyoma middle T genes, *EMBO J.,* 6, 1981, 1987.

374. Albino, A.P., Houghton, A.N., Eisinger, M., Lee, J.S., Kantor, R.R.S., Oliff, A.I., and Old, L.J., Class II histocompatibility antigen expression in human melanocytes transformed by Harvey murine sarcoma virus (Ha-MSV) and Kirsten MSV retroviruses, *J. Exp. Med.,* 164, 1710, 1986.

375. Wilson, L.D., Flyer, D.C., and Faller, D.V., Murine retroviruses control class I major histocompatibility antigen gene expression via a *trans* effect at the transcriptional level, *Mol. Cell. Biol.,* 7, 2406, 1987.

376. Morse, H.C., III, Tidmarsh, G.F., Holmes, K.L., Frederickson, T.N., Hartley, J.W., Pierce, J.H., Langdon, W.Y., Dailey, M.O., and Weissman, I.L., Expression of the 6C3 antigen on murine hematopoietic neoplasms. Association with expression of *abl, ras, fes, src, erb*B, and Cas NS-1 oncogenes but not with *myc, J. Exp. Med.,* 165, 920, 1987.

377. Maudsley, D.J. and Morris, A.G., Kirsten murine sarcoma virus abolishes interferon gamma-induced class II but not class I major histocompatibility antigen expression in a murine fibroblast line, *J. Exp. Med.,* 167, 706, 1988.

378. Graves, B.J., Eisenberg, S.P., Coen, D.M., and McKnight, S.L., Alternate utilization of two regulatory domains within the Moloney murine sarcoma virus long terminal repeat, *Mol. Cell. Biol.,* 5, 1959, 1985.

379. Auersperg, N. and Calderwood, G.A., Development of serum independence in Kirsten murine sarcoma virus-infected rat adrenal cells, *Carcinogenesis,* 5, 175, 1984.

380. Thomassen, D.G., Gilmer, T.M., Annab, L.A., and Barrett, J.C., Evidence for multiple steps in neoplastic transformation of normal and preneoplastic Syrian hamster embryo cells following transfection with Harvey murine sarcoma virus oncogene (v-Ha-*ras*), *Cancer Res.,* 45, 726, 1985.

381. Auersperg, N., Siemens, C.H., Krystal, G., and Myrdal, S.E., Modulation by normal serum factors of Kirsten murine sarcoma virus-induced transformation in adult rat cells infected in early passage, *Cancer Res.,* 46, 5715, 1986.

382. Green, P.L., Kaehler, D.A., and Risser, R., Clonal dominance and progression in Abelson murine leukemia virus lymphomagenesis, *J. Virol.,* 61, 2192, 1987.

383. Radinsky, R., Kraemer, P.M., Raines, M.A., Kung, H.-J., and Culp, L.A., Amplification and rearrangement of the Kirsten *ras* oncogene in virus-transformed BALB/c 3T3 cells during malignant tumor progression, *Proc. Natl. Acad. Sci. U.S.A.,* 84, 5143, 1987.

384. Smith, B.L. and Sager, R., Multistep origin of tumor-forming ability in Chinese hamster embryo fibroblast cells, *Cancer Res.,* 42, 389, 1982.

385. MacAuley, A., Auersperg, N., and Pawson, T., Expression of viral p21^{ras} during acquisition of a transformed phenotype by rat adrenal cortex cells infected with Kirsten murine sarcoma virus, *Mol. Cell. Biol.,* 6, 342, 1986.

386. Darfler, F.J., Shih, T.Y., and Lin, M.C., Revertants of Ha-MuSV-transformed MDCK cells express reduced levels of p21 and possess a more normal phenotype, *Exp. Cell Res.,* 162, 335, 1986.

387. Gilmer, T.M., Annab, L.A., Oshimura, M., and Barrett, J.C., Neoplastic transformation of normal and carcinogen-induced preneoplastic Syrian hamster embryo cells by the v-*src* oncogene, *Mol. Cell. Biol.,* 5, 1707, 1985.

388. Land, H., Parada, L.F., and Weinberg, R.A., Tumorigenic conversion of primary embryo fibroblasts requires at least two cooperating oncogenes, *Nature,* 304, 596, 1983.

389. Land, H., Parada, L.F., and Weinberg, R.A., Cellular oncogenes and multistep carcinogenesis, *Science,* 222, 771, 1983.

390. Mougneau, E., Lemieux, L., Rassoulzadegan, M., and Cuzin, F., Biological activities of v-*myc* and rearranged c-*myc* oncogenes in rat fibroblast cells in culture, *Proc. Natl. Acad. Sci. U.S.A.,* 81, 5758, 1984.

391. Glaichenhaus, N., Coopération entre oncogènes: fonction des oncogènes immortalisants, *Pathol. Biol.,* 34, 819, 1986.

392. Alema, S., Tato, F., and Boettiger, D., *myc* and *src* oncogenes have complementary effects on cell proliferation and expression of specific extracellular matrix components in definitive chondroblasts, *Mol. Cell. Biol.,* 5, 538, 1985.

393. Kahn, P., Fryberg, L., Brady, C., Stanley, I., Beug, H., Vennström, B., and Graf, T., v-*erbA* cooperates with sarcoma oncogenes in leukemic cell transformation, *Cell,* 45, 349, 1986.

394. Schwartz, R.C., Stanton, L.W., Riley, S.C., Marcu, K.B., and Witte, O.N., Synergism of v-*myc* and v-Ha-*ras* in the in vitro neoplastic progression of murine lymphoid cells, *Mol. Cell. Biol.,* 6, 3221, 1986.

395. Cleveland, J.L., Jansen, H.W., Bister, K., Fredrickson, T.N., Morse, H.C., III, Ihle, J.N., and Rapp, U.R., Interaction between *raf* and *myc* oncogenes in transformation *in vivo* and *in vitro, J. Cell. Biochem.,* 30, 195, 1986.

396. Blasi, E., Mathieson, B.J., Varesio, L., Cleveland, J.L., Borchert, P.A., and Rapp, U.R., Selective immortalization of murine macrophages from fresh bone marrow by a *raf/myc* recombinant murine retrovirus, *Nature,* 318, 667, 1985.

397. Smith, M.R., DeGudicibus, S.J., and Stacey, D.W., Requirement for c-*ras* proteins during viral oncogene transformation, *Nature,* 320, 540, 1986.

398. Schwab, M., Varmus, H.E., and Bishop, J.M., Human N-*myc* gene contributes to neoplastic transformation of mammalian cells in culture, *Nature,* 316, 160, 1985.

399. Wong, P.M.C., Humphries, R.K., Chen, T.R., and Eaves, C.J., Evidence for a multistep pathogenesis in the generation of tumorigenic cell lines from hemopoietic colonies exposed to Abelson virus *in vitro, Exp. Hematol.,* 15, 280, 1987.

400. Rohan, P. and Wainberg, M.A., Effect of prior inoculation with chemical carcinogens on development of avian retrovirus-induced neoplasia in chickens, *Br. J. Cancer,* 41, 130, 1980.

401. Hsiao, W.-L.W., Gattoni-Celli, S., and Weinstein, I.B., Oncogene-induced transformation of C3H 10T1/2 cells is enhanced by tumor promoters, *Science,* 226, 552, 1984.

402. Hsiao, W.-L.W., Wu, T., and Weinstein, I.B., Oncogene-induced transformation of a rat embryo fibroblast cell line is enhanced by tumor promoters, *Mol. Cell. Biol.,* 6, 1943, 1986.

403. Hsiao, W.-L.W., Lopez, C.A., Wu, T., and Weinstein, I.B., A factor present in fetal calf serum enhances oncogene-induced transformation of rodent fibroblasts, *Mol. Cell. Biol.,* 7, 3380, 1987.

404. Connan, G., Rassoulzadegan, M., and Cuzin, F., Focus formation in rat fibroblasts exposed to a tumour promoter after transfer of polyoma *plt* and *myc* oncogenes, *Nature,* 314, 277, 1985.

405. Yuspa, S.H., Kilkenny, A.E., Stanley, J., and Lichti, U., Keratinocytes blocked in phorbol ester-responsive early stage of terminal differentiation by sarcoma viruses, *Nature,* 314, 459, 1985.

406. Brown, K., Quintanilla, M., Ramsden, M., Kerr, I.B., Young, S., and Balmain, A., v-*ras* genes from Harvey and BALB murine sarcoma viruses can act as initiators of tw-stage mouse skin carcinogenesis, *Cell,* 46, 447, 1986.

407. Milo, G.E., Olsen, R.G., Weisbrode, S.E., and McCloskey, J.A., Feline sarcoma virus induced *in vitro* progression from premalignant to neoplastic transformation of human diploid cells, *In Vitro,* 16, 813, 1980.

408. Morris, A.G., Neoplastic transformation of mouse fibroblasts by murine sarcoma virus: a multi-step process, *J. Gen. Virol.,* 53, 39, 1981.

409. Jurdic, P., Bouabdelli, M., Moscovici, M.G., and Moscovici, C., Embryonic erythroid cells transformed by avian erythroblastosis virus may proliferate and differentiate, *Virology,* 144, 73, 1985.

410. Woods, C.M., Boyer, B., Vogt, P.K., and Lazarides, E., Control of erythroid differentiation: asynchronous expression of the anion transporter and the peripheral components of the membrane skeleton in AEV- and S13-transformed cells, *J. Cell Biol.,* 103, 1789, 1986.

411. Hines, D.L., Differentiation of Abelson murine leukemia virus-infected promonocytic leukemia cells, *Int. J. Cancer,* 36, 233, 1985.

412. Auersperg, N., Wan, M.W.C., Sanderson, R.A., Wong, K.S., and Mauldin, D., Morphological and functional differentiation of Kirsten murine sarcoma virus transformed rat adrenocortical cell lines, *Cancer Res.,* 41, 1763, 1981.

413. Wiebe, J.P., Myers, K.I., and Auersperg, N., Modification of steroidogenesis in rat adrenocortical cells transformed by Kirsten murine sarcoma virus, *Cancer Res.,* 47, 1325, 1987.

414. Bar-Sagi, D. and Feramisco, J.R., Microinjection of the *ras* oncogene protein into PC12 cells induces morphological differentiation, *Cell,* 42, 841, 1985.

415. Roberts, A.B., Roche, N.S., and Sporn, M.B., Selective inhibition of the anchorage-independent growth of *myc*-transfected fibroblasts by retinoic acid, *Nature,* 315, 237, 1985.

416. Flatow, U., Willingham, M.C., and Rabson, A.S., Butyrate prevents Harvey sarcoma virus focus formation but permits oncogene expression, *Cancer Lett.,* 22, 203, 1984.

417. Kopelovich, L., Rich, R.F., and Wallace, A.L., Hydrocortisone promotes the neodifferentiation of Kirsten murine sarcoma virus transformed human skin fibroblasts to adipose cells: relevance to oncogenic mechanisms, *Exp. Cell Biol.,* 54, 25, 1986.

418. Mitrani, E., Coffin, J., Boedtker, H., and Doty, P., Rous sarcoma virus is integrated but not expressed in chicken early embryonic cells, *Proc. Natl. Acad. Sci. U.S.A.,* 84, 2781, 1987.

419. Howlett, A.R., Cullen, B., Hertle, M., and Bissell, M.J., Tissue tropism and temporal expression of Rous sarcoma virus in embryonic avian limb *in ovo, Oncogene Res.,* 1, 255, 1987.

420. Pillemer, E., Whitlock, C., and Weissman, I.L., Transformation-associated proteins in murine B-cell lymphomas that are distinct from Abelson virus gene products, *Proc. Natl. Acad. Sci. U.S.A.,* 81, 4434, 1984.

421. Fischinger, P.J., Nomura, S., Peebles, P.T., Haapala, D.K., and Bassin, R.H., Reversion of murine sarcoma virus transformed mouse cells: variants without a rescuable sarcoma virus, *Science,* 176, 1033, 1972.

422. Boettiger, D., Reversion and induction of Rous sarcoma virus expression in virus transformed baby hamster kidney cells, *Virology,* 62, 522, 1974.

423. Krzyzek, R.A., Lau, A.F., Spector, D.H., and Faras, A.J., Post-transcriptional control of avian oncornavirus transforming gene sequences in mammalian cells, *Nature,* 269, 175, 1977.

424. Porzig, K.J., Robbins, K.C., and Aaronson, S.A., Cellular regulation of mammalian sarcoma virus expression: a gene regulation model for oncogenesis, *Cell,* 16, 875, 1979.

425. Whitlock, C.A., Ziegler, S.F., and Witte, O.N., Progression of the transformed phenotype in clonal lines of Abelson virus-infected lymphocytes, *Mol. Cell. Biol.,* 3, 596, 1983.

426. Norton, J.D., Cook, F., Roberts, P.C., Clewley, J.P., and Avery, R.J., Expression of Kirsten murine sarcoma virus in transformed nonproducer and revertant NIH/3T3 cells: evidence for cell-mediated resistance to a viral oncogene in phenotypic reversion, *J. Virol.,* 50, 439, 1984.

427. Catala, A., DNA methylation and transcriptional controls of proviral DNA in avian sarcoma virus-transformed mammalian cells, *Nucleic Acids Res.,* 14, 2481, 1986.

428. Chan, J.C., Keck, M.E., and Li, W., Monoclonal antibody detection of transformation associated protein (TAP) in ts110 Moloney murine sarcoma virus transformed 6M2 cells that are different from the mos gene product, *Biochem. Biophys. Res. Commun.,* 134, 1223, 1986.

429. Herzog, N.K., Bargmann, W.J., and Bose, H.R., Jr., Oncogene expression in reticuloendotheliosis virus-transformed lymphoid cell lines and avian tissues, *J. Virol.,* 57, 371, 1986.

430. Beug, H., Müller, H., Grieser, S., Doederlein, G., and Graf, T., Hematopoietic cells transformed in vitro by REV-T avian reticuloendotheliosis virus express characteristics of very immature lymphoid cells, *Virology,* 115, 295, 1981.

431. Mercola, D., Rundell, A., Westwick, J., and Edwards, S.A., Antisense RNA to the c-*fos* gene: restoration of density-dependent growth arrest in a transformed cell line, *Biochem. Biophys. Res. Commun.,* 147, 288, 1987.

432. Kawano, T., Taniguchi, S., Nakamatsu, K., Sadano, H., and Baba, T., Malignant progression of a transformed rat cell line by transfer of the v-*fos* oncogene, *Biochem. Biophys. Res. Commun.,* 149, 173, 1987.

433. Oshimura, M., Gilmer, T.M., and Barrett, J.C., Nonrandom loss of chromosome 15 in Syrian hamster tumours induced by v-Ha-*ras* plus v-*myc* oncogenes, *Nature,* 316, 636, 1985.

434. Vogt, M., Lesley, J., Bogenberger, J., Volkman, S., and Haas, M., Coinfection with viruses carrying the v-Ha-*ras* and v-*myc* oncogenes leads to growth factor independence by an indirect mechanism, *Mol. Cell. Biol.,* 6, 3545, 1986.

435. Straus, D.S. and Mohandas, T., Growth suppression of hybrids between transformed cells and normal fibroblasts in serum-free medium: correlation with retention of human chromosomes, *Somat. Cell Mol. Genet.,* 13, 587, 1987.

436. Zarbl, H., Latreille, J., and Jolicoeur, P., Revertants of v-*fos*-transformed fibroblasts have mutations in cellular genes essential for transformation by other oncogenes, *Cell,* 51, 357, 1987.

437. Klinken, S.P., Castilla, M.J., and Thorgeirsson, S.S., Effect of inhibitors of ornithine decarboxylase on retrovirus induced transformation of murine erythroid precursors *in vitro, Cancer Res.,* 46, 6246, 1986.

438. Beug, H. and Hayman, M.J., Temperature-sensitive mutants of avian erythroblastosis virus: surface expression of the *erbB* product correlates with transformation, *Cell,* 36, 963, 1984.

439. Milford, J.J. and Duran-Reynals, F., Growth of a chicken sarcoma virus in the chick embryo in the absence of neoplasia, *Cancer Res.,* 3, 578, 1943.

440. Dolberg, D.S. and Bissell, M.J., Inability of Rous sarcoma virus to cause sarcomas in the avian embryo, *Nature,* 309, 552, 1984.

441. Saule, S., Mérigaud, J.P., Al-Moustafa, A.-E.M., Ferré, F., Rong, P.M., Amouyel, P., Quatannens, B., Stéhelin, D., and Dieterlen-Lièvre, F., Heart tumors specifically induced in young avian embryos by the v-*myc* oncogene, *Proc. Natl. Acad. Sci. U.S.A.,* 84, 7982, 1987.

442. Miyaki, M., Akamatsu, N., Ono, T., and Sasaki, M.S., Susceptibility of skin fibroblasts from patients with retinoblastoma to transformation by murine sarcoma virus, *Cancer Lett.,* 18, 137, 1983.

443. Rhim, J.S., Trimmer, R., Huebner, R.J., Papas, T.S., and Gay, G., Differential susceptibility of human cells to transformation by murine and avian sarcoma viruses, *Proc. Soc. Exp. Biol. Med.,* 170, 350, 1982.

444. Rasheed, S., Rhim, J.S., and Gardner, E.J., Inherited susceptibility to retrovirus-induced transformation of Gardner syndrome cells, *Am. J. Hum. Genet.,* 35, 919, 1983.

445. Rhim, J.S. and Huebner, R.J., Neoplastic transformation induced by adeno 12-SV40 hybrid virus in skin fibroblasts from humans genetically predisposed to cancer, *Cancer Detect. Prevent.,* 6, 345, 1983.

446. Shimada, T., Dowjat, W.K., Gindhart, T.D., Lerman, M.I., and Colburn, N.H., Lifespan of basal cell nevus syndrome fibroblasts by transfection with mouse *pro* or v-*myc* genes, *Int. J. Cancer*, 39, 649, 1987.
447. Rabotti, G., Teutsch, B., Mariller, M., and Mongiat, F., Transformation de fibroblastes diploides humains avec production virale apres infection par des retrovirus aviaires, *C.R. Acad. Sci. Paris*, 297, 17, 1983.
448. McCoy, J.L., Fefer, A., McCoy, N.T., and Kirsten, W.H., Immunobiological studies of tumors induced by murine sarcoma virus (Kirsten), *Cancer Res.*, 32, 343, 1972.
449. Wainberg, M.A., Yu, M., Schwartz-Luft, E., and Israel, E., Cellular and humoral antitumor immune responsiveness in chickens bearing tumors induced by avian sarcoma virus, *Int. J. Cancer*, 19, 680, 1977.
450. Wainberg, M.A., Israel, E., and Yu, M., Immune selection of tumor cell variants in chickens bearing tumors induced by avian sarcoma viruses, *Cancer Res.*, 42, 1669, 1982.
451. Johnson, P.W., Baubock, C., and Roder, J.C., Transfection of a rat cell line with the v-Ki-*ras* oncogene is associated with enhanced susceptibility to natural killer cell lysis, *J. Exp. Med.*, 162, 1732, 1985.
452. Trimble, W.S., Johnson, P.W., Hozumi, N., and Roder, J.C., Inducible cellular transformation by a metallothionein-*ras* hybrid oncogene leads to natural killer cell susceptibility, *Nature*, 321, 782, 1986.
453. Greenberg, A.H., Egan, S.E., Jarolim, L., and Wright, J.A., NK sensitivity of H-*ras* transfected fibroblasts is transformation-independent, *Cell. Immunol.*, 109, 444, 1987.
454. Greenberg, A.H., Egan, S.E., Jarolim, L., Gingras, M.-C., and Wright, J.A., Natural killer cell regulation of implantation and early lung growth of H-*ras*-transformed 10T1/2 fibroblasts in mice, *Cancer Res.*, 47, 4801, 1987.
455. Halpern, M.S. and McMahon, S.B., The immune status of avian sarcoma virus-infected chickens as a determinant of sarcoma growth pattern and viral antigen expression, *J. Immunol.*, 138, 3014, 1987.

Chapter 3

CHRONIC RETROVIRUSES

I. INTRODUCTION

Chronic retroviruses (nonacute or "slow" viruses) are replication-competent, infectious agents that have been found to be associated with both malignant and nonmalignant diseases under natural conditions in many vertebrate species.[1] Usually, there is a long latency period between the infection and the clinical manifestation of the disease. Chronic retroviral infections are most frequently associated with nonmalignant diseases or may remain asymptomatic. Infections with chronic retroviruses may not occur in all mammalian species or in all genetic variants of a particular species. Infectious MuLV is by no means ubiquitous in feral mice (*Mus musculus*).[2] No horizontally transmitting, infectious retrovirus has been detected in rats, whose retroviruses are all of the endogenous (vertically transmitted) category.[3]

Morphologically, chronic retrovirus are classified into four types (A, B, C, and D), according to their electron microscopic characteristics.[4-6] In contrast to acute retroviruses, chronic retroviruses have a complete, nondefective genome and do not require helper viruses for replication. Chronic retroviruses do not possess specific transforming genes (oncogenes) and are not able to induce transformation in cultured cells.

Chronic retroviruses that have been found to be associated with the development of malignant diseases include type C viruses such as the avian leukemia viruses (ALVs),[7] murine leukemia viruses (MuLVs),[8] feline leukemia viruses (FeLVs),[9,10] and bovine leukemia viruses (BLVs),[11,12] as well as type C retroviruses associated with leukemia in nonhuman primates, and type B retroviruses such as the murine mammary tumor virus (MMTV). Prototypes of chronic viruses are the MuLVs, which were among the first known biological oncogenic agents in mammals and have been subjected to intensive study during the last few decades.[2,8,13,14] The role of chronic retroviruses in the etiology of human cancer remained controversial for many years, but a chronic retrovirus of human origin, the human T-cell lymphotropic virus type I (HTLV-I), also called adult T-cell leukemia virus (ATLV), has been recently implicated in the etiology of a relatively rare form of leukemia, the adult T-cell leukemia (ATL).[14-28] Another chronic retrovirus, the human immunodeficiency virus (HIV), has been recognized as the etiologic agent of a new epidemic disease, the acquired immune deficiency syndrome (AIDS).[29-38] A high prevalence of cancer, especially of Kaposi's sarcoma and lymphomas, is observed in AIDS patients. Both HTLV-I and HIV are transmitted horizontally, i.e., by contagion between infected individuals.

The transmission of murine retroviruses occurs primarily via germ line viral DNA integration in form of endogenous proviruses or through congenital infection by virions present either in the birth canal or in mammary secretions. Type C retroviruses are present in the mouse sperm and could be transmitted horizontally to the females during copulation and to the germ line of mice during penetration of ova.[39] Horizontal transmission is generally not considered to be an important mode of retrovirus infection in mice but well-documented examples of this type of infection have been observed in chronically viremic mice.[40] Horizontal transmission of retroviruses in mice results in a persistent infection with viremia and low levels of virus replication. External secretions of viremic mice, including saliva, semen, and uterine secretions, may contain high concentrations of infectious retroviruses but, paradoxically, transmission is not frequent and occurs only from viremic males to either males or females. Infection of female mice would occur by the venereal route. Horizontal transmission of other retroviruses in nonmurine species, for example, FeLV in cats, is also a relatively rare event that does not appear to have an important role in most cases of feline leukemia/lymphoma.[41] In any case retroviral infections are usually well tolerated and are frequently controlled by the immune system of the animal, which does not develop clinical signs of disease.

Infection of susceptible hosts with chronic retroviruses may result in the appearance of different types of nonmalignant diseases. Infection of mice early in life with MuLV can result in a spectrum of nonmalignant conditions, including graying due to dysfunction of melanocytes derived from the virus-infected melanoblasts.[42] Infection of cats by FeLV only rarely results in leukemia; far more prevalent are nonneoplastic diseases causally related to FeLV, including nonregenerative anemia, panleukopenia-like syndrome, thymic atrophy, hemolytic anemia, and glomerulonephritis, which are tightly associated with disturbances of the immune system of the infected animal.[43] MuLVs are capable of inducing in mice progressive neurodegenerative diseases associated with spongiform encephalomyelopathy, but the mechanisms by which these viruses cause neuronal degeneration remain unresolved.[44]

In principle, the spread of infections caused by chronic retroviruses may be controlled by preventive or therapeutic procedures. Protection against these infections could be achieved by vaccination using inactivated tumor cells or viruses, purified viral antigenic compounds, or recombinant vectors carrying defined genetic components of the particular retrovirus.[45] The therapeutic possibilities for the control of retroviral infections are very limited at present. An interesting approach to this end may be represented by the use of antisense RNA.[46]

II. STRUCTURE OF CHRONIC RETROVIRUSES

The virions of chronic retroviruses contain two copies of genomic RNA, which in MuLV are approximately 8000 bases in length, capped at the 5' end and polyadenylated at the 3' end.[8] The two copies of the retroviral RNA genome are single stranded and are joined at their 5' ends. The intracellular replication of chronic retroviruses proceeds via the synthesis of a DNA intermediate, the provirus, by the action of a specific enzyme, the virion-associated RNA-dependent DNA polymerase (reverse transcriptase). The proviral DNA of retroviruses can be integrated into the host cell genome and can be passed in this form onto subsequent generations of daughter cell. From its chromosomal location, proviral DNA can be transcribed by cellular enzymes to produce new progeny viral RNA as well as mRNAs that can encode viral proteins.

The genome of chronic retroviruses is composed of at least three structural genes in the sequence *gag-pol-env*, from 5' to 3'. Retroviruses that possess full-length sequences of these three genes are replication competent. The genes *gag* and *env* code for the core and envelope proteins of the virion, respectively, whereas the gene *pol* code for the enzyme reverse transcriptase. At both ends of the genome there are short repeated stretches of noncoding sequences, designated r, and unique sequences near the 5' and 3' termini, designated U5 and U3, respectively. The repeated sequences located at the terminal regions of the viral genome are arranged in a particular configuration to form the long terminal repeats (LTRs) which are situated at both ends of the integrated provirus. Thus, the typical structure of a chronic retrovirus provirus, integrated into the host cell genome, is composed of the following sequence, from 5' to 3': LTR-*gag-pol-env*-LTR. (Figure 1 in Chapter 2).

In addition to the essential structural genes, chronic retroviruses such as BLV and its close relatives, the human retroviruses HTLV-I, HTLV-II, and HIV, contain a genomic region with coding capacity between the *env* gene and the 3' LTR. In BLV this region, termed X or pX, is 1.8-kb long and is transcribed into an mRNA that is produced by a complex splicing mechanism which results in juxtaposition of the 5' end of the *env* gene and the two overlapping ORFs contained in the pX region.[47] The protein encoded by the BLV pX region has a molecular weight of 19-kDa and is a nuclear phosphoprotein but its function is unknown. In addition to a pX homologous region located between the *env* gene and the 3' LTR, the human HIV virus possesses another coding region, termed R or *tat*, situated between the structural genes *pol* and *env*. Both the pX and R regions have capacity for coding more than one protein product, which is due, at least in part, to differential RNA splicing mechanisms.

A. STRUCTURAL COMPONENTS OF CHRONIC RETROVIRUSES

The two full-genomic RNA molecules of chronic retroviruses are enclosed in a capsid and core particle made up primarily of products of the *gag* gene. The virion is surrounded by a lipid-containing membrane derived from the host cell during viral budding and this envelope also contains a glycoprotein product, derived from the *env* gene, which is required for infectivity. A nomenclature was proposed for the virion proteins associated with avian and murine retroviruses.[51] Recently, a revised standardized nomenclature was proposed for the proteins common to all retroviruses, based on their functions, enzymatic activities, and/or virion locations.[52]

Construction of molecular recombinants between different subgroups of avian sarcoma and leukosis retroviruses indicates that the host range determinant defining subgroup specificity is located within a region of the viral genome that includes most of the coding sequence for the *env* gene product gp85.[53] The primary structures of the protein products of the structural genes *gag* and *env* from several chronic retroviruses have been characterized. Microinjection techniques together with genetic and molecular analyses may be useful for establishing a correlation between retroviral polynucleotide structure and retroviral-encoded protein function.[50] Myristylation (covalent addition of the fatty acid myristic acid) of the *gag* protein product of mammalian type C and type D retroviruses at the amino-terminal glycine residue is apparently required for both the association with cellular membranes and the assembly into virions.[54] Mutants of Mason-Pfizer monkey virus (MPMV, a type D retrovirus isolated from a rhesus monkey mammary tumor) in which a codon for valine substitutes for that of glycine residue at the amino terminus of the *gag* product are completely noninfectious.[55]

Retroviruses possess a calcium binding site and this site, as determined by a specific radioimmunoassay, is represented by calmodulin.[56] All of the retroviruses tested contained calmodulin, including the following viruses: Kowakami-Theilen strain of FeLV, rhabdomyosarcoma virus 114 (RD-114), Rauscher MuLV, Balb-MuLV, New Zealand Black MuLV, gibbon ape leukemia virus (GaLV), and the human retrovirus HTLV-I. The function of calmodulin in retroviruses is unknown but calcium is involved in the assembly and disassembly of some viruses and calmodulin may be important in maintaining the structural integrity of retroviruses.

B. LONG TERMINAL REPEATS

Chronic retroviruses contain genetic regulatory elements and infection with these viruses can result in profound alterations in the regulation of host cell genomic functions. Retroviruses replicate through a double-stranded DNA intermediate, the provirus, which is integrated into the genome of the host cell. The provirus genome sequences are complementary to the RNA sequences of the respective virus, with the exception that there are long terminal repeats (LTRs) at both ends of the provirus. The LTRs are stretches of linear double-stranded DNA with terminally redundant sequences 300 to 1200 bp in length. They are synthesized from the viral RNA genome by the reverse transcriptase present in virions and are formed by duplication of the nonstructural segments of the retrovirus genome, containing the sequences 5'-U3-r-U5-3' (Figure 1 in Chapter 2). The detailed structure and nucleotide sequences of LTRs and adjacent genomic regions from 19 different type-C and type-B retroviruses have been determined and compared.[57] LTRs are efficient promoters for transcription carried out by the host cell RNA polymerase II.[58,59] At least two domains within retroviral LTRs are involved as regulation signals of virus transcription. Two elements contained in BLV LTR are involved in the regulation of gene expression.[60]

The transcriptional activity of chronic retrovirus LTRs depends partially on the cellular environment. Hormones and growth factors may have an important role in regulating this activity. Glucocorticoid response elements (GREs) composed of 17-nucleotide consensus sequences are present in the LTRs of both nonleukemogenic and T-cell leukemogenic MuLVs.[61] The pattern of expression of MuLV GREs varies according to cell type and is related to the spatial arrangement of GREs as well as to their precise sequence context.

Specific sequences contained in LTRs may be used as probes for the infection of cells with chronic retroviruses. For example, in contrast to sequences from the U5 region of FeLV LTR, sequences associated with the U3 region of FeLV LTR are not endogenous to domestic cats and can be used as evidence for exposure to FeLV.[62] Lymphosarcomas of virus-negative cats have no exogenous U3 sequences despite epidemiological evidence of an association of virus-negative leukemia with exposure to FeLV.

C. TRANSCRIPTIONAL ENHANCERS

In addition to LTRs and promoters, chronic retroviruses may possess another class of genomic regulatory elements, the enhancers or activators, which are able to increase the transcriptional activity of homologous and heterologous promoters located in *cis* position in a form which is relatively independent of distance and orientation. Although no nucleotide sequence homology has been recognized in different enhancers, they may share some particular organizational features and may be constituted by mosaics of multiple different and often redundant sequence motifs.

Transcriptional enhancers are contained in the LTRs of both chronic and acute retroviruses. The 5' boundary of the M-MuSV enhancer consists of only 53 bp which are required for the enhancement effect of the virus in mouse fibroblasts.[63] The molecular mechanisms of action of enhancer elements are unknown but they could act by interacting with specific protein factors.[64] Two enhancer regions contained within the U3 portion of RSV LTR are recognized by protein factors (EF-I and EF-II) that have been extracted from quail cell nuclei. Enhancer elements acting in a *cis* manner may be contained not only in LTR sequences but also in other regions of retroviruses, for example, within the *gag* gene.[65]

D. TRANSCRIPTIONAL SILENCERS

In addition to enhancers, there is evidence of the existence in the eukaryotic genome of DNA sequences able to function in either 5' or 3' orientation, with effects relatively independent of their position with respect to the affected promoter, but acting as transcriptional repressors, and for that reason such sequences have been called silencers.[66] An interaction between enhancer and silencer elements could play an important role in determining the expression of particular genes in both tissue-specific and developmentally regulated genetic programs. The possible role of silencers in the origin and development of malignant diseases produced by chronic transforming retroviruses or other oncogenic agents remains uncharacterized.

E. REVERSE TRANSCRIPTION OF RETROVIRAL GENOMES

Reverse transcription of the genome of retroviruses is essential for their integration into the host cell genome. This process is catalyzed by reverse transcriptase, an enzyme first detected in the Rauscher strain of MuLV (R-MuLV).[67,68] The enzyme leads to the production of circular DNA replication intermediates containing single or tandemly repeated LTR elements.[69] Circular DNAs containing tandem LTRs undergo an integration process (integrative recombination) in which short inverted repeat sequences at the LTR-LTR junction are recombined with host chromosomal DNA.[70] The process requires an endonuclease activity that is encoded by the 3'-terminal one third of the *pol* gene (the *pol-endo*) and is characterized by the deletion of two nucleotides on the U5 and U3 sides of the virus integration site and by duplication of four to six nucleotides at the host cell integration site. Reverse transcriptase activity is not an exclusive property of retroviruses since a similar activity is present in some DNA viruses, e.g., in the duck hepatitis virus.[71] Nucleotide sequences homologous to the reverse transcriptase sequences of MuLVs are present in the human hepatitis B virus and other related hepadnaviruses, suggesting that both types of viruses derived from a common ancestor.[72] Moreover, reverse transcriptase activity may be present in normal cells.

As other DNA polymerases, reverse transcriptase appears to be a metalloenzyme, with an obligatory zinc requirement for activity.[73] Reverse transcriptase of avian sarcoma and leukosis viruses is a multifunctional enzyme composed of α- and β-polypeptide chains. Three *pol* gene products have been identified in avian retroviral particles: the full-length 95-kDa β chain of reverse transcriptase and two proteolytic products of β, a 63-kDa reverse transcriptase α chain derived from the amino terminus of β, and a 32-kDa (pp32) endonuclease derived by proteolytic cleavage from its carboxyl terminus. The products of the *pol* gene from chronic retroviruses can be isolated from virus particles as an α monomer, a β-β homodimer, an α-β heterodimer, and a pp32 homodimer. The last three of these proteins possess endonuclease activity. The viral reverse transcriptase products can be associated as a complex involving a disulfide bond.[74] Expression vectors containing the entire *pol* gene and the region encoding pp32 have been constructed.[70,75,76] The pp32 protein possesses a Mg^{2+}- or Mn^{2+}-dependent DNA endonuclease activity. Avian retrovirus mutants with deletions in the pp32 region allowed to demonstrate that this region encodes function(s) essential for replication of the virus, while separate point mutations generated near the amino terminus of pp32 resulted in decreased replication and cell transformation.[77] Reverse transcriptase activity is essential for development of leukemia by exogenous retroviruses.[78] Activity of reverse transcriptase from R-MuLV, but not AMV, is inhibited by hemin *in vitro*.[79]

III. TRANSPOSABLE GENETIC ELEMENTS AND INSERTION SEQUENCES

The RNA-mediated movement of genetic information from one locus to another within the cellular genome is known as retroposition. Transposable genetic elements, including insertion elements, transposons, and retroposons are DNA sequences of viral or nonviral origin that can change their position within the genome and rearrange adjacent DNA. In their new location, these elements can give origin to either functional genes or nonfunctional DNA sequences called retropseudogenes. Transposable elements were originally studied in plants (maize) by classical genetic methods. The element *Cin4*, present in *Zea mays*, is a nonviral retrotransposon which contains two ORFs and has coding capacity for reverse transcriptase identified in plants.[80] Insertion of the *Cin4* element into the *A1* locus of the plant alters its transcription in comparison to other *A1* alleles without the insertion. Transposable genetic elements or transposons have been identified in bacteria, yeast, insects, and vertebrates.[81-90] Insertion of transposable elements into genes may cause unstable mutations.

Retroviral LTRs have sequence homology to cellular movable elements, including transposons, which indicates that these sequences may have a role in genomic processes related to DNA integration and/or transposition.[57,91-98] Retroviruses, as well as true eukaryotic transposons, such as the *Ty* elements of yeast and the *copia* family of elements found in *Drosophila*, are integrated into the cell genome by insertion mechanisms that are precise to the nucleotide level with respect to the viral or transposon DNA. In contrast, the site of insertion of these elements in the cell genome is random or semirandom and there is no discernible consensus recognition site or sequence for integration or transposition.[99] It may be hypothesized that the termini of the LTRs contain *cis*-acting recognition sequences for the enzyme(s) catalyzing integration.

Insertion of a *copia*-like transposable element into the specific *Drosophila* locus, *l(2)gl*, results in inactivation of the normal transcriptional activity of the gene.[100] The *l(2)gl* locus is a recessive gene and homozygous mutations at this locus are associated with the development of malignant neuroblastomas in the brain and tumors of the imaginal disc.[101] The *l(2)gl* locus may be considered not as a protooncogene, but as a tumor suppressor gene or antioncogene, whose deletion or functional inactivation may lead to a tumorigenic phenotype in the insect.[101,102]

A. INSERTION SEQUENCES
Although transposable genetic elements similar to those described in yeast and insects have

not been rigorously identified in mammals, a family of middle repetitive DNA elements described in the mouse may have similar or identical function.[104] These mouse elements show characteristics of both insertion sequences (ISs) and solitary retroviral LTRs and have been termed LTR-IS. They are about 500 bp in length, have 11 bp inverted repeats at their termini, and contain regulatory signals implicated in transcription by RNA polymerase II. There are about 500 LTR-IS per mouse haploid genome, interspersed among variable flanking regions of mouse DNA, and their structure suggests that they could be mobile in the genome and function as insertion mutagens. However, LTR-IS elements seem to be relatively stable within the genome. If LTR-IS elements are mobile, they do not rearrange frequently or may have lost their mobility during evolution. Consequently, LTR-IS may represent an evolutionary intermediate in retroviral evolution.

B. RETROPOSONS

LTR-ISs and other DNA sequences with potential transposable properties present in the mammalian genome are generically called retrotransposons or retroposons.[105-107] These elements are defined as dispersed repeated DNA sequences sharing common properties which imply that they are derived from RNA by processes involving reverse transcription. The possible role of such sequences, including the human *Alu* sequences, in normal developmental processes and/or oncogenic processes occurring in mammalian species is only partially understood.[108-112] Transposon-like elements that may show sequence homology to reverse transcriptases are present in human DNA.[113,114] Although the role of mobile elements in tumorigenic processes is not understood, the content of transposable repetitive elements such as IAPs and B2 sequences may be higher in tumor cells than in normal cells.[115]

IV. REPEATED DNA SEQUENCES IN THE MAMMALIAN GENOME

Although at least one third of various mammalian genomes is composed of families of repeated DNA sequences, the function of these sequences remains little understood.[11,116,117] Two different classes of mammalian interspersed and highly repeated sequences have been distinguished on the basis of size and relative abundance: short interspersed (SINE) repeated sequences with unit lengths under 500 bp, which are present in as many as hundreds of thousands of copies, and long interspersed (LINE) repeated sequences, which are several kbp in length and occur in the order of 10^4 times.[116] The presence or absence of LINE or SINE elements at a particular site of the genome could have profound effects on the contiguous DNA sequences, including effects on gene activity and structural changes such as deletion, duplication, and DNA rearrangements.

A. LINE SEQUENCES

The LINE family of repeated DNA sequences comprises, in the human genome, at least two members, the *Kpn* I family and the L2Hs family.[118] The latter family appears to have emerged only recently in evolution and is restricted to the human and gorilla genomes. The L2Hs family shows qualitative and quantitative polymorphisms which may reflect DNA sequence rearrangements, amplifications, and/or deletions. The presence of absence of a LINE element could potentially exert profound effects on contiguous DNA sequences, including effects on gene activity and generation of DNA rearrangements. Some members of the LINE DNA family may encode one or more proteins, and the putative product(s) of functional LINE genes may contain reverse transcriptase activity and nucleic acid binding domains.[119] Thus, at least some members of the LINE family may behave as retroviruses or retroposons in spite of the lack of LTRs in their nucleotide sequences.

The most intensively studied LINE is called LINE-1 or L1.[120] The consensus element of L1 is 6 to 7 kbp long and contains sequences with no coding potential at the 5′ and 3′ ends. However, a region of about 5 kbp is bracketed by the 5' and 3' L1 noncoding regions and is capable of coding for one or more proteins. In the mouse and human this region contains two ORFs, one 5' proximal ORF (ORF-1) about 1 kbp long and a 3' proximal ORF (ORF-2) about 4 kbp long. In addition, an adenine-rich region follows the 3' noncoding region and the entire element is often bordered by short direct repeats. However, most L1 elements differ from the consensus elements in a number of significant pathways including truncations, rearrangements, or deletions.[120] Few, if any, L1 transcripts are present in normal human or mouse cells but one L1 transcript was found in a human teratocarcinoma cell line exhibiting the carcinoma phenotype.[122]

L1 elements are abundant in the mammalian genome. The number of DNA copies of L1 elements may constitute up to 5% of the mammalian genome, which suggests some important beneficial function(s) for these elements.[120] L1-like elements are present even in invertebrates such as *Drosophila*, *Bombix*, and *Trypanosoma*. The function(s) of L1 elements in mouse or human cells is unknown but they may function as retroposons and could have some role during embryogenesis. The possible role of these elements in carcinogenic processes is unknown.

B. SINE SEQUENCES

A member of the mammalian SINE families of repeated DNA sequences is the human *Alu* family.[122] The 300,000 to 500,000 copies of the *Alu* family carried per haploid human genome are broadly distributed throughout the genome, representing between 3 to 6% of the total mass of DNA.[123] The human *Alu* sequences are approximately 300 bp in length and consist of two directly repeating monomeric units. The structural features of the *Alu* family of DNA sequences suggest that it derives from a large pool of precursors and not from a single precursor.[124] Individual *Alu* family repeats are usually surrounded by short direct repeats and terminate in a poly A-rich 3' end, which suggests that such members are dispersed by a mechanism involving an RNA intermediate. Consistent with this possibility, *Alu* family members are transcribed *in vitro* by RNA polymerase III, with the transcription initiation start site corresponding to the 5' end of the consensus *Alu* family sequence.[125] Several *Alu* members are transcribed by RNA polymerase II colinearly with protein coding sequences. Most nucleotides substitutions among the *Alu* members are transitions, rather than transversion, which may reflect evolutionary and functional conservations of the *Alu* DNA sequences.[123]

The *in vivo* transcription of *Alu* family members is complex. *Alu* transcripts are present in as much as 10% of human heterogeneous RNA and 7S RNA shows homology with *Alu* transcripts. Although most *Alu* repeats may represent pseudogenes, it is possible that one or more human *Alu* repeats may code for an as yet unidentified polypeptide product.[123] Interestingly, no *Alu* transcripts have been detected in HeLa cells. The reason for the transcriptional silence of *Alu* sequences in HeLa cells is unknown.

Another subgroup of the SINE superfamily of tandemly repeated DNA sequences contained in the human genome is represented by the *Mst* II family.[126] This family consists in a canonical structure composed of a 220-bp left arm joined to a 160-bp right arm by a 39-bp junction sequence. The *Mst* II family shows some similarities with variable tandem repeats of approximately 1.5-kb located downstream of the c-H-*ras*-1 protooncogene but its physiological role is unknown. Approximately 80 bp of the *Mst* II left arm occurs immediately adjacent to the tandem repeat that comprises the human homologue of the BK virus enhancer. A retroposon SINE sequence present in the human genome was found to be represented by dispersed DNA sequences homologous to part of the MMTV-like human endogenous retrovirus HERV-K.[127] The cloned sequence, SINE-R, was 630-bp in length and contained an adenine-rich tail at the 3' end. SINE-R elements are present at 4000 to 5000 copies per haploid human genome.

C. REITERATED DNA SEQUENCES AND HUMAN CANCER

The possible role of reiterated genomic sequences in human carcinogenic processes is little known. Comparison of reiterated DNA restriction fragments between primary human tumors and paired normal human tissues suggests the existence of qualitative and quantitative differences, and some of the reiterated sequences were found to be amplified in particular types of tumors.[128] The altered reiterated sequences detected in the human tumors were not character-ized. In an independent study, an L1 element was found to be inserted within the second intron of a c-*myc* protooncogene in the tumor tissue, but not the normal tissue, of a patient with a ductal adenocarcinoma of the breast.[129]

V. MECHANISMS OF CHRONIC RETROVIRUS-INDUCED TRANSFORMATION

The mechanisms by which chronic retroviruses may induce the malignant transformation of cells are little understood. By definition, chronic retroviruses have little oncogenic potential by themselves and may cause tumors only after long latency periods and acting through indirect mechanisms. Loss of immune competence which frequently accompanies infection by chronic retroviruses may be an important factor in the development of neoplastic diseases associated with these viruses. Although the oncogenic potential of different types of chronic retroviruses has been well documented in defined experimental systems *in vivo*, the role of these viruses in natural tumorigenic processes occurring in humans and other animal species is not totally clear. Chronic retroviruses are apparently unable to cause the direct transformation of normal cells into malignant cells *in vitro* and probably also *in vivo*, but they could act as indirect oncogenic agents or as cofactors in oncogenic processes, in association with other etiological agents.

Tumors associated with chronic retroviruses are of clonal origin, although individual cells may contain several copies of the provirus.[130] Persistent infection by a chronic retrovirus, or persistent expression of the retrovirus functions, may not always be required for malignant disease to develop. Lymphosarcomas and leukemias observed in cats are frequently associated with FeLV infection, but FeLVs are not detected in about 30% of the diseased animals. The presence of FeLV-associated membrane antigen in the virus-free cats with neoplasms could indicate a previous exposure to the virus.[131] However, this interpretation is complicated by the fact that normal cat cell DNA contains both sequences partially homologous to the genome of horizontally transmitted FeLV and information coding antigen against FeLV.[132,133] Thus, indirect mechanisms are most probably involved in FeLV-associated leukemogenesis. In any case, the general available evidence accumulated from the results obtained in many studies strongly suggests that multistage phenomena are probably always implicated in the oncogenic processes associated with infection by chronic retroviruses.

A. HOST GENETIC FACTORS

Host genetic factors are crucially important for determining the susceptibility of animals to infection by chronic retroviruses as well as for the possible induction of neoplastic diseases such as leukemias and lymphomas by these viruses.[134] The influence of host genetic factors in the susceptibility to lymphoid malignancies was initially demonstrated by the development of the highly susceptible AKR strain of mouse by selective inbreeding.[135] It was subsequently recognized that the leukemogenic agent in AKR mice is a retrovirus.[136] Different chronic retroviruses, including the Friend strain of MuLV (F-MuLV),[137] may be involved in the induction of hematopoietic malignancies in mice. Leukemias induced by F-MuLV or other chronic retroviruses evolve by multistage processes in which different stages from benignancy to full malignancy can be detected.[138]

The consequences of chronic retroviral infection are largely determined by the genetic constitution of the host. The host genes which can influence the development of retrovirus-induced leukemogenesis in mice can be divided into two groups: genes controlling the production and/or expression of the retrovirus in the host target cells and genes affecting the generation of immune responses to the virus or the expression of cell surface antigens.[134] Host genes controlling retrovirus production and/or expression include those coding for the specific cell surface receptor (*Rev*, which has been mapped to mouse chromosome 5), target cell availability (*S1* and *W*), virus replication (*Fv-1* on mouse chromosome 4 and *Fv-2* on mouse chromosome 9), and genes linked to the mouse MHC system (*H-2*). MHC genes are involved not only in controlling retrovirus production and/or expression but also in the immune responses to retroviruses and retrovirus-infected cells. However, genes nonlinked to *H-2*, like *Rfv-3* and *hr*, also participate in these responses. A dominant gene, termed *Akvr-1ʳ* or *Fv-4ʳ*, prevents viremia of AKR endogenous ecotropic virus and virus-mediated lymphoma in certain hybrid mice. This gene has been mapped to mouse chromosome 12 and its expression is linked to an ecotropic MuLV-related cell surface glycoprotein (gp70), which apparently interferes with the entry of related ecotropic virus into target cells.[139] Susceptibility of wild mice to exogenous infection with xenotropic leukemia viruses is controlled by a single dominant gene, *Sxv*, which maps to chromosome 1.[140] Susceptibility of BALB/c mice to develop F-MuLV-induced erythroleukemia depends on various DBA/2 genes.[141] In AKR mice, genes other than endogenous retroviruses, located on chromosomes 7 and 15, are involved in the predisposition to rapid onset of thymic lymphoma after inoculation with F-MuLV.[142]

The importance of the genetic constitution of the host in relation to oncogenic processes associated with chronic retroviruses is probably valid for all animal species, including primate species. The chronic retrovirus GaLV, isolated from a gibbon with chronic granulocytic leukemia, can induce leukemia by inoculation into young healthy gibbons but other primate and nonprimate animals are resistant to the leukemogenic potential of GaLV.[143] In general, humans are resistant to infection by nonhuman chronic retroviruses. Milk of dairy cows frequently contains infectious BLV,[144] and human cells can be infected by BLV *in vitro,* but there is no evidence that consumption of unpasteurized milk by people in many countries is associated with BLV infection. Genomic integration of BLV is not a factor in childhood acute lymphoblastic leukemia or non-Hodgkin's lymphoma, as demonstrated by the Southern blot technique using cloned BLV as a probe.[145] The factors responsible for the resistance of humans to infection by retroviruses of nonhuman origin have not been characterized but may include immune responses.

In general, the cellular and molecular mechanisms responsible for specific resistance to infection by chronic retroviruses are little understood. Mouse embryonal carcinoma cells, as normal mouse embryo cells from the preimplantation stage, are resistant to infection by chronic retroviruses such as MuLVs. The restriction of retrovirus expression in these cells may be due to a specific protein, called embryonal promoter-binding factor (EPBF), which binds to a consensus sequence (CCAAT) located 80 nucleotides upstream from the cap site.[146] The consensus sequence is highly conserved among murine retroviruses and has been shown by deletion and point mutation analyses to be essential for both LTR-mediated transcription and retrovirus infectivity.

B. CHANGES IN HOST GENOMIC FUNCTIONS

The insertion of chronic transforming viruses into the host cell genome may produce different changes in genomic functions, according to the site of integration in the chromosomes of the host cell. The site of viral integration is clonal, but would not be sequence specific, and a retrovirus may be integrated as a provirus into the host genome at many different locations.[57] However, the screening and analysis of DNA libraries for a large collection of retrovirus integration sites has indicated that integration does not occur at random, and that there are strongly preferred sites at which independent integrations occur at precisely the same nucleotide.[147] Monoclonality of provirus integration is observed for chronic retroviruses such as F-MuLV as early as a few weeks after infection, which suggests that malignant transformation induced by these viruses is initiated by a monoclonal or oligoclonal proliferation of nondifferentiated preneoplastic cells which precedes truly malignant cells by several months.[148] The integrated retrovirus can act as an insertion mutagen, determining the activation or inactivation of particular genetic loci in the host cell. In fact, it has suggested that retroviruses may be useful instruments for the genetic dissection of the various mammalian cell phenotypes.[149]

The retrovirus could be integrated into the cellular genome and could be expressed without regard to LTR sequences, with adjacent host DNA presumably supplying signals required for the expression of retroviral genetic information.[150] BLV, for example, may be integrated into different chromosomes and leukemogenesis associated with BLV infection would be largely, if not entirely, independent of the provirus integration site.[151-153] In patients with human T-cell leukemia/lymphoma, integration of the HTLV-I proviral genome is also clonal but apparently nonspecific.[154] HTLV-I provirus integration in the human tumor cells probably occurs at random sites. Thus, it is unlikely that the oncogenic properties of BLV and HTLV-I are associated with activation of specific protooncogenes. LTR sequences, however, are important for determining tissue selectivity of chronic transforming retroviruses like MuLVs.[155] Continued expression of viral functions is apparently not required for maintenance of a malignant phenotype in cells that were transformed as a consequence of BLV or HTLV-I infection.[151,156]

C. ALTERATION OF ENZYME ACTIVITIES

Various cellular enzymatic activities may be altered after infection with chronic transforming retroviruses. Infection of BALB/c mice with M-MuLV on the first day after birth results in a gradual enlargement of the spleen and induction of lymphoma within $1\frac{1}{2}$ to 3 months. Protein kinase C activity, assayed in extracts of spleen and thymus cells of the M-MuLV-infected animals, declines gradually during the development of lymphoma and is replaced by a Ca^{2+}/lipid-independent type of protein kinase.[157] However, the possible role of changes in cellular enzyme activities in relation to the development of tumors induced by chronic transforming retroviruses is not understood.

D. INDUCTION OF IMMUNOSUPPRESSION

An important component of the mechanisms involved in the pathogenicity, including the potential oncogenicity, of chronic retroviruses is the impairment of immune competence.[158] Induction of immunodepression by the infecting chronic retrovirus may rend the host unable to mount an efficient specific immune response against the virus, which may contribute to a more easier replication of the virus, further increasing the immunodepression and facilitating the persistence of the viral infection. Further, if the virus has an oncogenic potential, lowered immunologic surveillance and impaired immune reactions could favor the appearance of neoplastic diseases or could contribute to the dissemination of an already existent tumor. The mechanisms responsible for the genetic susceptibility or resistance of animals from different species, or different individuals from the same species, to chronic retroviral infections are probably very complex. Immune responses of the host may greatly influence the course and consequence of chronic retrovirus infection.[159] Most frequently, animals infected with chronic retroviruses develop humoral and cellular immune responses against these viruses.

1. Feline Acquired Immunodeficiency Syndrome

Cats infected with FeLV may develop an efficient production of antibodies directed to both mature viruses in the serum and cells infected with the virus, which may terminate their infection after a brief viremic episode.[160] In contrast, cats that become persistently infected after exposure to FeLV develop only very low levels of specific antivirus antibodies. Reactivation of latent FeLV infection from myelomonocytic and lymphoid cells of cats immune to FeLV is suppressed by the immune system of the host but can be altered by adrenal corticosteroid hormones *in vivo* and *in vitro*.[161] Persistently viremic cats can suffer from FeLV-related diseases that include bone marrow-suppressive disorders, lymphoproliferative and myeloproliferative cancers, and secondary infectious diseases due to the immunosuppressive effects of FeLV.[162,163] Loss of T-cell associated, immune competence-induced FeLV may lead to a feline acquired immunodeficiency syndrome (FAIDS), a syndrome similar to human AIDS.[43] A particular FeLV strain (FeLV-FAIDS) has been detected at high concentrations and principally as unintegrated viral DNA in the bone marrow of cats with FAIDS.[164] A replication-defective variant of FeLV associated with the development of FAIDS has been cloned and sequenced.[165] Cats inoculated at 8 weeks of age or younger develop an acute disease within 6 months, whereas older cats develop a more chronic disease course marked by an asymptomatic or prodromal period of 1 or more years, similar to that found in human AIDS.

2. Mechanisms of Immunosuppression Induced by Chronic Retroviruses

A component of the retroviral transmembrane envelope protein, termed p15E, is immunosuppressive in that it inhibits immune responses of lymphocytes, monocytes, and macrophages.[166] p15E has been conserved among murine and feline retroviruses and has also been found in the transmembrane envelope proteins of the human retroviruses HTLV-I and HTLV-II. Moreover, a p15E-related protein is normally present in the human blood and is increased in some leukemic patients.[167] This protein is probably encoded by endogenous retroviral genomes.

The severe pathological consequences of HIV infection are closely related to the potent immunosuppressive properties of the virus. These properties depend, at least in part, on the binding of the large envelope protein gp120 of the virus to the CD4 molecule which probably represents the HIV receptor on the surface of lymphocytes.[168] The mechanisms of HIV-associated pathogenicity are discussed in detail in Section XII.

E. EXPRESSION OF MHC ANTIGENS

The major histocompatibility complex (MHC) of the cellular genome is directly involved in controlling the synthesis of specific antigens expressed on the cell surface of normal and transformed cells and plays an essential role in immunoregulatory phenomena. This complex is represented by the H-2 gene complex in the mouse and the HLA complex in the human. The H-2 complex, located on mouse chromosome 17, and the HLA complex, located on human chromosome 6, have been divided into class I and class II genes on the basis of structural and functional similarities.[169] Class I genes of mouse H2 and human HLA complexes encode glycoprotein products which are expressed in noncovalent association with β_2-microglobulin on the surface of nucleated cells. In the mouse, the MHC class I products are represented by H2K, H-2D/H-2L, Qa-2,3, and Tla specificities. In the human, the class I products are represented by HLA-A, -B, and -C specificities. In addition to serving as target molecules in allogeneic graft rejection, these antigens are essential for the recognition and destruction of neoplastic and virus-infected cells by the cytotoxic T cells of the host immune system.[170]

Marked alterations in the quantitative expression of MHC antigens on the cell surface may be associated with infection and/or transformation by chronic retroviruses. Transformation of murine thymocytes after infection with by radiation leukemia virus (RadLV) is associated with reduced expression of class I H-2 antigens encoded by MHC genes in the tumor cells, which is apparently due to increased methylation and rearrangement of MHC DNA.[171] In contrast, M-MuLV-infected cells express significantly increased levels of H-2 antigens on the cell surface.[172] As a reflection of their increased level of H-2 class I antigen expression, M-MuLV-infected cells are efficiently lysed by M-MuLV-specific cytotoxic T lymphocytes. The increased levels of H-2 gene expression occurring in M-MuLV-infected cells are associated with increased steady-state levels of H-2 and β_2-microglobulin mRNA transcripts as a consequence of a direct activation of the respective cellular genes by the virus or a virus product.[173] Interestingly, the simultaneous infection of these cells with an acute retrovirus (M-MuSV carrying the v-*mos* oncogene) results in inhibition of the enhanced expression of H-2 antigens on the cell surface.

F. INTERACTION WITH CHEMICAL CARCINOGENS

Chronic retroviruses are generally unable to transform cultured cells by themselves but they are capable of facilitating chemical carcinogenesis *in vitro* in various types of cells. Transformation is not observed in Fischer rat embryo cell cultures infected with R-MuLV or treated with MCA alone, but it readily occurs when the R-MuLV infected cells are treated with the carcinogen.[174] NRK cells are highly resistant to the transforming action of a variety of carcinogens, but they become chemically transformable after being productively infected with M-MuLV.[175] Moreover, integration of only one M-MuLV proviral DNA into the cellular genome is sufficient for this change in the response of NRK to chemical carcinogens. Interestingly, randomly isolated foci of the cells transformed by identical procedures exhibit a striking degree of heterogeneity regarding their morphology, growth rate, saturation density, serum requirement, virus release, and response to interferon. The mechanisms involved in the early phenotypic diversification of transformed cells cloned from the same original population are unknown.

Chemical carcinogens can potentiate tumorigenic processes induced by chronic retroviruses *in vivo*. Administration of NMU is highly effective in rendering resistant adult cats susceptible to FeLV infection and subsequent development of thymic lymphosarcoma.[176] Benzo(a)pyrene (BP) exerts a potentiating effect on F-MuSV-induced leukemogenesis in mice.[177] Exposure of mice to BP results in a time-dependent increased incidence of leukemia among animals subsequently injected with very low doses of F-MuLV. Caffeine, an inhibitor of DNA repair, further enhances the potentiating effect of BP on F-MuLV-induced feline leukemia, which suggests that the initial step of the BP-associated potentiation process is probably linked to the DNA damage produced by the carcinogen and that inhibition of DNA repair processes may facilitate the pathogenic action of the chronic retrovirus. Treatment of the normal mouse mammary epithelial cell line C57MG with both DMBA and MMTV results in transformation of the cells, as indicated by an increased tumorigenicity in athymic mice and the ability of cells to grow in soft agar.[178] However, no synergistic or potentiating effect of chemical carcinogen on chronic retrovirus-induced tumorigenesis is observed MMTV-induced mammary tumorigenesis in C3H mice treated with DMBA.[179] Thus, different retroviruses may use different pathways for the induction of neoplastic diseases, and the influence of chemical carcinogens or other exogenous and endogenous factors may be variable according to the retrovirus and the physiologic conditions of the animal.

G. ROLE OF ASSOCIATED RETROVIRUSES

Coinfection with two or more different types of chronic retroviruses may occur under either natural or experimental conditions and may result in potentiation or reduction of the individual pathogenicities of the involved viruses. At least in some cases, infection with a given retrovirus can induce protection against infection by another retrovirus. Intrathymic injection of SMX-1 (a dualtropic MuLV derived from M-MuLV virus stocks) induced protection of AKR mice from developing MuLV-accelerated leukemia and spontaneous leukemia.[180] Most probably, this protection is due to mechanisms involving some aspect of viral interference.

The complex mechanisms involved in malignant diseases associated with chronic retrovirus infection may be exemplified by mouse leukemia induced by F-MuLV.[181] This leukemia is originated by a multistage process. The early stage of the disease is associated with a marked increase in the number of erythroid cells in the bone marrow and spleen. These cells retain the ability to differentiate terminally to mature erythrocytes, have little or no self-renewal capability, are nontumorigenic *in vivo*, and cannot give rise to cell lines in culture. The late stage of the disease begins 3 to 4 weeks after infection and is characterized by the appearance of cells that are tumorigenic *in vivo* and capable of growing as permanent cell lines in culture.

The original isolate of F-MuLV, FV-A, causes anemia and a rapid enlargement of the spleen, while a subsequently isolated virus, FV-P, derived from a stock of FV-A, can cause an increase in the number of mature erythrocytes (polycytemia).[181] Both FV-A and FV-P are complexes of a replication-defective spleen focus-forming virus, SFFV, and a replication-competent F-MuLV. The SFFV component of FV-A and FV-P is responsible for the induction of spleen foci, erythroid proliferation, and splenomegaly associated with the early stages of Friend leukemia in adult mice and, furthermore, many of the properties of the late stages of the disease are specified by SFFV. Replicating SFFV may exist for years in mouse bone marrow cultures and is associated with the generation of growth factor-independent cell lines, several of which can produce tumors *in vivo*. Interestingly, growth factor-dependent and -independent cells may coexist in the same long-term cultures, which may indicate that a subpopulation of stem cells is able to escape irreversible transformation by SFFV.[182]

H. ROLE OF THE DELETION OF RETROVIRAL SEQUENCES

Replication-defective viruses derived from chronic retroviruses may be capable of inducing malignant disease in an acute manner despite the fact that they do not contain oncogenes. For example, the myeloproliferative leukemia virus (MPLV), derived from *in vivo* passage of F-MuLV clone 57, is capable of inducing in an acute form (2 to 3 weeks after inoculation) a myeloproliferative disorder that affects all major lineages in adult mice of different strains.[183] A comparison of F-MuLV and MPLV indicates that the MPLV genome is derived from F-MuLV with conservation of *gag* and *pol* regions and that it contains a deleted and rearranged *env* region.[184] Replication-incompetent retrovirus particles (helper virus-free particles) containing genomes that express the *env* gene (gp52) of SFFV are capable of inducing transformation of bone marrow cells *in vitro* and, after direct i.v. introduction of the vector into animals, can induce fully malignant erythroid disease *in vivo*.[185,186]

VI. ROLE OF LTRs AND ENHANCERS IN TRANSFORMATION INDUCED BY CHRONIC RETROVIRUSES

The pathogenetic effects of chronic retroviruses, including neoplastic transformation, crucially depend on the presence of nucleotide sequences such as LTRs and enhancers that can act as effective stimulators of the transcriptional activity of both viral and cellular genes. A high level of retrovirus replication in a tissue is not sufficient for inducing transformation. High levels of virus replication may be required only transiently during an early preleukemic stage of MuLV-induced disease.[187]

A. EFFECTS OF LTRs

The LTRs contained at both ends of retroviral proviruses contain nucleotide sequences required for viral integration, replication, and expression. LTRs can act as strong short-range promoters of transcription for the neighbor viral or cellular genes and are thus important in determining the possible pathological consequences of viral infection. LTRs also contain sequences with enhancer effects capable of stimulating the transcription of genes located relatively far from the site of insertion of the provirus. Neoplastic changes may result from the insertion of promoters elements and transcriptional enhancers contained in LTRs when proviral integration occurs near cellular sequences with potential capability for inducing the transformed phenotype. As a consequence, the adjacent cellular sequences could be expressed at high levels in inappropriate site and/or time. U3 tandem direct repeat sequences within the LTR of MuLVs are primary determinants of their leukemogenic potential.[188] Such sequences are both necessary and sufficient to confer some leukemogenic potential to MuLV, although *env* 3'-end sequences are required for the expression of a fully leukemic phenotype. The transcriptional activity of LTRs plays a crucial role in determining the target cell and tissue specificity for retroviral-associated oncogenesis.[189] However, the tissue tropism and target specificity of leukemogenic murine retroviruses is also determined, at least in part, by viral sequences outside the LTR, in particular by sequences within the *env* or *pol-env* region.[187,190,191]

B. EFFECTS OF ENHANCERS

Enhancer sequences have been associated not only with RNA viruses but also with DNA viruses with oncogenic potential (SV40, BKV, polyoma virus, adenovirus) and are also present in the eukaryotic genome. These sequences are able to enhance gene expression by an as yet undefined *cis*-acting regulatory mechanism. Enhancers are less restricted by position than classical promoters and play an important role in regulation of gene expression.[192,193] The function of enhancers appears to be controlled by *trans*-acting factors. In contrast to promoter elements, the enhancers may act in any orientation and at a distance from the gene whose expression is being modulated. Some enhancer-like sequences, called silencers, may be responsible not for activation but for repression of transcription of particular genes.

The role of viral and cellular enhancers in oncogenic processes is little understood. In general, there exists a correlation between LTR transcriptional activity, LTR-induced enhancement of mRNA transcription, and retroviral oncogenic potential.[194] This phenomenon is probably related to the presence within LTR of enhancer sequences. The promoter and the enhancer are interacting but functionally distinct elements that form parts of the transcriptional control regions of genes transcribed by RNA polymerase II.[195] At least some promoters are inactive in the absence of an enhancer element. According to a model, the LTR enhancer of RSV is located entirely within the LTR U3 region and 5' to the promoter of the same region.[196] Factors depending on the host cell may be importantly involved in the regulation of retrovirus expression through the activity of LTR-associated enhancers. Murine embryonal carcinoma cells are refractory to infection by retroviruses because retroviral LTR enhancers have little activity in these cells.[197]

Enhancers may be characterized by cell specificity. For example, an enhancer element contained in a lymphotropic papovavirus (LPV) possesses a very restricted tissue range, being active in all human cells of the hematopoietic tissues tested, but not in cells of fibroblast or epithelial origin.[198] The direct repeat in U3, which in the case of M-MuLV has been shown to have the properties of a transcriptional enhancer, is a determinant of disease specificity in nondefective MuLVs.[199] A small number of nucleotide differences within the viral transcription signals which may interact with nuclear, sequence-specific DNA binding proteins may underlie the different types of neoplastic diseases induced by F-MuLV and M-MuLV. It is well known that M-MuLV induces T-cell lymphomas after injection into NFS mice, whereas the nondefective F-MuLV induces primarily erythroleukemias. The specific leukemogenic properties of certain chronic retroviruses seems to depend on enhancers located within the viral LTR.[199-201] LTR sequences of retroviruses associated with both human and bovine leukemia (HTLV and BLV, respectively) contain enhancer elements, the activities of which would depend on the presence of virus-associated *trans*-acting factors. Recognition sites for such factors could also be present within the regulatory regions of genes that govern lymphocyte growth, which would explain the leukemogenic potential of these viruses.[202]

BLV LTRs appear to be unusual promoter units, functioning in a cell type-specific manner and possessing sequences, on both the 5' and 3' sides of the RNA start site, that can influence the expression of cellular genes.[203] The chromosomal site of integration of enhancer retroviral elements with enhancer activity may exert a strong influence on the rate of transcriptional activation of particular genes.[204] Regulation of LTR function is susceptible to environmental stimuli, including the influences of hormones and cellular growth factors.

VII. INSERTIONAL ACTIVATION OF PROTOONCOGENES

Retroviruses may integrate preferentially close to DNase I-hypersensitive sites that are expressed in some but not all cells.[205] Analysis of DNA libraries has revealed the presence of strongly preferred sites for retrovirus integration, with independent integrations occurring precisely at the same nucleotide.[147] Chronic retroviruses could act as "insertion mutagens" through their random integration in the genome of the host cell.[206] Deletion of regulatory sequences produced by retrovirus insertion could result in activation or deregulation of the cellular gene. Chronic retroviruses can also activate protooncogenes, or putative protooncogenes, through a promoter insertion mechanism.[207-212] In this case, the virus LTR is inserted near the 5′ end of a protooncogene, or a putative protooncogene, and the promoter sequence of the LTR is used to stimulate transcription of the gene. In addition, as discussed previously in this chapter, some genetic elements contained within the proviral LTR may act not as promoters with a short-range effect but may display enhancer effects on relatively remote DNA sequences.

A. ALTERATION OF THE C-*MYC* GENE

Both avian and murine lymphomas associated with chronic retrovirus infection may exhibit insertional alteration of the c-*myc* protooncogene. Deregulation of c-*myc* expression as a consequence of retroviral insertion may contribute to the lymphomagenic process.

1. Chicken Bursal Lymphomas

Bursal lymphomas induced by ALVs in chickens are frequently associated with proviral insertions in the region 5′ to the c-*myc* gene coding sequences, which may result in transcriptional activation of c-*myc* gene expression. Downstream LTRs of the integrated proviruses may act as efficient promoters when the upstream LTR is deleted, which could explain the observation that only deleted proviruses are found to be inserted upstream and in the same orientation to the c-*myc* protooncogene in B-cell lymphomas of chickens.[213] Integration of an ALV provirus adjacent to c-*myc* would then result in increased expression of this protooncogene promoted by the 3′ LTR of the integrated provirus. Newly integrated ALV proviral sequences may affect the structure of chromatin in surrounding cellular sequences.[214] However, in 3 out of 5 cell lines derived from ALV-induced bursal lymphomas no viral LTR sequences were found to be associated with c-*myc* mRNA, but a 30- to 60-fold increase in the level of c-*myc* transcripts was detected in these cells.[215] These results suggest that in some cases the retroviral LTR may act not as a promoter but as an enhancer of transcription. Moreover, the LTR promoter function may not be required for maintenance of the transformed phenotype in tissue culture. In one exceptional chicken bursal lymphoma (LL6), provirus insertion occurred not on the 5′ side of the c-*myc* gene but downstream of the c-*myc* coding sequences.[216] The cells from this tumor expressed increased levels of a hybrid transcript, consisting of c-*myc* sequences at the 5′ end and viral sequences at the 3′ end. The LL6 provirus was apparently the result of intrachromosomal recombination between two proviruses that were integrated 3′ to the c-*myc* gene. The recombination was associated with an internal proviral deletion as well as with deletion of intervening cellular DNA sequences. However, no transcripts could be detected within a 20-kb region downstream of the LL6 provirus, and the question of whether the additional chromosomal alterations contributed to LL6-associated tumorigenesis remained unresolved.

Another chronic retrovirus capable of inducing B-cell lymphomas is the chicken syncytial virus (CSV), a member of the reticuloendotheliosis virus (REV) group. In all of 22 B-cell lymphomas induced in chickens with CSV, the virus was found to be integrated upstream from the second c-*myc* exon and 70% of these insertion sites were clustered in a 0.5-kb region immediately preceding the exon.[217,218] In these tumors, the CSV proviruses were all arranged in the same transcriptional orientation as c-*myc*, bearing a strong resemblance to ALV proviruses involved in c-*myc* activation in chicken B-cell lymphomas. The integrated CSV provirus has a deletion of 80% the viral genes but retains two intact LTRs. Deletion of proviral sequences may be important for the oncogenic potential of chronic retroviruses. Elevated levels of c-*myc* expression are found in CSV-induced chicken bursal lymphomas, probably as a consequence of increased c-*myc* transcription stimulated by the 3′ LTR of CSV.

In addition to bursal B-cell lymphomas, REV infection in chicken may result in the development of T-cell lymphomas resembling the herpesvirus-induced Marek's disease.[219] The molecular characterization of the REV-induced chicken T-cell lymphomas indicated that in all of 14 tumors analyzed the c-*myc* locus was interrupted by REV proviral insertions occurring upstream of the protooncogene coding exons.[220]

2. Murine Lymphomas

Proviral insertion near protooncogenes does not appear to be quantitatively important in murine leukemias and lymphomas, in comparison to avian bursal lymphomas. In one study only 7 of 59 MuLV-induced mouse T-cell leukemias exhibited provirus insertion near the c-*myc*, *pim*-1, or *Mlvi*-1 loci.[221] Of 18 T-cell lymphomas induced in BALB/c mice by the Soule strain of MuLV, 2 were found to be associated with rearrangement of the c-*myc* gene, but in none of these neoplasms a proviral insertion occurred near the c-*myc* promoter.[222,223] Of 61 lymphomas induced in rats or mice by inoculation of MuLV, 5 showed alterations adjacent to the c-*myc* gene and in 2 of them MuLV proviruses were found to be integrated adjacent to the same protooncogene.[224] Retroviral integration near the mouse c-*myc* gene was detected in 10 to 20% of AKR lymphomas induced in mice by the retrovirus MCF 247.[225] A rearranged c-*myc* gene was not contained in 80 to 90% of the tumors analyzed in the latter study after integration of the retrovirus and no evidence was found of viral integration near several other protooncogenes (c-H-*ras*, c-K-*ras*, c-*abl*, c-*myb*, c-*erb*-A, c-*erb*-B, and c-*mos*).

Different mechanisms may be involved in activation of the c-*myc* protooncogene in specific types of tumors associated with chronic retroviruses, such as T-cell lymphomas induced in mice by MuLV. In approximately 45% of MuLV-induced early developing T-cell lymphomas in mice, integration of the proviruses occurred near c-*myc*, and, from 33 lymphomas with proviral integration in the c-*myc* domain, 29 insertions were localized upstream of the first exon, in a region spanning less than 2kb, and 4 integrations within the first exon.[226] In 95% of these lymphomas the transcriptional orientation was opposite to the transcriptional direction of c-*myc*. Proviral integration in the c-*myc* domain was associated with increased c-*myc* mRNA levels (up to 30-fold). Enhanced c-*myc* mRNA levels were also found in some lymphomas without proviral integration near c-*myc* but in a few of these lymphomas c-*myc* mRNA transcripts were hardly detectable. Some murine T-cell lymphomas are characterized by the presence of a variant (6;15) translocation and in such cases the proviral inserts occur in a locus, termed *pvt*-1, which is located at least 72 kb from the c-*myc* promoters.[227] It is conceivable that in these cases an altered *pvt*-1 locus may lead to lymphoid cell neoplasia via long-range effects on c-*myc* expression.

In R-MuLV-induced murine B-cell lymphomas the virus could either induce transformation of a stem cell that undergoes further differentiation and becomes blocked at various stages of development or transform B cells at various stages of differentiation. In these tumors the c-*myc* gene is rearranged at one particular stage in B cell development, which implicates a developmentally regulated alteration of the protooncogene.[228] The tumors induced by R-MuLV are clonal in origin but the mechanisms responsible for their development, including the possible participation of c-*myc* and/or other cellular oncogenes, are not understood. It is not known if integration of the virus near c-*myc* is required for the development of such tumors.

A retrovirus related to radiation leukemia virus (RadLV/VL3) is capable of inducing lymphomas upon inoculation into rats. Although integration of this virus takes place in most cases apparently at random sites, a few tumors display insertion of an either full length or deleted provirus adjacent to the c-*myc* protooncogene.[229] However, this particular site of integration does not necessarily reflect a viral induction of radiation-induced leukemogenesis since the presence of a provirus at specific site can lead to an *in vitro* growth advantage independently of a lymphomagenic process.

Leukemogenesis that follows intrathymic injection of mink cell focus virus (MCFV) in young adult mice occurs through several stages. Specific proviral integrations in the c-*myc* locus were detected in 15% of early clonal populations of thymocytes and in up to 65% of late-developing thymomas and frank leukemias.[230] These findings suggest that c-*myc* activation occurs both early and late in leukemogenesis by the same mechanism of proviral insertion. However, blot hybridization experiments showed that on the average there is only a twofold elevation of the steady-state c-*myc* mRNA levels in the MCFV-induced thymomas as compared to the levels in normal thymocytes.[231] Such an increase does not appear to be sufficient for thymomas induction, although a shift in c-*myc* promoter usage was detected in virtually all thymomas tested. It seems likely that in addition to c-*myc* other as yet uncharacterized genes are activated to produce the malignant phenotype in chronic retrovirus-induced lymphomas. Further studies are required for a proper evaluation of c-*myc* gene dysfunction in oncogenic processes associated with infection by chronic retroviruses.

3. Rat Thymomas

A minority of thymomas induced in rats by chronic retroviruses is associated with insertional activation of c-*myc*. Only 1 of 24 thymomas induced in Fischer rats by M-MuLV contained a provirus integrated adjacent to the c-*myc* protooncogene.[232] In another study, 2 of 17 M-MuLV-induced rat thymomas contained rearrangements of c-*myc*.[233] Interestingly, in one of these two tumors the observed rearrangement of c-*myc* was not due to the insertion of an intact M-MuLV provirus but was associated with a homologous recombination event that occurred between sequences of two proviruses integrated on the same chromosome, one of which was inserted near the c-*myc* protooncogene.

4. Feline Leukemia

Tumor cells from spontaneous feline leukemia have been examined for structural abnormality and expression of the c-*myc* gene.[234] Of 12 spontaneous leukemia cases, 4 exhibited some abnormality of c-*myc*. From these four cases, one case showed a DNA rearrangement in the 5′ portion of the c-*myc* locus associated with integration of an FeLV genome. Another case had a newly inserted v-*myc* oncogene which was transduced by FeLV, and two additional cases exhibited structural abnormalities of the c-*myc* gene not directly related to FeLV insertion. No structural abnormalities of c-*myc* were detected in the remaining 8 cases of feline leukemia.

B. ALTERATION OF THE C-*MYB* GENE

Rearrangement in the c-*myb* locus of BALB/c plasmacytoid lymphosarcomas and myelomonocytic tumors may be associated with the insertion of M-MuLV at the 5′ end of the c-*myb* protooncogene.[235-237] Disruption of the c-*myb* gene by viral insertional mutagenesis in mouse myeloid cells may result in truncated c-*myb* proteins that could play a role in neoplastic transformation of myeloid cells.[238,239] Activation of the c-*myb* protooncogene by inserted retroviruses could also be accomplished by exon deletion and/or replacement which may remove a regulatory domain of the normal gene.[236] The viral integration may result in the initiation of transcription within M-MuLV viral sequences and replacement of the c-*myb* amino-terminal sequences by *gag* sequences.[240] In any case, deregulation of c-*myb* gene expression by retrovirus insertion in the murine system may represent a situation which is similar to that observed in the avian system by transduction of a v-*myb* oncogene which contains deleted coding sequences at both ends of the respective cellular gene.

Among a series of ten murine myeloid leukemia cell lines induced by nondefective MuLVs, only one (NSF-60) was found to have a rearrangement of the c-*myb* locus due to integration of the retrovirus into the region of the gene corresponding to the sixth exon of the avian c-*myb* locus, resulting in the production of a truncated RNA.[241] The properties of these cells supported the concept that the c-*myb* protooncogene is involved in the control of normal differentiation of hematopoietic cells.

C. ALTERATION OF THE C-K-*RAS* GENE

Newborn NFS/n mice inoculated with F-MuLV rapidly develop erythroleukemia and die within 8 to 14 weeks. The mechanisms of F-MuLV-induced leukemia are unknown but at least in some cases F-MuLV integration is associated with altered patterns of activation of protooncogenes. From 12 different cellular oncogenes examined in F-MuLV-transformed cells, only c-K-*ras* transcripts were expressed at higher levels than in normal mouse bone marrow.[242] The murine bone marrow-derived cell line 416B exhibits 25- to 30-fold overexpression of c-K-*ras* protooncogene, which is apparently due to integration of F-MuLV proviral DNA within this gene.[243] In another study of F-MuLV-induced mouse erythroleukemia no increased expression of c-K-*ras* or c-H-*ras* was detected in the tumor cells but, in contrast, increased levels of normal (2.3 kb) and short (1.8 kb) c-*myc* transcripts were found in both early preleukemic and late leukemic phases of the disease, as compared to normal erythroid cells.[244]

D. ALTERATION OF THE C-*ERB*-B GENE

The type of tumor induced by chronic retroviruses would depend, at least in part, on the protooncogene that is altered by insertion of a viral promoter. For example, the chronic retroviruses ALVs induce lymphoid leukosis when the cellular oncogene c-*myc* is activated by insertion of the viral LTR but they induce erythroblastosis when a different protooncogene, c-*erb*-B, is activated by a similar mechanism.[245] The c-*erb*-B gene is highly homologous to the EGF receptor gene. The truncated EGF receptor proteins produced in ALV-induced chicken erythroblastosis contain a small extracellular glycosylated domain, a transmembrane hydrophobic region, and a cytoplasmic domain with tyrosine-specific kinase activity.[246]

In ALV-induced erythroblastosis, the ALV integration sites are clustered 5′ to the first exon of the c-*erb*-B protooncogene at the region where homology to v-*erb*-B starts, and the ALV proviruses are full-length and orientated in the same transcriptional direction as c-*erb*-B.[247] The transcripts are initiated in the 5′ LTR of the integrated provirus and contain truncated portions of the avian c-*erb*-B gene as well as viral *gag* and *env* sequences that are generated by splicing processes.[248] Insertion of ALV into the c-*erb*-B locus serves to create a complex transcription unit in which at least eight different mRNAs can be generated from a single primary transcript by alternative RNA processing.[249] The c-*erb*-B protooncogene may be transduced in ALV-induced erythroblastosis.[250]

Helper viruses of acute retroviruses may act as transducers of c-*erb*-B-derived sequences. The RSV-associated helper virus RAV-1 may occasionally transduce the c-*erb*-B gene in chickens that have dominant genes for susceptibility to RAV-1-induced erythroblastosis.[251] The induction of angiosarcomas by a new AEV retrovirus transducing c-*erb*-B-derived sequences has also been reported.[252] Hence, acute and chronic retroviruses would utilize a common pathway for transformation. It is not known, however, whether qualitative and/or quantitative alterations in the expression of the c-*erb*-B gene are responsible, or even required, for the neoplastic transformation of cells infected by chronic retroviruses.

E. ACTIVATION OF THE *PIM*-1 GENE

In a significant number of M-MuLV-induced mouse T-cell lymphomas, the proviruses are integrated in the vicinity or inside the transcriptional unit of a putative protooncogene, *pim*-1, causing enhanced transcription of this cellular gene.[253,254] M-MuLV frequently induces oligoclonal T-cell lymphomas in mice by proviral insertion near c-*myc* of *pim*-1 in the independent clones.[255] Activation of these genes may occur after proviral insertion, and clonal selections during tumor progression are frequently marked by acquisition of new proviral integrations.

1. The Murine *pim* Genes

The *pim*-1 gene is located on mouse chromosome 17, within the *t* complex which affects a variety of developmental and genetic processes including male fertility, embryonic development, and meiotic transmission.[256] The murine *pim*-1 gene has been cloned and sequenced, and it has been shown that it codes for a protein of 313 amino acids whose primary structure shows extensive homology with protein kinases.[257] However, it is not known whether the *pim*-1 protein functions effectively as a serine/threonine or a tyrosine kinase. Two DNA sequences homologous to *pim*-1, termed *pim*-2 and *pim*-3, have been assigned to mouse chromosomes 6 and 16, respectively.[257] Proviral integration near *pim*-2 and *pim*-3 has not been detected.

The role of *pim*-1 activation in mouse and the origin and development of mouse lymphomas is not understood. Whereas 31 out of 66 BALB/c mice which developed lymphomas within 6 months after injection with M-MuLV during the newborn period contained a provirus integrated in the *pim*-1 region, only 5 out of 64 mice which developed the disease after more than 6 months had proviral insertions near *pim*-1. The majority (60%) of proviral integrations in these lymphomas occurred in the 3′ region of the *pim*-1 transcription unit.

2. The Human *pim*-1 Gene

A homologue of the murine *pim*-1 gene is located on human chromosome region 6p21.[258] The human *pim*-1 gene has been cloned and sequenced.[259,260] It codes for a 313-amino acid protein of 35.6 kDa which is 94% homologous to the deduced amino acid sequence of murine *pim*-1. All the mouse *pim*-1 residues which are homologous to protein kinase are conserved in the human *pim*-1 protein. As its mouse counterpart, the human *pim*-1 protein shows clear structural homology with protein sequences of the catalytic domain of protein kinases. However, from the deduced amino acid sequence it cannot be predicted whether the protein possesses tyrosine- or threonine/serine-specific kinase activity, since it shows homology with members of both groups of kinases.

Elevated levels of 3.2-kb transcripts of human *pim*-1 are expressed in the erythroleukemia cell line K562, which contains a cytogenetically demonstrable rearrangement in the 6p21 region.[258] Although the short arm of chromosome 6 is involved in various translocations observed in human leukemias, the possible role of this gene in human malignant diseases is not understood.

F. ALTERATION OF *INT* GENES

In female BR6 mice a mammary tumor incidence of over 90% occurs after several pregnancies as a result of milk-borne infection with MMTV. A high percentage of the mice mammary tumors contain an acquired MMTV provirus in either of three defined integration regions, *int*-1, *int*-2, and *int*-3.[261-263] Proviral MMTV insertion at *int*-1 and *int*-2 loci are also observed in a number of transplanted mammary tumors of the GR mouse strain which exhibit endogenous MMTV provirus expression.[264] MMTV provirus insertion at *int* loci is accompanied by expression of specific RNA transcripts from these loci.[265-268]

1. The *int*-1 Gene

The gene *int*-1 contains four exons capable of coding a 41-kDa protein of 370 amino acids.[269,270] As many as five species of *int*-1 protein, ranging in apparent MW from 36 to 44 kDa, are generated by the sequential addition of N-linked carbohydrates to a primary *int*-1 translation product from which an amino-terminal signal sequence is removed.[271,272] The structure of the *int*-1 protein, as deduced from the nucleotide sequence of the four exons of the *int*-1 gene, shows no obvious homology to proteins encoded by known cellular oncogenes but suggests that the *int*-1 protein may be located at the level of a plasma membrane and that the protein may be secreted. There are no differences in nucleotide sequences between the known exons of the normal and a proviral activated *int*-1 allele.[270] Activation of *int*-1 should be attributed to an enhancer action of MMTV insertion rather than to a promoter insertion effect of the provirus since the majority of viral insertions occur downstream and away from the *int*-1 gene.[269]

The *int*-1 gene is located on the distal third of mouse chromosome 15 and a sequence homologous to this gene has been mapped to human chromosome 12, at region 12q13.[273-275] The nucleotide sequence of the human *int*-1 gene has been determined and a very high degree of homology was found between the predicted amino acid sequences of the human and mouse *int*-

1-encoded proteins.[276] There is evidence that the human analog to the mouse *int*-1 locus may be activated in some human mammary carcinomas.[277,278]

DNA sequences related to *int*-1 are highly conserved during evolution. A *Drosophila melanogaster* homologue of the murine *int*-1 gene has been isolated and cDNA clones of this gene indicated that the deduced protein product contains 468 amino acids and is 54% identical to the murine *int*-1 sequence, with all 23 cysteine residues conserved.[279,280] Expression of the *Drosophila int*-1 gene is observed in early embryos and in larval and pupal stages but is barely detected in adult tissues of the insect. The *int*-1 gene of *Drosophila* is identical to the segmental polarity gene *wingless* of the insect, whose product contributes to cooperative decisions made by groups of cells, possibly through a gradient of positional information, in individual segments or in imaginal discs.[281] The putative protein product of the *Drosophila int*-1/*wingless* gene is a diffusible extracellular factor. According to the animal species and the target cell, the *int*-1 gene product could have differentiating or transforming activities. The *wingless* gene is developmentally regulated in *Drosophila* and zygotic-lethal or viable mutants of this gene have important consequences in the development of the insect.

2. The *int*-2 Gene

The *int*-2 gene is located on mouse chromosome 7 and an MMTV provirus is early integrated there in about 50% of all BR6 mammary tumors examined, whether hormone dependent or independent.[266] The sequence, topography, and protein coding potential of the mouse *int*-2 gene have been characterized.[282] The *int*-2 gene sequence comprises 7869 bp of DNA and encodes for a protein of 245 amino acids with an estimated 27-kDa mol wt. Nucleotide sequences related to the mouse *int*-2 gene are present in DNAs from human, monkey, cat, rat, mink, and hamster, but are apparently absent in lower vertebrates and invertebrates, including chicken, *Xenopus*, and yeast.[283]

The human *int*-2 gene is located on human chromosome region 11q13,[283,284] and the progesterone receptor has been mapped to the same human chromosome region.[285] Since progesterone action and breast cancer have been linked by many clinical and experimental studies, it is possible that the physical proximity of the *int*-2 locus with the progesterone receptor locus may have biological significance. However, no evidence for amplification or rearrangement of the *int*-2 locus has been obtained from the study of primary human breast tumors. Although the mechanism of *int*-2 transforming potential is unknown, it is interesting that the product of this gene shows partial homology with fibroblast growth factors (FGFs), especially with basic FGF.[286] The *int*-2 gene, as well as the *hst* gene which is also structurally related to the FGF gene, are located on the same human chromosome band, 11q13.[284] These two genes possibly derive from a common ancestor by duplication and they were found to be coamplified in a melanoma from eight primary human melanomas examined.

3. The *int*-3 Gene

A third *int* gene, termed *int*-3, has been identified in the cellular genome of a colony of *Mus musculus* designated Czech II.[263,287] The *int*-3 gene is located on mouse chromosome 17 and MMTV insertion at this site activates expression of a 2.4-kb species of RNA from a previously silent cellular gene. Expression of the three putative transforming *int* genes would be under hormone control during the early stages of the disease, until the acquisition of autonomous, hormone-independent growth potential by the tumor tissue.

4. Expression of *int* Genes in Normal Tissues

The genes *int*-1 and *int*-2 are independently regulated during mouse development and may have a central role in mouse embryogenesis.[288] Gene *int*-2 is apparently not expressed in normal adult mouse tissues, and *int*-1 expression is restricted to the testis of sexually mature mice, more specifically to postmeiotic germ cells undergoing differentiation from round spermatids into mature spermatozoa.[289] In mouse embryos (11 to 15 d after conception), *int*-1 expression is restricted to the developing central nervous system in regions of the neural tube other than the telencephalon.[289,290] Expression of *int-2* is observed in embryonic and extraembryonic tissues of the mouse and may have a role in developmental processes including migration of early mesodermal cells and induction of the otocyst.[291]

5. Oncogenic Potential of *int* Genes

It is not known if *int-1*, *int-2*, and *int-3* are true protooncogenes, but the mouse and human *int* genes show no structural homology with known cellular or viral oncogenes. A genomic fragment containing the entire protein-encoding domain of the mouse *int-1* gene has been inserted into a retroviral shuttle vector and after one round of virus replication a recombinant proviral DNA containing a correctly spliced copy of *int-1* was recovered.[292] High level of expression of *int-1* in NIH/3T3 cells or other established fibroblast cell lines did not lead to morphological neoplastic transformation. These results suggest that either *int-1* is not a true protooncogene or that the biological effects of activated *int-1* may be limited to certain cell types, perhaps mammary gland cells only. The oncogenic potential of the *int-1* gene on mammary cells is suggested by the demonstration that infection of a mouse mammary epithelial cell line with a retrovirus vector carrying an intact coding sequence for *int-1* protein produces several changes in morphology and growth control that are characteristic of neoplastic transformation.[293] Around half of mammary tumors that arise spontaneously in BR6 mice infected with MMTV express both *int-1* and *int-2* genes, which suggests that these genes may act cooperatively in the development of mice carcinomas.[294] However, about 10% of these spontaneous mouse mammary tumors express neither gene. Moreover, mouse mammary tumors induced by a chemical carcinogen (DMBA) may or may not be associated with activation of endogenous MMTV sequences, but may be independent of *int-1* and *int-2* gene activation.[295] It is thus clear that chemical carcinogens can induce mammary tumors in mice through more than one pathway. These results indicate that *int-1* or *int-2* gene expression is not absolutely required for mice mammary carcinogenesis and that other loci, including *int-3*, as well as other mechanisms may contribute to the origin and development of these tumors. Additional studies are required for a better knowledge of the normal functions of *int* genes and their possible role in oncogenic processes.

G. ALTERATION OF THE *LCK/LSK/TCK* GENE

The LSTRA murine thymoma cell line was induced by M-MuLV and probably contains the M-MuLV sequences inserted upstream of a gene called *lck*, *lsk*, or *tck*.[296] This gene is located at the distal end of mouse chromosome 4 and a homologous gene has been mapped to human chromosome 1, at region 1p32-p35, near a site of frequent structural abnormalities in human lymphomas and neuroblastomas. The *lck* gene codes a protein of 56 kDa, $p56^{lck}$, which is a tyrosine-specific protein kinase closely related to the kinases coded by the members of the *src* oncogene family.[297] The $p56^{lck}$ protein is expressed at low levels in murine T cells. DNA sequences positioned 5' to the *lck* locus, containing AUG codons, significantly reduce the *in vivo* efficiency of $p56^{lck}$ translation from the normal mRNA.[298] LSTRA cells contain an elevated level of tyrosine kinase activity which is apparently related to rearrangement and overexpression of the *lck* gene.[299] The $p56^{lck}$ protein is encoded in LSTRA cells by a hybrid mRNA which contains at the 5' end sequences identical to the 5' end of the M-MuLV genome.[300] The three- to ninefold increases in transcriptional expression of this gene in LSTRA cells would thus result from retroviral promoter insertion. Translational activation of the *lck* gene may occur when the 5' translational control region of the gene is deleted or rearranged by insertion of a provirus.[298]

H. ALTERATION OF *MLVI* GENES

A putative protooncogene family, defined for its activation upon chronic retrovirus insertion and termed *Mlvi* (Moloney leukemia virus insertion site) was identified in the murine genome. A homologous gene family exists in the human genome.

1. Rodent *Mlvi* Genes

In rat thymomas at least five independent DNA regions have been identified as common sites for M-MuLV provirus integration: *Mlvi*-1, *Mlvi*-2, *Mis*-1 (= RMo*Int*-1), and c-*myc*.[224,301-305] Proviral integration site *Mis*-1 in rat thymomas corresponds to the *pvt*-1 translocation breakpoint in murine plasmacytomas.[306] M-MuLV-induced DNA rearrangements in *Mlvi*-1 and *Mlvi*-2 may occur together in the same population of tumor cells, which suggests that a synergism of these two provirus insertion events may be important in tumor induction and progression.[303] The *Mlvi*-2 locus may show polymorphism in rats due to the presence or absence of a long (>5 kb) interspersed repeated DNA element of the LINE family.[307] Although the biological significance of this polymorphic change is unknown, the insertion of LINE sequences could potentially exert profound effects on the contiguous DNA sequences, including effects on gene activity and structural changes such as deletion, duplication, and other DNA rearrangements. In mice, both sequences homologous to *Mlvi*-1 and *Mlvi*-2 map to chromosome 15, a chromosome which contains two protooncogenes, c-*myc* and c-*sis*, and which is frequently involved in chromosome aberrations observed in murine thymic lymphomas.[308,309] However, *Mlvi*-2 sequences are not homologous to either c-*myc* or c-*sis* sequences, and *Mlvi*-2 maps proximal to both protooncogenes on chromosome 15.

Another locus implicated in insertional mutagenesis in the rat is RMo*Int*-1 or *Mis*-1; this locus and is associated with the development of rat thymic leukemia induced by M-MuLV.[305] The *Mis*-1 gene has been assigned to rat chromosome 15 and aberrations of this chromosome have been described frequently. Rat *Mis*-1 gene appears to be a homologue of the murine gene *pvt*-1, which is located on mouse chromosome 15 and may be involved in the development of plasmacytomas.[227,310-312]

2. Human *Mlvi* Genes

Human sequences homologous to rat *Mlvi* have been identified. Insertion of an *Alu* SINE DNA sequence has been detected in the human homologue of the *Mlvi*-2 locus in 1 B-cell lymphoma of 59 DNA samples derived from either normal tissues or hematopoietic neoplasms examined for rearrangements in the *Mlvi*-2 locus.[313] Since normal tissue from the individual whose B-cell lymphoma gave rise to the cell line with the polymorphic *Mlvi*-2 locus was not available, nor was there any access to his relatives, it could not be determined whether the transposition of the *Alu* sequence represented a somatic event possibly related to tumor induction or a germ-line event that occurred earlier in evolution and continues segregating in the human population.

I. INSERTIONAL ALTERATION OF OTHER PUTATIVE PROTOONCOGENES

Several other loci, which may be considered as putative protooncogenes, have been found to be involved in chronic retrovirus insertion associated with malignant diseases occurring in rodent species.

1. Alteration of the *Fis*-1 Locus

A common proviral integration region on mouse chromosome 7, *Fis*-1, was detected in 4 of 35 F-MuLV-induced lymphomas and myelogenous leukemias.[314] The F-MuLV proviruses identified in the *Fis*-1 region appear to be intact and nonrecombinant. The *Fis*-1 locus is linked to *int*-2, but molecular studies have demonstrated that both loci are separated by at least 25 to 30 kb and that provirus insertions in the *Fis*-1 region do not result in induction of *int*-2 mRNA expression.[315]

2. Alteration of the *fim* Loci

Two other F-MuLV integration sites are represented by the loci *fim*-1 and *fim*-2.[316] These loci are different from *Fis*-1 and were found to be involved in virus insertions occurring in 5% (*fim*-

1) and 15% (*fim*-2) of 42 F-MuLV-induced murine myeloblastic primary leukemias or leukemic cell lines. No rearrangement of the *Fis* locus was detected in the 42 leukemias examined in this study.

3. Alteration of the *Dsi*-1 Locus

A region of chromosomal DNA, *Dsi*-1, was found to be involved in proviral insertion occurring in 3 of 24 M-MuLV-induced rat thymomas.[232] In one of these tumors, a provirus was also integrated adjacent to the protooncogene c-*myc*. *Dsi*-1 is located on mouse chromosome 4 and is probably different from known protooncogenes and other proviral integration regions described previously.

4. Alteration of the *Gin*-1 Locus

T-cell leukemia induced in mice by inoculation of Gross passage A MuLV is frequently (28%) associated with integration of the virus at a locus designated *Gin*-1.[317] The normal function of this locus is unknown.

5. Alteration of the *Evi*-1 Locus

AKXD-23 recombinant inbred mice (a strain derived from crosses between the highly leukemogenic AKR/J strain and the low leukemogenic strain DBA/2J) develop myeloid tumors at a high frequency. AKXD-23 myeloid tumors are monoclonal and their DNA contains somatically acquired proviruses.[318] A common site of ecotropic viral integration, present in the myeloid tumors occurring in AKXD-23 mice, was designated *Evi*-1. Few *Evi*-1 rearrangements were detected in the DNA of T- or B-cell tumor, which indicates that the putative proto-oncogene *Evi*-1 may be specifically involved in myeloid hematopoietic processes. DNA of T-cell lymphomas occurring in AKXD-23 mice contains rearrangements not at *Evi*-1, but at other loci (c-*myc*, *Fis*-1, *pim*-1, *pvt*-1, *Mlvi*-1, and *Mlvi*-2).[319]

J. INSERTIONAL ACTIVATION OF OTHER GENES

Genes other than protooncogenes may be activated by the insertion of chronic retrovirus genomes. For example, the GALV-infected T-cell line MLA-144, originally established from a gibbon ape lymphosarcoma, constitutively produces IL-2 and this line contains two GALV insertions in the IL-2 gene, one in the 3′ untranslated region and the other 1200 bp 5′ to the gene.[320] It is thus likely that one or both of these viral insertions is (are) involved in activation of IL-2 gene expression.

Provirus insertion occurring during the intrauterine life may result in embryonic mutations.[321] Infection of mouse embryos with M-MuLV has yielded several mouse substrains with stable germ line integration of retroviral DNA at distinct chromosome loci, termed *Mov* loci.[322] Flanking host DNA sequences can have an effect on provirus expression and, conversely, inserted viral DNA may affect the expression of adjacent host cell genes. Four different *Mov* loci have been mapped and localized in the mouse genome by somatic cell hybrid analysis followed by *in situ* hybridization.[323] *Mov* loci can be used to identify genes that are expressed only at the specific time of proviral integration.

K. CONCLUSION

Many tumors induced in avian and rodent species by different chronic retroviruses are associated with an insertional activation of host genome integration regions which may be represented by known protooncogenes or other genes with a hypothetical oncogenic potential. The functions of nonprotooncogene genes involved in proviral integrations are little understood but their study may contribute to the identification of cellular genes involved in growth control or important metabolic functions. The frequency of provirus integration in the protooncogene and nonprotooncogene loci described until present is variable, according to the virus and the animal species; in some cases, for example, in MuLV-induced murine leukemias, the frequency is rather low. Other identified or unidentified loci could be involved in such instances, but the function of these putative loci is unknown. The general validity of an insertional mechanism for tumors induced by chronic retroviruses in different animal species is not apparent at present. Mechanisms other than insertional activation of neighbor genes may be responsible for the potential oncogenicity of chronic retroviruses.

VIII. NONINSERTIONAL MECHANISMS OF PATHOGENICITY ASSOCIATED WITH CHRONIC RETROVIRUSES

Chronic retroviruses could induce malignant diseases through an activation of protooncogenes or other cellular genes by mechanisms not depending on insertional mutagenesis. However, only limited evidence exists supporting this possibility. In addition, nononcogene or oncogene-derived sequences contained in the genome of chronic retroviruses could contribute to the pathogenic effects of these viruses. Disturbances in the immune system are importantly involved in the mechanisms of pathogenicity associated with infection by chronic retroviruses. In particular, immunosuppression conditioned by exogenous and/or endogenous factors may crucially determine the consequence of chronic retrovirus infection, including the possible occurrence of neoplastic diseases.

A. NONINSERTIONAL ACTIVATION OF PROTOONCOGENES

Altered expression of protooncogenes may occur in cells infected by chronic retroviruses through mechanisms not involving retrovirus insertion. Enhanced expression of c-*myc* found in murine lymphomas associated with MuLV infection may involve mechanisms other than promoter insertion.[223] The increased levels of c-*myc* mRNA found in some of these tumors could involve an enhancer effect via the viral LTR. Elevated levels of c-*myc* transcripts have been found in both the preleukemic and leukemic stages of F-MuLV associated erythroleukemias without apparent structural alteration of the protooncogene.[244] The Friend leukemia cells may contain, despite the lack of c-*myc* gene rearrangement, a 2.3-kb c-*myc* mRNA which initiated an intron 1 at a promoter called P3.[324] This mRNa has a longer half-life than the normal c-*myc* mRNA but its possible role in F-MuLV-associated leukemogenesis is unknown.

Elevated levels of c-*myc* gene expression have been detected in bovine lymphosarcomas associated with BLV infection, but no rearrangement or amplification of the c-*myc* gene was found in these tumors.[325] Furthermore, BLV proviral DNA does not appear to have preferred sites of integration in these tumors. The mechanism of c-*myc* increased transcriptional activity in the bovine tumors could not be elucidated. Activation of c-*myc* expression in the tumor cells was apparently not due to the action of *trans*-activating protein produced by the pX region of BLV (a region situated between the *env* gene and the 3' LTR), since pX-specific transcripts were not detected in polyadenylated RNA from uncultured tumors associated with BLV. Moreover, no evidence of a cellular transcript initiated from the 3' LTR of the BLV proviral DNA was detected in the tumors. Lack of enhanced expression of the c-*myc* gene in bovine tumors associated with BLV infection was reported in independent studies.[152,153]

ANLL induced in mice by F-MuLV can be divided into two distinct stages based on the growth properties of the leukemia cells.[326] In the early stage (stage I disease) of leukemia, the blast cells are unable to grow outside their normal hematopoietic environment (bone marrow or spleen), whereas in the late stage of leukemia (stage II disease), leukemia cells can grow at any site in the mouse and will form continuous cell lines *in vitro*. The genetic basis for this progression from restricted and unrestricted cell growth is unknown but the possible participation of an activation of protooncogenes in the progression of the malignant disease is suggested by the experimental observation that F-MuLV-infected cells can proliferate in culture in the absence of growth factors when they are superinfected with A-MuLV, which carries the v-*abl* oncogene.[326] It is possible that activation of the c-*abl* protooncogene may have a similar effect but no direct proof exists in favor of this possibility.

B. REARRANGEMENT OF THE P53 CELLULAR GENE

Rearrangement of the p53 cellular gene may occur in some erythroleukemic cells transformed by F-MuLV.[327] The p53 rearrangement may occur *in vivo* during the progression of F-MuLV-induced erythroleukemia. As a consequence of the rearrangement, a DNA deletion of approximately 3.0 kb removes exon 2 coding sequence of the p53 gene, which results in the synthesis of a truncated p53 protein of 44 kDa (p44) in which the amino-terminal residues of normal p53 are missing.[328] The truncated protein is unusually stable and accumulates to high levels intracellularly in the nucleus but its role in F-MuLV-induced transformation is not understood. Two tumor cell populations may coexist in F-MuLV-induced mouse erythroleukemia: one containing a normal p53 gene and the other containing rearranged p53 genes.[181] These cell clones arise as the result of independent transformation events but the selective advantage of those containing p53 gene rearrangement is not clear. p53 could be considered as a tumor suppressor gene.

C. STIMULATION OF GROWTH FACTOR SYNTHESIS

Unregulated synthesis of growth factors can contribute to the expression of a transformed phenotype or may induce the appearance of this phenotype. Infection of specific fibroblastic cell lines which produce low levels of CSF-2 activity with murine retroviruses results in large increases in CSF-2 production.[329] The murine erythroleukemia cell line IW32, which derives by F-MuLV-induced transformation, constitutively synthesizes considerable amounts of erythropoietin, a hormone involved in the formation of erythrocytes. IW32 cells contain, in addition to a normal erythropoietin gene, a rearranged and amplified erythropoietin gene which is more sensitive to DNase I than is the normal gene.[330] Thus, the rearranged erythropoietin gene is probably the active one in IW32 cells. However, this activation is apparently not associated with F-MuLV provirus insertion near the gene.

D. INFLUENCE OF RETROVIRUS-SPECIFIC SEQUENCES

Subgenomic sequences contained in chronic retroviruses may be responsible for the oncogenic potential of these viruses. Certain strains of the GaLV can infect gibbons without causing leukemia, and it has been shown that leukemia-specific RNA sequences are present in GaLV genomes that are isolated from animals with leukemia but are absent in GaLV strains isolated from animals free of clinical symptoms of leukemia.[331]

It has been suggested that *env* gene and LTR determine the biological properties of different chronic retroviruses.[332] Putative viral enhancers in the U3 region would play two roles in the process of leukemogenesis: in the diseases induced by F-MuLV and R-MuLV the viral enhancers would act by increasing transcription of the generated MCF virus, whereas in thymic lymphomas the enhancers would activate the expression of protooncogenes or other cellular genes.

Inoculation of high-virulence F-MuLV into mice results in an early phase of hemolytic anemia, followed at later stages by splenomegaly and low reticulocyte counts associated with the development of erythroleukemia. Studies on molecular recombination between high- and low-virulence strains of F-MuLV indicate that the early hemolytic anemia and the late erythroleukemia are separate pathological effects mediated by distinct viral gene sequences, namely, *pol-env* sequences and LTR-*gag* sequences, respectively.[333]

E. TRANSDUCTION OF ONCOGENES BY CHRONIC RETROVIRUSES

Chronic retroviruses are characterized by the absence of v-*onc* genes but, sporadically, some of these retroviruses can act as oncogene transducers. Naturally occurring variants of FeLV have been described which contain the oncogenes *fes*, *fms*, *fgr*, *abl*, *sis*, *kit*, or *myc*.[334] Among the variants of FeLV which contain oncogenes, all are derived from feline fibrosarcomas except those that contain *myc*. Among 31 lymphomas occurring naturally in cats, 16 were positive for FeLV, and 2 of them showed evidence for the presence of unaltered *myc* gene sequences.[335] Similar findings have been reported by other authors.[234,336,337] FeLV carrying the *myc* gene can act as an infectious virus since it may contain all the regulatory sequences necessary for its expression and packing in mammalian cells. However, FeLVs transducing the *myc* gene arise *de novo* in individual cases of cat tumors such as thymic lymphosarcomas and are not excreted and transmitted to other cats.[338] Thus, these oncogene-transducing viruses are not involved in a horizontal transmission of cancer. This virus is capable of inducing thymic lymphosarcomas 14 to 20 weeks after inoculation into kittens but, intriguingly, it is unable to transform leukocytes from peripheral blood, spleen, or thymus *in vitro*.[334] Embryonic feline fibroblasts infected with *myc*-carrying FeLV undergo marked alterations in growth patterns *in vitro* but are not fully transformed and do not form tumors when inoculated subcutaneously into athymic mice.

The nucleotide sequences of a transduced *myc* gene from a defective FeLV were determined and it was found that the entire c-*myc* coding sequence was represented in FeLV *myc* and that the transduced oncogene was expressed as a *gag-myc* fusion protein. However, the transduced *myc* gene lacked a potential phosphorylation site at amino acid 343 in the putative DNA-binding domain of the protein.[339] These results suggest that qualitative changes could be responsible for activation of c-*myc* products.

Leukemias can be produced in chicken by injection of the RSV-associated virus RAV-1, which does not usually transduce oncogenes. RAV-1 viruses can act as insertional mutagens and can induce erythroleukemia by their integration into the c-*erb*-B protooncogene.[340] Moreover, some of the RAV-1 viruses recovered from these leukemias have been found to transduce the c-*erb*-B protooncogene. These c-*erb*-B-containing retroviruses are not able to transform fibroblasts, however. It seems unlikely that oncogenes transduced by chronic transforming retroviruses can act as acute oncogenic agents under natural conditions.

F. IMMUNE DEPRESSION AND STIMULATION

It is well known that immunodepressed humans and other animals are predisposed to different forms of cancer.[341] Infection by different types of chronic retroviruses, including avian retroviruses as well as mammalian retroviruses such as MuLV, FeLV, and HIV, is commonly associated with a loss of immune competence, which may facilitate the occurrence of neoplastic diseases. The possibility also exists that not depression but stimulation of the immune system by chronic retrovirus infection can contribute to the development of neoplasms. During the preleukemic period in either AKR or BALB/c mice inoculated with M-MuLV, there exists a population of T cells that can proliferate in response to virus-specific gp71 antigen *in vitro*.[342] Since viral infection of specifically immune T cells *in vitro* can give rise to T-cell lines, it is possible that specifically immune cells can acquire autonomous growth and contribute to chronic retrovirus-induced leukemogenesis *in vivo*.

G. HOST CELL DNA DAMAGE

Damage to the host cell DNA is a common mechanism of action of chemical carcinogens and is also a possible mechanism for transformation induced by chronic retrovirus infection. Lymphocytes carrying endogenous or exogenous M-MuLV are more susceptible to spontaneous as well as chemically induced SCEs compared with controls.[343] SCEs are used for the detection of clastogenic and mutagenic agents and are considered to be an index of DNA damage and repair at the chromosomal level. However, transformation induced by chronic retroviruses may be independent of mutational events. Carcinogen-induced mutations at two separate genetic loci in Fischer rat embryo cells were not enhanced by R-MuLV infection in spite of the fact that this infection profoundly affects the expression of transformation.[344]

H. EPIGENETIC CHANGES INDUCED BY CHRONIC RETROVIRUSES

Although the mechanisms responsible for transformation induced by chronic retroviruses remain unknown, there is evidence that some epigenetic, regulatory phenomena may be of crucial importance for the expression of the malignant phenotype. F-MuLV-transformed leukemic stem cells of mice display clear malignant growth kinetics when proliferating in the spleen of the leukemic mice but revert to normal self-renewal and differentiation when grown in the spleen of irradiated syngeneic hosts in spite of a continuous expression of the virus.[345]

IX. HUMAN RETROVIRUSES

Human retroviruses are replication-competent, infectious viruses, represented by two classes of agents: the T-cell lymphotropic viruses (HTLVs) and the human immunodeficiency viruses (HIVs).[14-38] HTLVs and HIVs exhibit some structural similarities and affect primarily helper T lymphocytes; however, HTLVs and HIVs are essentially different in many characteristics. HTLVs (HTLV-I and HTLV-II) have some unusual features that can be used to distinguish them from other replication-competent, infectious chronic retroviruses of mice and chicken. Such features include lack of chronic viremia in infected individuals, absence of common proviral integration sites in the chromosomes of tumor cells, *trans*-activation of HTLV LTR-directed transcription in infected cells, and ability to immortalize T-cells *in vitro*.[346] HTLVs are morphologically similar to type-C retroviruses and are associated with the development of T-cell neoplasms occurring in humans and other primates. HTLV-I is closely associated with adult T-cell leukemia/lymphoma (ATL). HIVs (HIV-1 and HIV-2) include the retroviruses formerly called human T-cell lymphotropic virus III (HTLV-III), lymphadenopathy-associated virus (LAV), and AIDS-associated retrovirus (ARV).[347] HIVs are etiologically associated with the acquired immune deficiency syndrome (AIDS) and other nonmalignant human diseases characterized by profound alteration in the immune mechanisms of the organism. HIVs are morphologically similar to type-D retroviruses and are members of the Lentivirinae subfamily of retroviruses, resembling visna virus and equine infectious anemia viruses of ungulate mammals.[36,37,348-351] Lentiviruses may cause cytopathic effects *in vitro* and are able to produce chronic debilitating diseases *in vivo*. It has been hypothesized that HTLVs and HIVs probably originated from Africa, spreading to the U.S., the Caribbean, Japan, Europe, and other parts of the world.[32] However, this point is still under discussion and the precise origin and evolution of human retroviruses is unknown.

X. HTLV-I

HTLV-I is a human retrovirus that was isolated in the U.S. from patients with T-cell leukemia/lymphoma.[352-356] A related or identical virus, ATLV, was isolated in Japan from patients with ATL, a relatively rare form of leukemia which affect predominantly adults.[357-361] Both isolates, HTLV-I and ATLV may represent strains of the same virus since only a few structural differences exist between both isolates of the virus.[362,363] Another HTLV-I virus was isolated from an African ATL patient and the molecular cloning and characterization of this isolate indicated that the African virus is similar, but not identical, to other HTLV-I isolates.[364] Different strains of the HTLV-I virus may be distributed among different parts of the world.

HTLV-I is a T-cell lymphotropic virus and is an infectious, exogenous agent since its nucleotide sequences are present in the DNA of neoplastic T cells but not in the DNA of nonneoplastic B cells from the same patient.[365] The malignant cells observed in ATL are in most cases helper T cells that exhibit a highly lobulated nucleus. ATL is a neoplasm of mature T-cells frequently associated with with hypercalcemia and skin lesions.[366] The prognosis of this disease is rather poor. HTLV-I has been transmitted *in vitro* by cocultivation and by cell-free filtrates not only into human T lymphocytes but also into nonlymphoid human cells, including fibroblasts and epithelial cells as well as an osteogenic sarcoma cell line.[367-371] Moreover, there is no species specificity in the *in vitro* transmission of HTLV-I since rat and rabbit cells can be infected with the virus.

A. EPIDEMIOLOGY OF HTLV-I INFECTION

ATL has an uneven geographical distribution, being endemic in southwestern Japan, the Caribbean, central Africa, and other areas of the world.[372-380] Most patients with adult T-cell leukemia have antibodies to HTLV.[385] Virological studies have confirmed the results of seroepidemiological surveys which indicate that HTLV-I infection is distributed in different geographical areas of the world.[386,387] Prevalence of HTLV-I infection in geographically distinct areas of the U.S. is rather low (0.025%).[388] The majority (98 to 99%) of HTLV-I-infected persons will have no signs or symptoms of disease but the carrier state should not be considered innocuous, as these individuals may remain infectious and may have progression to more obvious disease, including subclinical (preleukemic), chronic (smoldering), and acute (suba-cute) ATL.[389]

HTLV-I would be etiologically associated only with ATL and not with other diseases such as mycosis fungoides/Sézary's syndrome, T-cell hairy cell leukemia, AIDS, or multiple sclerosis.[390] However, proviral HTLV-I genomes have been isolated from the peripheral blood lymphocytes of patients with chronic neurological diseases classified as multiple sclerosis.[391,392] Neurological diseases such as tropical spastic paraparesis and chronic progressive myelopathy may be etiologically associated with HTLV-I infection.[392,393] Chronic progressive myelopathy is characterized by the gradual progression of spastic paraparesis without evidence of spinal cord compression or motor neuron involvement and is clustered in geographic areas from several tropical countries including India, Africa, Central and South America, and the Caribbean islands.

Sera of individuals infected with HTLV-I react predominantly with the viral core polypep-tides p24 and p19 as well as with a 68-kDa glycoprotein, gp68, which is probably a precursor to the viral envelope polypeptide, gp46.[394,395] Monoclonal antibodies generated against particu-lar components of the HTLV-I virion such as the p24 internal core protein may be useful as diagnostic probes for the identification of HTLV-I infected cells.[396]

Antibodies against HTLV-I structural proteins p24, p19, and p15 range from modest to high titers not only in the leukemia patients but also in their close relatives and in normal unrelated people from the same region in Japan and other countries,[354,372,373,378,380,384,397] although the average antibody titers are higher in ATL patients than in normal sera.[381] In Japan, the Kyushu district has the highest anti-HTLV seropositivity incidence among 64 blood centers tested in 8 districts of the country (about 8% of the population), and the frequency of seropositivity increases with age (up to 15%).[383] In Venezuela, a tropical country facing the Caribbean, the overall prevalence of natural HTLV-I antibodies is 6.8% but the distribution of positive individuals varies between 1 and 15% for different geographical areas of the country.[384] High rates of antibody positivity are present in apparently healthy young Venezuelan children, which indicates that the infection can occur very early in life. In contrast to the high prevalence of HTLV-I infection among Venezuelan Indians, the virus is apparently not endemic in the aborigine populations from Brazil.[398]

Antibodies to HTLV-I antigens are frequent in certain groups of persons, such as hemophili-acs and patients with AIDS.[399,400] The prevalence of HTLV-I antibodies in untransfused patients with a variety of malignant diseases other than ATL is significantly higher compared to age- and sex-matched general population.[401] These results suggest that, as may occur with other viruses, development of cancer may contribute to expression of latent HTLV-I infection. Parasitic infections may also promote HTLV-I infection or may favor the expression or proliferation of HTLV-I viruses in the host.[402]

Unlike other animal retroviruses, HTLV-I is not lysed by normal human serum and is resistant to human complement, which may explain the infectivity and persistence of HTLV-I in human populations.[403] HTLV-I is not inherited with the genome but is acquired by contagion during life either congenitally, sexually, by blood transfusion, or through other mechanisms which remain poorly characterized. The predominant natural transmission routes of HTLV-I in humans are unknown but both a transmission from parents to children and between spouses have been suggested.[404] HTLV-I antigens have been detected in the milk from some HTLV-I seropositive mothers,[405] which suggests the possibility of a horizontal transmission of the virus from mothers to infants. Epidemiologic evidence suggesting the natural milk-borne transmission of HTLV-I from mother to child in humans is supported by experimental data obtained in virus-infected female rabbits.[406]

B. ETIOLOGICAL ROLE OF HTLV-I IN ATL

Almost all patients with ATL studied in Japan and other countries have HTLV-I proviral DNA in the blood cells, whereas the viral genome is usually absent in the cells of seropositive healthy individuals or in patients with myeloid leukemia or patients subjected to blood transfusion who were positive for antibody against HTLV-I antigen.[407] In general, HTLV-I is associated only with acute or subacute ATL, not with other types of leukemia and lymphoma, although some patients with T-cell malignant lymphoma are positive for the presence of HTLV-I proviral DNA. In addition, it has been suggested that HTLV-I infection may contribute by an indirect mechanism to the development of B-cell chronic lymphocytic leukemia.[408] The tumor cells from B-CLL patients with this type of leukemia would be originated as a consequence of an antigen-committed B cell responding to HTLV-I infection.

The existence of ATL not associated with HTLV-I has been reported in Japan, where 5 out of 69 ATL patients were negative for anti-HTLV-I antibody in the serum and did not show integration of the HTLV-I genome into chromosomal DNA of leukemic cells.[409] There were no clear differences between the clinical, hematologic, cytopathologic, and immunologic features of HTLV-I-positive and HTLV-I-negative ATL. Furthermore, the chromosome abnormalities found in HTLV-I-associated ATL were similar to those found in HTLV-I-negative ATL.[410] These findings indicate that, at least in some cases, and in a way similar to that of EBV in Burkitt's lymphoma, the causative agent of ATL may not be HTLV-I. Thus, ATL may not be universally defined as an HTLV-I-induced T-cell malignancy and HTLV-I infection is not sufficient nor necessary for the development of ATL. However, it has been demonstrated that, in a way which is also similar to that of EBV in relation to human B lymphocytes, *in vitro* transmission of HTLV-I frequently results in immortalization of recipient human T lymphocytes. Most probably, HTLV-I infection is involved, in concert with other oncogenic factors, in the etiology of the majority of cases of ATL.

C. STRUCTURE AND EXPRESSION OF HTLV-I

The complete nucleotide sequence of the HTLV-I provirus genome integrated in human leukemia cell DNA has been determined and it was predicted that genome would code for 48-, 99-, and 54-kDa proteins, corresponding to *gag*, *pol*, and *env* products, respectively.[361] The precursor of HTLV-I *gag* products is a protein of 53-kDa which is processed into three mature *gag* proteins, p19, p24, and p15, in this order, from the 5′ end of the *gag* gene.[411] The *gag* protein of both HTLV-I and HTLV-II is modified by the addition of fatty acid (myristylation),[412] but the biological significance of this posttranslational modification is not understood. The LTR nucleotide sequences of American and Japanese isolates of HTLV-I exhibit only a few differences, which reinforce the concept that these isolates are strains of the same virus.[363]

In addition to *gag*, *pol*, and *env*, which are common to all other chronic retroviruses, the HTLV genome contains a 1.5-kb region, called region X, *pX*, *tax*, or *tat*-I (for *trans*-acting transcriptional activator), which is located between the *env* gene and the 3′ LTR. Thus, the genomic structure of an HTLV-I provirus consists of the following sequence, from 5′ to 3′: LTR-*gag-pol-env-pX/tax*-LTR. The *pX/tax* region of HTLV-I can be divided into a 5′ nonconserved region and a 3′ highly conserved region designated *lor* (for long open reading frame).[413,414] HTLV-I *pX/tax* region contains four ORFs, enumerated I to IV, each defined by an initiation and a termination codon.[361] Thus, the *pX* region of HTLV-I may code for four proteins.

The *pX/tax* region of HTLV-I is expressed as a subgenomic mRNA of 2.1 kb which may be formed by double splicing in the cells infected with the virus.[415] A protein of 40 to 42 kDa, termed p40^x, p42, TaI, *tat*, or Tax, encoded by the *pX/tax* region of HTLV-I, is produced in HTLV-I-infected cells and may be present in the serum of patients with ATL.[346,416-420] The Tax protein is essential for the replication cycle of HTLV-I.[421] The biological effects of Tax have not been determined, but this protein may act as a *trans*-acting factor that activates transcription from the LTR of HTLV-I.[414,420] It has been suggested that an enhancer sequence within the HTLV-I LTR is responsible, at least in part, for transcriptional *trans*-activation mediated by the Tax viral product.[422] Distinct regulatory sequences located within the upstream sequences required for Tax-associated *trans*-activation of HTLV-I LTR have been chemically synthesized and cloned upstream of the basal HTLV-I promoter.[423] The level of *trans*-transcription inducible by Tax was greatly increased when repeats of these regulatory sequences were present in the upstream control region.

In addition to Tax, at least two other proteins are encoded by the *pX* region of the HTLV-I genome, namely, the phosphoproteins, p27^{x-III} and p21^{x-III}, which are encoded by ORF III of region *pX/tax*.[424] A 2.1-kb *pX* mRNA of HTLV-I encodes the three proteins, Tax, p27^{x-III}, and p21^{xIII}, by different initiation codons, but the last two proteins are not involved in *trans*-activation of the unintegrated LTR.[425] The localization of these proteins may also be different. Whereas Tax and p27^{x-III} are localized in the nucleus of HTLV-I-infected cells and is tightly bound to nuclear components, pp21^{x-III} is found only in the soluble fraction after subcellular fractionation. The functions of the *pX/tax* gene products are unknown but the nuclear association of pp27^{x-III} suggests its possible involvement in regulation of gene expression. In addition, there is evidence that p27^{x-III} controls the level of *gag* mRNA by posttranscriptional modulation.[426] Tax, p27^{x-III}, and p21^{x-III} are not expressed in leukemic cells immediately after their isolation from ATL patients, but anomalous amounts of these proteins are expressed by the cells after 2-d culture. The *pX/tax* gene of HTLV-I has been cloned and the Tax protein was produced by constructed plasmids expressed in *Escherichia coli*.[427] A genomic region homologous to the *pX/tax* region of HTLV-I is contained in the chronic retrovirus BLV, which is involved in bovine leukemia. The *pX* region of BLV is also located between the *env* gene and the 3′ end of the BLV provirus and is expressed in the tumor cells as a 2.1-kb RNA transcript.[428] The level of HTLV-I expression may be altered by environmental factors. Tumor promoters such as the phorbol ester TPA may induce HTLV-I expression through their interaction with a 230-bp segment located on the U3 region of the virus LTR.[429]

D. MECHANISMS OF HTLV-I-ASSOCIATED ONCOGENICITY

The mechanisms involved in HTLV-I-associated leukemogenesis are unknown.[26] HTLV-I antigen may be expressed in leukemic cells of patients with acute ATL *in vitro* but it is not expressed in human leukemic cells *in vivo*.[430] Continuous expression of HTLV-I antigens does not seem to be required for maintenance of a malignant phenotype in HTLV-I-infected cells. Since only a small minority of HTLV-I-carrying subjects will develop the neoplastic disease, other factors, either endogenous or exogenous, must be crucially involved in the etiology of the disease. HTLV-I transcripts are present in long-term cultured T lymphocytes from ATL patients but are usually not expressed in the fresh primary leukemic cells of these patients.[431] These results indicate that expression of the viral genes is not required for the maintenance of the neoplastic state *in vivo*.

1. Expression of Protooncogenes

HTLV-I-induced activation of one or more protooncogene in human lymphoid cells should be considered as a possible mechanism for the origin and/or development of human T-cell leukemia associated with HTLV. The human protooncogene c-*sis* was found to be active in a cell line, HUT-102, derived from a cutaneous T-cell lymphoma and infected with HTLV-I.[432] A cDNA clone of c-*sis* from HUT-102 cells induced transformation of NIH/3T3 cells. However, it is unlikely that activation of c-*sis* is involved in the pathogenesis of HTLV-associated ATL since expression of c-*sis* is not found in the majority of HTLV-transformed cells. The possible role of other protooncogenes in HTLV-I-associated leukemogenesis is not understood.

2. Integration Site of the HTLV-I Genome

Experimental infection of normal cord blood and peripheral blood lymphocytes with purified HTLV-I results in progression from polyclonality to monoclonality within 4 to 6 weeks.[433] The integration site of the provirus genome in HTLV-I-associated malignancies is monoclonal,[434] but, as determined in 35 patients with ATL, it is nonspecific.[154] Apparently, HTLV-I provirus integration in the human tumor cells occurs at random sites, and a mechanism of insertional mutagenesis for explaining the potential oncogenicity of HTLV-I is unlikely. Consequently, other types of mechanisms must be discussed. The analysis of the T-cell receptor gene rearrangement may be used as an approach for the elucidation of the clonality and the mechanisms of leukemogenesis of HTLV-I-positive cell lines in ATL.[435]

3. Expression of Cellular Antigens

Interference with the expression of cellular antigens at the cell surface is another possible mechanism for the oncogenicity of chronic retroviruses. The HTLV-I *env* gene shows homology with the coding regions for the extracellular domains of class I HLA genes.[436] Moreover, HTLV induces altered HLA alloantigen expression in the infected cells.[437] Apparently, the viral proteins have HLA-like determinants that may appear at the lymphocyte surface when the provirus is transcribed.

4. Chromosome Abnormalities

A diversity of chromosome abnormalities is observed in fresh and cultured cells from patients with HTLV-associated T-cell leukemia/lymphoma.[438] Some of these abnormalities are apparently nonrandom, including a 6q deletion near the locus of the c-*myb* protooncogene but the possible significance of this alteration is not understood. In a series of 18 patients with ATL studied in Japan, the most frequent chromosomal abnormalities were trisomy 3 and trisomy 7.[439] In this series, the more aggressive the clinical course of ATL, the more complex the numerical and structural chromosomal abnormality. The chromosome abnormalities found in HTLV-I-positive ATL are similar to those found in HTLV-I negative ATL,[410] which reinforces the idea that the causative agent of ATL may not always be HTLV-I and that infection by this virus is not essential for the development of the disease.

5. Growth Factors

IL-2, initially called T-cell growth factor,[440] is a cytokine which allows an indefinite growth of mature human T lymphocytes in culture after lectin/antigen activation.[441-445] The roles of IL-2 and its cellular receptor in HTLV-I-associated leukemogenesis have been the focus of many research reports. The leukemic cells from ATL patients exhibit striking heterogeneity in both the production of IL-2 and the response to this cytokine.[446] HTLV-I-infected cells and HTLV-I virions are both able to induce the proliferation of T colony-forming cells in the absence of exogenous IL-2.[447] The loss of exogenous requirement for IL-2 may define an early event of HTLV-I infection.

The role of the IL-2 receptor in HTLV-I-associated ATL is not clear. The IL-2 receptor is represented by a multichain molecular complex which is involved in the control of normal and malignant T-cell proliferation.[448-454] HTLV-I-infected human umbilical cord blood T lymphocytes can be propagated in culture indefinitely and exhibit a diminished requirement for IL-2; these cells may have an increased density of IL-2 receptors and often become completely independent of the exogenous supply of IL-2.[455] A short sequence of homology exists between the envelope protein of HTLV-I (amino acids 20 to 27) and the sequence of IL-2.[456] This homology raises the possibility that HTLV-I can interact directly with the IL-2 receptor on the cell surface, generating an IL-2-like signal within the lymphocyte. Several HTLV-I-infected T-cell lines may not contain IL-2 mRNA, which suggests that immortalization of these cells by HTLV-I may sometimes occur by mechanisms that bypass the IL-2/IL-2 receptor system.[457]

Exogenous IL-2 augments IL-2 receptor expression in leukemic cells from ATL patients, although IL-2 do not induce proliferation of these cells.[458] Constitutive expression of the IL-2 receptor is observed in rat lymphoid cell lines producing HTLV-I.[459] IL-2 receptors are also expressed constitutively in HTLV-I-infected human T cells, and, paradoxically, stimulation of these cells with PHA or PMA results in inhibition of IL-2 receptor gene transcription.[460] Deregulation of the IL-2 receptor gene was found in the tumor cells of patients with ATL associated with HTLV-I infection. These findings suggest that HTLV-I may act by stimulating the T-cell-specific growth factor system. One of the products of HTLV-I, the Tax protein, can induce expression of IL-2 and IL-2 receptors in some, but not all human T-cell lines.[461,462] The mechanism of regulation of IL-2 receptor expression by the Tax protein remains unclear but may involve the binding of the Tax protein to specific nucleotide sequences at the DNA level.[463] HTLV-I can also infect normal mature B cells *in vitro,* where it induces the expression of IL-2 receptors.[464] HTLV-I infection converts B cells into Ig-secreting cells, without affecting their proliferation.

Peripheral leukemic cells from ATL patients do not usually grow as cell lines in the presence of IL-2, but in a few cases the leukemic T cells can be grown in the presence of the interleukin.[435] In some cases the evidence indicates the operation of an autocrine mechanism involving IL-2 in the pathogenesis of ATL.[465] However, extremely low levels of IL-2 transcripts are detected in HTLV-I-positive human T-cell lines, and IL-2 is not expressed in fresh leukemic cells from patients with T-cell leukemia.[17] A simple autostimulation model involving IL-2 and its cellular receptor is probably not realistic for T-cell leukemogenesis in general. The available evidence indicates that abnormalities in production of IL-2 and/or expression of IL-2 receptors may not be essential for HTLV-I-associated leukemogenesis.[466]

The possibility that some protein(s) encoded by HTLV-I act by mechanisms similar to those of growth factors or oncogene protein products should be considered. The p28 HTLV-I-associated antigen, encoded by a 28S mRNA, has an associated protein kinase activity,[467] but its possible role in transformation is not understood. HTLV-I shows DNA sequence homologies with the 5′ flanking region of the gene coding for human IL-2.[468,469] The region of homology, represented by the consensus sequence TGGANNGNANCCAA, is also shared by sequences contained in the flanking regions of the c-*myc* and c-*fos* protooncogenes, whose protein products are also involved in the control of hematopoietic cell proliferation.[469] The presence of a consensus sequence in these viral and cellular genomes suggests the existence of common mechanisms related to the control of cell proliferation, which could contribute to the formation of immortal T-cell clones.

The *pX/tax* gene of HTLV-I and HTLV-II contains a region coding for a 38-amino acid sequence in the Tax protein product which shows highly significant homology (40%) with murine IL-3.[470] If the similarity between different amino acids is taken into account, the homology increases to a level of about 60%. This homology suggests that the biological functions of the retroviral Tax product may be related to those exerted by IL-3 in leukemogenic processes. Interleukins other than IL-2 could have a role in certain symptoms observed in HTLV-I-associated leukemogenesis. ATL cells express IL-1 mRNA and protein, and IL-1 is capable of enhancing IL-2 receptor expression.[471] Moreover, IL-1 may represent the osteoclast activating factor described in ATL-associated hypercalcemia. Another growth factor synthesized by human T cells immortalized by HTLV-I and HTLV-II is PDGF.[472] However, these cells do not express PDGF receptors and the possible role of PDGF in their growth is not understood.

6. Transforming Properties of HTLV-I Products

The protein products from the *pX/tax* region of the HTLV-I genome would be good candidates for the transforming properties associated with this virus.[415] According to the results of *in vitro* mutagenesis, the presence of a functional *pX/tax* gene is essential for HTLV-I replication.[473] In the absence of a functional *pX/tax* gene, approximately 100-fold lower levels of viral mRNA are transcribed. Protein products from the *pX/tax* region of HTLV-I are present in the serum of ATL patients.[316,416] In HTLV-I-transformed human lymphocytes the Tax protein has a short half-life (approximately 120 min) and a significant fraction of the protein is located in the nucleus, which suggests a possible role of Tax in the regulation of genomic functions.[474-476] The precise role of the protein products of HTLV-I *pX/tax* region in neoplastic transformation of human lymphoid cells *in vivo* is difficult to evaluate at present. Since little or no Tax protein is present in fresh leukemic cells from patients, this protein would be involved in the initiation but probably not the maintenance of transformation.[421] The results obtained in some experimental studies, especially in studies performed with transgenic mice, suggest that the Tax protein may have an oncogenic potential.[477] Transgenic mice that express the protein under the control of HTLV-I LTR develop mesenchymal tumors. These results indicate that the Tax protein may function in some cases in a manner similar to that of oncogene products. In any case, the precise role of the Tax protein in relation to human leukemogenic processes remains unknown.

7. Immunosuppressive Properties of HTLV-I

The retroviral transmembrane envelope protein p15E of HTLV-I and HTLV-II is immunosuppressive in that it inhibits immune responses of lymphocytes, monocytes, and macrophages. A region of p15E has been conserved among murine and feline retroviruses as well as in a putative envelope protein encoded by an endogenous type-C human retroviral DNA.[166] Human cancerous effusions contain p15E-related proteins that inhibit the responses of human monocytes to chemotactic stimuli, and p15E-related proteins have been identified in human malignant cells and in the plasma of leukemic patients. A synthetic peptide, termed CKS-17, corresponding to the p15E region, inhibits the proliferation of an IL-2-dependent murine cytotoxic T-cell line as well as alloantigen-stimulated proliferation of murine and human lymphocytes.[166] CKS-17 inhibits the effector phase of monocyte-associated cytotoxicity and the mechanism of this inhibition appears to involve the inactivation of IL-1.[478] These results suggest that the 15E protein may be responsible, at least in part, for the immunosuppressive properties of HTLV-I and HTLV-II. P15E would exert its immunosuppressive effect by inactivating IL-1, which would eliminate the stimulus for IL-2 production.

E. SIMIAN T-CELL LEUKEMIA VIRUSES

Antibodies to HTLV-I-related viruses as well as HTLV-I-like retroviral particles have been detected in troops of monkeys (*Macaca fuscata*) widely distributed through Japan and in other species of monkeys of the Old World, but not in Prosimians or monkeys of New World origin.[479,480] DNA sequences homologous to HTLV-I provirus, as well as type C virus particles and reverse transcriptase, were detected in cell lines established from several different species of monkeys which were positive for antibodies cross-reacting with HTLV-I.[481,482] Gene-specific probes hybridized efficiently with *gag, pol, env, pX/tax,* and LTR sequences of HTLV-I but the restriction map indicated the existence of some differences between HTLV-I and their simian homologues, the simian T-cell leukemia viruses (STLVs).[483] The overall nucleotide sequence homology between the 3′ half of an STLV isolated from a pig-tailed monkey and HTLV-I was 90%.[484] Serological and biochemical studies indicate that HTLV-I and STLVs are distinct viruses.[485] An HTLV-I-like virus isolated from a T-cell line established from a seropositive baboon (*Papio cynocephalus*) had DNA sequences that were related to but distinct from HTLV-I and HTLV-II.[486] However, STLVs are very similar to each other and also to HTLV-I of human origin (90 to 95% homology), which suggests the existence of a common ancestor of simian and human retroviruses. STLVs are species specific and sequence variations occurring between the viruses of different species of monkeys are larger than those observed between monkeys and humans. The genetic constitution of STLVs is the same of that of HTLV-I, with the genes LTR-*gag-pol-env-pX*-LTR in the direction 5′ to 3′.

Transfusion of blood from an anti-HTLV positive female monkey (*Macaca mulatta*) to a seronegative male monkey of the same species resulted in the seroconversion of the recipient, and HTLV antigens and type-C virus particles were detected in cultured lymphocytes from the seroconverted monkey.[487] A direct transmission of HTLV-like viruses from simians to humans seems unlikely.

In a manner similar to that of its human counterpart, all STLV isolates can immortalize monkey lymphocytes *in vitro*, which suggests that STLV may have leukemogenic properties in monkeys. In fact, lymphomas occurring in macaques have been associated with a virus of the STLV family. Antibodies to membrane antigens of HTLV-infected cells were found in 11 of 13 macaques with malignant lymphoma or lymphoproliferative disease but were present in only 7 of 95 of healthy macaques.[488] A higher incidence of lymphoma or leukemia has been observed among STLV-infected monkeys than among uninfected animals. A case of spontaneous leukemia in an African green monkey (*Cercopithecus aethiops*) that showed clinicopathological features similar to that of human ATL was found to be associated with a subtype of simian retrovirus, termed STLV-I.[489,490] This case of simian leukemia was detected among 31 adult African green monkeys that were seropositive for STLV-I and a preleukemic state was found in 5 other monkeys from this group. The leukemic and preleukemic monkeys contained integrated STLV-I provirus genomes in their lymphocytes. STLV provirus and antibodies were also detected in a captive 24-year-old female gorilla with non-Hodgkin's lymphoma.[491] This gorilla had antibodies against the virus at least 4 years prior to the development of lymphoma and at the time of lymphoma she was also seropositive for other viruses (CMV, EBV, and Yaba virus).

F. CONCLUSION

Adult T-cell leukemia/lymphoma (ATL) is a relatively rare type of hematologic malignancy which occurs with increased incidence in particular geographical areas from different parts of the world including Japan, the Caribbean, and Central Africa. Evidence based on seroepidemiological studies suggests an association between HTLV-I infection and ATL. In addition, studies with transgenic mice suggest an oncogenic potential for products from the *pX/tax* region of the HTLV-I genome. There is no definitive proof, however, for an etiological relationship between the HTLV-I infection and the development of ATL. Most individuals infected with the virus do not develop ATL and some cases of typical ATL are not associated at all with HTLV-I infection, which indicates that the virus is not sufficient nor necessary for the development of ATL. Thus, although HTLV-I infection may play an important role in the etiology of most cases of ATL, other exogenous and/or endogenous factors which remain largely unidentified, must be crucially involved in ATL leukemogenesis.

XI. HTLV-II

Human T-cell leukemia virus type II (HTLV-II) was isolated from the spleen cells of a patient with a benign form of a T-cell variant of hairy-cell leukemia and was characterized thereafter.[492-494] Hairy-cell leukemia is a rare human lymphoid neoplasm which typically involves cells of the B lineage, but rarely occurs as a T lymphocytic variant.[495] A permanent cell line, termed *Mo*, was established from primary culture of splenic tissue from the original case used for HTLV-II isolation. HTLV-II was also isolated from a T-cell line established from a patient with hemophilia-A and pancytopenia.[496] IgG antibody titers against HTLV-II were detected in the serum from one patient with leukopenic chronic T cell leukemia mimicking hairy cell leukemia.[497]

HTLV-II infects both human B and T cells *in vitro* but transforms only T cells, which acquire an indefinite growth potential.[498] The possible role of HTLV-II in human malignancies is unclear but it appears to be associated with less aggressive subtypes of leukemia than those forms associated with HTLV-I.[499] In any case, HTLV-II would be associated only with the rare T-cell variant of hairy cell leukemia, not with the usual B-cell form of the disease. Since HTLV-II has been isolated from only a few cases of leukemia, its pathogenicity would be rather low.

A. STRUCTURE OF HTLV-II

Results of studies with molecular hybridization techniques indicate strong conservation of nucleotide sequences between HTLV-I and HTLV-II.[500] The complete nucleotide sequence of an HTLV-II provirus molecularly cloned from a patient with hairy-cell leukemia has been determined and the virus was found to be replication competent.[501] The HTLV-II provirus has a genetic structure which is similar to that of HTLV-I, with the following gene sequence from 5′ to 3′: LTR-*gag-pol-env-pX/tax*-LTR. The coding regions of the HTLV-II provirus show on average about 60% homology with those of HTLV-I at the nucleotide level. However, a higher degree of homology is found when the *pX/tax* sequences of HTLV-I and HTLV-II are compared.

B. PROTEIN PRODUCTS OF HTLV-II

The LTR of HTLV-II has overall general features which are similar to those of HTLV-I LTR, but the respective sequences differ markedly throughout most of their length.[502-504] The major antigen of HTLV-II is a glycoprotein whose precursor is 486 amino acids long. The predicted amino acid sequences of HTLV-I and HTLV-II *env* proteins are very similar, which provides an explanation for the antigenic cross-reactivity observed among different members of the HTLV retrovirus family by procedures that assay for the viral envelope glycoprotein.[505] The *pX/tax* region of HTLV-II is expressed in HTLV-II-infected cells in form of a 37- to 38-kDa protein termed p38 ^{x}, p37^{xII}, *tat-2*, or Tax-2.[226,230,240] The possible role of p38^x/Tax-2 in transformation is not understood, but there is evidence that the *pX/tax* gene of HTLV-II acts by a mechanism involving *trans*-activation of other genes. The product of the *trans*-activator *pX/tax* gene of HTLV-II is capable of inducing IL-2 receptor and IL-2 cellular gene expression,[506] which would contribute to the mechanisms of the hypothetical HTLV-II-induced human leukemogenesis.

C. CONCLUSION

HTLV-II is a human retrovirus related to but distinct from HTLV-I. The general genetic structure of HTLV-II is similar to that of HTLV-I but the average homology between the two viruses is only 60%. One of the products encoded by the genome of this HTLV-II, the protein p38^x/Tax-2, may have transforming potential. The virus has been detected in a few cases of the rare T-cell variant of human hairy cell leukemia. The possible role of HTLV-II in this disease or in other human hematologic malignancies is not known.

XII. HIV AND THE ACQUIRED IMMUNE DEFICIENCY SYNDROME

Specific chronic retroviruses are associated with a new epidemic disease, the human acquired immune deficiency syndrome (AIDS). One of these viruses, the lymphadenopathy-associated virus (LAV), was isolated in France from the lymph node of a patient with lymphadeno-pathy.[507-510] A second virus isolate, HTLV-III, was described in the U.S.[511-514] Similar or identical virus isolates were later described in AIDS patients from Zaire, Africa, and San Francisco.[515,516] The nucleotide sequences of some retrovirus isolates associated with AIDS were determined.[517-520] The different isolates would represent variants of the same virus and at least some of these isolates may be identical. Recently, these AIDS-associated retrovirus isolates have been collectively designated human immunodeficiency viruses (HIVs).

HIVs are etiologically associated with AIDS.[29-38] This syndrome has been observed with increasing frequency since 1981, when an unprecedented occurrence of Kaposi's sarcoma, non-Hodgkin's lymphomas, and opportunistic infections such as *Pneumocystis carinii*-associated pneumonia, was observed, especially among homosexual and bisexual men but also in other groups of individuals including i.v. drug users and patients transfused with blood.[33-37,521-537] Heterosexual partners of AIDS patients as well as infants born to HIV-infected mothers were also found to be at risk of developing AIDS.[538] Since 1983 the number of children diagnosed as having AIDS has risen dramatically.[539]

A. CLINICAL AND BIOLOGICAL CHARACTERISTICS OF AIDS

The clinical characteristics of AIDS are closely related to a severe alteration of the immune mechanisms, especially those associated with cellular immunity.

1. The AIDS Syndrome

The symptoms of AIDS include localized or generalized lymphadenopathy, splenomegaly, neutropenia, lymphopenia, anemia, fever, weight loss, fatigue, skin disorders, diarrhea, thrombocytopenia, chronic infections including the gingiva, opportunistic infections, and chronic wasting disease. In addition, AIDS patients are prone to develop neoplastic diseases such as Kaposi's sarcoma and non-Hodgkin's lymphomas and may show neurologic disturbances, especially encephalitic syndromes. The immunologic features of AIDS include depletion of T4+ helper/inducer lymphocytes, follicular hyperplasia, hypergammaglobulinemia, circulating immune complexes, impaired interferon production, and progressive atrophy of lymphoid tissues. Patients with AIDS frequently develop life-threatening infections with one or more opportunistic pathogens, including *Pneumocystis carinii*, *Cryptococcus neoformans*, *Toxoplasma gondii*, *Candida albicans*, *Mycobacterium tuberculosis*, *Mycobacterium avium-intracellulare*, and several DNA viruses (EBV, CMV, HSV, adenoviruses, and papovariruses). Most patients with AIDS die within the first 3 years of the disease. The pathological characteristics of AIDS, observed in post-mortem examination, have been described in detail.[540]

2. Pediatric AIDS

AIDS is occurring in children with a dramatically increasing incidence. AIDS in children has special characteristics.[539] The predominant risk factor for AIDS in infants is represented by an HIV-infected mother. While many HIV-infected adults remain asymptomatic, most children infected with the virus develop AIDS-associated symptomatology. Opportunistic infections by *P. carinii* or other agents occurring in HIV-infected children have a very poor prognosis. A wide range of neurological abnormalities is observed in most children with AIDS. In addition, an AIDS embryopathy associated with microcephaly and other dysmorphic congenital abnormalities is frequently observed in children born from HIV-infected mothers. HIV infection in children is associated not with T-cell defects but with dysfunction of lymphocytes including poor responses to B-cell mitogens *in vitro* and poor *in vivo* antibody responses to protein and carbohydrate antigens. These children do not mount adequate antibody responses to infecting pathogens. Treatment of AIDS occurring in children is limited to some symptomatic actions including hyperimmune HIV-gamma globulin and glucocorticoids.

3. AIDS-Associated Neoplastic Diseases

Kaposi's sarcoma, frequently observed in immunosuppressed patients,[341,541] is characterized by red or violaceous cutaneous lesions which provide a most visible symptom of the fundamental disease. Generally considered as an angiosarcoma of endothelial cell origin, Kaposi's sarcoma is a multifocal neoplasm which occurs in the form of subcutaneous palpable and painless nodules or pigmented plaques of the skin or oral mucosa. Such tumors often have a rather benign clinical course. Visceral Kaposi's sarcoma is fairly common among AIDS patients but the subcutaneous location of the lesions make difficult a diagnosis by endoscopic biopsy procedures. The typical lesion is characterized by an infiltration of spindle-shaped cells accompanied by proliferation of small, incompletely formed blood vessels which appear to be lined by very large cells with the histological characteristics of endothelium.

AIDS patients are at high risk of developing Kaposi's sarcoma and other malignant diseases.[341,541-544] During the last decades Kaposi's sarcoma was frequently observed in Central Africa, where it followed an indolent course, with many patients surviving for 10 or more years. Since 1981 atypical and more aggressive form of the tumor appeared in the same region of Africa, and it was demonstrated that a high proportion of the patients with this form of the tumor are seropositive for HIV; in contrast, only a minority of patients with the classic, more benign form of Kaposi's sarcoma are positive.[545] Thus, an etiologic association between HIV infection and atypical Kaposi's sarcoma is strongly suspected. However, the exact relationship between HIV infection and Kaposi's sarcoma in Africa is not totally clear. In a recent study, only three of nine patients from Tanzania with severe, locally aggressive forms of Kaposi's sarcoma were seropositive for HIV, and none had evidence of AIDS or the AIDS-related syndrome.[546] Moreover, the evidence implicating altered immunity in the aggressive forms of Kaposi's sarcoma in Africans in the absence of HIV infection was not clear in this clinical study. Viruses other than HIV or nonviral factors may play an important role in the development of Kaposi's sarcoma.

Other malignant diseases that may be observed with increased frequency in patients with AIDS include a diversity of lymphomas (primary central nervous system lymphoma, high-grade non-Hodgkin lymphomas, undifferentiated Burkitt's type lymphomas, and immunoblastic lymphomas).[542,544] The exact role of HIV in the pathogenesis of these malignancies is not clear. Burkitt's lymphomas occurring in AIDS patients may be characterized by atypical chromosome translocations such as t(2;8) and are associated with EBV infection but are negative for HIV-related sequences.[547] Thus, HIV is not directly involved in the development of these lymphomas.

4. Neurologic Manifestations of AIDS

Neurologic dysfunction occurs frequently in AIDS.[549] Approximately 60% of AIDS patients have neurologic symptoms and up to 90% of the total AIDS patients may show neurologic lesions at autopsy. HIV has been shown to be neurotropic and was found to be etiologically associated with encephalopathy in both adults and children.[550] Support to an etiologic relationship of HIV infection and AIDS leukoencephalopathy is given by *in situ* molecular hybridization studies which indicate the association of HIV with lesions of the white matter.[551] Subacute encephalitis (AIDS encephalopathy or dementia complex), the most common neurologic manifestation of AIDS, is characterized by poor memory, inability to concentrate, apathy, and psychomotor retardation. Focal motor abnormalities and behavioral changes may also occur. The neurologic symptoms usually progress rapidly and a full-blown dementia complex may develop within 1 year. In addition, several distinct, previously unexplained neurologic syndromes (subacute encephalitis, vacuolar myelopathy, aseptic meningitis, and peripheral neuropathy) may appear as components of the AIDS symptomatic complex.

5. The AIDS-Related Complex

The prodromes of AIDS, frequently designated as "pre-AIDS" syndrome, may include nonspecific symptoms such as night sweats, unexplained weight loss, wasting, and diarrhea. A lymphadenopathy syndrome (LAS) with unexplained chronic lymphadenopathy and leukopenia with diminished number of circulating helper T lymphocytes may form part of the AIDS-related complex of organic alterations. In addition, HIV infection should be considered in high-risk persons with an acute febrile mononucleosis-like illness, since this clinical picture may represent an acute form of AIDS retrovirus infection.[552]

6. Immunologic Abnormalities in AIDS

Peripheral T lymphocytes which are the cells involved in cellular immune mechanisms may be classified into two subsets that exhibit distinct biochemical and functional characteristics depending on the expression of either T4 (OKT4+) or T8 (OKT8+) surface glycoproteins.[553] CD4+ (T4+) lymphocytes recognize antigen on target cells in association with class II MHC molecules and contain the majority of helper T cells, whereas CD8+ (T8+) cells recognize antigen on targets bearing class I MHC molecules and contain the majority of cytotoxic and suppressor T cells.[554] Patients with AIDS usually have a severe immune deficiency with a reversal of the ratio of helper-inducer (T4+) to suppressor-cytotoxic (T8+) subsets of T lymphocytes in the peripheral blood, impairment of delayed cutaneous hypersensitivity reactions, and decreased responsiveness of T lymphocytes to *in vitro* stimulation by specific mitogenic agents.

The structural gene of the CD4 (T4) protein resides on the short arm of human chromosome 12, at region 12p12-pter.[555] The available evidence indicates that the CD4 molecule is the receptor for HIV on the lymphocyte surface. HIV interacts largely with CD4+ cells and the virus infection can be specifically inhibited by using monoclonal antibodies against the CD4 molecule.[556] In addition, portions of the HIV envelope not directly involved in binding to the CD4 molecule, in particular the second conserved domain of the HIV gp120 envelope protein, may be necessary for the initiation of productive viral infection.[557] As determined by the study of specific mutants, the gp120 protein may have an essential role in internalization events subsequent to the virus interaction with the CD4 receptor on the surface of T lymphocytes, including penetration and endocytosis of the viral particle. The loss of marked reduction in CD4 receptor expression observed in HIV-1-infected helper T lymphocytes is an indirect effect of viral infection and replication.[558] CD4+/CD8+ lymphocyte ratios have been found to be significantly lower in homosexual patients with AIDS associated with Kaposi's sarcoma.[543] These patients have a higher prevalence of antigen HLA-DR5 and exhibit high antibody titers to antigens of DNA viruses (EBV and HCMV).

7. Asymptomatic HIV Infection

Many individuals with HIV infection do not develop AIDS within the first few years after infection and, moreover, some of them will never develop the disease at all. The main outcome of seroepidemiological studies is that HIV infection is most often asymptomatic.[37] Whether or not cofactors or host susceptibility factors increase the risk of developing AIDS in infected persons is unclear at present. Cells of the mononuclear phagocyte system may have an important role in the pathogenesis of AIDS.[559] These cells may harbor HIV infection in both peripheral blood and bone marrow as well as in target organs such as brain, lungs, lymph nodes, and skin. Mononuclear phagocytes that have been infected by HIV do not undergo significant cytopathic changes, suggesting that they may be important viral reservoirs. These cells may also promote the slow, persistent nature of HIV infections by escaping host immunologic surveillance mechanisms. Functional abnormalities occurring in the HIV-infected mononuclear macrophages may be partially responsible for the severe immunosuppression characteristic of AIDS and AIDS-related disorders.

B. EPIDEMIOLOGY OF HIV INFECTION

Epidemiological data initially suggested the existence of an infectious etiologic agent of AIDS.[521-529] The agent was subsequently recognized as the HIV retrovirus which is transmitted by different types of intimate contact. HIV infection is occurring in the present decade at a worldwide level and is following an apparently inexorable spreading process. The reported incidence of AIDS is continually increasing throughout the world.[537]

1. Routes of HIV Transmission

HIV is a highly infectious agent which can be experimentally transmitted to human lymphocytes obtained from cord blood, peripheral blood, or bone marrow. HIV has been isolated from peripheral blood, semen, saliva, and tears.[33] Although many routes of natural transmission of HIV infection have been discussed, including insects, the data accumulated in the last years strongly support the concept that transmission of HIV occurs only through blood (during transfusion or in i.v. drug use), during sexual activity (either homosexual or heterosexual), and during perinatal events (from HIV-infected mothers).[534] HIV may be transmitted from infected women to their offspring by three possible routes: to the fetus *in utero* through the maternal circulation, to the infant during labor and delivery by inoculation of blood and/or other infected fluids, and to the infant shortly after birth through breast milk infected with the virus. Whereas homosexual contacts between men were the predominant form of HIV transmission in the initial years of the AIDS epidemic, heterosexual transmission of HIV is becoming the more common form of spread of this infection in the recent years.[538,560] Between 10 and 70% of female and male partners of heterosexuals with HIV infection are HIV antibody positive.

2. Seroepidemiological and Virological Studies

Seropositivity for HIV is found in most patients with pre-AIDS and it is also frequently found in clinically normal mothers of juvenile AIDS patients, in juvenile AIDS, and in adult AIDS with Kaposi's sarcoma or with opportunistic infections.[528,561] Antibodies to HIV are present in the majority of patients with either AIDS or pre-AIDS, in hemophiliacs and blood donors, and in certain groups of persons such as i.v. drug abusers and homosexual men.[514,528,562-566] Immunologic methods with variable degrees of specificity and sensitivity have been used for the detection of HIV, including enzyme-linked immunosorbant assays (ELISA) and radioimmunoprecipitation tests. Synthetic peptides derived from conserved domains of different HIVs can be used in sensitive and specific immunoassays that detect antibodies in sera from patients infected with HIV-1 or HIV-2 and can also be used for the detection of the simian virus STLV-III.[567] Moreover, single amino acid substitutions can be made in the reactive domain of HIV-1 to create immunodiagnostic antigens that are increasingly or decreasingly strain specific. A simple cell-based test can also serve to detect antibodies to both HIV-1 and HIV-2.[568]

Different percentages of seropositivity for HIV or HIV-related viruses may be found in different human populations, according to the geographic region, the predominant type of virus, and the method used for virus detection. Frequent positivity for HIV-related antibodies was reported in alcoholic patients with hepatitis as well as in patients with acute malarial infections.[569,570] Relatively high rate of seropositivity for HIV-related antigen was also detected in healthy rural populations and Amazonian Indians living in Venezuela.[571] However, these results were not confirmed by other investigators who used more specific methods for HIV detection (immunofluorescence, Western blot hybridization, and radioimmunoprecipitation).[572] HIV infection is apparently not endemic among Brazilian Indians, whereas the population of Rio de Janeiro showed a relatively high prevalence (0.34%) of seropositivity among apparently normal individuals.[398] HIV did probably not evolve in native populations of South America. HIV-related DNA sequences have been detected in various insects from Central Africa but not in similar insects from the area of Paris.[573] The isolation and characterization of putative HIV-like retroviruses which are apparently endemic in nonclassical AIDS risk populations may contribute to a better understanding and definition of the whole group of HIV-like retroviruses.

The application of highly sensitive and specific techniques may contribute to elucidate controversial epidemiological and clinical aspects related to HIV infection. Measurement of circulating anti-HIV antibodies is an indicator of a past encounter with the virus but the method is not appropriate for determining the presence of HIV sequences in the infected cells and for directly assessing HIV load. A sensitive solution hybridization technique may be applied to the detection and quantitation of HIV in blood cells.[574] Cells to be probed are dissolved in concentrated guanine thiocyanate and the solubilized HIV target RNA is hybridized directly with an RNA probe which contains the HIV *pol* gene. RNA-RNA hybrids are precipitated and collected on membranes after unhybridized probe is destroyed with RNAse. The presence and quantitation of HIV proviral DNA in the same cells can be determined by a minor variation of the technique.

C. HIV-RELATED HUMAN RETROVIRUSES

Retroviruses related to, but distinct from, the original HIV isolate have been identified recently. At least some of these viruses are capable of inducing a disease which is clinically similar or identical to AIDS.

1. HIV-2

A retrovirus distantly related to HIV was isolated by the end of 1985 from the peripheral blood lymphocytes of two West-African patients with AIDS.[575,576] The new virus, termed HIV-2 or LAV-2 in contradistinction to the classic HIV virus (HIV-1, LAV-1, or HTLV-III), is a distinct human retrovirus. HIV-2 has been identified in AIDS patients from West Africa, Europe, and other parts of the world.[577] The virus exhibits tropism for CD4+ lymphocytes, being capable of inducing in the infected cells cytopathic effects similar to those caused by HIV-1. The clinical picture associated with HIV-2 infection would be similar or identical to that of AIDS induced by HIV-1.[578] However, the exact role of HIV-2 in the AIDS epidemic in Africa and other geographical areas of the world is not known as yet. In a recent study of the clinical, hematologic, and immunologic status in HIV-2-infected prostitutes from Dakar, Senegal, it was concluded that HIV-2 is a sexually transmitted agent that produces immunologic alterations with a persistent viral infection but the infected prostitutes did not show signs of immunosuppression similar to those observed in HIV-1-infected persons.[579] Thus, the pathogenic potential of HIV-2 appears to differ from that of HIV-1, and the latter virus should be considered as the true etiologic agent of the AIDS pandemic.

The entire genome of HIV-2 has been sequenced.[580] The overall organization of the 9.5-kb HIV-2 genome is very similar to that of HIV-1. However, HIV-2 exhibits only 42% general nucleotide sequence homology to HIV-1. HIV-1 and HIV-2 cannot be considered as strains of the same virus but as distinct retroviruses and they probably diverged from a common ancestor well before the present AIDS epidemic. The structural study of HIV-1 and HIV-2 suggests that they may have derived from a common ancestor as recently as 40 years ago.[581] HIV-2 displays an antigenic relationship to the STLV-III retrovirus isolated from African monkeys with or without SAIDS. The very close structural relationship between HIV-2 and the simian virus suggest that they may have evolutionarily diverged recently and that a transmission from nonhuman primates to humans may have occurred.[577] In contrast, a close simian relative to HIV-1 has not been found as yet. Another HIV isolate of West African origin, termed SBL-6669, is closely related to HIV-2 and is associated with immunodeficiency disease.[582]

2. HTLV-4

Another chronic retrovirus, HTLV-IV or HTLV-4, is related to the simian virus STLV-III and infects apparently healthy people in West Africa.[583,584] Restriction map and partial nucleotide sequence studies indicate that HTLV-4 and STLV-III isolated from African green monkey may not be independent virus isolates.[585] In contrast to HIV-1 and HIV-2, HTLV-4 does not appear to be associated with immunodeficiency-related disorders and its biological characteristics are different from those of HIVs.

D. GENETIC STRUCTURE AND PROTEIN PRODUCTS OF HIV

Nucleic acid hybridization analysis showed that HIV-1 genome organization and sequences are partially homologous to those of HTLV-I and HTLV-II, but that HIV-1 is a distinct human retrovirus.[586] HIV-1 has been cloned in molecular vectors, the proviral genome has been analyzed, and the complete nucleotide sequences (9,213-9,749 bp), including the LTR, have been characterized.[518-520,587-590] The molecular clones represent different isolates from the provirus integrated into the productively infected human T cells. The results establish that HIV-1 has no strong nucleotide sequence homology with previously characterized animal and human retroviruses and that different virus isolates display significant genetic heterogeneity. HIV-1 is in several aspects different from HTLV-I and HTLV-II. As stated before, HTLV-I and HTLV-II are members of the Oncovirinae subfamily of retroviruses, with morphological similitude to type C retroviruses. They are capable of immortalizing T cells and are associated with T-cell malignant diseases in humans and other primates. In contrast, HIV-1 is more closely related to the Lentivirinae subfamily of retroviruses, which includes the visna virus and other infectious viruses of ungulate (hoofed) mammals.[348,349]

1. HIV-1-Specific ORFs

The basic genetic structure of the HIV-1 provirus includes the genes *gag*, *pol*, and *env* as well as the 5' and 3' LTR sequences contained in all chronic retroviruses. However, in addition to these genes the HIV-1 genome contains two genomic ORF regions which would correspond to novel genes. One of them, termed ORF-2, *lor*, *tat*-III, or E', is located at the 3' end of the genome, between *env* and the 3' LTR, and the other, termed ORF-1, *sor*, or P', is located between *pol* and *env*. Transcripts of the latter two genes are processed as spliced subgenomic RNAs in the cells infected by HIV-1,[592] but the functions of the putative protein products of these two genetic regions are little understood. A region of HIV-1 containing *env-lor* sequences has been cloned in and expressed from a molecular vector.[592] A protein product of *tat*-III ORF is a 14-kDa polypeptide that may act as a *trans*-activator which increases the levels of steady-state mRNA transcribed from the viral LTR promoter.[593,594] An additional gene in the HIV-1 genome is necessary for replication of the virus and acts posttranscriptionally to relieve negative regulation of the mRNA for the virion capsid and envelope proteins.[595]

Four genes contained in the ORF-1 and ORF-2 regions of HIV-1 have been termed *tat* (transcriptional/translational *trans*-activator), *art* (antirepression *trans*-activator) or *trs* (trans-acting regulator of splicing), *sor* (short open reading frame), and 3' *orf* (3' open reading frame), which encode for protein products of different molecular weight.[596] The functions of the products of these genes are only partially understood. Genes *tat* and *art* are essential for replication, *sor* is not essential for replication or cytopathic effects, and 3' *orf* encodes for a 27-kDa protein which is not essential for replication. Sequences from the 5' *env* gene would not be directly responsible for cytopathic effects but may be required for virus replication. The complex *in vivo* behavior of HIV-1, which is characterized by persistent infection in the human host, would depend at least in part on the regulatory control of viral RNA splicing and translation.[597]

2. HIV-1 Reverse Transcriptase

The *pol* gene of HIV-1 has been cloned and expressed in *Escherichia coli*, which resulted in the appearance of reverse transcriptase activity in the bacterial extracts.[598] The extracts contained two virus-related polypeptides of 66 kDa (p66) and 51 kDa (p51), which would correspond to processed forms of HIV-1-derived reverse transcriptase. A third form of *pol*-derived HIV-1 protein of 34 kDa (p34) would possess integrase/endonuclease activity. Antibodies against reverse transcriptase p66/p51 proteins have been detected in about 80% of 700 HIV-antibody-positive sera.[599]

Inhibition of HIV-1 reverse transcriptase activity may be useful for understanding the mechanisms of HIV-1-associated pathogenicity as well as for the therapy of HIV-1-induced human diseases; 90 analogues of suramin, a known reverse transcriptase inhibitor, have been developed and tested for their ability to inhibit HIV-1 reverse transcriptase activity.[600] Of the compounds tested, 24 were superior to suramin in the reverse transcriptase inhibition assay but no clear relationship was found between the chemical structure and the different kinetic types of enzyme inhibitors.

3. Homologies of HIV Protein Products

The carboxyl-terminal region of the HIV *env* protein contains an hexapeptide sequence that is homologous to a portion of the IL-2 protein which is complementary to the IL-2 receptor.[601,602] Although the detected region of homology is small, it may be significant because it coincides with the portion of IL-2 predicted to bind the IL-2 receptor. The primary amino acid sequence of a stretch of 25 residues (positions 91-116) of the middle portion of the 27-kDa 3'*orf* protein (p27$^{3'-orf}$) of HIV-1 shares structural homology with both an intracytoplasmic phosphorylation domain of the human IL-2 receptor and the ATP-binding site of the catalytic subunit of cAMP-dependent protein kinase as well as with the kinases of the *src* family of oncogenes.[603] The biological significance of these homologies is not understood but they suggest that the p27$^{3'-orf}$ protein could serve functions similar to those of cellular kinases.

4. Genetic Heterogeneity of HIV-1

A characteristic feature of HIV-1 is its genomic heterogeneity, which occurs to varying degrees in different viral isolates.[604-608] The molecular characterization of an HIV isolated from a Zairian AIDS patient indicated that the LTR, ORF-1, carboxy-terminal *env* gene domain, and ORF-2 had less than 6% difference in nucleotide sequence when compared to other HIV isolates including HTLV-III, LAV-1, and ARV-2.[609] However, approximately 15% difference in nucleotide sequence was noted in the amino-terminal domain of the *env* gene. The detailed comparison of the Zairian isolate with other HIV isolates demonstrated that the nucleotide differences existing among different isolates are clustered and that the *env* gene is composed of constant and variable regions. Some of the variable regions are characterized by small deletions and insertions and a high degree of amino acid substitutions. The significance of sequence variation in HIV *env* gene remains to be established but sequence differences in this region are likely to affect the immunogenicity of the virus, and perhaps also its host range (cell type or species). Viral *env* glycoproteins are usually the targets of protective immune responses.

Most patients appear to be infected with only one of two predominant forms of the virus at any one time. Variation in the structure of HIV-1 envelopes may affect the antigenic properties of the virus to a degree that make it difficult to design and develop effective diagnostic, therapeutic, and preventive measures for the virus. The development of vaccines must especially circumvent obstacles related to the broad spectrum of genomic variability of the virus.[610] If the frequency of mutation of the retrovirus is high, the virus may escape from a vaccine-induced host immune response. Moreover, vaccination is not likely to benefit HIV carriers because nearly all of these carriers have active antiviral immunity.[611] A therapeutic approach to human diseases associated with HIV infection is also difficult, although there are several steps of the viral lifecycle that can be profited from therapeutic strategies.[612]

E. HIV EXPRESSION

HIV LTR contains enhancer elements and is involved in the regulation of HIV gene expression and replication. Different classes of T-cell mitogens (the lectin PHA, the phorbol ester PMA, the calcium ionophore ionomycin, and the *tat*-1 *trans*-activator of HTLV-I) may act in either an isolated or synergistic manner to regulate HIV-1 gene expression via the HIV-1 LTR.[613] Sodium butyrate, which is believed to alter chromatin structure, can activate LTR-directed HIV-1 expression.[614] Thus, the HIV-1 LTR may be regulated like a T-cell activation gene.

High level of HIV expression in certain human T-cell lines may be attributed, at least in part, to a virus-encoded *trans*-activator protein, termed *tat, tat*-3, or *tat*-III.[615] Sequences in the HIV LTR that respond to *tat* have been localized to the mRNA start site, between nucleotides -17 and 80 (TAR region).[616] Nuclear extracts from human T cells infected with HIV contain a factor that stimulates transcription specifically from the HIV LTR promoter, but it is not known whether this factor is identical to the virus-encoded *tat* protein.[617] The *tat* gene of HIV-1 is apparently not involved in the regulation of translational processes.[618] In any case, the *trans*-activator is probably important for regulating the level of expression of HIV in the infected lymphocytes. Lack of HIV expression during the long latency period that precedes overt AIDS or AIDS-related complex may be due, at least in part, to transcriptional inactivation of the virus genome by methylation of LTR cytosine residues.[619]

F. MECHANISMS OF HIV-ASSOCIATED PATHOGENICITY

The fundamental question concerning the mechanism by which HIV exerts its cytopathic effects and induces AIDS remains unanswered. It is generally accepted that the pathogenic effects of HIV are mainly or completely due to the induction of immunosuppression. The molecular mechanisms involved in HIV-induced immunosuppression are little known but they include as an important component a profound depletion of CD4+ (helper/inducer) lymphocytes. However, it has been suggested that AIDS does not result solely from a progressive depletion of the HIV-infected CD4+ lymphocyte subset but that the virus triggers an autoimmune response in the immune system of the infected individual and that the syndrome develops as a consequence of a kind of "host vs. host" reaction.[620] In any case, the pathogenesis of full-blown AIDS would include the operation of many different primary and secondary abnormalities and the exact role of HIV (or HIV-related viruses) in the development of AIDS is not totally clear.

1. The HIV Receptor

The CD4 antigen on the surface of OKT4+ human lymphocytes has been identified as an essential component of the receptor for HIV.[556,621] The gp120 envelope protein of HIV-1 directly interacts with the CD4 protein of helper T cells.[622] The marked immunosuppressive properties of HIV depends on the initial binding of the large envelope protein gp120 of the virus to the CD4 molecule.[168] The CD4 molecule is a nonpolymorphic surface protein expressed in CD4+ cells as an antigen which shows partial sequence identity to immunoglobulins. Soluble, secreted forms of CD4 produced by transfection of mammalian cells (CHO cells) with vectors encoding versions of the CD4 molecule lacking its transmembrane and cytoplasmic domains results in prevention of HIV-1 infection of CD4+ cells *in vitro*.[623] This neutralizing effect may result from the saturation of virion-associated gp120 with soluble receptor molecules, thus interfering with the adsorption of virus to the cells. The neutralizing effect of soluble CD4 on HIV-1 infection may be applied, in principle, for therapeutic intervention in AIDS and other HIV-1-associated diseases.

2. Activation of T-Cells

Activation of sequences contained in the LTR of HIV may be important in the pathogenesis of HIV-associated diseases. HIV LTR can induce a marked *trans*-activation of transcription of heterologous genes.[624] Although human T cells derived from peripheral blood lymphocytes can efficiently bind HIV without previous activation and the early phase of viral infection does not require activation of T cells, the extent of viral replication is directly related to T-cell activation. Gene expression directed by the HIV LTR increases in response to T-cell activation signals.[625] Moreover, the effects of T-cell activation and of the HIV-encoded *tat trans*-activator are multiplicative. Analysis of mutations and deletions of the HIV LTR revealed that the region corresponding to T-cell activation signals is located at positions -105 to -80 and that these sequences are composed of two direct repeats which are homologous to the core transcriptional enhancer elements of the SV40 genome and that function as the HIV enhancer.

3. Integration of Proviral HIV DNA

HIV is more a cytopathic virus than an oncogenic virus and, in contrast to HTLV-I and HTLV-II, it persists in both integrated and unintegrated forms in the chronically infected cells. Proviral HIV DNA is integrated at multiple sites in the infected cells, which indicates that the cell population is polyclonal with respect to the site of HIV integration.[588]

4. Cofactors in the Etiology of AIDS

Since only a fraction of those individuals infected with HIV develop AIDS, it is evident that other endogenous and/or exogenous factors, in addition to HIV infection, are of crucial importance in the etiology of the disease. Many different factors may contribute to determine the fate of HIV infection in particular individuals. The exact place of HIV itself among all of these factors is still uncertain. In any case, it is clear that the severely impaired function of immune system is centrally involved in the pathogenesis of AIDS-associated neoplasms.

5. Associated Viral Infections

The possible role of EBV, HCMV, and other DNA viruses in AIDS and Kaposi's sarcoma remains undetermined. HCMV-associated retinitis has been described in AIDS patients.[626] There is evidence that patients with AIDS or AIDS-related disorders have a defect in the regulation of EBV-infected B cells, which results in the circulation of abnormally high numbers of these cells.[627] The possibility has been suggested that HIV or HIV-related viruses may have a role in the induction of EBV-positive Burkitt's lymphoma in Africa. DNA viruses from different families (papovaviruses, adenoviruses, and herpesviruses) can stimulate the expression of HIV.[628,629] An EBV immediate early gene product, *Bam*HI *MLF1*, is able to stimulate the expression of a heterologous gene linked to the HIV promoter.[630] Activation of HIV expression by products of EBV may be biologically significant in relation to disease development. It is thus possible that infections with unrelated viruses can alter the expression of HIV in HIV-infected individuals, triggering the conversion of a persistent asymptomatic HIV infection to a productive cytolytic, symptomatic infection.

6. Hormones and Growth Factors

Hormones and growth factors may have an important role in the development of AIDS, but information in relation to this possibility is limited. An important consequence of HIV-induced damage to infected lymphoid cells may be the deficient production of cytokines that would otherwise help in the elimination of the virus. Treatment of cells with a combination of TNF-α and IFN-γ greatly reduces their susceptibility to infection with HIV and suppresses the production of HIV mRNA and core protein p24 as well as the production of infectious HIV.[631] CSF-2 and IFN-γ, may modify the pathogenic properties of HIV.[632]

The role of the T-cell-specific growth factor IL-2 and its receptor in AIDS development is unclear. Expression of the α chain of the IL-2 receptor (IL-2R α) may be regulated by a nuclear protein, HIVEN86A, which specifically binds to both the enhancer element of the HIV-1 LTR and a 12-bp sequence present in the 5′ regulatory region of the IL-2R α gene.[633] These findings suggest that the normal action of an inducible nuclear DNA binding protein involved in the regulation of IL-2R α gene expression can be subverted by the HIV-1 provirus to promote activation of retroviral gene transcription. T cells from patients with AIDS produce adequate amounts of IL-2 in response to lectin stimulation but their response to exogenously supplied IL-2 is severely impaired and a significantly diminished expression of IL-2 receptors is observed in these cells following lectin stimulation.[634] Significantly elevated levels of soluble IL-2 receptors have been found in the majority of HIV-infected individuals, including patients with

AIDS, AIDS-related complex, and HIV-positive lymphadenopathy syndrome.[635-637] Soluble IL-2 receptors could have an immunoregulatory role in patients with AIDS or lymphoid malignancies.

Although T helper lymphocytes of HIV-infected persons may be capable of producing adequate amounts of IL-2 as a response to mitogenic stimulation, they may have a defective response to a soluble antigenic stimulus.[638] As stated previously, a region of the human IL-2 protein which was predicted to be a contact point with the IL-2 receptor contains a hexapeptide that is homologous to an amino acid sequence from the carboxy-terminal region of the HIV envelope protein.[601,602] The homologous hexapeptide sequence was found to inhibit the biological activity of human IL-2 in a murine spleen cell proliferation assay. These results suggest a possible mechanism by which HIV may cause significant immunosuppression that may lead to the development of AIDS.

7. Oncogene-Like Properties of HIV Products

The protein product of the 3′ *orf* gene contained in the HIV genome exhibits some features in common with oncogene protein products.[639] Recombinant HIV p27[3′-orf] protein produced by genetically manipulated *Escherichia coli* is myristylated and is phosphorylated by protein kinase C at a residue close to the amino terminus, in a manner similar to that of the *src* oncogene kinase. Moreover, the purified recombinant bacterial protein shows GTP-binding and GTPase and autophosphorylation activities in a manner similar to that of the *ras* oncogene product.

8. Oncogenic Potential of HIV

The mechanisms responsible for the putative oncogenic properties of AIDS-associated retroviruses are, as those of other chronic transforming retroviruses, little understood. Usually, no evidence for HIV DNA is detected in Kaposi's sarcoma tumor specimens, which indicates that HIV can only be indirectly involved in the pathogenesis of this tumor.[36] Kaposi's sarcoma may be polyclonal even within the same lesion and the tumor cells have a tendency to a diversity of chromosomal rearrangements.[640] Chromosome instability and clonal changes were found in lymph node biopsies from three out of seven patients with AIDS or AIDS-related complex.[641] Karyotypically abnormal AIDS-associated lymphadenopathies may represent prelymphomatous proliferations. The enlarged lymph nodes of these patients are frequently associated with EBV infection and show translocations or rearrangements of the c-*myc* protooncogene locus, but no HIV sequences are detectable in these lesions.[642] Thus, HIV does not seem to have a direct role in AIDS-associated lymphomagenesis.

The immunosuppressive action of HIV infection is probably an important factor in determining the high frequency of neoplastic processes occurring in AIDS. Probably due to the profound defect of T-cell-associated immunity, AIDS patients may have high numbers of EBV-infected B cells and increased levels of EBV-associated antigens in the circulation, which may predispose them to the development of EBV-containing lymphomas.[627,643]

The possible participation of protooncogenes in the mechanisms of HIV-associated oncogenicity is suggested by the fact that angiosarcomatous tumors are produced in nude mice by NIH/3T3 cells transfected with DNA from Kaposi's sarcoma occurring in patients with AIDS.[644] The histopathologic features of the nude mouse tumors are similar to those of Kaposi's sarcoma. Although it is conceivable that these tumors are induced by a cascade of phenomena that could include the activation of protooncogenes, no significant homology with several oncogenes (N-*ras*, v-H-*ras*, v-K-*ras*, v-*sis*, v-*src*, and v-*fes*) was identified in the tumor cells.

G. HIV-RELATED AND NONHUMAN TYPE D RETROVIRUSES

Clinical and experimental studies with monkeys have indicated the existence of retroviral-induced diseases with characteristics similar to that of human AIDS.[645-650] The subfamily of type D retroviruses detected in nonhuman primates (New and Old World monkeys) contain three exogenous and two endogenous viruses. The typical type D exogenous viruses of nonhuman primates include the Mason-Pfizer monkey virus (MPMV) and two serotypes of simian AIDS retroviruses (SRV-1 and SRV-2) detected in macaque monkeys.

1. Simian AIDS

The immunosuppressive properties of type D retroviruses in macaque monkeys are well documented.[649] MPMV was initially shown to be immunopathogenic in newborn rhesus monkeys (*Macaca mulatta*).[651] The majority of rhesus monkeys inoculated with the virus develop clinical signs of immunosuppression and hematological abnormalities and die with severe signs of immunosuppression. A syndrome of acquired immune deficiency, similar to human AIDS, was identified in rhesus monkeys (*Macaca mulatta*).[646] A group of closely related type D retroviruses appear to be the etiologic agents of simian AIDS (SAIDS).[652,653] SAIDS is characterized by generalized lymphadenopathy, splenomegaly, weight loss, diarrhea, hepatitis, fever, neutropenia, lymphopenia, anemia, and other symptoms including tumors (lymphomas and fibrosarcomas).[647] Fatal SAIDS frequently includes wasting, necrotizing gingivitis (noma), septicemia, and opportunistic infections. SAIDS can be transmitted in rhesus monkeys by inoculation of supernatants of homogenates of various tissues. Intravenous injection of SRV-1 to juvenile rhesus monkeys may result in development of SAIDS after 2 to 4 weeks.

SRV-1 isolated from transfected cells transfected with a cloned SRV-1 genome was shown to be infectious and pathogenic, resulting in disease in monkeys that followed the same time and mortality as disease induced by uncloned, *in vitro* cultivated virus isolated from diseased animals.[654] These results unequivocally demonstrate that a type D retrovirus (SRV-1) causes a fatal immunosuppressive syndrome (SAIDS) in rhesus monkeys. Experimental induction of SAIDS by inoculation of juvenile rhesus monkeys with SRV-1 can be prevented by immunization with a vaccine containing Formalin-killed SRV-1 plus an adjuvant.[655]

In addition to SAIDS, two neoplasms, retroperitoneal fibromatosis and subcutaneous fibrosarcomas, have been found in macaques infected with SRV viruses.[649] Only SRV-2 is found in association with retroperitoneal fibromatosis, and about 35% of SRV-2-infected macaques develop this disease. Subcutaneous fibrosarcoma is found in association with both SRV-1 and SRV-2, but less than 5% of the infected monkeys develop the disease.

2. Structure of Nonhuman Primate Type D Retroviruses

The isolation, molecular cloning, and nucleotide sequences of nonhuman primate retroviruses has been reported.[652-654,656,657] The genomes of these viruses are typical of chronic retroviruses, with LTRs and three structural genes (*gag, pol,* and *env*) but without oncogene sequences. However, in addition to the essential components of all chronic retroviruses, the genome of nonhuman primate type D retroviruses contains a large separate gene, *prt*, which codes for the protease function of the virus. The *prt* gene resides in a particular ORF situated between the *gag* and *pol* genes. Nonhuman primate type D retroviruses are not immunologically related to HIV-1.[658]

3. HIV-Related Viruses in Nonhuman Primates

Chronic retroviruses other than MPMV and SRVs may be associated with nonhuman primate diseases.[649,650] A new lentivirus, termed MnIV (WPRC-1), related to HIV-1 with respect to molecular weight, antigenic cross-reaction, and amino acid sequence has been isolated from a lymph node from a macaque (*Macaca nemestrina*) that died with malignant lymphoma.[659] The MnIV virus is distinct from retroviruses associated with human AIDS. The pathogenicity of this virus remains to be characterized.

Other HIV-related viruses were detected in healthy wild-caught African green monkeys (*Cercopithecus aethiops*) and asymptomatic asymptomatic sooty mangabeys (*Cercocebus atys*).[660,661] The HIV-related retrovirus isolated from African green monkeys show detectable homology with HIV, especially in the genomic regions *pol*, *gag*, and 3′ *orf*.[662,663] A virus found in African green monkeys and classified as simian T-lymphotropic virus type 3 (STLV-3 or STLV-III), also called simian immunodeficiency virus (SIV), has the same general genomic structure as the human virus HIV-1.[664] However, SIV is closely related not to HIV-1 but to HIV-2, and some species of monkeys may develop SAIDS after SIV infection.[577,665] The authenticity of the isolate STLV-III, derived from African green monkeys, and HTLV-IV, derived from humans, has been questioned.[666] They could be derived from cell cultures infected with an SIV isolate ($SIV_{Mac-251}$) derived from a macaque.

4. Effects of Inoculation of HIV to Nonhuman Primates

The chimpanzee (*Pan troglodytes*) is highly susceptible to HIV infection, developing persistent viremia after infusion of plasma from AIDS patients and a transient clinical syndrome of lymphadenopathy and immunologic impairment, which suggests that this animal may provide a model for the study of human AIDS.[667,668] However, after more than 2 years of clinical observation, experimentally infected chimpanzees had not developed a fatal disease comparable to human AIDS.[648]

H. SUMMARY

There may be little doubt that HIV and HIV-related retroviruses are crucially involved in the etiology and pathogenesis of AIDS and AIDS-related conditions. The main result of infection with these viruses is a depletion of CD4+ (helper/inducer) lymphocytes. However, the mechanisms of HIV-associated pathogenicity are complex and factors other than virus infection are probably important for the full development of AIDS.

XIII. CONCLUSION

Chronic retroviruses are infectious, nondefective viruses characterized by the absence of specific transforming sequences (oncogenes). Although these agents have limited oncogenic potential, they are capable of inducing tumors in different mammalian species, including primates, under defined experimental conditions. Some animal species are rather resistant to the tumorigenic action of these viruses. Chronic retroviruses may have a role in the etiology of spontaneous (nonexperimental) tumors when they act on susceptible hosts and in concert with other etiologic agents.

Tumors associated with retroviruses are usually clonal in origin, but individual tumor cells may contain several copies of the provirus. Multistage phenomena are crucially involved in the tumorigenic processes associated with chronic retroviruses. Several cellular genes could be activated, and perhaps other genes could be inactivated, at different periods of the complex oncogenic processes associated with these viruses. Alteration of particular cellular genes, which may or may not correspond to protooncogenes, may occur by insertion of chronic retrovirus proviruses at particular genomic sites. This alteration may represent an important mechanism for the tumorigenic processes occurring in certain murine species infected by chronic retroviruses. Noninsertional alterations in the expression of protooncogenes or other cellular genes could also have a role in the leukemogenic and lymphomagenic processes associated with retroviral infection in murine species. Further studies are required for a better characterization of the molecular mechanisms related to such phenomena. In any case, it may be accepted that chronic retroviruses have no intrinsic oncogenic capability and that these viruses are associated with neoplastic diseases only through indirect mechanisms.

Human chronic retroviruses include the human T-cell lymphotropic viruses type I and type II (HTLV-I and HTLV-II) as well as the human immunodeficiency viruses type 1 and type 2 (HIV-1 and HIV-2). HTLVs may be involved in the etiology of two relatively rare hematologic neoplasms: HTLV-I in adult T-cell leukemia (ATL) and HTLV-II in the T-cell variety of human hairy leukemia. However, at least some patient with typical ATL are free from HTLV-I infection and only a few cases of human hairy T-cell leukemia have been found to be associated with HTLV-II infection. HIV-1 and HIV-2 are etiologically associated with the worldwide epidemic disease AIDS as well as with the AIDS-related complex. Since only a minority of the individuals infected with either HTLV or HIV viruses will develop the respective disease, factors other than viral infection must be importantly involved in the development of the diseases that have been found to be associated with these retroviruses.

REFERENCES

1. Ihle, J.N., Charman, H., and Gilden, R.V., Comparative biology of mammalian retroviruses, *Cancer Biol. Rev.*, 1, 133, 1980.
2. Gardner, M.B., Naturally occurring leukaemia viruses in wild mice: how good a model for humans?, *Cancer Surv.*, 6, 55, 1987.
3. Rasheed, S., Retroviruses and oncogenes in rats, in *Retroviruses and Human Pathology*, Gallo, R.C., Stehelin, D., and Varnier, O.E., Eds., Humana Press, Clifton, NJ, 1985, 153.
4. Bernhard, W., The detection and study of tumor viruses with the electron microscope, *Cancer Res.*, 20, 712, 1960.
5. Dalton, A.J., Further analysis of the detailed structure of type B and C particles, *J. Natl. Cancer Inst.*, 48, 1095, 1972.
6. Dalton, A.J., RNA tumor viruses — terminology and ultrastructural aspects of virion morphology and replication, *J. Natl. Cancer Inst.*, 49, 323, 1972.
7. Hanafusa, H., Cell transformation by RNA tumor viruses, in *Comprehensive Virology*, Vol. 10, Fraenkel-Conrat, H. and Wagner, R., Eds., Plenum Press, New York, 1977, 401.
8. Goff, S.P., The genetics of murine leukemia viruses, *Curr. Top. Microbiol. Immunol.*, 112, 45, 1984.
9. Essex, M.E., Feline leukemia: a naturally occurring cancer of infectious origin, *Epidemiol. Rev.*, 4, 189, 1982.
10. Hardy, W.D., Jr., Feline retroviruses, *Adv. Viral Oncol.*, 5, 1, 1985.
11. Wittmann, W. and Liebermann, H., Enzootische Rinderleukose, *Arch. Geschwulstforsch.*, 50, 686, 1980.
12. Burny, A., Bruck, H., Chantrene, H., Cleuter, Y., Dekegel, D., Ghysdael, J., Kettmann, R., Lellercq, M., Leunen, J., Mammerickx, M., and Portelle, D., Bovine leukemia virus: molecular biology and epidemiology, in *Viral Oncology*, Klein, G., Ed., Raven Press, New York, 1980, 231.
13. Gross, L., Viral etiology of leukemia and lymphomas in mice. A brief historical survey and present status, *Zentralbl. Bakteriol. Hyg.*, 220, 57, 1972.
14. Gallo, R.C. and Reitz, M.S., Jr., Human retroviruses and adult T-cell leukemia-lymphoma, *J. Natl. Cancer Inst.*, 69, 1209, 1982.
15. Blayney, D.W., Jaffe, E.S., Fisher, R.I., Schechter, G.P., Cossman, J., Robert-Guroff, M., Kalyanaraman, V.S., Blattner, W.A., and Gallo, R.C., The human T-cell leukemia/lymphoma virus, lymphoma, lytic bone lesions, and hypercalcemia, *Ann. Int. Med.*, 98, 144, 1983.
16. Yoshida, M., Human leukemia virus associated with adult T-cell leukemia, *Jpn. J. Cancer Res.*, 74, 777, 1983.
17. Broder, S., Bunn, P.A., Jaffe, E.S., Blattner, W., Gallo, R.C., Wong-Staal, F., Waldmann, T.A., and DeVita, V.T., T-cell lymphoproliferative syndrome associated with human T-cell leukemia/lymphoma virus, *Ann. Int. Med.*, 100, 543, 1984.
18. Sarin, P.S. and Gallo, R.C., Human T-lymphotropic retroviruses in adult T-cell leukemia-lymphoma and acquired immune deficiency syndrome, *J. Clin. Immunol.*, 4, 415, 1984.
19. Gallo, R.C. and Wong-Staal, F., Current thoughts on the viral etiology of certain human cancers, *Cancer Res.*, 44, 2742, 1984.
20. Sarin, P.S. and Gallo, R.C., Retroviruses in human T-cell malignancies, *Cancer Invest.*, 2, 467, 1984.
21. Hinuma, Y., Retrovirus in adult T-cell leukemia, *Progr. Med. Virol.*, 30, 156, 1984.
22. Sugamura, K. and Hinuma, Y., Human retrovirus in adult T-cell leukemia/lymphoma, *Immunol. Today*, 6, 83, 1985.
23. Hinuma, Y., Natural history of the retrovirus associated with a human leukemia, *BioEssays*, 3, 205, 1985.
24. Hunsmann, G. and Hinuma, Y., Human adult T-cell leukemia virus and its association with disease, *Adv. Viral Oncol.*, 5, 147, 1985.
25. Robert-Guroff, M., Markham, P.D., Popovic, M., and Gallo, R.C., Isolation, characterization, and biological effects of the first human retroviruses: the human T-lymphotropic retrovirus family, *Curr. Top. Microbiol. Immunol.*, 115, 7, 1985.

26. Wong-Staal, F., Some perspectives on the molecular mechanism of *in vitro* transformation and *in vivo* leukemogenesis by HTLV, *Curr. Top. Microbiol. Immunol.,* 115, 211, 1985.

27. Wantzin, G.L., The isolation of human T-cell leukemia lymphoma virus I, *Eur. J. Haematol.,* 38, 97, 1987.

28. Yoshida, M., Expression of the HTLV-1 genome and its association with a unique T-cell malignancy, *Biochim. Biophys. Acta,* 907, 145, 1987.

29. Broder, S. and Gallo, R.C., A pathogenic retrovirus (HTLV-III) linked to AIDS, *N. Engl. J. Med.,* 311, 1292, 1984.

30. Wong-Staal, F. and Gallo, R.C., The family of human T-lymphotropic leukemia viruses: HTLV-I as the cause of adult T-cell leukemia and HTLV-III as the cause of acquired immunodeficiency syndrome, *Blood,* 65, 253, 1985.

31. Gallo, R.C., The human T-cell leukemia/lymphotropic retroviruses (HTLV) family: past, present, and future, *Cancer Res.,* 45, 4524s, 1985.

32. Wong-Staal, F. and Gallo, R.C., Human T-lymphotropic retroviruses, *Nature,* 317, 395, 1985.

33. Curran, J.W., Morgan, W.M., Hardy, A.M., Jaffe, H.W., Darrow, W.W., and Dowdle, W.R., The epidemiology of AIDS: current status and future prospects, *Science,* 229, 1352, 1985.

34. Blattner, W.A. and Gallo, R.C., Human T-cell leukemia/lymphoma viruses: clinical and epidemiologic features, *Curr. Top. Microbiol. Immunol.,* 115, 67, 1985.

35. Gallo, R.C. and Wong-Staal, F., A human T-lymphotropic retrovirus (HTLV-III) as the cause of the acquired immunodeficiency syndrome, *Ann. Int. Med.,* 103, 679, 1985.

36. Gallo, R.C., Sarngadharan, M.G., Popovic, M., Shaw, G.M., Hahn, B., Wong-Staal, F., Robert-Guroff, M., Salahuddin, S.Z., and Markham, P.D., HTLV-III and the etiology of AIDS, *Prog. Allergy,* 37, 1, 1986.

37. Montagnier, L., Lymphadenopathy associated virus: its role in the pathogenesis of AIDS and related diseases, *Prog. Allergy,* 37, 46, 1986.

38. Gallo, R.C., Human tumor and immunodeficiency viruses, *AIDS Res. Hum. Retrovir.,* 3 (Suppl. 1), 187, 1988.

39. Levy, J.A., Joyner, J., and Borenfreund, E., Mouse sperm can horizontally transmit type C viruses, *J. Gen. Virol.,* 51, 439, 1980.

40. Portis, J.L., McAtee, F.J., and Hayes, S.F., Horizontal transmission of murine retroviruses, *J. Virol.,* 61, 1037, 1987.

41. Schneider, R., Feline malignant lymphoma: environmental factors and the occurrence of this viral cancer in cats, *Int. J. Cancer,* 10, 345, 1972.

42. Morse, H.S., III, Yetter, R.A., Stimpfling, J.H., Pitts, O.M., Fredrickson, T.N., and Hartley, J.W., Greying with age in mice: relation to expression of murine leukemia viruses, *Cell,* 41, 439, 1985.

43. Olsen, R.G., Lewis, M.G., Lafrado, L.J., Mathes, L.E., Hafter, K., and Sharpee, R., Feline leukemia virus: current status of the feline induced immune depression and immunoprevention, *Cancer Metast. Rev.,* 6, 234, 1987.

44. Bilello, J.A., Pitts, O.M., and Hoffman, P.M., Characterization of a progressive neurodegenerative disease induced by a temperature-sensitive Moloney murine leukemia virus infection, *J. Virol.,* 59, 234, 1986.

45. Earl, P.L., Moss, B., Morrison, R.P., Wehrly, K., Nishio, J., and Chesebro, B., T-lymphocyte priming and protection against Friend leukemia by vaccina-retrovirus *env* gene recombinant, *Science,* 234, 728, 1986.

46. To, R.Y.-L., Booth, S.C., and Neiman, P.E., Inhibition of retroviral replication by anti-sense RNA, *Mol. Cell. Biol.,* 6, 4758, 1986.

47. Rice, N.R., Simek, S.L., Dubois, G.C., Showalter, S.D., Gilden, R.V., and Stephens, R.M., Expression of the bovine leukemia virus X region in virus-infected cells, *J. Virol.,* 61, 1577, 1987.

48. Eisenman, R.N. and Vogt, V.M., The biosynthesis of oncovirus proteins, *Biochim. Biophys. Acta,* 473, 187, 1978.

49. Coffin, J.M., Structure, replication and recombination of retrovirus genome: some unifying hypotheses, *J. Gen. Virol.,* 42, 1, 1979.

50. Stacey, D.W., Microinjection studies of retroviral polynucleotides, *Curr. Top. Microbiol. Immunol.,* 123, 23, 1986.

51. August, J.T., Bolognesi, D.P., Fleissner, E., Gilden, R.V., and Nowinski, R.C., A proposed nomenclature for the virion proteins of oncogenic RNA viruses, *Virology,* 60, 595, 1974.

52. Leis, J., Baltimore, D., Bishop, J.M., Coffin, J., Fleissner, E., Goff, S.P., Oroszlan, S., Robinson, H., Skalka, A.M., Temin, H.M., and Vogt, V., Standardized and simplified nomenclature for proteins common to all retroviruses, *J. Virol.,* 62, 1808, 1988.

53. Bova, C.A., Manfredi, J.P., and Swanstrom, R., *env* genes of avian retroviruses: nucleotide sequence and molecular recombinants define host range determinants, *Virology,* 152, 343, 1986.

54. Rein, A., McClure, M.R., Rice, N.R., Luftig, R.B., and Schultz, A.M., Myristylation site in Pr65[gag] is essential for virus particle formation by Moloney murine leukemia virus, *Proc. Natl. Acad. Sci. U.S.A.,* 83, 7246, 1986.

55. Rhee, S.S. and Hunter, E., Myristylation is required for intracellular transport but not for assembly of D-type retrovirus capsids, *J. Virol.,* 61, 1045, 1987.

56. Lewis, M.G., Chang, J.Y., Olsen, R.G., and Fertel, R.H., Identification of calmodulin activity in purified retroviruses, *Biochem. Biophys. Res. Commun.,* 141, 1077, 1986.

57. Chen, H.R. and Barker, W.C., Nucleotide sequences of the retroviral long terminal repeats and their adjacent regions, *Nucleic Acids Res.,* 12, 1767, 1984.

58. Ostrowski, M.C., Berard, D., and Hager, G.L., Specific transcriptional initiation *in vitro* on murine type C retrovirus promoters, *Proc. Natl. Acad. Sci. U.S.A.,* 78, 4485, 1981.

59. Mitsialis, S.A., Manley, J.L., and Guntaka, R.V., Localization of active promoters for eucaryotic RNA polymerase II in the long terminal repeat of avian sarcoma virus DNA, *Mol. Cell. Biol.,* 3, 811, 1983.

60. Derse, D. and Casey, J.W., Two elements in the bovine leukemia virus long terminal repeat that regulate gene expression, *Science,* 231, 1437, 1986.

61. Celander, D., Hsu, B.L., and Haseltine, W.A., Regulatory elements within the murine leukemia virus enhancer regions mediate glucocorticoid responsiveness, *J. Virol.,* 62, 1314, 1988.

62. Casey, J.W., Roach, A., Mullins, J.I., Burck, K.B., Nicolson, M.O., Gardner, M.B., and Davidson, N., The U3 portion of feline leukemia virus DNA identify horizontally acquired proviruses in leukemic cats, *Proc. Natl. Acad. Sci. U.S.A.,* 78, 7778, 1981.

63. Schulze, F., Boehnlein, E., and Gruss, P., Mutational analyses of the Moloney murine sarcoma virus enhancer, *DNA,* 4, 193, 1985.

64. Sealey, L. and Chalkley, R., At least two nuclear proteins bind specifically to the Rous sarcoma virus long terminal repeat enhancer, *Mol. Cell. Biol.,* 7, 787, 1987.

65. Arrigo, S., Yun, M., and Beemon, K., *cis*-Acting regulatory elements within *gag* genes of avian retroviruses, *Mol. Cell. Biol.,* 7, 388, 1987.

66. Brand, A.H., Breeden, L., Abraham, J., Sternglanz, R., and Nasmyth, K., Characterization of a "silencer" in yeast: a DNA sequence with properties opposite to those of a transcriptional enhancer, *Cell,* 41, 41, 1985.

67. Baltimore, D., An RNA-dependent DNA polymerase in virions of RNA tumor viruses, *Nature,* 226, 1209, 1970.

68. Baltimore, D., RNA-dependent synthesis of DNA by virions of mouse leukemia virus, *Cold Spring Harbor Symp. Quant. Biol.,* 35, 843, 1970.

69. Skalka, A.M. and Leis, J., Retroviral DNA integration, *BioEssays,* 1, 206, 1984.

70. Cobrink, D., Katz, R., Terry, R., Skalka, A.M., and Leis, J., Avian sarcoma and leukosis virus *pol*-endonuclease recognition of the tandem long terminal repeat junction: minimum site required for cleavage is also required for viral growth, *J. Virol.,* 61, 1999, 1987.

71. Summers, J. and Mason, W.S., Replication of the genome of a hepatitis B-like virus by reverse transcription of an RNA intermediate, *Cell,* 29, 403, 1982.

72. Miller, R.H., Close evolutionary relatedness of the hepatitis B virus and murine leukemia virus polymerase gene sequences, *Virology,* 164, 147, 1988.

73. Poiesz, B.J., Seal, G., and Loeb, L.A., Reverse transcriptase: correlation of zinc content with activity, *Proc. Natl. Acad. Sci. U.S.A.,* 71, 4892, 1974.

74. Hu, S.C., Court, D.L., Zweig, M., and Levin, J.G., Murine leukemia virus *pol* gene products: analysis with antisera generated against reverse transcriptase and endonuclease fusion proteins expressed in *Escherichia coli, J. Virol.,* 60, 267, 1986.

75. Roth, M.J., Tanese, N., and Goff, S.P., Purification and characterization of murine retroviral reverse transcriptase expressed in *Escherichia coli, J. Biol. Chem.,* 260, 9326, 1985.

76. Alexander, F., Leis, J., Soltis, D.A., Crowl, R.M., Danho, W., Poonian, M.S., Pan, Y.-C.E., and Skalka, A.M., Proteolytic processing of avian sarcoma and leukosis viruses *pol-endo* recombinant proteins reveals another *pol* gene domain, *J. Virol.,* 61, 534, 1987.

77. Hippenmeyer, P.J. and Grandgenett, D.P., Mutants of the Rous sarcoma virus reverse transcriptase gene are nondefective in early replication events, *J. Biol. Chem.,* 260, 8250, 1985.

78. Wu, A.M., Ting, R.C.Y., and Gallo, R.C., RNA-directed DNA polymerase and virus-induced leukemia in mice, *Proc. Natl. Acad. Sci. U.S.A.,* 70, 1298, 1973.

79. Tsutsui, K. and Mueller, G.C., Hemin inhibits virion-associated reverse transcriptase of murine leukemia virus, *Biochem. Biophys. Res. Commun.,* 149, 628, 1987.

80. Schwarz-Sommer, Z., Leclercq, L., Göbel, E., and Saedler, H., Cin4, an insert altering the structure of the *A1* gene in *Zea mays*, exhibits properties of nonviral retrotransposons, *EMBO J.,* 6, 3873, 1987.

81. Nevers, P. and Saedler, H., Transposable genetic elements as agents of gene instability and chromosomal rearrangements, *Nature,* 268, 109, 1977.

82. Calos, M.P. and Miller, J.H., Transposable elements, *Cell,* 20, 579, 1980.

83. Starlinger, P., IS elements and transposons, *Plasmid,* 3, 241, 1980.

84. Strobel, E., Mobile dispersed repeated DNA elements in the *Drosophila* genome, *Fed. Proc. Fed. Am. Soc. Exp. Biol.,* 41, 2656, 1982.

85. Starlinger, P., Transposable elements, *Trends Biochem. Sci.,* 9, 125, 1984.

86. Finnegan, D.J., Transposable elements in eukaryotes, *Int. Rev. Cytol.,* 93, 281, 1985.

87. Starlinger, P., Transposable elements in plants, *Biol. Chem. Hoppe-Seyler,* 366, 931, 1985.

88. Peterson, P.A., Transposon-induced events at gene loci, *BioEssays,* 3, 199, 1985.

89. Hull, R. and Covey, S.N., Genome organization and expression of reverse transcribing elements: variations and a theme, *J. Gen. Virol.,* 67, 1751, 1986.
90. Weiner, A.M., Deininger, P.L., and Efstratiadis, A., Nonviral retroposons: genes, pseudogenes, and transposable elements generated by the reverse flow of genetic information, *Annu. Rev. Biochem.,* 55, 631, 1986.
91. Shimotono, K., Mizutani, S., and Temin, H.M., Sequence of retrovirus provirus resembles that of bacterial transposable elements, *Nature,* 285, 550, 1980.
92. Ju, G. and Skalka, A.M., Nucleotide sequence analysis of the long terminal repeat (LTR) of avian retroviruses: structural similarities with transposable elements, *Cell,* 22, 379, 1980.
93. Swanstrom, R., DeLorbe, W.J., Bishop, J.M., and Varmus, H.E., Nucleotide sequence of cloned unintegrated avian sarcoma virus DNA: viral DNA contains direct and inverted repeats similar to those in transposable elements, *Proc. Natl. Acad. Sci. U.S.A.,* 78, 124, 1981.
94. Temin, H., Function of the retrovirus long terminal repeat, *Cell,* 28, 3, 1982.
95. Ju, G., Hishinuma, F., and Skalka, A.M., Nucleotide sequence analysis of avian retroviruses: structural similarities with transposable elements, *Fed. Proc. Fed. Am. Soc. Exp. Biol.,* 41, 2659, 1982.
96. Shiba, T. and Saigo, K., Retrovirus-like particles containing RNA homologous to the transposable element *copia* in *Drosophila melanogaster*, *Nature,* 302, 119, 1983.
97. Kugimiya, W., Ikenaga, H., and Saigo, K., Close relationship between the long terminal repeats of avian leukosis-sarcoma virus and *copia*-like movable genetic elements of *Drosophila*, *Proc. Natl. Acad. Sci. U.S.A.,* 80, 3193, 1983.
98. Mount, S.M. and Rubin, G.M., Complete nucleotide sequence of the *Drosophila* transposable element copia: homology between copia and retroviral proteins, *Mol. Cell. Biol.,* 5, 1630, 1985.
99. Panganiban, A.T., Retroviral DNA integration, *Cell,* 42, 5, 1985.
100. Lützelschwab, R., Müller, G., Wälder, B., Schmidt, O., Fürbass, R., and Mechler, B., Insertion mutation inactivates the expression of the recessive oncogene *lethal(2)giant larvae* of *Drosophila melanogaster*, *Mol. Gen. Genet.,* 204, 58, 1986.
101. Gateff, E., Malignant neoplasms of genetic origin in *Drosophila melanogaster*, *Science,* 200, 1448, 1978.
102. Opper, M., Schuler, G., and Mechler, B.M., Hereditary suppression of *lethal (2) giant larvae* malignant tumor development in *Drosophila* by gene transfer, *Oncogene,* 1, 91, 1987.
103. Gateff, E. and Mechler, B.M., Tumor-suppressor genes of *Drosophila melanogaster*, *Crit. Rev. Oncogenesis,* 1(2), 221, 1989.
104. Wirth, T., Schmidt, M., Baumruker, T., and Horak, I., Evidence for mobility of a new family of mouse middle repetitive DNA elements (LTR-IS), *Nucleic Acids Res.,* 12, 3603, 1984.
105. Rogers, J., Retroposons defined, *Nature,* 301, 460, 1983.
106. Rogers, J.H., The origin and evolution of retroposons, *Int. Rev. Cytol.,* 93, 187, 1985.
107. Temin, H.M., Reverse transcription in the eukaryotic genom: retroviruses, pararetroviruses, retrotransposons, and retrotranscripts, *Mol. Cell. Evol.,* 2, 455, 1985.
108. Jagadeeswaran, P., Forget, B.G., and Weisman, S.M., Short interspersed repetitive DNA elements in eucaryotes: transposable DNA elements generated by reverse transcription of RNA pol III transcripts?, *Cell,* 26, 141, 1981.
109. Calabretta, B., Robberson, D.L., Barrera-Saldana, H.A., Lambrou, T.P., and Sauders, G.F., Genome instability in a region of human DNA enriched in *Alu* repeat sequences, *Nature,* 296, 219, 1982.
110. Davidson, E.H. and Posakony, J.W., Repetitive sequence transcripts in development, *Nature,* 297, 633, 1982.
111. Jelinek, W.R. and Schmid, C.W., Repetitive sequences in eukaryotic DNA and their expression, *Annu. Rev. Biochem.,* 51, 813, 1982.
112. Baltimore, D., Retroviruses and retrotransposons: the role of reverse transcription in shaping the eukaryotic genome, *Cell,* 40, 481, 1985.
113. Paulson, K.E., Deka, N., Schmid, C.W., Misra, R., Schindler, C.W., Rush, M.G., Kadyk, L., and Leinwand, L., A transposon-like element in human DNA, *Nature,* 316, 359, 1985.
114. Flügel, R.M., Maurer, B., Bannert, H., Rethwilm, A., Schnitzler, P., and Darai, G., Nucleotide sequence analysis of a cloned DNA fragment from human cells reveals homology to retrotransposons, *Mol. Cell. Biol.,* 7, 231, 1987.
115. Grigoryan, M.S., Kramerov, D.A., Tulchinsky, E.M., Revasova, E.S., and Lukanidin, E.M., Activation of putative transposition intermediate formation in tumor cells, *EMBO J.,* 4, 2209, 1985.
116. Singer, M.F., Highly repeated sequences in mammalian genomes, *Int. Rev. Cytol.,* 76, 67, 1982.
117. Hardman, N., Structure and function of repetitive DNA in eukaryotes, *Biochem. J.,* 234, 1, 1986.
118. Musich, P.R. and Dykes, R.J., A long interspersed (LINE) DNA exhibiting polymorphic patterns in human genomes, *Proc. Natl. Acad. Sci. U.S.A.,* 83, 4854, 1986.
119. Fanning, T. and Singer, M., The LINE-1 DNA sequences in four mammalian orders predict proteins that conserve homologies to retrovirus proteins, *Nucleic Acids Res.,* 15, 2251, 1987.
120. Fanning, T.G. and Singer, M.F., LINE-1: a mammalian transposable element, *Biochim. Biophys. Acta,* 910, 203, 1987.

121. Skowronski, J. and Singer, M.F., Expression of a cytoplasmic LINE-1 transcript is regulated in a human teratocarcinoma cell line, *Proc. Natl. Acad. Sci. U.S.A.,* 82, 6050, 1985.
122. Schmid, C.W. and Jelinek, W.R., The *alu* family of dispersed repetitive sequences, *Science,* 216, 1065, 1982.
123. Kariya, Y., Kato, K., Hayashizaki, Y., Himeno, S., Tarui, S., and Matsubara, K., Revision of consensus sequence of human *Alu* repeats — a review, *Gene,* 53, 1, 1987.
124. Bains, W., The multiple origins of human Alu sequences, *J. Mol. Evol.,* 23, 189, 1986.
125. Paulson, K.E. and Schmid, C.W., Transcriptional inactivity of Alu repeats in HeLa cells, *Nucleic Acids Res.,* 14, 6145, 1986.
126. Mermer, B., Colb, M., and Krontiris, T.G., A family of short, interspersed repeats is associated with tandemly repetitive DNA in human genome, *Proc. Natl. Acad. Sci. U.S.A.,* 84, 3320, 1987.
127. Ono, M., Kawakami, M., and Takezawa, T., A novel human nonviral retroposon derived from an endogenous retrovirus, *Nucleic Acids Res.,* 15, 8725, 1987.
128. Baskin, F., Grossman, A., Bhagat, S.G., Burns, D., Davis, R.M., Warmoth, L.A., and Rosenberg, R.N., Frequent alterations of specific reiterated DNA sequence abundances in human cancer, *Cancer Genet. Cytogenet.,* 28, 163, 1987.
129. Morse, B., Rothberg, P.G., South, V.J., Spandorfer, J.M., and Astrin, S.M., Insertional mutagenesis of the *myc* locus by a LINE-1 sequence in a human breast carcinoma, *Nature,* 333, 87, 1988.
130. Tsichlis, P.N., Oncogenesis by Moloney murine leukemia virus, *Anticancer Res.,* 7, 171, 1987.
131. Hardy, W.D., Jr., McClelland, A.J., Zuckerman, E.E., Snyder, H.W., Jr., MacEwen, E.G., Francis, D., and Essex, M., Development of virus non-producer lymphosarcomas in pet cats exposed to FeLV, *Nature,* 288, 90, 1980.
132. Niman, H.L., Akhavi, M., Gardner, M.B., Stephenson, J.R., and Roy-Burman, P., Differential expression of two distinct endogenous retrovirus genomes in developing tissues of the domestic cat, *J. Natl. Cancer Inst.,* 64, 587, 1980.
133. Koshy, R., Gallo, R.C., and Wong-Staal, F., Characterization of the endogenous feline leukemia virus-related DNA sequences in cats and attempts to identify exogenous viral sequences in tissues of virus-negative leukemic animals, *Virology,* 103, 434, 1980.
134. Blank, K.J. and Klyczek, K.K., Host genetic control of retrovirus-induced leukemogenesis in the mouse: direct genetic and epistatic effects, *J. Leukocyte Biol.,* 40, 479, 1986.
135. Furth, J., Seibold, H.R., and Rathbone, R.R., Experimental studies on lymphomatosis of mice, *Am. J. Cancer,* 19, 521, 1933.
136. Gross, L., "Spontaneous" leukemia developing in C3H mice following inoculation, in infancy, with AK-leukemic extracts or AK-embryos, *Proc. Soc. Exp. Biol. Med.,* 76, 27, 1951.
137. Friend, C., Cell-free transmission in adult Swiss mice of a disease having the characteristics of a leukemia, *J. Exp. Med.,* 105, 307, 1957.
138. Wendling, F., Moreau-Gachelin, F., and Tambourin, P., Emergence of tumorigenic cells during the course of Friend virus leukemias, *Proc. Natl. Acad. Sci. U.S.A.,* 78, 3614, 1981.
139. Dandekar, S., Rossitto, P., Pickett, S., Mockli, G., Bradshaw, H., Cardiff, R., and Gardner, M., Molecular characterization of the *Akvr-1* restriction gene: a defective endogenous retrovirus-borne gene identical to *Fv-4^r, J. Virol.,* 61, 308, 1987.
140. Kozak, C.A., Susceptibility of wild mouse cells to exogenous infection with xenotropic leukemia viruses: control by a single dominant locus on chromosome 1, *J. Virol.,* 55, 690, 1985.
141. Ruscetti, S., Matthai, R., and Potter, M., Susceptibility of BALB/c mice carrying various DBA/2 genes to development of Friend murine leukemia virus-induced erythroleukemia, *J. Exp. Med.,* 162, 1579, 1985.
142. Silver, J., Genetic study of lymphoma induction by Friend murine leukemia virus in crosses involving AKR mice, *J. Natl. Cancer Inst.,* 77, 793, 1986.
143. Kawakami, T.G., Kollias, G.V., Jr., and Holmberg, C., Oncogenicity of gibbon type-C myelogenous leukemia virus, *Int. J. Cancer,* 25, 641, 1980.
144. Ferrer, J.F., Kenyon, S.J., and Gupta, P., Milk of dairy cows frequently contains a leukemogenic virus, *Science,* 213, 1014, 1981.
145. Bender, A.P., Robison, L.L., Kashmiri, S.V.S., McClain, K.L., Woods, W.G., Smithson, W.A., Heyn, R., Finlay, J., Schuman, L.M., Renier, C., and Gibson, R., No involvement of bovine leukemia virus in childhood acute lymphoblastic leukemia and non-Hodgkin's lymphoma, *Cancer Res.,* 48, 2919, 1988.
146. Flamant, F., Gurin, C.C., and Sorge, J.A., An embryonic DNA-binding protein specific for the promoter of the retrovirus long terminal repat, *Mol. Cell. Biol.,* 7, 3548, 1987.
147. Shih, C.-C., Stoye, J.P., and Coffin, J.M., Highly preferred targets for retrovirus integration, *Cell,* 53, 531, 1988.
148. Sola, B., Heard, J.-M., Fichelson, S., Martial, M.-A., Pozo, F., Bordereaux, D., and Gisselbrecht, S., Monoclonal proliferation of Friend murine leukemia virus-transformed myeloblastic cells occurs early in the leukemogenic process, *Mol. Cell. Biol.,* 5, 1009, 1985.
149. King, W., Patel, M.D., Lobel, L.I., Goff, S.P., and Nguyen-Huu, M.C., Insertion mutagenesis of embryonal carcinoma cells by retroviruses, *Science,* 228, 554, 1985.

150. Luciw, P.A., Oppermann, H., Bishop, J.M., and Varmus, H.E., Integration and expression of several molecular forms of Rous sarcoma virus DNA used for transfection of mouse cells, *Mol. Cell. Biol.,* 4, 1260, 1984.

151. Kettmann, R., Deschamps, J., Cleuter, Y., Couez, D., Burny, A., and Marbaix, G., Leukemogenesis by bovine leukemia virus: proviral DNA integration and lack of RNA expression of viral long terminal repeat and 3′ proximate cellular sequences, *Proc. Natl. Acad. Sci. U.S.A.,* 79, 2465, 1982.

152. Kettmann, R., Deschamps, J., Couez, D., Claustriaux, J., Palm, R., and Burny, A., Chromosome integration domain for bovine leukemia provirus in tumors, *J. Virol.,* 47, 146, 1983.

153. Gregoire, D., Couez, D., Deschamps, J., Heuertz, S., Hors-Cayla, M.-C., Szpirer, J., Szpirer, C., Burny, A., Huez, G., and Kettmann, R., Different bovine leukemia virus-induced tumors harbor the provirus in different chromosomes, *J. Virol.,* 50, 275, 1984.

154. Seiki, M., Eddy, R., Shows, T.B., and Yoshida, M., Nonspecific integration of the HTLV provirus genome into adult T-cell leukaemia cells, *Nature,* 309, 640, 1984.

155. Rosen, C.A., Haseltine, W.A., Lenz, J., Ruprecht, R., and Cloyd, M.W., Tissue selectivity of murine leukemia virus infection is determined by long terminal repeat sequences, *J. Virol.,* 55, 862, 1985.

156. Hoshino, H., Esumi, H., Miwa, M., Shimoyama, M., Minato, K., Tobinai, K., Hirose, M., Watanabe, S., Inada, N., Kinoshita, K., Kamihira, S., Ichimaru, M., and Sugimura, T., *Proc. Natl. Acad. Sci. U.S.A.,* 80, 6061, 1983.

157. Wolfson, M., Aboud, M., Ofir, R., Weinstein, Y., and Segal, S., Modulation of protein kinase C and Ca^{2+} lipid-independent protein kinase in lymphoma induced by Moloney murine leukemia virus in BALB/c mice, *Int. J. Cancer,* 37, 589, 1986.

158. Virelizier, J.L., Mechanisms of immunodepression induced by viruses: possible role of infected macrophages, *Biomedicine,* 22, 255, 1975.

159. Herberman, R.B., Holden, H.T., Ting, C.-C., Lavrin, D.L., and Kirchner, H., Cell-mediated immunity to leukemia virus- and tumor-associated antigens in mice, *Cancer Res.,* 36, 615, 1976.

160. Lutz, H., Pedersen, N., Higgins, J., Hübscher, U., Troy, F.A., and Theilen, G.H., Humoral immune reactivity to feline leukemia virus and associated antigens in cats naturally infected with feline leukemia virus, *Cancer Res.,* 40, 3642, 1980.

161. Rojko, J.L., Hoover, E.A., Quackenbush, S.L., and Olsen, R.G., Reactivation of latent feline leukaemia virus infection, *Nature,* 298, 385, 1982.

162. Perryman, L.E., Hoover, E.A., and Yohn, D.S., Immunologic reactivity of the cat: immunosuppression in experimental feline leukemia, *J. Natl. Cancer Inst.,* 49, 1357, 1972.

163. Cockerell, G.L., Hoover, E.A., and Krakowka, S., Lymphocyte mitogen reactivity and enumeration of circulating B- and T-cells during feline leukemia virus infection in the cat, *J. Natl. Cancer Inst.,* 57, 1995, 1976.

164. Mullins, J.I., Chen, C.S., and Hoover, E.A., Disease-specific and tissue-specific production of unintegrated feline leukaemia virus variant DNA in feline AIDS, *Nature,* 319, 333, 1986.

165. Overbaugh, J., Donahue, P.R., Quackenbush, S.L., Hoover, E.A., and Mullins, J.I., Molecular cloning of a feline leukemia virus that induced fatal immunodeficiency disease in cats, *Science,* 239, 906, 1988.

166. Cianciolo, G.J., Copeland, T.D., Oroszlan, S., and Snyderman, R., Inhibition of lymphocyte proliferation by a synthetic peptide homologous to retroviral envelope proteins, *Science,* 230, 453, 1985.

167. Jacquemin, P.C., Strijckmans, P., and Thiry, L., Study of the expression of a glycoprotein of retroviral origin in the plasma of patients with hematologic disorders and in the plasma of normal individuals, *Blood,* 64, 832, 1984.

168. Mann, D.L., Lasane, F., Popovic, M., Arthur, L.O., Robey, W.G., Blattner, W.A., and Newman, M.J., HTLV-III large envelope protein (gp120) suppresses PHA-induced lymphocyte blastogenesis, *J. Immunol.,* 238, 2640, 1987.

169. Flavell, R.A., Allen, H., Burkly, L.C., Sherman, D.H., Waneck, G.L., and Widera, G., Molecular biology of the H-2 histocompatibility complex, *Science,* 233, 437, 1986.

170. Festenstein, H., The biological consequences of altered MHC expression on tumours, *Br. Med. Bull.,* 43, 217, 1987.

171. Meruelo, D., Kornreich, R., Rossomando, A., Pampeno, C., Boral, A., Silver, J.L., Buxbaum, J., Weiss, E.H., Devlin, J.J., Mellor, A.L., Flavell, R.A., and Pellicer, A., Lack of class I H-2 antigens in cells transformed by radiation leukemia virus is associated with methylation and rearrangement of H-2 DNA, *Proc. Natl. Acad. Sci. U.S.A.,* 83, 4504, 1986.

172. Flyer, D.C., Burakoff, S.J., and Faller, D.V., Retrovirus-induced changes in major histocompatibility complex antigen expression influenced susceptibility to lysis by cytotoxic T lymphocytes, *J. Immunol.,* 135, 2287, 1985.

173. Wilson, L.D., Flyer, D.C., and Faller, D.V., Murine retroviruses control class I major histocompatibility antigen gene expression via a *trans* effect at the transcriptional level, *Mol. Cell. Biol.,* 7, 2406, 1987.

174. Price, P.J., Suk, W.A., and Freeman, A.E., Type C RNA tumor viruses as determinants of chemical carcinogenesis: effects of sequence of treatment, *Science,* 177, 1033, 1972.

175. Hassan, Y., Wolfson, M., and Aboud, M., Phenotypic heterogeneity in 3-methylcholanthrene-induced transformation of normal rat kidney cells infected with Moloney murine leukemia virus, *Cell Biol. Int. Rep.,* 10, 19, 1986.

176. Schaller, J.P., Mathes, L.E., Hoover, E.A., and Olsen, R.G., Enhancement of feline leukemia virus-induced leukemogenesis in cats exposed to methylnitrosourea, *Int. J. Cancer,* 24, 700, 1979.

177. Raikow, R.B., Okuwenick, J.P., Buffo, M.J., Jones, D.L., Brozovich, B.J., Seeman, P.R., and Koval, T.M., Potentiating effect of benzo(a)pyrene and caffeine on Friend viral leukemogenesis, *Carcinogenesis,* 2, 1, 1981.

178. Howard, D.K., Schlom, J., and Fisher, P.B., Chemical carcinogen-mouse mammary tumor virus interactions in cell transformation, *In Vitro,* 19, 58, 1983.

179. Smith, G.H., Arthur, L.A., and Medina, D., Evidence of separate pathways for viral and chemical carcinogenesis in C3H/StWi mouse mammary glands, *Int. J. Cancer,* 26, 373, 1980.

180. Stockert, E., O'Donnell, P.V., Obata, Y., and Old, L.J., Inhibition of AKR leukemogenesis by SMX-1, a dualtropic murine leukemia virus, *Proc. Natl. Acad. Sci. U.S.A.,* 77, 3720, 1980.

181. Chow, V., Ben-David, Y., Bernstein, A., Benchimol, S., and Mowat, M., Multistage Friend erythroleukemia: independent origin of tumor clones with normal or rearranged p53 cellular oncogenes, *J. Virol.,* 61, 2777, 1987.

182. Greenberger, J.S., Daugherty, C., Sakakeeny, M.A., Braun, J., Pierce, J.H., Eckner, R.J., and FitzGerald, T.J., Friend virus-infected long-term bone marrow cultures produce colony stimulating factor dependent and independent granulocyte-macrophage progenitor cells for over four years *in vitro, Leukemia Res.,* 11, 51, 1987.

183. Wendling, F., Varlet, P., Charon, M., and Tambourin, P., MPLV: a retrovirus complex inducing an acute myeloproliferative leukemic disorder in adult mice, *Virology,* 149, 242, 1986.

184. Penciolelli, J.F., Wendling, F., Robert-Lezenes, J., Barque, J.P., Tambourin, P., and Gisselbrecht, S., Genetic analysis of myeloproliferative leukemia virus, a novel acute leukemogenic replication-defective retrovirus, *J. Virol.,* 61, 579, 1987.

185. Wolff, L. and Ruscetti, S., Malignant transformation of erythroid cells *in vivo* by introduction of a nonreplicating retrovirus vector, *Science,* 228, 1549, 1985.

186. Wolff, L., Tambourin, P., and Ruscetti, S., Induction of the autonomous stage of transformation in erythroid cells infected with SFFV: helper virus is not required, *Virology,* 152, 272, 1986.

187. Evans, L.H., and Morrey, J.D., Tissue-specific replication of Friend and Moloney murine leukemia viruses in infected mice, *J. Virol.,* 61, 1350, 1987.

188. DesGroseillers, L. and Jolicoeur, P., The tandem direct repeats within the long terminal repeat of murine leukemia viruses are the primary determinant of their leukemogenic potential, *J. Virol.,* 52, 945, 1984.

189. Short, M.K., Okenquist, S.A., and Lenz, J., Correlation of leukemogenic potential of murine retroviruses with transcriptional tissue preference of the viral long terminal repeats, *J. Virol.,* 61, 1067, 1987.

190. Ishimoto, A., Adachi, A., Sakai, K., and Matsuyama, M., Long terminal repeat of Friend-MCF virus contains the sequence responsible for erythroid leukemia, *Virology,* 141, 30, 1985.

191. Wolff, L. and Ruscetti, S., Tissue tropism of a leukemogenic murine retrovirus is determined by sequences outside the long terminal repeats, *Proc. Natl. Acad. Sci. U.S.A.,* 83, 3376, 1986.

192. Rogers, B.L. and Saunders, G.F., Transcriptional enhancers play a major role in gene expression, *BioEssays,* 4, 62, 1986.

193. Lang, J.C. and Spandidos, D.A., The structure and function of eukaryotic enhancer elements and their role in oncogenesis, *Anticancer Res.,* 6, 437, 1986.

194. Cullen, B.R., Raymond, K., and Ju, G., Transcriptional activity of avian retroviral long terminal repeats directly correlates with enhancer activity, *J. Virol.,* 53, 515, 1985.

195. Khoury, G. and Gruss, P., Enhancer elements, *Cell,* 33, 313, 1983.

196. Cullen, B.R., Raymond, K., Berg, P.E., and Ju, G., Functional analysis of the transcription control region located within the avian retroviral long terminal repeat, *Mol. Cell. Biol.,* 5, 438, 1985.

197. Taketo, M. and Tanaka, M., A cellular enhancer of retrovirus gene expression in embryonal carcinoma cells, *Proc. Natl. Acad. Sci. U.S.A.,* 84, 3748, 1987.

198. Mosthaf, L., Pawlita, M., and Gruss, P., A viral enhancer element specifically active in human haematopoietic cells, *Nature,* 315, 597, 1985.

199. Li, Y., Golemis, E., Hartley, J.W., and Hopkins, N., Disease specificity of nondefective Friend and Moloney murine leukemia viruses is controlled by a small number of nucleotides, *J. Virol.,* 61, 693, 1987.

200. Lenz, J., Celander, D., Crowther, R.L., Patarca, R., Perkins, D.W., and Haseltine, W.A., Determination of the leukaemogenicity of a murine retrovirus by sequences within the long terminal repeat, *Nature,* 308, 467, 1984.

201. Weber, F. and Schaffner, W., Enhancer activity correlates with the oncogenic potential of avian retroviruses, *EMBO J.,* 4, 949, 1985.

202. Rosen, C.A., Sodroski, J.G., Kettman, R., and Haseltine, W.A., Activation of enhancer sequences in type II human T-cell leukemia virus and bovine leukemia virus long terminal repeats by virus-associated *trans*-acting regulatory factors, *J. Virol.,* 57, 738, 1986.

203. Derse, D., Caradonna, S.J., and Casey, J.W., Bovine leukemia virus long terminal repeat: a cell type-specific promoter, *Science,* 227, 317, 1985.

204. Yoshimura, F.K. and Chaffin, K., Different activities of viral enhancer elements before and after stable integration of transfected DNAs, *Mol. Cell. Biol.,* 7, 1296, 1987.

205. Vijaya, S., Steffen, D.L., and Robinson, H.L., Acceptor sites for retroviral integrations map near DNase I-hypersensitive sites in chromatin, *J. Virol.,* 60, 683, 1986.

206. Varmus, H.E., Quintrell, N., and Ortiz, S., Retroviruses as mutagens: insertion and excision of a nontransforming provirus alter expression of a resident transforming provirus, *Cell,* 25, 23, 1981.
207. Neel, B.G., Hayward, W.S., Robinson, H.L., Fang, J., and Astrin, S.M., Avian leukosis virus-induced tumors have common proviral integration sites and synthesize discrete new RNAs: oncogenesis by promoter insertion, *Cell,* 23, 323, 1981.
208. Hayward, W.S., Neel, B.G., and Astrin, S.M., Activation of a cellular *onc* gene by promoter insertion in ALV-induced lymphoid leukosis, *Nature,* 290, 475, 1981.
209. Fung, Y-K.T., Fadly, A.M., Crittenden, L.B., and Kung, H.-J., On the mechanism of retrovirus-induced avian lymphoid leukosis: deletion and integration of the proviruses, *Proc. Natl. Acad. Sci. U.S.A.,* 78, 3418, 1981.
210. Etkind, P.R. and Sarkar, N.H., Integration of new endogenous mouse mammary tumor virus proviral DNA at common sites in the DNA of mammary tumors of C3Hf mice and hypomethylation of the endogenous mouse mammary tumor virus proviral DNA in C3Hf mammary tumors and spleens, *J. Virol.,* 45, 114, 1983.
211. Mölders, H., Defesche, J., Müller, D., Bonner, T.I., Rapp, U.R., and Müller, R., Integration of transfected LTR sequences into the c-*raf* proto-oncogene: activation by promoter insertion, *EMBO J.,* 4, 693, 1985.
212. Nusse, R., The activation of cellular oncogenes by retroviral insertion, *Trends Genet.,* 2, 244, 1986.
213. Cullen, B.R., Lomedico, P.T., and Ju, G., Transcriptional interference in avian retroviruses: implications for the promoter insertion model of leukaemogenesis, *Nature,* 307, 241, 1984.
214. Schubach, W. and Groudine, M., Alteration of c-*myc* chromatin structure by avian leukosis virus integration, *Nature,* 307, 702, 1984.
215. Linial, M. and Groudine, M., Transcription of three c-*myc* exons is enhanced in chicken bursal lymphoma cell lines, *Proc. Natl. Acad. Sci. U.S.A.,* 82, 53, 1985.
216. Nottenburg, C., Stubblefield, E., and Varmus, H.E., An aberrant avian leukosis virus provirus inserted downstream from the chicken c-*myc* coding sequence in a bursal lymphoma results from intrachromosomal recombination between two proviruses and deletion of cellular DNA, *J. Virol.,* 61, 1828, 1987.
217. Swift, R.A., Shaller, E., Witter, R.L., and Kung, H.-J., Insertional activation of c-*myc* by reticuloendotheliosis virus in chicken B lymphoma: nonrandom distribution and orientation of the proviruses, *J. Virol.,* 54, 869, 1985.
218. Swift, R.A., Boerkoel, C., Ridgway, A., Fujita, D.J., Dogdson, J.B., and Kung, H.-J., B-lymphoma induction by reticuloendotheliosis virus: characterization of a mutated chicken syncytial virus provirus involved in c-*myc* activation, *J. Virol.,* 61, 2084, 1987.
219. Witter, R., Sharma, J.M., and Fadly, A.M., Nonbursal lymphomas induced by nondefective reticuloendotheliosis virus, *Avian Pathol.,* 15, 467, 1986.
220. Isfort, R., Witter, R.L., and Kung, H.-J., c-*myc* activation in an unusual retrovirus-induced avian T-lymphoma resembling Marek's disease: proviral insertion 5' of exon one enhances the expression of an intron promoter, *Oncogene Res.,* 2, 81, 1987.
221. Wirschubsky, Z., Tsichlis, P., Klein, G., and Sumegi, J., Rearrangement of c-*myc*, *pim*-1 and *Mlvi*-1 and trisomy of chromosome 15 in MCF- and Moloney-MuLV-induced murine T-cell leukemias, *Int. J. Cancer,* 38, 739, 1986.
222. Adams, J.M., Gerondakis, S., Webb, E., Mitchell, J., Bernard, O., and Cory, S., Transcriptionally active DNA region that rearranges frequently in murine lymphoid tumors, *Proc. Natl. Acad. Sci. U.S.A.,* 79, 6966, 1092.
223. Corcoran, L.M., Adams, J.M., Dunn, A.R., and Cory, S., Murine T lymphomas in which the cellular *myc* oncogene has been activated by retroviral insertion, *Cell,* 37, 113, 1984.
224. Steffen, D., Proviruses are adjacent to c-*myc* in some murine leukemia virus-induced lymphomas, *Proc. Natl. Acad. Sci. U.S.A.,* 81, 2097, 1984.
225. Li, Y., Holland, C.A., Hartley, S.W., and Hopkins, N., Viral integration near c-*myc* in 10-20% of MCF 247-induced AKR lymphomas, *Proc. Natl. Acad. Sci. U.S.A.,* 81, 6808, 1984.
226. Selten, G., Cuypers, H.T., Zijlstra, M., Melief, C., and Berns, A., Involvement of c-*myc* in MuLV-induced T cell lymphomas in mice: frequency and mechanisms of activation, *EMBO J.,* 3, 3215, 1984.
227. Graham, M., Adams, J.M., and Cory, S., Murine T lymphomas with retroviral inserts in the chromosomal 15 locus for plasmacytoma variant translocations, *Nature,* 314, 740, 1985.
228. Balachandran, R., Reddy, E.P., Dunn, C.Y., Aaronson, S.A., and Swan, D.C., Immunoglobulin synthesis and gene rearrangements in lymphoid cells transformed by replication-competent Rauscher murine leukemia virus: transformation of B cells at various stages of differentiation, *EMBO J.,* 3, 3199, 1984.
229. Janowski, M., Merregaert, J., and Reddy, P., Retroviruses in radiation-induced lymphomas, *Leukemia Res.,* 10, 833, 1986.
230. O'Donnell, P.V., Fleissner, E., Lonial, H., Koehne, C.F., and Reicin, A., Early clonality and high-frequency proviral integration into the c-*myc* locus in AKR leukemias, *J. Virol.,* 55, 500, 1985.
231. Reicin, A., Yang, J.-Q., Marcu, K.B., Fleissner, E., Koehne, C.F., and O'Donnell, P.V., Deregulation of the c-*myc* oncogene in virus-induced thymic lymphomas in AKR/J mice, *Mol. Cell. Biol.,* 6, 4088, 1986.
232. Vijaya, S., Steffen, D.L., Kozak, C., and Robinson, H.L., *Dsi-1*, a region with frequent proviral insertions in Moloney murine leukemia virus-induced rat thymomas, *J. Virol.,* 61, 1164, 1987.

233. Lazo, P.A. and Tsichlis, P.N., Recombination between two integrated proviruses, one of which was inserted near c-*myc* in a retrovirus-induced rat thymoma: implications for tumor progression, *J. Virol.,* 62, 788, 1988.

234. Miura, T., Tsujimoto, H., Fukasawa, M., Kodama, T., Shibuya, M., Hasegawa, A., and Hayami, M., Structural abnormality and over-expression of the *myc* gene in feline leukemias, *Int. J. Cancer,* 40, 564, 1987.

235. Shen-Ong, G.L.C., Potter, M., Mushinski, J.F., Lavu, S., and Reddy, E.P., Activation of the c-*myb* locus by viral insertional mutagenesis in plasmacytoid lymphosarcomas, *Science,* 226, 1077, 1984.

236. Lavu, S. and Reddy, E.P., Structural organization and nucleotide sequence of mouse c-*myb* oncogene: activation in ABPL tumors is due to viral integration in an intron which resulsts in the deletion of the 5' coding sequences, *Nucleic Acids Res.,* 14, 5309, 1986.

237. Shen-Ong, G.L.C. and Wolff, L., Moloney murine leukemia virus-induced myeloid tumors in adult BALB/c mice: requirement of c-*myb* activation but lack of v-*abl* involvement, *J. Virol.,* 61, 3721, 1987.

238. Shen-Ong, G.L.C., Morse, H.C., III, Potter, M., and Mushinski, J.F., Two modes of c-*myb* activation in virus-induced mouse myeloid tumors, *Mol. Cell. Biol.,* 6, 380, 1986.

239. Gonda, T.J., Cory, S., Sobieszczuk, P., Holtzman, D., and Adams, J.M., Generation of altered transcripts by retroviral insertion within c-*myb* gene in two murine monocytic leukemias, *J. Virol.,* 61, 2754, 1987.

240. Rosson, D., Dugan, D., and Reddy, E.P., Aberrant splicing events that are induced by proviral integration: implications for *myb* oncogene activation, *Proc. Natl. Acad. Sci. U.S.A.,* 84, 3171, 1987.

241. Weinstein, Y., Ihle, J.N., Lavu, S., and Reddy, E.P., Truncation of the c-*myb* gene by a retroviral integration in an interleukin 3-dependent myeloid leukemia cell line, *Proc. Natl. Acad. Sci. U.S.A.,* 83, 5010, 1986.

242. Oliff, A., Oliff, I., Schmidt, B., and Famulari, N., Isolation of immortal cell lines from the first stage of murine leukemia virus-induced leukemia, *Proc. Natl. Acad. Sci. U.S.A.,* 81, 5464, 1984.

243. George, D.L., Glick, B., Trusko, S., and Freeman, N., Enhanced c-Ki-*ras* expression associated with Friend virus integration in a bone marrow-derived mouse cell line, *Proc. Natl. Acad. Sci. U.S.A.,* 83, 1651, 1986.

244. Robert-Lezenes, J., Moreau-Gachelin, F., Wendling, F., Tambourin, P., and Tavitian, A., Expression of c-*ras* and c-*myc* oncogenes in murine erythroleukemias induced by Friend viruses, *Leukemia Res.,* 8, 975, 1984.

245. Fung, Y.-K.T., Lewis, W.G., Crittenden, L.B., and Kung, H.-J., Activation of the cellular oncogene c-*erbB* by LTR insertion: molecular basis for induction of erythroblastosis by avian leukosis virus, *Cell,* 33, 357, 1983.

246. Lax, I., Kris, R., Sasson, I., Ullrich, A., Hayman, M.J., Beug, H., and Schlessinger, J., Activation of c-*erbB* in avian leukosis virus-induced erythroblastosis leads to the expression of a truncated EGF receptor kinase, *EMBO J.,* 4, 3179, 1985.

247. Raines, M.A., Lewis, W.G., Crittenden, L.B., and Kung, H.-J., c-*erbB* activation in avian leukosis virus-induced erythroblastosis: clustered integration sites and the arrangement of provirus in the c-*erbB* alleles, *Proc. Natl. Acad. Sci. U.S.A.,* 82, 2287, 1985.

248. Nilsen, T.W., Maroney, P.A., Goodwin, R.G., Rottman, F.M., Crittenden, L.B., Raines, M.A., and Kung, H.-J., c-*erbB* activation in ALV-induced erythroblastosis: novel RNA processing and promoter insertion result in expression of an amino-truncated EGF receptor, *Cell,* 41, 719, 1985.

249. Goodwin, R.G., Rottman, F.M., Callaghan, T., Kung, H.-J., Maroney, P.A., and Nilsen, T.W., c-*erbB* activation in avian leukosis virus-induced erythroblastosis: multiple epidermal growth factor receptor mRNAs are generated by alternative RNA processing, *Mol. Cell. Biol.,* 6, 3128, 1986.

250. Miles, B.D. and Robinson, H.L., High-frequency transduction of c-*erbB* in avian leukosis virus-induced erythroblastosis, *J. Virol.,* 54, 295, 1985.

251. Robinson, H.L., Miles, B.D., Catalano, D.E., Briles, W.E., and Crittenden, L.B., Susceptibility to *erbB*-induced erythroblastosis is a dominant trait in 151 chickens, *J. Virol.,* 55, 617, 1985.

252. Tracy, S.E., Woda, B.A., and Robinson, H.L., Induction of an angiosarcoma by a c-*erbB* transducing virus, *J. Virol.,* 54, 304, 1985.

253. Cuypers, H.T., Selten, G., Quint, W., Zijlstra, M., Maandag, E.R., Boelens, W., van Wezenbeek, P., Melief, C., and Berns, A., Murine leukemia virus-induced T-cell lymphomagenesis: integration of proviruses in a distinct chromosomal region, *Cell,* 37, 141, 1984.

254. Selten, G., Cuypers, H.T., and Berns, A., Proviral activation of the putative oncogene *Pim*-1 in MuLV induced T-cell lymphomas, *EMBO J.,* 4, 1793, 1985.

255. Cuypers, H.T.M., Selten, G.C., Zijlstra, M., de Goede, R.E., Melief, C.J., and Berns, A.J., Tumor progression in murine leukemia virus-induced T-cell lymphomas: monitoring clonal selections with viral and cellular probes, *J. Virol.,* 60, 230, 1986.

256. Hilkens, J., Cuypers, H.T., Selten, G., Kroezen, V., Hilgers, J., and Berns, A., Genetic mapping of *Pim-1* putative oncogene to mouse chromosome 17, *Somat. Cell Mol. Genet.,* 12, 81, 1986.

257. Selten, G., Cuypers, H.T., Boelens, W., Robanus-Maandag, E., Verbeek, J., Domen, J., van Beveren, C., and Berns, A., The primary structure of the putative oncogene *pim*-1 shows extensive homology with protein kinases, *Cell,* 46, 603, 1986.

258. Nagarajan, L., Louie, E., Tsujimoto, Y., ar-Rushdi, A., Hueber, K., and Croce, C.M., Localization of the human *pim* oncogene (*PIM*) to a region of chromosome 6 involved in translocations in acute leukemias, *Proc. Natl. Acad. Sci. U.S.A.,* 83, 2556, 1986.

259. Zakout-Houri, R., Hazum, S., Givol, D., and Telerman, A., The cDNA sequence and gene analysis of the human *pim* oncogene, *Gene*, 54, 105, 1987.

260. Domen, J., von Lindern, M., Hermans, A., Breuer, M., Grosveld, G., and Berns, A., Comparison of the human and mouse *PIM*-1 cDNAs: nucleotide sequence and immunological identification of the *in vitro* synthesized *PIM*-1 protein, *Oncogene Res.*, 1, 103, 1987.

261. Peters, G., Brookes, S., Smith, R., and Dickson, C., Tumorigenesis by mouse mammary tumor virus: evidence for a common region for provirus integration in mammary tumors, *Cell*, 33, 369, 1983.

262. Ponta, H., Günzburg, W.H., Salmons, B., Groner, B., and Herrlich, P., Mouse mammary tumour virus: a proviral gene contributes to the understanding of eukaryotic gene expression and mammary tumorigenesis, *J. Gen. Virol.*, 66, 931, 1985.

263. Gallahan, D., Kozak, C., and Callahan, R., A new common integration region (*int-3*) for mouse mammary tumor virus on mouse chromosome 17, *J. Virol.*, 61, 218, 1987.

264. Mester, J., Wagenaar, E., Sluyser, M., and Nusse, R., Activation of *int*-1 and *int*-2 mammary oncogenes in hormone-dependent and -independent mammary tumors of GR mice, *J. Virol.*, 61, 1073, 1987.

265. Nusse, R., van Ooyen, A., Cox, D., Fung, Y.-K.T., and Varmus, H., Mode of proviral activation of a putative mammary oncogene (*int*-1) on mouse chromosome 15, *Nature*, 307, 131, 1984.

266. Peters, G., Lee, A.E., and Dickson, C., Activation of cellular gene by mouse mammary tumour virus may occur early in mammary tumour development, *Nature*, 309, 273, 1984.

267. Dickson, C., Smith, R., Brookes, S., and Peters, G., Tumorigenesis by mouse mammary tumor virus: proviral activation of a cellular gene in the common integration region *int*-2, *Cell*, 37, 529, 1984.

268. Gray, D.A., Jackson, D.P., Percy, D.H., and Morris, V.L., Activation of *int*-1 and *int*-2 loci in GRf mammary tumors, *Virology*, 154, 271, 1986.

269. van Ooyen, A. and Nusse, R., Structure and nucleotide sequence of the putative mammary oncogene *int*-1; proviral insertions leave the protein-encoding domain intact, *Cell*, 39, 233, 1984.

270. Fung, Y.-K.T., Shackleford, G.M., Brown, A.M.C., Sanders, G.S., and Varmus, H.E., Nucleotide sequence and expression *in vitro* of cDNA derived from mRNA of *int*-1, a provirally activated mouse mammary oncogene, *Mol. Cell. Biol.*, 5, 3337, 1985.

271. Brown, A.M.C., Papkoff, J., Fung, Y.K.T., Shackleford, G.M., and Varmus, H.E., Identification of protein products encoded by the proto-oncogene *int*-1, *Mol. Cell. Biol.*, 7, 3971, 1987.

272. Papkoff, J., Brown, A.M.C., and Varmus, H.E., The *int*-1 proto-oncogene products are glycoproteins that appear to enter the secretory pathway, *Mol. Cell. Biol.*, 7, 3978, 1987.

273. van 't Veer, L.J., van Kessel, A.G., van Heerikhuizen, H., van Ooyen, A., and Nusse, R., Molecular cloning and chromosomal assignment of the human homolog of *int*-1, a mouse gene implicated in mammary tumorigenesis, *Mol. Cell. Biol.*, 4, 2532, 1984.

274. Adolph, S., Bartram, C.R., and Hameister, H., Mapping of the oncogenes *Myc*, *Sis*, and *int-1* to the distal part of mouse chromosome 15, *Cytogenet. Cell Genet.*, 44, 65, 1987.

275. Arheden, K., Mandahl, N., Strömbeck, B., Isaksson, M., and Mitelman, F., Chromosome localization of the human oncogene INT1 to 12q13 by *in situ* hybridization, *Cytogenet. Cell Genet.*, 47, 86, 1988.

276. van Ooyen, A., Kwee, V., and Nusse, R., The nucleotide sequence of the human *int*-1 mammary oncogene: evolutionary conservation of coding and noncoding sequences, *EMBO J.*, 4, 2905, 1985.

277. Lane, M.-A., Sainten, A., and Cooper, G.M., Activation of related transforming genes in mouse and human mammary carcinomas, *Proc. Natl. Acad. Sci. U.S.A.*, 78, 5185, 1981.

278. Becker, D., Lane, M.-A., and Cooper, G.M., Identification of an antigen associated with transforming genes of human and mouse mammary carcinomas, *Proc. Natl. Acad. Sci. U.S.A.*, 79, 3315, 1982.

279. Rijsewijk, F., Scheuermann, M., Wagenaar, E., Parren, P., Weigel, D., and Nusse, R., The *Drosophila* homolog of the mouse mammary oncogene *int*-1 is identical to the segment polarity gene *wingless*, *Cell*, 50, 649, 1987.

280. Uzvölgyi, E., Kiss, I., Pitt, A., Arsenian, S., Ingvarsson, S., Udvardy, A., Hamada, M., Klein, G., and Sümegi, J., *Drosophila* homolog of the murine *Int-1* protooncogene, *Proc. Natl. Acad. Sci. U.S.A.*, 85, 3034, 1988.

281. Baker, N.E., Molecular cloning of sequences from *wingless*, a segment polarity gene in *Drosophila*: the spatial distribution of a transcript in embryos, *EMBO J.*, 6, 1765, 1987.

282. Moore, R., Casey, G., Brookes, S., Dixon, M., Peters, G., and Dickson, C., Sequence, topography and protein coding potential of mouse *int*-2: a putative oncogene activated by mouse mammary tumor virus, *EMBO J.*, 5, 919, 1986.

283. Casey, G., Smith, R., McGillivray, D., Peters, G., and Dickson, C., Characterization and chromosome assignment of the human homolog of *int*-2, a potential proto-oncogene, *Mol. Cell. Biol.*, 6, 502, 1986.

284. Adelaide, J., Mattei, M.-G., Marics, I., Raybaud, F., Planche, J., De Lapeyriere, O., and Birnbaum, D., Chromosomal localization of the *hst* oncogene and its co-amplification with the *int*.2 oncogene in a human melanoma, *Oncogene*, 2, 413, 1988.

285. Law, M.L., Kao, F.T., Wei, Q., Hartz, J.A., Greene, G.L., Zarucki-Schulz, T., Conneely, O.M., Jones, C., Puck, T.T., O'Malley, B.W., and Horwitz, K.B., The progesterone receptor gene maps to human chromosome band 1q13, the site of the mammary oncogene *int*-2, *Proc. Natl. Acad. Sci. U.S.A.*, 84, 2877, 1987.

286. Dickson, C. and Peters, G., Potential oncogene products related to growth factors, *Nature*, 326, 833, 1987.

287. Gallahan, D. and Callahan, R., Mammary tumorigenesis in feral mice: identification of a new *int* locus in mouse mammary tumor virus (Czech II)-induced mammary tumors, *J. Virol.*, 61, 66, 1987.

288. Jakobovits, A., Shackleford, G.M., Varmus, H.E., and Martin, G.R., Two proto-oncogenes implicated in mammary carcinogenesis, *int-1* and *int-2*, are independently regulated during mouse development, *Proc. Natl. Acad. Sci. U.S.A.*, 83, 7806, 1986.

289. Shackleford, G.M. and Varmus, H.E., Expression of the proto-oncogene *int*-1 is restricted to postmeiotic male germ cells and the neural tube of mid-gestational embryos, *Cell*, 50, 89, 1987.

290. Wilkinson, D.G., Bailes, J.A., and McMahon, A.P., Expression of the proto-oncogene *int*-1 is restricted to specific neural cells in the developing mouse embryo, *Cell*, 50, 79, 1987.

291. Wilkinson, D.G., Peters, G., Dickson, C., and McMahon, A.P., Expression of the FGF-related proto-oncogene *int-2* during gastrulation and neurulation in the mouse, *EMBO J.*, 7, 691, 1988.

292. Rijsewijk, F.A.M., van Lohuizen, M., van Ooyen, A., and Nusse, R., Construction of a retroviral cDNA version of the *int*-1 mammary oncogene and its expression *in vitro*, *Nucleic Acids Res.*, 14, 693, 1986.

293. Brown, A.M.C., Wildin, R.S., Prendergast, T.J., and Varmus, H.E., A retrovirus vector expressing the putative mammary oncogene *int*-1 causes partial transformation of a mammary epithelial cell line, *Cell*, 46, 1001, 1986.

294. Peters, G., Lee, A.E., and Dickson, C., Concerted activation of two potential proto-oncogenes in carcinomas induced by mouse mammary tumour virus, *Nature*, 320, 628, 1986.

295. Knepper, J.E., Medina, D., and Butel, J.S., Activation of endogenous MMTV proviruses in murine mammary cancer induced by chemical carcinogen, *Int. J. Cancer*, 40, 414, 1987.

296. Marth, J.D., Disteche, C., Pravtcheva, D., Ruddle, F., Krebs, E.G., and Perlmutter, R.M., Localization of a lymphocyte-specific protein tyrosine kinase gene (*lck*) at a site of frequent chromosomal abnormalities in human lymphomas, *Proc. Natl. Acad. Sci. U.S.A.*, 83, 7400, 1986.

297. Voronova, A.F., Buss, J.E., Patschinsky, T., Hunter, T., and Sefton, B.M., Characterization of the protein apparently responsible for the elevated tyrosine protein kinase activity in LSTRA cells, *Mol. Cell. Biol.*, 4, 2705, 1984.

298. Marth, J.D., Overell, R.W., Meier, K.E., Krebs, E.G., and Perlmutter, R.M., Translational activation of the *lck* proto-oncogene, *Nature*, 332, 171, 1988.

299. Marth, J.D., Peet, R., Krebs, E.G., and Perlmutter, R.M., A lymphocyte-specific protein-tyrosine kinase gene is rearranged and overexpressed in the murine T cell lymphoma LSTRA, *Cell*, 43, 393, 1985.

300. Voronova, A.F. and Sefton, B.M., Expression of a new tyrosine protein kinase is stimulated by retrovirus promoter insertion, *Nature*, 319, 682, 1986.

301. Tsichlis, P.N., Strauss, P.G., and Hu, L.F., A common region for proviral DNA integration in MoMuLV-induced rat thymic lymphomas, *Nature*, 302, 445, 1983.

302. Lemay, G. and Jolicoeur, P., Rearrangement of a DNA sequence homologous to a cell-virus junction fragment in several Moloney murine leukemia virus-induced rat thymomas, *Proc. Natl. Acad. Sci. U.S.A.*, 81, 38, 1984.

303. Tsichlis, P.N., Straus, P.G., and Lohse, M.A., Concerted DNA rearrangements in Moloney murine leukemia virus-induced thymomas: a potential synergistic relationship in oncogenesis, *J. Virol.*, 56, 258, 1985.

304. Tsichlis, P.N., Lohse, M.A., Szpirer, C., Szpirer, J., and Levan, G., Cellular DNA regions involved in the induction of rat thymic lymphomas (*Mlvi-1*, *Mlvi-2*, *Mlvi-3*, and c-*myc*) represent independent loci as determined by their chromosomal map location in the rat, *J. Virol.*, 56, 938, 1985.

305. Jolicoeur, P., Villeneuve, L., Rassart, E., and Kozak, C., Mouse chromosomal mapping of a murine leukemia virus integration region (*Mis-1*) first identified in rat thymic leukemia, *J. Virol.*, 56, 1045, 1985.

306. Villeneuve, L., Rassart, E., Jolicoeur, P., Graham, M., and Adams, J.M., Proviral integration site *Mis*-1 in rat thymomas corresponds to the *pvt*-1 translocation breakpoint in murine plasmacytomas, *Mol. Cell. Biol.*, 6, 1834, 1986.

307. Economou-Pachnis, A., Lohse, M.A., Furano, A.V., and Tsichlis, P.N., Insertion of long interspersed repeated elements at the *Igh* (immunoglobulin heavy chain) and *Mlvi-2* (Moloney leukemia virus integration 2) loci of rats, *Proc. Natl. Acad. Sci. U.S.A.*, 82, 2857, 1985.

308. Tsichlis, P.N., Strauss, P.G., and Kozak, C.A., Cellular DNA region involved in induction of thymic lymphomas (*Mlvi-2*) maps to mouse chromosome 15, *Mol. Cell. Biol.*, 4, 997, 1984.

309. Kozak, C.A., Straus, P.G., and Tsichlis, P.N., Genetic mapping of a cellular DNA region involved in induction of thymic lymphomas (*Mlvi-1*) to mouse chromosome 15, *Mol. Cell. Biol.*, 5, 894, 1985.

310. Cory, S., Graham, M., Webb, E., Corcoran, L., and Adams, J.M., Variant (6;15) translocations in murine plasmacytomas involve a chromosome 15 locus at least 72 kb from the c-*myc* oncogene, *EMBO J.*, 4, 675, 1985.

311. Banerjee, M., Wiener, F., Spira, J., Babonits, M., Nilsson, M.-G., Sumegi, J., and Klein, G., Mapping of the c-*myc*, *pvt*-1 and immunoglobulin kappa genes in relation to the mouse plasmacytoma-associated variant (6;15) translocation breakpoint, *EMBO J.*, 4, 3183, 1985.

312. Gough, N., Chromosomal translocation and the c-*myc* gene: paradigm lost?, *Trends Genet.*, 1, 63, 1985.

313. Economou-Pachnis, A. and Tsichlis, P.N., Insertion of an Alu SINE in the human homologue of the *Mlvi-2* locus, *Nucleic Acids Res.*, 13, 8379, 1985.

314. Silver, J. and Kozak, C., Common proviral integration region on mouse chromosome 7 in lymphomas and myelogenous leukemias induced by Friend murine leukemia virus, *J. Virol.,* 57, 526, 1986.

315. Silver, J. and Buckler, C.E., A preferred region for integration of Friend murine leukemia virus in hematopoietic neoplasms is closely linked to the *Int-2* oncogene, *J. Virol.,* 60, 1156, 1986.

316. Sola, B., Fichelson, S., Bordereaux, D., Tambourin, P.E., and Gisselbrecht, S., *fim-1* and *fim-2*: two new integration regions of Friend murine leukemia virus in myeloblastic leukemias, *J. Virol.,* 60, 718, 1986.

317. Villemur, R., Monczak, Y., Rassart, E., Kozak, C., and Jolicoeur, P., Identification of a new common provirus integration site in Gross passage A murine leukemia virus-induced mouse thymoma DNA, *Mol. Cell. Biol.,* 7, 512, 1987.

318. Mucenski, M.L., Taylor, B.A., Ihle, J.N., Hartley, J.W., Morse, H.C., III, Jenkins, N.A., and Copeland, N.G., Identification of a common ecotropic viral integration site, *Evi-1*, in the DNA of AKXD murine myeloid tumors, *Mol. Cell. Biol.,* 8, 301, 1988.

319. Mucenski, M.L., Gilbert, D.J., Taylor, B.A., Jenkins, N.A., and Copeland, N.G., Common sites of viral integration in lymphomas arising in AKXD recombinant inbred mouse strains, *Oncogene Res.,* 2, 33, 1987.

320. Holbrook, N.J., Gulino, A., Durand, D., Lin, Y., and Crabtree, G.R., Transcriptional activity of the gibbon ape leukemia virus in the interleukin 2 gene of MLA 144 cells, *Virology,* 159, 178, 1987.

321. Jaenisch, R., Breindl, M., Harbers, K., Jähner, D., and Löhler, J., Retroviruses and insertional mutagenesis, *Cold Spring Harbor Symp. Quant. Biol.,* 50, 439, 1985.

322. Jaenisch, R., Jähner, D., Nobis, P., Simon, I., Löhler, J., Harbers, K., and Grotkopp, D., Chromosomal position and activation of retroviral genomes inserted into the germ line of mice, *Cell,* 24, 519, 1981.

323. Münke, M., Harbers, K., Jaenisch, R., and Francke, U., Chromosomal mapping of four different integration sites of Moloney murine leukemia virus including the locus for alpha 1 (I) collagen in mouse, *Cytogenet. Cell Genet.,* 43, 140, 1986.

324. Ray, D., Meneceur, P., Tavitian, A., and Robert-Lezenes, J., Presence of a c-*myc* transcript initiated in intron 1 in Friend erythroleukemia cells and in other murine cell types with no evidence of c-*myc* gene rearrangement, *Mol. Cell. Biol.,* 7, 940, 1987.

325. Gupta, P., Kashmiri, S.V.S., Erisman, M.D., Rothberg, P.G., Astrin, S.M., and Ferrer, J.F., Enhanced expression of the c-*myc* gene in bovine leukemia virus-induced bovine tumors, *Cancer Res.,* 46, 6295, 1986.

326. Oliff, A., Agranovsky, O., McKinney, M.D., Murty, V.V.V.S., and Bauchwitz, R., Friend murine leukemia virus-immortalized myeloid cells are converted into tumorigenic cell lines by Abelson leukemia virus, *Proc. Natl. Acad. Sci. U.S.A.,* 82, 3306, 1985.

327. Mowat, M., Cheng, A., Kimura, N., Bernstein, A., and Benchimol, S., Rearrangements of the cellular p53 gene in erythroleukaemic cells transformed by Friend virus, *Nature,* 314, 633, 1985.

328. Rovinski, B., Munroe, D., Peacock, J., Mowat, M., Bernstein, A., and Benchimol, S., Deletion of 5'-coding sequences of the cellular p53 gene in mouse erythroleukemia: a novel mechanism of oncogene regulation, *Mol. Cell. Biol.,* 7, 847, 1987.

329. Koury, M.J. and Pragnell, I.B., Retroviruses induce granulocyte-macrophage colony stimulating activity in fibroblasts, *Nature,* 299, 638, 1982.

330. McDonald, J., Beru, N., and Goldwasser, E., Rearrangement and expression of erythropoietin genes in transformed mouse cells, *Mol. Cell. Biol.,* 7, 365, 1987.

331. Sun, L. and Kawakami, T.G., Oncogenicity of gibbon retrovirus determined by leukemia-specific genomic sequences, *Virology,* 114, 261, 1981.

332. Vogt, M., Haggblom, C., Swift, S., and Haas, M., Envelope gene and long terminal repeat determine the different biological properties of Rauscher, Friend, and Moloney mink cell focus-inducing virus, *J. Virol.,* 55, 184, 1985.

333. Sitbon, M., Sola, B., Evans, L., Nishio, J., Hayes, S.F., Nathanson, K., Garon, C.F., and Chesebro, B., Hemolytic anemia and erythroleukemia, two distinct pathogenic effects of Friend MuLV: mapping of the effects to different regions of the viral genome, *Cell,* 47, 851, 1986.

334. Bonham, L., Lobelle-Rich, P.A., Henderson, L.A., and Levy, L.S., Transforming potential of a *myc*-containing variant of feline leukemia virus *in vitro* in early-passage feline cells, *J. Virol.,* 61, 3072, 1987.

335. Mullins, J.I., Brody, D.S., Binari, R.C., Jr., and Cotter, S.M., Viral transduction of c-*myc* gene in naturally occurring feline leukaemias, *Nature,* 308, 856, 1984.

336. Neil, J.C., Hughes, D., McFarlane, R., Wilkie, N.M., Onions, D.E., Lees, G., and Jarrett, O., Transduction and rearrangement of the *mycv* gene by feline leukaemia virus in naturally occurring T-cell leukaemias, *Nature,* 308, 814, 1984.

337. Levy, L.S., Gardner, M.B., and Casey, J.W., Isolation of a feline leukaemia provirus containing the oncogene *myc* from a feline lymphosarcoma, *Nature,* 308, 853, 1984.

338. Onions, D., Lees, G., Forrest, D., and Neil, J., Recombinant feline viruses containing the *myc* gene rapidly produce clonal tumors expressing T-cell antigen receptor gene transcripts, *Int. J. Cancer,* 40, 40, 1987.

339. Braun, M.J., Deininger, P.L., and Casey, J.W., Nucleotide sequence of a transduced *myc* gene from a defective feline leukemia provirus, *J. Virol.,* 55, 177, 1985.

340. Beug, H., Hayman, M.J., Raines, M.B., Kung, H.J., and Vennström, B., Rous-associated virus 1-induced erythroleukemic cells exhibit a weakly transformed phenotype *in vitro* and release c-*erbB*-containing retroviruses unable to transform fibroblasts, *J. Virol.,* 57, 1127, 1986.

341. Penn, I., Why do immunosuppressed patients develop cancer?, *Crit. Rev. Oncogenesis,* 1, 27, 1989.

342. Ihle, J.N., Lee, J.C., Enjuanes, L., Cicurel, L., Horak, I., and Pepersack, L., Chronic immunostimulation as a possible mechanism in type-C viral leukemogenesis, *Cold Spring Harbor Conf. Cell Prolif.,* 7, 1049, 1980.

343. Majone, F., Montaldi, A., Ronchese, F., De Rossi, A., Chieco-Bianchi, L., and Levis, A.G., Sister chromatid exchanges induced *in vivo* and *in vitro* by chemical carcinogens in mouse lymphocytes carrying endogenized Moloney leukemia virus, *Carcinogenesis,* 4, 33, 1983.

344. Mishra, N.K., Pant, K.J., Wilson, C.M., and Thomas, F.O., Carcinogen-induced mutations at two separate genetic loci are not enhanced by leukaemia virus infection, *Nature,* 266, 548, 1977.

345. Matioli, G., Friend leukemic mouse stem cell reversion to normal growth in irradiated hosts, *J. Reticuloendothel. Soc.,* 14, 380, 1973.

346. Lee, T.H., Coligan, J.E., Sodroski, J.G., Haseltine, W.A., Salahuddin, S.Z., Wong-Staal, F., Gallo, R.C., and Essex, M., Antigens encoded by the 3'-terminal region of human T-cell leukemia virus: evidence for a functional gene, *Science,* 226, 57, 1984.

347. Fauci, A.S., The human immunodeficiency virus: infectivity and mechanisms of pathogenesis, *Science,* 239, 617, 1988.

348. Gonda, M.A., Wong-Staal, F., Gallo, R.C., Clements, J.E., Narayan, O., and Gilden, R.V., Sequence homology and morphologic similarity of HTLV-III and Visna virus, a pathogenic lentivirus, *Science,* 227, 173, 1985.

349. Alizon, M. and Montagnier, L., Lymphadenopathy/AIDS virus: genetic organization and relationship to animal lentiviruses, *Anticancer Res.,* 6, 403, 1986.

350. Jeffreys, D., Virological aspects of AIDS, *Clin. Immunol. Allergy,* 6, 627, 1986.

351. Soto-Aguilar, M.C. and Deshazo, R.D., Human retroviruses and the acquired immunodeficiency syndrome. I. Virology update, *J. Allergy Clin. Immunol.,* 81, 619, 1988.

352. Poiesz, B.J., Ruscetti, F.W., Gazdar, A.F., Bunn, P.A., Minna, J.D., and Gallo, R.C., Detection and isolation of type C retrovirus particles from fresh and cultured lymphocytes of a patient with cutaneous T-cell lymphoma, *Proc. Natl. Acad. Sci. U.S.A.,* 77, 7415, 1980.

353. Reitz, M.S., Jr., Poiesz, B.J., Ruscetti, F.W., and Gallo, R.C., Characterization and distribution of nucleic acid sequences of a novel type C retrovirus isolated from neoplastic human T lymphocytes, *Proc. Natl. Acad. Sci. U.S.A.,* 78, 1887, 1981.

354. Poiesz, B.J., Ruscetti, F.W., Reitz, M.S., Kalyanaraman, V.S., and Gallo, R.C., Isolation of a new type C retrovirus (HTLV) in primary uncultured cells of a patient with Sezary T-cell leukaemia, *Nature,* 294, 268, 1981.

355. Kalyanaraman, V.S., Sarngadharan, M.G., Poiesz, B., Ruscetti, F.W., and Gallo, R.C., Immunological properties of a type C retrovirus isolated from cultured human T-lymphoma cells and comparison to other mammalian retroviruses, *J. Virol.,* 38, 906, 1981.

356. Rho, H.M., Poiesz, B., Ruscetti, F.W., and Gallo, R.C., Characterization of the reverse transcriptase from a new retrovirus (HTLV) produced by a human cutaneous T-cell lymphoma cell line, *Virology,* 112, 355, 1981.

357. Hinuma, Y., Nagata, K., Hanaoka, M., Nakai, M., Matsumoto, T., Kinoshita, K., Shirakawa, S., and Miyoshi, I., Adult T-cell leukemia: antigen in an ATL cell line and detection of antibodies to the antigen in human sera, *Proc. Natl. Acad. Sci. U.S.A.,* 78, 6476, 1981.

358. Miyoshi, I., Kubonishi, I., Yoshimoto, S., Akagi, T., Ohtsuki, Y., Shiraishi, Y., Nagata, K., and Hinuma, Y., Type C virus particles in a cord T-cell line derived by co-cultivating normal human cord leukocytes and human leukaemic cells, *Nature,* 294, 770, 1981.

359. Yoshida, M., Miyoshi, I., and Hinuma, Y., Isolation and characterization of retrovirus from cell lines of human adult T-cell leukemia and its implication in the disease, *Proc. Natl. Acad. Sci. U.S.A.,* 79, 2031, 1982.

360. Seiki, M., Hattori, S., and Yoshida, M., Human adult T-cell leukemia virus: molecular cloning of the provirus DNA and the unique terminal structure, *Proc. Natl. Acad. Sci. U.S.A.,* 79, 6899, 1982.

361. Seiki, M., Hattori, S., Hirayama, Y., and Yoshida, M., Human adult T-cell leukemia virus: complete nucleotide sequence of the provirus genome integrated in leukemia cell, *DNA,* 80, 3618, 1983.

362. Popovic, M., Reitz, M.S., Jr., Sarngadharan, M.G., Robert-Guroff, M., Kalyanaraman, V.S., Nakao, Y., Miyoshi, I., Minowada, J., Yoshida, M., Ito, Y., and Gallo, R.C., The virus of Japanese adult T-cell leukaemia is a member of the human T-cell leukaemia virus group, *Nature,* 300, 63, 1982.

363. Josephs, S.F., Wong-Staal, F., Manzari, V., Gallo, R.C., Sodroski, J.G., Trus, M.D., Perkins, D., Patarca, R., and Haseltine, W.A., Long terminal repeat structure of an American isolate of type I human T-cell leukemia virus, *Virology,* 139, 340, 1984.

364. Hahn, B.H., Shaw, G.M., Popovic, M., Lo Monico, A., Gallo, R.C., and Wong-Staal, F., Molecular cloning and analysis of a new variant of human T-cell leukemia virus (HTLV-1b) from an African patient with adult T-cell leukemia-lymphoma, *Int. J. Cancer,* 34, 613, 1984.

365. Gallo, R.C., Mann, D., Broder, S., Ruscetti, F.W., Maeda, M., Kalyanaraman, V.S., Robert-Guroff, M., and Reitz, M.S., Jr., Human T-cell leukemia-lymphoma virus (HTLV) is in T but not B lymphocytes from a patient with cutaneous T-cell lymphoma, *Proc. Natl. Acad. Sci. U.S.A.,* 79, 5680, 1982.

366. Swerdlow, S.H., Habeshaw, J.A., Rohatiner, A.Z.S., Lister, T.A., and Stansfeld, A.G., Caribbean T-cell lymphoma/leukemia, *Cancer,* 54, 687, 1984.

367. Clapham, P., Nagy, K., Cheingsong-Popov, R., Exley, M., and Weiss, R.A., Productive infection and cell-free transmission of human T-cell leukemia virus in a nonlymphoid cell line, *Science,* 222, 1125, 1983.

368. Hayami, M., Tsujimoto, H., Komuro, A., Hinuma, Y., and Fujiwara, K., Transmission of adult T-cell leukemia virus from lymphoid cells to non-lymphoid cells associated with cell membrane fusion, *Jpn. J. Hum. Genet.,* 75, 99, 1984.

369. Miyamoto, K., Tomita, N., Ishii, A., Nishizaki, T., Kitajima, K., Tanaka, T., Nakamura, T., Watanabe, S., and Oda, T., Transformation of ATLA-negative leukocytes by blood components from anti ATLA-positive donors *in vitro, Int. J. Cancer,* 33, 721, 1984.

370. Ho, D.D., Rota, T.R., and Hirsch, M.S., Infection of human endothelial cells by human T-lymphotropic virus type I, *Proc. Natl. Acad. Sci. U.S.A.,* 81, 7588, 1984.

371. Hoxie, J.A., Matthews, D.M., and Cines, D.B., Infection of human endothelial cells by human T-cell leukemia virus type I, *Proc. Natl. Acad. Sci. U.S.A.,* 81, 7591, 1984.

372. Robert-Guroff, M., Nakao, Y., Notake, K., Ito, Y., Sliski, A., and Gallo, R.C., Natural antibodies to human retrovirus HTLV in a cluster of Japanese patients with adult T cell leukemia, *Science,* 215, 975, 1982.

373. Kalyanaraman, V.S., Sarngadharan, M.G., Nakao, Y., Ito, Y., Aoki, T., and Gallo, R.C., Natural antibodies to the structural core protein (p24) of the human T-cell leukemia (lymphoma) retrovirus found in sera of leukemia patients in Japan, *Proc. Natl. Acad. Sci. U.S.A.,* 79, 1653, 1982.

374. Blattner, W.A., Kalyanaraman, V.S., Robert-Guroff, M., Lister, T.A., Galton, D.A.G., Sarin, P.S., Crawford, M.H., Catovsky, D., Greaves, M., and Gallo, R.C., The human type-C retrovirus, HTLV, in Blacks from the Caribbean region, and relationship to adult T-cell leukemia/lymphoma, *Int. J. Cancer,* 30, 257, 1982.

375. Blattner, W.A., Gibbs, W.N., Saxinger, C., Robert-Guroff, M., Clark, J., Lofters, W., Hanchard, B., Campbell, M., and Gallo, R.C., Human T-cell leukaemia/lymphoma virus-associated lymphoreticular neoplasia in Jamaica, *Lancet,* 2, 61, 1983.

376. Blayney, D.W., Blattner, W.A., Robert-Guroff, M., Jaffe, E.S., Fisher, R.I., Bunn, P.A., Jr., Patton, M.G., Rarick, H.R., and Gallo, R.C., The human T-cell leukemia-lymphoma virus in the Southeastern United States, *JAMA,* 250, 1048, 1983.

377. Blayney, D.W., Jaffe, E.S., Blattner, W.A., Cossman, J., Robert-Guroff, M., Longo, D.L., Bunn, P.A., Jr., and Gallo, R.C., The human T-cell leukemia/lymphoma virus associated with American adult T-cell leukemia/lymphoma, *Blood,* 62, 401, 1983.

378. Yamamoto, N., Schneider, J., Koyanagi, Y., Hinuma, Y., and Hunsmann, G., Adult T-cell leukemia (ATL) virus-specific antibodies in ATL patiens and healthy virus carriers, *Int. J. Cancer,* 32, 281, 1983.

379. Hunsmann, G., Schneider, J., Schmitt, J., and Yamamoto, N., Detection of serum antibodies to adult T-cell leukemia virus in non-human primates and in people from Africa, *Int. J. Cancer,* 32, 329, 1983.

380. Schüpbach, J., Kalyanaraman, V.S., Sarngadharan, M.G., Nakao, Y., Ito, Y., and Gallo, R.C., Antibodies against three purified structural proteins of the human type-c retrovirus, HTLV, in Japanese adult T-cell leukemia patients, healthy family members, and unrelated normals, *Int. J. Cancer,* 32, 583, 1983.

381. Schüpbach, J.D., Kalyanaraman, V.S., Sarngadharan, M.G., Blattner, W.A., and Gallo, R.C., Antibodies against three purified proteins of the human type C retrovirus, human T cell leukemia/lymphoma virus, in adult T cell leukemia lymphoma patients and healthy Blacks from the Caribbean, *Cancer Res.,* 43, 886, 1983.

382. Saxinger, W., Blattner, W.A., Levine, P.H., Clark, J., Biggar, R., Hoh, M., Moghissi, J., Jacobs, P., Wilson, L., Jacobson, R., Crookes, R., Strong, M., Ansari, A.A., Dean, A.G., Nkrumah, F.K., Mourali, N., and Gallo, R.C., Human T-cell leukemia virus (HTLV-I) antibodies in Africa, *Science,* 225, 1473, 1984.

383. Maeda, Y., Furukawa, M., Takehara, Y., Yoshimura, K., Miyamoto, K., Matsuura, T., Morishima, Y., Tajima, K., Okochi, K., and Hinuma, Y., Prevalence of possible adult T-cell leukemia virus-carriers among volunteer blood donors in Japan: a nation-wide study, *Int. J. Cancer,* 33, 717, 1984.

384. Merino, F., Robert-Guroff, M., Clark, J., Biondo-Bracho, M., Blattner, W.A., and Gallo, R.C., Natural antibodies to human T-cell leukemia/lymphoma virus in healthy Venezuelan population, *Int. J. Cancer,* 34, 501, 1984.

385. Kalyanaraman, V.S., Sarngadharan, M.G., Bunn, P.A., Minna, J.D., and Gallo, R.C., Antibodies in human sera reactive against an internal structural protein of human T-cell lymphoma virus, *Nature,* 294, 271, 1981.

386. Popovic, M., Sarin, P.S., Robert-Guroff, M., Kalyanaraman, V.S., Mann, D., Minowada, J., and Gallo, R.C., Isolation and transmission of human retrovirus (human T-cell leukemia virus), *Science,* 219, 856, 1983.

387. Haynes, B.F., Miller, S.E., Palker, T.J., Moore, J.O., Dunn, P.H., Bolognesi, D.P., and Metzgar, R.S., Identification of human T cell leukemia virus in a Japanese patient with adult T cell leukemia and cutaneous lymphomatous vasculitis, *Proc. Natl. Acad. Sci. U.S.A.,* 80, 2054, 1983.

388. Williams, A.E., Fang, C.T., Slamon, D.J., Poiesz, B.J., Sandler, S.G., Darr, W.F., II, Shulman, G., McGowan, E.I., Douglas, D.K., Bowman, R.J., Peetoom, F., Kleinman, S.H., Lenes, B., and Dodd, R.Y., Seroprevalence and epidemiological correlates of HTLV-I infection in U.S. blood donors, *Science,* 240, 643, 1988.

389. Kim, J.H. and Durack, D.T., Manifestations of human T-lymphotropic virus type I infection, *Am. J. Med.,* 84, 919, 1988.

390. Karpas, A., Malik, K., and Lida, J., Studies of human retroviruses in relation to adult T-cell leukaemia, acquired immune deficiency syndrome, and multiple sclerosis, *Arch. Virol.,* 95, 237, 1987.

391. Reddy, E.P., Mettus, R.V., DeFreitas, E., Wroblewska, Z., Cisco, M., and Koprowski, H., Molecular cloning of human T-cell lymphotropic virus type I-like proviral genome from the peripheral lymphocyte DNA of a patient with chronic neurologic disorders, *Proc. Natl. Acad. Sci. U.S.A.,* 85, 3599, 1988.

392. Bhagavati, S., Ehrlich, G., Kula, R.W., Kwok, S., Sninsky, J., Udani, V., and Poiesz, B.J., Detection of human T-cell lymphoma/leukemia virus type I DNA and antigen in spinal fluid and blood of patients with chronic progressive myelopathy, *N. Engl. J. Med.,* 318, 1141, 1988.

393. Jacobson, S., Raine, C.S., Mingioli, E.S., and McFarlin, D.E., Isolation of an HTLV-1-like retrovirus from patients with tropical spastic paraparesis, *Nature,* 331, 540, 1988.

394. Schneider, J., Yamamoto, N., Hinuma, Y., and Hunsmann, G., Precursor polypeptides of adult T-cell leukaemia virus: detection with antisera against isolated polypeptides gp68, p24 and p19, *J. Gen. Virol.,* 65, 2249, 1984.

395. Lee, T.H., Coligan, J.E., Homma, T., McLane, M.F., Tachibana, N., and Essex, M., Human T-cell leukemia virus-associated antigens: identity of the major antigens recognized after virus infection, *Proc. Natl. Acad. Sci. U.S.A.,* 81, 3856, 1984.

396. Palker, T.J., Scearce, R.M., Miller, S.E., Popovic, M., Bolognesi, D.P., Gallo, R.C., and Haynes, B.F., Monoclonal antibodies against human T cell leukemia-lymphoma virus (HTLV) p24 internal core protein: use as diagnostic probes and cellular localization of HTLV, *J. Exp. Med.,* 159, 1117, 1984.

397. Gotoh, Y.-I., Sugamura, K., and Hinuma, Y., Healthy carriers of a human retrovirus, adult T-cell leukemia virus (ATLV): demonstration by clonal culture of ATLV-carrying T cells from peripheral blood, *Proc. Natl. Acad. Sci. U.S.A.,* 79, 4780, 1982.

398. Andrada-Serpa, M.J., Dobbin, J.A., Gomes, P., Linhares, D., Azevedo, J.G., Hendriks, J., Clayden, S.A., Rumjanek, V.M., and Tedder, R.S., Incidence of retroviruses in some Brazilian groups, *Immunol. Lett.,* 18, 15, 1988.

399. Essex, M., McLane, M.F., Lee, T.H., Tachibana, N., Mullins, J.I., Kreiss, J., Kasper, C.K., Poon, M.-C., Landay, A., Stein, S.F., Francis, D.P., Cabradilla, C., Lawrence, D.N., and Evatt, B.L., Antibodies to human T-cell leukemia virus membrane antigens (HTLV-MA) in hemophiliacs, *Science,* 221, 1061, 1983.

400. Essex, M., McLane, M.F., Lee, T.H., Falk, L., Howe, W.S., Mullins, J.I., Cabradilla, C., and Francis, D.P., Antibodies to cell membrane antigens associated with human T-cell leukemia virus in patients with AIDS, *Science,* 220, 859, 1983.

401. Asou, N., Kumagai, T., Uekihara, S., Ishii, M., Sato, M., Sakai, K., Nishimura, H., Yamaguchi, K., and Takatsuki, K., HTLV-I seroprevalence in patients with malignancy, *Cancer,* 58, 903, 1986.

402. Tajima, K., Fujita, K., Tsukidate, S., Oda, T., Tominaga, S., Suchi, T., and Hinuma, Y., Seroepidemiological studies on the effects of filarial parasites on infestation of adult T-cell leukemia virus in the Goto Islands, Japan, *Jpn. J. Cancer Res.,* 74, 188, 1983.

403. Hoshino, H., Tanaka, H., Miwa, M., and Okada, H., Human T-cell leukaemia virus is not lysed by human serum, *Nature,* 310, 324, 1984.

404. Tajima, K., Tominaga, S., and Suchi, T., Clinico-epidemiological analysis of adult T-cell leukemia, *Gann Monogr.,* 28, 197, 1982.

405. Kinoshita, K., Hino, S., Amagasaki, T., Ikeda, S., Yamada, Y., Suzuyama, J., Momita, S., Toriya, K., Kamihira, S., and Ichimaru, M., Demonstration of adult T-cell leukemia virus antigen in milk from three sero-positive mothers, *Jpn. J. Cancer Res.,* 75, 103, 1984.

406. Uemura, Y., Kotani, S., Yoshimoto, S., Fujishita, M., Yamashita, M., Ohtsuki, Y., Taguchi, H., and Miyoshi, I., Mother-to-offspring transmission of human T cell leukemia virus type I in rabbits, *Blood,* 69, 1255, 1987.

407. Yamaguchi, K., Seiki, M., Yoshida, M., Nishimura, H., Kawano, F., and Takatsuki, K., The detection of human T cell leukemia virus proviral DNA and its application for classification and diagnosis of T cell malignancy, *Blood,* 63, 1235, 1984.

408. Mann, D.L., DeSantis, P., Mark, G., Pfeifer, A., Newman, M., Gibbs, N., Popovic, M., Sarngadharan, M.G., Gallo, R.C., Clark, J., and Blattner, W., HTLV-I-associated B-cell CLL: indirect role for retrovirus in leukemogenesis, *Science,* 236, 1103, 1987.

409. Shimoyama, M., Kagami, Y., Shimotohno, K., Miwa, M., Minato, K., Tobinai, K., Suemasu, K., and Sugimura, T., Adult T-cell leukemia/lymphoma not associated with human T-cell leukemia virus type I, *Proc. Natl. Acad. Sci. U.S.A.,* 83, 4524, 1986.

410. Shimoyama, M., Abe, T., Miyamoto, K., Minato, K., Tobinai, K., Nagoshi, H., Matsunaga, M., Nomura, T., Tsubota, T., Ohnoshi, T., Kimura, I., and Suemasu, K., Chromosome aberrations and clinical features of adult T cell leukemia-lymphoma not associated with human T cell leukemia virus type I, *Blood,* 69, 984, 1987.

411. Hattori, S., Kiyokawa, T., Imagawa, K., Shimizu, F., Hashimura, E., Seiki, M., and Yoshida, M., Identification of *gag* and *env* gene products of human T-cell leukemia virus (HTLV), *Virology,* 136, 338, 1984.

412. Ootsuyama, Y., Shimotohno, K., Miwa, M., Oroszlan, S., and Sugimura, T., Myristylation of *gag* protein in human T-cell leukemia virus type-I and type-II, *Jpn. J. Cancer Res.,* 76, 1132, 1985.

413. Haseltine, W.A., Sodroski, J., Patrarca, R., Briggs, D., Perkins, D., and Wong-Staal, F., Structure of 3' terminal region of type II human T lymphotropic virus: evidence for new coding region, *Science,* 225, 419, 1984.

414. Yoshida, M. and Seiki, M., Recent advances in the molecular biology of HTLV-1: *trans*-activation of viral and cellular genes, *Annu. Rev. Immunol.,* 5, 541, 1987.

415. Wachsman, W., Shimotohno, K., Clark, S.C., Golde, D.W., and Chen, I.S.Y., Expression of the 3' terminal region of human T-cell leukemia viruses, *Science,* 226, 177, 1984.

416. Kiyokawa, T., Seiki, M., Imagawa, K., Shimizu, F., and Yoshida, M., Identification of a protein (p40^x) encoded by a unique sequence *pX* of human T-cell leukemia virus type I, *Jpn. J. Cancer Res.,* 75, 747, 1984.

417. Shimotohno, K., Miwa, M., Slamon, D.J., Chen, I.S.Y., Hoshino, H., Takano, M., Fujino, M., and Sugimura, T., Identification of new gene products coded from X regions of human T-cell leukemia viruses, *Proc. Natl. Acad. Sci. U.S.A.,* 82, 302, 1985,

418. Sodroski, J., Rosen, C., Goh, W.C., and Haseltine, W., A transcriptional activator protein encoded by the x-*lor* region of the human T-cell leukemia virus, *Science,* 228, 1430, 1985.

419. Cann, A.J., Rosenblatt, J.D., Wachsman, W., Shah, N.P., and Chen, I.S.Y., Identification of the gene responsible for human T-cell leukaemia virus transcriptional regulation, *Nature,* 318, 571, 1985.

420. Seiki, M., Inoue, J., Takeda, T., Hikikoshi, A., Sato, M., and Yoshida, M., The p40^x of human T-cell leukemia virus type I is a *trans*-acting activator of viral gene transcription, *Jpn. J. Cancer Res.,* 76, 1127, 1985.

421. Felber, B.K., Paskalis, H., Kleinman-Ewing, C., Wong-Staal, F., and Pavlakis, G.N., The pX protein of HTLV-I is a transcriptional activator of its long terminal repeats, *Science,* 229, 675, 1985.

422. Fujisawa, J., Seiki, M., Sato, M., and Yoshida, M., A transcriptional enhancer sequence of HTLV-I is responsible for *trans*-activation mediated by p40^x of HTLV-I, *EMBO J.,* 5, 713, 1986.

423. Brady, J., Jeang, K.-T., Duvall, J., and Khoury, G., Identification of p40x-responsive regulatory sequences within the human T-cell leukemia virus type I long terminal repeat, *J. Virol.,* 61, 2175, 1987.

424. Kiyokawa, T., Seiki, M., Iwashita, S., Imagawa, K., Shimizu, F., and Yoshida, M., p27t^{x-III} and p21^{x-III}, proteins encoded by the *pX* sequence of human T-cell leukemia virus type I, *Proc. Natl. Acad. Sci. U.S.A.,* 82, 8359, 1985.

425. Nagashima, K., Yoshida, M., and Seiki, M., A single species of *pX* mRNA of human T-cell leukemia virus type I encodes *trans*-activator p40^x and two other phosphoproteins, *J. Virol.,* 60, 394, 1986.

426. Inoue, J., Seiki, M., and Yoshida, M., The second pX product p27^{x-III} of HTLV-1 is required for gag gene expression, *FEBS Lett.,* 209, 187, 1986.

427. Sánchez, A., Richardson, M.A., Yoshida, M., and Furuichi, Y., Synthesis in *Escherichia coli* of the HTLV-I *trans*-acting protein p40^x, *Virology,* 161, 555, 1987.

428. Mamoun, R.Z., Astier-Gin, T., Kettmann, R., Deschamps, J., Rebeyrotte, N., and Guillemain, B.J., The pX region of the bovine leukemia virus is transcribed as a 2.1-kilobase mRNA, *J. Virol.,* 54, 625, 1985.

429. Fujii, M., Nakamura, M., Ohtani, K., Sugamura, K., and Hinuma, Y., 12-*O*-tetradecanoylphorbol-13-acetate induces the enhancer function of human T-cell leukemia virus type I, *FEBS Lett.,* 223, 299, 1987.

430. Hoshino, H., Esumi, H., Miwa, M., Shimoyana, M., Minato, K., Tobinai, K., Hirose, M., Watanabe, S., Inada, N., Kinoshita, K., Kamihira, S., Ichimaru, M., and Sugimura, T., Establishment and characterization of 10 cell lines derived from patients with adult T-cell leukemia, *Proc. Natl. Acad. Sci. U.S.A.,* 80, 6061, 1983.

431. Franchini, G., Wong-Staal, F., and Gallo, R.C., Human T-cell leukemia virus (HTLV-I) transcripts in fresh and cultured cells of patients with adult T-cell leukemia, *Proc. Natl. Acad. Sci. U.S.A.* 81, 6207, 1984.

432. Clarke, M.F., Westin E., Schmidt, D., Josephs, S.F., Ratner, L., Wong-Staal, F., Gallo, R.C., and Reitz, M.S., Jr., Transformation of NIH 3T3 cells by a human c-*sis* cDNA clone, *Nature,* 308, 464, 1984.

433. de Rossi, A., Aldovini, A., Franchini, G., Mann, D., Gallo, R.C., and Wong-Staal, F., Clonal selection of T lymphocytes infected by cell-free human T-cell leukemia/lymphoma virus type I: parameters of virus integration and expression, *Virology,* 143, 640, 1985.

434. Yoshida, M., Seiki, M., Yamaguchi, K., and Takatsuki, K., Monoclonal integration of human T-cell leukemia provirus in all primary tumors of adult T-cell leukemia suggests causative role of human T-cell leukemia virus in the disease, *Proc. Natl. Acad. Sci. U.S.A.,* 81, 2534, 1984.

435. Maeda, M., Shimizu, A., Ikuta, K., Okamoto, H., Kashihara, M., Uchiyama, T., Honjo, T., and Yodoi, J., Origin of human T-lymphotrophic virus I-positive T cell lines in adult T cell leukemia: analysis of T cell receptor gene rearrangement, *J. Exp. Med.,* 162, 2169, 1985.

436. Clarke, M.F., Gelmann, E.P., and Reitz, M.S., Jr., Homology of human T-cell leukaemia virus envelope gene with class I HLA gene, *Nature,* 305, 60, 1983.

437. Mann, D.L., Popovic, M., Sarin, P., Murray, C., Reitz, M.S., Strong, D.M., Haynes, B.F., Gallo, R.C., and Blattner, W.A., Cell lines producing human T-cell lymphoma virus show altered HLA expression, *Nature,* 305, 58, 1983.

438. Whang-Peng, J., Bunn, P.A., Knutsen, T., Kao-Shan, C.S., Broder, S., Jaffe, E.S., Gelmann, E., Blattner, W., Lofters, W., Young, R.C., and Gallo, R.C., Cytogenetic studies in human T-cell lymphoma virus (HTLV)-positive leukemia-lymphoma in the United States, *J. Natl. Cancer Inst.,* 74, 357, 1985.

439. Sanada, I., Tanaka, R., Kumagai, E., Tsuda, H., Nishimura, H., Yamaguchi, K., Kawano, F., Fujiwara, H., and Takatsuki, K., Chromosomal aberrations in adult T cell leukemia: relationship to the clinical severity, *Blood,* 65, 649, 1985.

440. Morgan, D.A., Ruscetti, F.W., and Gallo, R.C., Selective *in vitro* growth of T lymphocytes from normal human bone marrows, *Science,* 193, 107, 1976.

441. Ruscetti, F.W. and Gallo, R.C., Human T-lymphocyte growth factor: regulation of growth and function of T lymphocytes, *Blood,* 57, 379, 1981.

442. Cantrell, D.A. and Smith, K.A., The interleukin-2 T-cell system: a new cell growth model, *Science,* 224, 1312, 1984.

443. Sarin, P.S. and Gallo, R.C., Human T-cell growth factor (TCGF), *Crit. Rev. Immunol.,* 4, 279, 1984.

444. Farrar, W.L., Cleveland, J.L., Beckner, S.K., Bonvini, E., and Evans, S.W., Biochemical and molecular events associated with interleukin 2 regulation of lymphocyte proliferation, *Immunol. Rev.,* 92, 49, 1986.

445. Pimentel, E., *Hormones, Growth Factors, and Oncogenes,* CRC Press, Boca Raton, FL, 1987.

446. Arima, N., Daitoku, Y., Yamamoto, Y., Fujimoto, K., Ohgaki, S., Kojima, K., Fukumori, J., Matsushita, K., Tanaka, H., and Onoue, K., Heterogeneity in response to interleukin 2 and interleukin 2-producing ability of adult T cell leukemic cells, *J. Immunol.,* 138, 3069, 1987.

447. Dodon, M.D. and Gazzolo, L., Loss of interleukin-2 requirement for the generation of T colonies defines an early event of human T-lymphotropic virus type I infection, *Blood,* 69, 12, 1987.

448. Waldmann, T.A., The structure, function, and expression of interleukin-2 receptors on normal and malignant lymphocytes, *Science,* 232, 727, 1986.

449. Diamantstein, T. and Osawa, H., The interleukin-2 receptor, its physiology and a new approach to a selective immunosuppressive therapy by anti-interleukin-2 receptor monoclonal antibodies, *Immunol. Rev.,* 92, 5, 1986.

450. Greene, W.C. and Leonard, W.J., The human interleukin-2 receptor, *Annu. Rev. Immunol.,* 4, 69, 1986.

451. Greene, W.C., Depper, J.M., Krönke, M., and Leonard, W.J., The human interleukin-2 receptor: analysis of structure and function, *Immunol. Rev.,* 92, 29, 1986.

452. Greene, W.C., Leonard, W.J., Depper, J.M., Nelson, D.L., and Waldmann, T.A., The human interleukin-2 receptor: normal and abnormal expression in T cells and in leukemias induced by the human T-lymphotropic retroviruses, *Ann. Int. Med.,* 105, 560, 1986.

453. Yodoi, J. and Uchiyama, T., IL-2 receptor dysfunction and adult T-cell leukemia, *Immunol. Rev.,* 92, 135, 1986.

454. Waldmann, T.A., The role of the multichain IL-2 receptor complex in the control of normal and malignant T-cell proliferation, *Environ. Health Perspect.,* 75, 11, 1987.

455. Popovic, M., Lange-Wantzin, G., Sarin, P.S., Mann, D., and Gallo, R.C., Transformation of human umbilical cord blood T cells by human T-cell leukemia/lymphoma virus, *Proc. Natl. Acad. Sci. U.S.A.,* 80, 5402, 1983.

456. Kohtz, D.S., Altman, A., Kohtz, J.D., and Puszkin, S., Immunological and structural homology between human T-cell leukemia virus type I envelope glycoprotein and a region of human interleukin-2 implicated in binding the beta receptor, *J. Virol.,* 62, 659, 1988.

457. Arya, S.K., Wong-Staal, F., and Gallo, R.C., T-cell growth factor gene: lack of expression in human T-cell leukemia-lymphoma virus-infected cells, *Science,* 223, 1086, 1984.

458. Hori, T., Uchiyama, T., Umadome, H., Tamori, S., Tsudo, M., Araki, K., and Uchino, H., Dissociation of interleukin-2-mediated cell proliferation and interleukin-2 receptor upregulation in adult T-cell leukemia cells, *Leukemia Res.,* 10, 1447, 1986.

459. Yodoi, J., Okada, M., Tagaya, Y., Teshigawara, K., Fukui, K., Ishida, N., Ikuta, K-I., Maeda, M., Honjo, T., Osawa, H., Diamantstein, T., Tateno, M., and Toshiki, T., Rat lymphoid cell lines producing human T cell leukemia virus. II. Constitutive expression of rat interleukin 2 receptor, *J. Exp. Med.,* 161, 924, 1985.

460. Krönke, M., Leonard, W.J., Depper, J.M., and Greene, W.C., Deregulation of interleukin-2 receptor gene expression in HTLV-I-induced adult T-cell leukemia, *Science,* 228, 1215, 1985.

461. Inoue, J., Seiki, M., Taniguchi, T., Tsuru, S., and Yoshida, M., Induction of interleukin 2 receptor gene expression by p40^x encoded by human T-cell leukemia virus type 1, *EMBO J.,* 5, 2883, 1986.

462. Siekevitz, M., Feinberg, M.B., Holbrook, N., Wong-Staal, F., and Greene, W.C., Activation of interleukin 2 and interleukin 2 receptor (Tac) promoter expression by the trans-activator (*tat*) gene product of human T-cell leukemia virus, type I, *Proc. Natl. Acad. Sci. U.S.A.,* 84, 5389, 1987.

463. Ruben, S., Poteat, H., Tan, T.-H., Kawakami, K., Roeder, R., Haseltine, W., and Rosen, C.A., Cellular transcription factors and regulation of IL-2 receptor gene expression by HTLV-I *tax* gene product, *Science,* 241, 89, 1988.

464. Tomita, S., Ambrus, J.L., Jr., Volkman, D.J., Longo, D.L., Mitsuya, H., Reitz, M.S., Jr., and Fauci, A.S., Human T cell leukemia/lymphoma virus I infection and subsequent cloning of normal human B cells: direct responsiveness of cloned cells to recombinant interleukin 2 by differentiation in the absence of enhanced proliferation, *J. Exp. Med.,* 162, 393, 1985.

465. Arima, N., Daitoku, Y., Ohgaki, S., Fukumori, J., Tanaka, H., Yamamoto, Y., Fujimoto, K., and Onoue, K., Autocrine growth of interleukin 2-producing leukemic cells in a patient with adult T cell leukemia, *Blood,* 68, 779, 1986.

466. Katoh, T., Harada, T., Morikawa, S., and Wakutani, T., IL-2- and IL-2-R-independent proliferation of T-cell lines from adult T-cell leukemia/lymphoma patients, *Int. J. Cancer,* 38, 265, 1986.

467. Kobayashi, N., Koyanagi, Y., Yamamoto, N., Hinuma, Y., Sato, H., Okochi, K., and Hatanaka, M., 28,000-dalton polypeptide (p28) of adult T-cell leukemia associated antigen encoded by 24S mRNA of human T-cell leukemia virus has an associated protein kinase activity, *J. Biol. Chem.,* 259, 11162, 1984.

468. Holbrook, N.J., Lieber, M., and Crabtree, G.R., DNA sequence of the 5′ flanking region of the human interleukin 2 gene: homologies with adult T-cell leukemia virus, *Nucleic Acids Res.,* 12, 5005, 1984.

469. Renan, M.J., Sequence homologies in the control regions of c-*myc,* c-*fos,* HTLV and the interleukin-2 receptor, *Cancer Lett.,* 69, 69, 1985.

470. Gojobori, T., Aota, S., Inoue, T., and Shimotohno, K., A sequence homology between the pX genes of HTLV-I/II and the murine IL-3 gene, *FEBS Lett.,* 208, 231, 1986.

471. Wano, Y., Hattori, T., Matsuoka, M., Takatsuki, K., Chua, A.O., Gubler, U., and Greene, W.C., Interleukin 1 gene expression in adult T cell leukemia, *J. Clin. Invest.,* 80, 911, 1987.

472. Pantazis, P., Sariban, E., Bohan, C.A., Antoniades, H.N., and Kalyanaraman, V.S., Synthesis of PDGF by cultured T cells transformed with HTLV-I and II, *Oncogene,* 1, 285, 1987.

473. Chen, I.S.Y., Slamon, D.J., Rosenblatt, J.D., Shah, N.P., Quan, S.G., and Wachsman, W., The *x* gene is essential for HTLV replication, *Science,* 229, 54, 1985.

474. Goh, W.C., Sodroski, J., Rosen, C., Essex, M., and Haseltine, W.A., Subcellular localization of the product of the long open reading frame of human T-cell leukemia virus type I, *Science,* 227, 1227, 1985.

475. Slamon, D.J., Press, M.F., Souza, L.M., Murdock, D.C., Cline, M.J., Golde, D.W., Gasson, J.C., and Chen, I.S.Y., Studies on the putative transforming protein of the type I human T-cell leukemia virus, *Science,* 228, 1427, 1985.

476. Kiyokawa, T., Kawaguchi, T., Seiki, M., and Yoshida, M., Association of the *pX* gene product of human T-cell leukemia virus type-I with nucleus, *Virology,* 147, 462, 1985.

477. Nerenberg, M., Hinrichs, S.H., Reynolds, R.K., Khoury, G., and Jay, G., The *tat* gene of human T-lymphotropic virus type 1 induces mesenchymal tumors in transgenic mice, *Science,* 237, 1324, 1987.

478. Kleinerman, E.S., Lachman, L.B., Knowles, R.D., Snyderman, R., and Cianciolo, G.J., A synthetic peptide homologous to the envelope proteins of retroviruses inhibits monocyte-mediated killing by inactivating interleukin 1, *J. Immunol.,* 139, 2329, 1987.

479. Miyoshi, I., Yoshimoto, S., Fujishita, M., Ohtsuki, Y., Taguchi, H., Shiraishi, Y., Akagi, T., and Minezawa, M., Isolation in culture of a type C virus from a Japanese monkey seropositive to adult T-cell leukemia-associated antigens, *Jpn. J. Cancer Res.,* 74, 323, 1983.

480. Hayami, M., Komuro, A., Nozawa, K., Shotake, T., Ishikawa, K., Yamamoto, K., Ishida, T., Honjo, S., and Hinuma, Y., Prevalence of antibody to adult T-cell leukemia virus-associated antigens (ATLA) in Japanese monkeys and other non-human primates, *Int. J. Cancer,* 33, 179, 1984.

481. Komuro, A., Watanabe, T., Miyoshi, I., Hayami, M., Tsujimoto, H., Seiki, M., and Yoshida, M., Detection and characterization of simian retroviruses homologous to human T-cell leukemia virus type I, *Virology,* 138, 373, 1984.

482. Tsujimoto, H., Komuro, A., Iijima, K., Miyamoto, J., Ishikawa, K., and Hayami, M., Isolation of simian retroviruses closely related to human T-cell leukemia virus by establishment of lymphoid cell lines from various non-human primates, *Int. J. Cancer,* 35, 377, 1985.

483. Fukasawa, M., Tsujimoto, H., Ishikawa, K.-I., Miura, T., Ivanoff, B., Cooper, R.W., Frost, E., Delaporte, E., Mingle, J.A.A., Grant, F.C., and Hayami, M., Human T-cell leukemia virus type I isolates from Gabon and Ghana: comparative analysis of proviral genomes, *Virology,* 161, 315, 1987.

484. Watanabe, T., Seiki, M., Tsujimoto, H., Miyoshi, I., Hayami, M., and Yoshida, M., Sequence homology of the simian retrovirus genome with human T-cell leukemia virus type I, *Virology,* 144, 59, 1985.

485. Yamamoto, N., Okada, M., Hinuma, Y., Hirsch, F.W., Chosa, T., Schneider, J., and Hunsmann, G., Human adult T-cell leukaemia virus is distinct from a similar isolate of Japanese monkeys, *J. Gen. Virol.,* 65, 2259, 1984.

486. Guo, H.-G., Wong-Staal, F., and Gallo, R.C., Novel viral sequences related to human T-cell leukemia virus in T cells of a seropositive baboon, *Science,* 223, 1195, 1984.

487. Miyoshi, I., Fujishita, M., Yoshimoto, S., Kubonishi, I., Taguchi, H., Ohtsuki, Y., and Tanioka, Y., Transmission of monkey retrovirus similar to human T-cell leukemia virus by blood transfusion, *Jpn. J. Cancer Res.,* 75, 479, 1984.

488. Homma, T., Kanki, P.J., King, N.W., Jr., Hunt, R.D., O'Connell, M.J., Letvin, N.L., Daniel, M.D., Desrosiers, R.C., Yang, C.S., and Essex, M., Lymphoma in macaques: association with virus of human T lymphotrophic family, *Science,* 225, 716, 1984.

489. Tsujimoto, H., Seiki, M., Nakamura, H., Watanabe, T., Sakakibara, I., Sasagawa, A., Honjo, S., Hayami, M., and Yoshima, M., Adult T-cell leukemia-like disease in monkey naturally infected with simian retrovirus related to human T-cell leukemia virus type I, *Jpn. J. Cancer Res.,* 76, 911, 1985.

490. Tsujimoto, H., Noda, Y., Ishiwaka, K., Nakamura, H., Fukasawa, M., Sakakibara, I., Sasagawa, A., Honjo, S., and Hayami, M., Development of adult T-cell leukemia-like disease in African green monkey associated with clonal integration of simian T-cell leukemia virus type I, *Cancer Res.,* 47, 269, 1987.

491. Srivastava, B.I.S., Wong-Staal, F., and Getchell, J.P., Human T-cell leukemia virus I provirus and antibodies in a captive gorilla with non-Hodgkin's lymphoma, *Cancer Res.,* 46, 4756, 1986.

492. Kalyanaraman, V.S., Sarngadharan, M.G., Robert-Guroff, M., Miyoshi, I., Blayney, D., Golde, D., and Gallo, R.C., A new type of human T-cell leukemia virus (HTLV-II) associated with a T-cell variant of hairy cell leukemia, *Science,* 218, 571, 1982.

493. Reitz, M.S., Jr., Popovic, M., Haynes, B.F., Clark, S.C., and Gallo, R.C., Relatedness by nucleic acid hybridization of new isolates of human T-cell leukemia-lymphoma virus (HTLV) and demonstration of provirus in uncultured leukemic blood cells, *Virology,* 126, 688, 1983.

494. Chen, I.S.Y., McLaughlin, J., Gasson, J.C., Clark, S.C., and Golde, D.W., Molecular characterization of genome of a novel human T-cell leukaemia virus, *Nature,* 305, 502, 1983.

495. Golde, D.W., Jacobs, A.D., Glaspy, J.A., and Champlin, R.E., Hairy-cell leukemia: biology and treatment, *Semin. Hematol.,* 23 (Suppl. 1), 3, 1986.

496. Kalyanaraman, V.S., Narayanan, R., Feorino, P., Ramsey, R.B., Palmer, E.L., Chorba, T., McDougal, S., Getchell, J.P., Holloway, B., Harrison, A.K., Cabradilla, C.D., Telfer, M., and Evatt, B., Isolation and characterization of a human T cell leukemia virus type II from a hemophilia-A patient with pancytopenia, *EMBO J.,* 4, 1455, 1985.

497. Sohn, C.C., Blayney, D.W., Misset, J.L., Mathé, G., Flandrin, G., Moran, E.M., Jensen, F.C., Winberg, C.D., and Rappaport, H., Leukopenic chronic T cell leukemia mimicking hairy cell leukemia: association with human retroviruses, *Blood,* 67, 949, 1986.

498. Chen, I.S.Y., Quan, S.G., and Golde, D.W., Human T-cell leukemia virus type II transforms normal human lymphocytes, *Proc. Natl. Acad. Sci. U.S.A.,* 80, 7006, 1983.

499. Wachsman, W., Golde, D.W., and Chen, I.S.Y., Hairy cell leukemia and human T cell leukemia virus, *Semin. Oncol.,* 11, 446, 1984.

500. Shaw, G.M., Gonda, M.A., Flickinger, M.A., Hahn, B.H., Gallo, R.C., and Wong-Staal, F., Genomes of evolutionarily divergent members of the human T-cell leukemia virus family (HTLV-I and HTLV-II) are highly conserved, especially in pX, *Proc. Natl. Acad. Sci. U.S.A.,* 81, 4544, 1984.

501. Shimotohno, K., Takahashi, Y., Shimizu, N., Gojobori, T., Golde, D.W., Chen, I.S.Y., Miwa, M., and Sugimura, T., Complete nucleotide sequence of an infectious clone of human T-cell leukemia virus type II: an open reading frame for the protease gene, *Proc. Natl. Acad. Sci. U.S.A.,* 82, 3101, 1985.

502. Sodroski, J., Patrarca, R., Perkins, D., Briggs, D., Lee, T.-H., Essex, M., Coligan, J., Wong-Staal, F., Gallo, R.C., and Haseltine, W.A., Sequence of the envelope glycoprotein gene of type II human T lymphotropic virus, *Science,* 225, 421, 1984.

503. Gelmann, E.P., Franchini, G., Manzari, V., Wong-Staal, F., and Gallo, R.C., Molecular cloning of a unique human T-cell leukemia virus (HTLV-II$_{Mo}$), *Proc. Natl. Acad. Sci. U.S.A.,* 81, 993, 1984.

504. Sodroski, J., Trus, M., Perkins, D., Patarca, R., Wong-Staal, F., Gelmann, E., Gallo, R., and Haseltine, W.A., Repetitive structure in the long-terminal-repeat element of a type II human T-cell leukemia virus, *Proc. Natl. Acad. Sci. U.S.A.,* 81, 4617, 1984.

505. Lee, T.H., Coligan, J.E., McLane, M.F., Sodroski, J.G., Popovic, M., Wong-Staal, F., Gallo, R.C., Haseltine, W., and Essex, M., Serological cross-reactivity between envelope gene products of type I and type II human T-cell leukemia virus, *Proc. Natl. Acad. Sci. U.S.A.,* 81, 7579, 1984.

506. Greene, W.C., Leonard, W.J., Wano, Y., Svetlik, P.B., Peffer, N.J., Sodroski, J.G., Rosen, C.A., Goh, W.C., and Haseltine, *Trans*-activator gene of HTLV-II induces IL-2 receptor and IL-2 cellular gene expression, *Science,* 232, 877, 1986.

507. Barré-Sinoussi, F., Chermann, J.C., Rey, F., Nugeyre, M.T., Chamaret, S., Gruest, J., Dauguet, C., Axler-Blin, C., Brun-Vézinet, F., Rouzioux, C., Rozenbaum, W., and Montagnier, L., Isolation of a T-lymphotropic retrovirus from a patient at risk for acquired immune deficiency syndrome (AIDS), *Science,* 220, 868, 1983.

508. Rey, M.A., Spire, B., Dormont, D., Barré-Sinoussi, F., Montagnier, L, and Chermann, J.C., Characterization of the RNA dependent DNA polymerase of a new human T lymphotropic retrovirus (lymphadenopathy associated virus), *Biochem. Biophys. Res. Commun.,* 121, 126, 1984.

509. Vilmer, E., Rouzioux, C., Brun, F., Fisher, A., Chermann, J., Barré-Sinoussi, F., Gazengelc, F., Dauguet, C., Manigne, P., and Griscelli, C., Isolation of a new lymphotropic retrovirus from two siblings with haemophilia B, one with AIDS, *Lancet,* i, 753, 1984.

510. Chermann, J.C., Barré-Sinoussi, F., Dauguet, C., Brun-Vézinet, F., Rouzioux, C., Rozenbaum, W., and Montagnier, L., Isolation of a new retrovirus in a patient at risk for acquired immunodeficiency syndrome, *Antibiot. Chemother.,* 32, 48, 1984.

511. Popovic, M., Sarngadharan, M.G., Read, E., and Gallo, R.C., Detection, isolation, and continuous production of cytopathic retroviruses (HTLV-III) from patients with AIDS and pre-AIDS, *Science*, 224, 497, 1984.
512. Gallo, R.C., Salahuddin, S.Z., Popovic, M., Shearer, G.M., Kaplan, M., Haynes, B.F., Palker, T.J., Redfield, R., Oleske, J., Safai, B., White, G., Foster, P., and Markham, P.D., Frequent detection and isolation of cytopathic retroviruses (HTLV-III) from patients with AIDS and at risk for AIDS, *Science*, 224, 500, 1984.
513. Schüpbach, J., Popovic, M., Gilden, R.V., Gonda, M.A., Sarngadharan, M.G., and Gallo, R.C., Serological analysis of a subgroup of human T-lymphotropic retroviruses (HTLV-III) associated with AIDS, *Science*, 224, 503, 1984.
514. Sarngadharan, M.G., Popovic, M., Bruch, L., Schupbach, J., and Gallo, R.C., Antibodies reactive with human T-lymphotropic retroviruses (HTLV-III) in the serum of patients with AIDS, *Science*, 224, 506, 1984.
515. Ellrodt, A., Barre-Sinoussi, F., Le Bras, P., Nugeyre, M.T., Palazzo, L., Rey, F., Brun-Vezinet, F., Rouzioux, C., Segond, P., Caquet, R., Montagnier, L., and Chermann, J.C., Isolation of a human T-lymphotropic retrovirus (LAV) from Zairain married couple, one with AIDS, one with prodromes, *Lancet*, i, 1383, 1984.
516. Levy, J.A., Hoffman, A.D., Kramer, S.M., Landis, J.A., Shimabukuro, J.M., and Oshiro, L.S., Isolation of lymphocytopathic retroviruses from San Francisco patients with AIDS, *Science*, 225, 840, 1984.
517. Wain-Hobson, S., Sonigo, P., Danos, O., Cole, S., and Alizon, M., Nucleotide sequence of the AIDS virus, LAV, *Cell*, 40, 9, 1985.
518. Ratner, I., Haseltine, W., Patrarca, R., Livak, K.J., Starcich, B., Josephs, S.F., Doran, E.R., Rafalski, J.S., Whitehorn, E.A., Baumeister, K., Ivanoff, L., Petteway, S.R., Pearson, M.L., Lautenberger, J.A., Ppas, T.S., Ghrayeb, J., Chang, N.T., Gallo, R.C., and Wong-Staal, F., Complete nucleotide sequence of the AIDS virus, HTLV-III, *Nature*, 313, 277, 1985.
519. Sanchez-Pescador, R., Power, M.D., Barr, P.J., Steimer, K.S., Stempien, M.M., Brown-Shimer, S.L., Ges, W.W., Renard, A., Randolph, A., Levy, J.A., Dina, D., and Luciw, P.A., Nucleotide sequence and expression of an AIDS-associated retrovirus (ARV-2), *Science*, 227, 484, 1985.
520. Muesing, M.A., Smith, D.H., Cabradilla, C.D., Benton, C.V., Lasky, L.A., and Capon, D.J., Nucleic acid structure and expression of the human AIDS/lymphadenopathy retrovirus, *Nature*, 313, 450, 1985.
521. Francis, D.P., Curran, J.W., and Essex, M., Epidemic acquired immune deficiency syndrome: epidemiologic evidence for a transmissible agent, *J. Natl. Cancer Inst.*, 71, 1, 1983.
522. Gottlieb, M.S., Groopman, J.E., Weinstein, W.M., Fahey, J.L., and Detels, R., The acquired immunodeficiency syndrome, *Ann. Int. Med.*, 99, 208, 1983.
523. Leavitt, R.D., Searching for the cause of the acquired immune deficiency syndrome, *Eur. J. Microbiol.*, 3, 79, 1984.
524. Fauci, A.S., Macher, A.M., Longo, D.L., Lane, H.C., Rook, A.H., Masur, H., and Gelmann, E.P., Acquired immunodeficiency syndrome: epidemiologic, clinical, immunologic, and therapeutic considerations, *Ann. Int. Med.*, 100, 92, 1984.
525. Wofsy, C.B. and Mills, J., The acquired immune deficiency syndrome: an international health problem of increasing importance, *Klin. Wochenschr.*, 62, 512, 1984.
526. Sinkovics, J.G., Gyorkey, F., Melnick, J.L., and Gyorkey, P., Acquired immune deficiency syndrome (AIDS): speculations about its etiology and comparative immunology, *Rev. Infect. Dis.*, 6, 745, 1984.
527. Barrett, D.J., Characterization of the acquired immune deficiency syndrome at the cellular and molecular level, *Mol. Cell. Biochem.*, 63, 3, 1984.
528. Broder, S. and Gallo, R.C., A pathogenic retrovirus (HTLV-III) linked to AIDS, *N. Engl. J. Med.*, 311, 1292, 1984.
529. Landesman, S.H., Ginzburg, H.M., and Weiss, S.H., The AIDS epidemic, *N. Engl. J. Med.*, 312, 521, 1985.
530. Fauci, A.S. and Lane, H.C., The acquired immunodeficiency syndrome (AIDS): an update, *Int. Arch. Allergy Appl. Immunol.*, 77, 81, 1985.
531. Fauci, A.S., Masur, H., Gelmann, E.P., Markhan, P.D., Hahn, B.H., and Lane, H.C., The acquired immunodeficiency syndrome: an update, *Ann. Int. Med.*, 102, 800, 1985.
532. Pien, F.D., HTLV-III infection: a clinical approach to diagnosis and treatment of the "AIDS virus", *Postgrad. Med.*, 80, 135, 1986.
533. Lifson, A.R., Ancelle, R.A., Brunet, J.B., and Curran, J.W., The epidemiology of AIDS worldwide, *Clin. Immunol. Allergy*, 6, 441, 1986.
534. Friedland, G.H. and Klein, R.S., Transmission of the human immunodeficiency virus, *N. Engl. J. Med.*, 317, 1125, 1987.
535. Biggar, R.J., AIDS and HIV infection: estimates of the magnitude of the problem worldwide in 1985/1986, *Clin. Immunol. Immunopathol.*, 45, 297, 1987.
536. Piot, P. and Caraël, M., Epidemiological and sociological aspects of HIV-infection in developing countries, *Br. Med. Bull.*, 44, 68, 1988.
537. Piot, P., Plummer, F.A., Mhalu, F.S., Lamboray, J.-L., Chin, J., and Mann, J.M., AIDS: an international perspective, *Science*, 239, 573, 1988.
538. Piot, P., Kreiss, J.K., Ndinya-Achola, J.O., Ngugi, E.N., Simonsen, J.N., Cameron, D.W., Taelman, H., and Plummer, F.A., Heterosexual transmission of HIV, *AIDS*, 1, 199, 1987.

539. Novick, B.E. and Rubinstein, A., AIDS — the pediatric perspective, *AIDS*, 1, 3, 1987.

540. Waisman, J., Rotterdam, H., Niedt, G.N., Lewin, K., and Racz, P., AIDS: an overview of the pathology, *Pathol. Res. Pract.*, 182, 729, 1987.

541. Penn, I., Kaposi's sarcoma in immunosuppressed patients, *J. Clin. Lab. Immunol.*, 12, 1, 1983.

542. Dorfman, R.F., Kaposi's sarcoma revisited, *Hum. Pathol.*, 15, 1013, 1984.

543. Marmor, M., Friedman-Kien, A.E., Zolla-Pazner, S., Stahl, R.E., Rubinstein, P., Laubenstein, L., William, D.C., Klein, R.J., and Spigland, I., Kaposi's sarcoma in homosexual men, *Ann. Int. Med.*, 100, 809, 1984.

544. Volberding, P.A., Kaposi's sarcoma, B-cell lymphoma and other AIDS-associated tumours, *Clin. Immunol. Allergy*, 6, 569, 1986.

545. Bayley, A.C., Downing, R.G., Cheingson-Popov, R., Tedder, R.S., Dalgleish, A.G., and Weiss, R.A., HTLV-III serology distinguishes atypical and endemic Kaposi's sarcoma in Africa, *Lancet*, 1, 359, 1985.

546. Craighead, J., Moore, A., Grossman, H., Ershler, W., Frattini, U., Saxinger, C., Hess, U., and Ngowi, F., Pathogenetic role of HIV infection in Kaposi's sarcoma of Equatorial East Africa, *Arch. Pathol. Lab. Med.*, 112, 259, 1988.

547. Rechavi, G., Ben-Bassat, I., Berkowicz, M., Martinowitz, U., Brok-Símoni, F., Neumann, Y., Vansover, A., Gotlieb-Stematsky, T., and Ramot, B., Molecular analysis of Burkitt's leukemia in two hemophilic brothers with AIDS, *Blood*, 70, 1713, 1987.

548. Biggar, R.J., Horm, J., Goedert, J.J., and Melbye, M., Cancer in a group at risk of acquired immunodeficiency syndrome (AIDS) through 1984, *Am. J. Epidemiol.*, 126, 578, 1987.

549. Ho, D.D., Pomerantz, R.J., and Kaplan, J.C., Pathogenesis of infection with human immunodeficiency virus, *N. Engl. J. Med.*, 317, 278, 1987.

550. Shaw, G.M., Harper, M.E., Hahn, B.H., Epstein, L.G., Gajdusek, D.C., Price, R.W., Navia, B.A., Petito, C.K., O'Hara, C.J., Cho, E.-S., Oleske, J.M., Wong-Staal, F., and Gallo, R.C., HTLV-III infection in brains of children and adults with AIDS encephalopathy, *Science*, 227, 177, 1985.

551. Rostad, S.W., Sumi, S.M., Shaw, C.-M., Olson, K., and McDougall, J.K., Human immunodeficiency virus (HIV) infection in brains with AIDS-related leukoencaphalopathy, *AIDS Res.*, 3, 363, 1987.

552. Cooper, D.A., Gold, J., Maclean, P., Donovan, B., Finlayson, R., Barnes, T.G., Michelmore, H.M., Brooke, P., and Penny, R., Acute retrovirus infection: definition of a clinical illness associated with seroconversion, *Lancet*, 1, 537, 1985.

553. Reinherz, E.L., Kung, P.C., Goldstein, G., Levy, R.H., and Scholssman, S.F., Discrete stages of human intrathymic differentiation: analysis of normal thymocytes and leukemic lymphoblasts on T-cell lineage, *Proc. Natl. Acad. Sci. U.S.A.*, 77, 1588, 1980.

554. Hood, L., Kronenberg, M., and Hunkapiller, T., T cell antigen receptors and the immunoglobulin supergene family, *Cell*, 40, 225, 1985.

555. Isobe, M., Huebner, K., Maddon, P.J., Littman, D.R., Axel, R., and Croce, C.M., The gene encoding the T-cell surface protein T4 is located on human chromosome 12, *Proc. Natl. Acad. Sci. U.S.A.*, 83, 4399, 1986.

556. Klatzmann, D., Champagne, E., Chamaret, S., Gruest, J., Guétard, D., Hercend, T., Gluckman, J.C., and Montagnier, L., T-lymphocyte T4 molecule behaves as the receptor for human retrovirus LAV, *Nature*, 312, 767, 1984.

557. Willey, R.L., Smith, D.H., Laski, L.A., Theodore, T.S., Earl, P.L., Moss, B., Capon, D.J., and Martin, M.A., *In vitro* mutagenesis identifies a region within the envelope gene of the human immunodeficiency virus that is critical for infectivity, *J. Virol.*, 62, 139, 1988.

558. Stevenson, M., Meier, C., Mann, A.M., Chapman, N., and Wasiak, A., Envelope glycoprotein of HIV induces interference and cytolysis resistance in CD4⁺ cells: mechanism for persistence in AIDS, *Cell*, 53, 483, 1988.

559. Roy, S. and Wainberg, M.A., Role of the mononuclear phagocyte system in the development of acquired immunodeficiency syndrome (AIDS), *J. Leukocyte Biol.*, 43, 91, 1988.

560. Redfield, R.R., Markham, P.D., Salahuddin, S.Z., Sarngadharan, M.G., Bodner, A.J., Folks, T.M., Ballou, W.R., Wright, D.C., and Gallo, R.C., Frequent transmission of HTLV-III among spouses of patients with AIDS-related complex and AIDS, *JAMA*, 253, 1571, 1985.

561. Safai, B., Sarngadharan, M.G., Groopman, J.E., Arnett, K., Popovic, M., Sliski, A., Schupbach, J., and Gallo, R.C., Seroepidemiological studies of human T-lymphotropic retrovirus type III in acquired immunodeficiency syndrome, *Lancet*, i, 1438, 1984.

562. Jaffe, H.W., Francis, D.P., McLane, M.F., Cabradilla, C., Curran, J.W., Kilbourne, B.W., Lawrence, D.N., Haverkos, H.W., Spira, T.J., Dodd, R.Y., Gold, J., Armstrong, D., Ley, A., Groopman, J., Mullins, J., Lee, T.H., and Essex, M., Transfusion-associated AIDS: serologic evidence of human T-cell leukemia virus infection of donors, *Science*, 223, 1309, 1984.

563. Gazzard, B.G., Shanson, D.C., Farthing, C., Lawrence, A.G., Tedder, R.S., Cheingsong-Popov, R., Dalgleish, A., and Weiss, R.A., Clinical findings and serological evidence of HTLV-III infection in homosexual contacts of patients with AIDS and persistent generalised lymphadenopathy in London, *Lancet*, ii, 480, 1984.

564. Goedert, J.J., Sarngadharan, M.G., Biggar, R.J., Weiss, S.L., Winn, D.M., Grossman, R.J., Greene, M.H., Bodner, A.J., Mann, D.L., Strong, D.M., Gallo, R.C., and Blattner, W.A., Determinants of retrovirus (HTLV-III) antibody and immunodeficiency conditions in homosexual men, *Lancet*, ii, 11, 1984.

565. Kitchen, L.W., Barin, F., Sullivan, J.L., McLane, M.F., Brettler, D.B., Levine, P.H., and Essex, M., Aetiology of AIDS: antibodies to human T-cell leukaemia virus (type III) in haemophiliacs, *Nature,* 312, 367, 1984.

566. Goedert, J.J., Sarngadharan, M.G., Eyster, M.E., Weiss, S.H., Bodner, A.J., Gallo, R.C., and Blattner, W.A., Antibodies reactive with human T cell leukemia viruses in the serum of hemophiliacs receiving factor VIII concentrate, *Blood,* 65, 492, 1985.

567. Gnann, J.W., McCormick, J.B., Mitchell, S., Nelson, J.A., and Oldstone, M.B.A., Synthetic peptide immunoassay distinguishes HIV type 1 and HIV type 2 infections, *Science,* 237, 1346, 1987.

568. Karpas, A., Hayhoe, F.G.J., Hill, F., Anderson, M., Tenant-Flower, M., Howard, L., and Oates, J.K., Use of Karpas HIV cell test to detect antibodies to HIV-2, *Lancet,* 2, 132, 1987.

569. Volsky, D.J., Wu, Y.T., Stevenson, M., Dewhurst, S., Sinangil, F., Merino, F., Rodriguez, L., and Godoy, G., Antibodies to HTLV-III/LAV in Venezuelan patients with acute malarial infection, *N. Engl. J. Med.,* 314, 647, 1986.

570. Mendenhall, C.L., Roselle, G.A., Grossman, C.J., Rouster, S.D., Weesner, R.E., and Dumaswala, U., False positive tests for HTLV-III antibodies in alcoholic patients with hepatitis, *N. Engl. J. Med.,* 314, 921, 1986.

571. Rodriquez, L., Dewhurst, S., Sinangil, F., Merino, F., Godoy, G., and Volsky, D.J., Antibodies to HTLV-III/LAV among aboriginal Amazonian Indians in Venezuela, *Lancet,* 2, 1098, 1985.

572. Azocar, J., Martinez, C., McLane, M.F., Allan, J., and Essex, M., Lack of endemic HIV infection in Venezuela, *AIDS Res. Hum. Retrovir.,* 3, 107, 1987.

573. Becker, J.-L., Hazan, U., Nugeyre, M.-T., Rey, F., Spire, B., Barré-Sinoussi, F., Georges, A., Teulières, L., and Chermann, J.-C., Infection de cellules d'insectes en culture par le virus HIV, agent du SIDA, et mise en évidence d'insectes d'origine africaine contaminés par ce virus, *C.R. Acad. Sci. Paris,* 303, 303, 1986.

574. Pellegrino, M.G., Lewin, M., Meyer, W.A., III, Lanciotti, R.S., Bhaduri-Hauck, L., Volsky, D.J., Sakai, K., Folks, T.M., and Gillespie, D., A sensitive solution hybridization technique for detecting RNA in cells: application to HIV in blood cells, *BioTechniques,* 5, 452, 1987.

575. Clavel, F., Brun-Vézinet, F., Guétard, D., Chamaret, S., Laurent, C., Rouizioux, C., Rey, M., Katlama, C., Rey, F., Champelinaud, J.L., Nina, J.S., Mansinho, K., Santos-Ferreira, M.-O., Klatzmann, D., and Montagnier, L., LAV type II: un second rétrovirus associé au SIDA en Afrique de l'Ouest, *C.R. Acad. Sci. Paris,* 302, 485, 1986.

576. Clavel, F., Guyader, M., Guétard, D., Sallé, M., Montagnier, L., and Alizon, M., Molecular cloning and polymorphism of the human immune deficiency virus type 2, *Nature,* 324, 691, 1986.

577. Clavel, F., HIV-2, the West African AIDS virus, *AIDS,* 1, 135, 1987.

578. Brun-Vézinet, F., Rey, M.A., Katlama, C., Girard, P.M., Roulot, D., Yeni, P., Lenoble, L., Clavel, F., Alizon, M., Gadelle, S., Madjar, J.J., and Harzic, M., Lymphadenopathy-associated virus type 2 in AIDS and AIDS-related complex: clinical and virological features in four patients, *Lancet,* 1, 128, 1987.

579. Marlink, R.G., Ricard, D., M'Boup, S., Kanki, P.J., Romet-Lemonne, J.-L., N'Doye, I., Diop, K., Simpson, M.A., Greco, F., Chou, M-J., Degruttola, V., Hsieh, C.-C., Boye, C., Barin, F., Denis, F., McLane, M.F., and Essex, M., Clinical, hematologic, and immunologic cross-sectional evaluation of individuals exposed to human immunodeficiency virus type 2 (HIV-2), *AIDS Res. Hum. Retrovir.,* 4, 137, 1988.

580. Guyader, M., Emerman, M., Sonigo, P., Clavel, F., Montagnier, L., and Alizon, M., Genome organization and transactivation of the human immunodeficiency virus type 2, *Nature,* 326, 662, 1987.

581. Smith, T.F., Srionivasan, A., Schochetman, G., Marcus, M., and Myers, G., The phylogenetic history of immunodeficiency viruses, *Nature,* 333, 573, 1988.

582. Albert, J., Bredberg, U., Chiodi, F., Böttiger, B., Fenyö, E.M., Norrby, E., and Biberfeld, G., A new human retrovirus isolate of West African origin (SBL-6669) and its relationship to HTLV-IV, LAV-II, and HTLV-IIIB, *AIDS Res. Hum. Retrovir.,* 3, 3, 1987.

583. Kornfeld, H., Riedel, N., Viglianti, G.A., Hirsch, V., and Mullins, J.I., Cloning of HTLV-4 and its relation to simian and human immunodeficiency viruses, *Nature,* 326, 610, 1987.

584. Kanki, P.J., M'Boup, S., Ricard, D., Barin, F., Denis, F., Boye, C., Sangare, L., Travers, K., Albaum, M., Marklink, R., Romet-Lemonne, J.-L., and Essex, M., Human T-lymphotropic virus type 4 and the human immunodeficiency virus in West Africa, *Science,* 236, 827, 1987.

585. Hahn, B.H., Kong, L.I., Lee, S.-W., Kumar, P., Taylor, M.E., Arya, S.K., and Shaw, G.M., Relation of HTLV-4 to simian and human immunodeficiency-associated viruses, *Nature,* 330, 184, 1987.

586. Arya, S.K., Gallo, R.C., Hahn, B.H., Shaw, G.M., Popovic, M., Salahuddin, S.Z., and Wong-Staal, F., Homology of genomes of AIDS-associated virus genomes of human T-cell leukemia viruses, *Science,* 225, 927, 1984.

587. Hahn, B.H., Shaw, G.M., Arya, S.K., Popovic, M., Gallo, R.C., and Wong-Staal, F., Molecular cloning and characterization of the HTLV-III virus associated with AIDS, *Nature,* 312, 166, 1984.

588. Shaw, G.M., Hahn, B.H., Arya, S.K., Groopman, J.E., Gallo, R.C., and Wong-Staal, F., Molecular characterization of human T-cell leukemia (lymphotropic) virus type III in the acquired immune deficiency syndrome, *Science,* 226, 1165, 1984.

589. Starcich, B., Ratner, L., Josephs, S.F., Okamoto, T., Gallo, R.C., and Wong-Staal, F., Characterization of long terminal repeat sequences of HTLV-III, *Science,* 227, 538, 1985.

590. Rabson, A.B. and Martin, M.A., Molecular organization of the AIDS retrovirus, *Cell,* 40, 477, 1985.

591. Rabson, A.B., Daugherty, D.F., Venkatesan, S., Boulukos, K.E., Benn, S.I., Folks, T.M., Feorino, P., and Martin, M.A., Transcription of novel open reading frames of AIDS retrovirus during infection of lymphocytes, *Science,* 229, 1388, 1985.

592. Chang, N.T., Chanda, P.K., Barone, A.D., McKinney, S., Rhodes, D.P., Tam, S.H., Shearman, C.W., Huang, J., Chang, T.W., Gallo, R.C., and Wong-Staal, F., Expression in *Escherichia coli* of open reading frame gene segments of HTLV-III, *Science,* 228, 93, 1985.

593. Wright, C.M., Felber, B.K., Paskalis, H., and Pavlakis, G.N., Expression and characterization of the *trans*-activator of HTLV-III/LAV virus, *Science,* 234, 988, 1986.

594. Peterlin, B.M., Luciw, P.A., Barr, P.J., and Walker, M.D., Elevated levels of mRNA can account for the *trans*-activation of human immunodeficiency virus, *Proc. Natl. Acad. Sci. U.S.A.,* 83, 9734, 1986.

595. Sodroski, J., Goh, W.C., Rosen, C., Dayton, A., Terwilliger, E., and Haseltine, W., A second post-transcriptional *trans*-activator gene required for HTLV-III replication, *Nature,* 321, 412, 1986.

596. Terwilliger, E., Sodroski, J.G., Rosen, C.A., and Haseltine, W.A., Effects of mutations within the 3′ *orf* open reading frame region of human T-cell lymphotropic virus type III (HTLV-III/LAV) on replication and cytopathogenicity, *J. Virol.,* 60, 754, 1986.

597. Feinberg, M.B., Jarrett, R.F., Aldovini, A., Gallo, R.C., and Wong-Staal, F., HTLV-III expression and production involve complex regulation at the levels of splicing and translation of viral RNA, *Cell,* 46, 807, 1986.

598. Farmerie, W.G., Loeb, D.D., Casavant, N.C., Hutchison, C.A., III, Edgell, M.H., and Swanstrom, R., Expression and processing of the AIDS virus reverse transcriptase in *Escherichia coli, Science,* 236, 305, 1987.

599. DeVico, A.L., Di Marzo Veronese, F., Lee, S.L., Gallo, R.C., and Sarngadharan, M.G., High prevalence of serum antibodies to reverse transcriptase in HIV-1-infected individuals, *AIDS Res. Hum. Retrovir.,* 4, 17, 1988.

600. Jentsch, K.D., Hunsmann, G., Hartmann, H., and Nickel, P., Inhibition of human immunodeficiency virus type I reverse transcriptase by suramin-related compounds, *J. Gen. Virol.,* 68, 2183, 1987.

601. Weigent, D.A., Hoeprich, P.D., Bost, K.L., Brunk, T.K., Reiher, W.E., III, and Blalock, J.E., The HTLV-III envelope protein contains a hexapeptide homologous to a region of interleukin-2 that binds to the interleukin-2 receptor, *Biochem. Biophys. Res. Commun.,* 139, 367, 1986.

602. Reiher, W.E. III, Blalock, J.E., and Brunck, T.K., Sequence homology between acquired immunodeficiency syndrome virus envelope protein and interleukin 2, *Proc. Natl. Acad. Sci. U.S.A.,* 83, 9188, 1986.

603. Samuel, K.P., Seth, A., Konopka, A., Lautenberger, J.A., and Papas, T.S., The 3′-orf protein of human immunodeficiency virus shows structural homology with the phosphorylation domain of human interleukin-2 receptor and the ATP-binding site of the protein kinase family, *FEBS Lett.,* 218, 81, 1987.

604. Hahn, B.H., Gonda, M.A., Shaw, G.M., Popovic, M., Hoxie, J.A., Gallo, R.C., and Wong-Staal, F., Genomic diversity of the acquired immune deficiency syndrome virus HTLV-III: different viruses exhibit greatest divergence in their envelope genes, *Proc. Natl. Acad. Sci. U.S.A.,* 82, 4813, 1985.

605. Wong-Staal, F., Shaw, G.M., Hahn, B., Salahuddin, S.Z., Popovic, M., Markham, P., Redfield, R., and Gallo, R.C., Genomic diversity of human T-lymphotropic virus type III (HTLV-III), *Science,* 229, 759, 1985.

606. Benn, S., Rutlegde, R., Folks, T., Gold, J., Baker, L., McCormick, J., Feorino, P., Piot, P., Quinn, T., and Martin, M., Genomic heterogeneity of AIDS retroviral isolates from North America and Zaire, *Science,* 230, 949, 1985.

607. Hahn, B., Shaw, G.M., Taylor, M.E., Redfield, R.R., Markham, P.D., Salahuddin, S.Z., Wong-Staal, F., Gallo, R.C., Parks, E.S., and Parks, W.P., Genetic variation in HTLV-III/LAV over time in patients with AIDS or at risk for AIDS, *Science,* 232, 1548, 1986.

608. Coffin, J.M., Genetic variation in AIDS viruses, *Cell,* 46, 1, 1986.

609. Srinivasan, A., Anand, R., York, D., Ranganathan, P., Feorino, P., Schochetman, G., Curran, J., Kalyanaraman, V.S., Luciw, P.A., and Sanchez-Pescador, R., Molecular characterization of human immunodeficiency virus from Zaire: nucleotide sequence analysis identifies conserved and variable domains in the envelope gene, *Gene,* 52, 71, 1987.

610. Francis, D.P. and Petricciani, J.C., The prospects for and pathways toward a vaccine for AIDS, *N. Engl. J. Med.,* 313, 1586, 1985.

611. Duesberg, P.H., Retroviruses as carcinogens and pathogens: expectations and reality, *Cancer Res.,* 47, 1199, 1987.

612. Mitsuya, H. and Broder, S., Strategies for antiviral therapy in AIDS, *Nature,* 325, 773, 1987.

613. Siekevitz, M., Josephs, S.F., Dukovich, M., Peffer, N., Wong-Staal, F., and Greene, W.C., Activation of the HIV-1 LTR by T cell mitogens and the trans-activator protein of HTLV-I, *Science,* 238, 1575, 1987.

614. Bohan, C., York, D., and Srinivasan, A., Sodium butyrate activates human immunodeficiency virus long terminal repeat-directed expression, *Biochem. Biophys. Res. Commun.,* 148, 899, 1987.

615. Arya, S.K., Guo, C., Josephs, S.F., and Wong-Staal, F., *trans*-Activator gene of human T-lymphotropic virus type III (HTLV-III), *Science,* 229, 69, 1985.

616. Rosen, C.A., Sodroski, J.G., and Haseltine, W.A., The location of *cis*-acting regulatory sequences in the human T-cell lymphotropic virus type III (HTLV-III/LAV) long terminal repeat, *Cell,* 41, 813, 1985.

617. Okamoto, T. and Wong-Staal, F., Demonstration of virus-specific transcriptional activator(s) in cells infected with HTLV-III by an *in vitro* cell-free system, *Cell,* 47, 29, 1986.
618. Rice, A.P. and Mathews, M.B., Transcriptional but not translational regulation of HIV-1 by the *tat* gene product, *Nature,* 332, 551, 1988.
619. Bednarik, D.P., Mosca, J.D., and Raj, N.B.K., Methylation as a modulator of expression of human immunodeficiency virus, *J. Virol.,* 61, 1253, 1987.
620. Ziegler, J.L. and Stites, D.P., Hypothesis: AIDS is an autoimmune disease directed at the immune system and triggered by a lymphotropic retrovirus, *Clin. Immunol. Immunopathol.,* 41, 305, 1986.
621. Dalgleish, A.G., Beverley, P.C.L., Clapham, P.R., Crawford, D.H., Greaves, M.F., and Weiss, R.A., The CD4 (T4) antigen is an essential component of the receptor for the AIDS retrovirus, *Nature,* 312, 763, 1984.
622. Jameson, B.A., Rao, P.E., Kong, L.I., Hahn, B.H., Shaw, G.M., Hood, L.E., and Kent, S.B.H., Location and chemical synthesis of a binding site for HIV-1 on the CD4 protein, *Science,* 240, 1335, 1988.
623. Smith, D.H., Byrn, R.A., Marsters, S.A., Gregory, T., Groopman, J.E., and Capon, D.J., Blocking of HIV-1 infectivity by a soluble, secreted form of the CD4 antigen, *Science,* 238, 1704, 1987.
624. Sodroski, J., Rosen, C., Wong-Staal, F., Salahuddin, S.Z., Popovic, M., Arya, S., Gallo, R.C., and Haseltine, W.A., *trans*-Acting transcriptional regulation of human T-cell leukemia virus type III long terminal repeat, *Science,* 227, 171, 1985.
625. Tong-Starksen, S.E., Luciw, P.A., and Peterlin, B.M., Human immunodeficiency virus long terminal repeat responds to T-cell activation signals, *Proc. Natl. Acad. Sci. U.S.A.,* 84, 6845, 1987.
626. Friedman, A.H., Orellana, J., Freeman, W.R., Luntz, M.H., Starr, M.B., Tapper, M.L., Spigland, I., Rotterdam, H., Mesa Tejada, kR., Braunhut, S., Mildvan, D., and Mathur, U., Cytomegalovirus retinitis: a manifestation of the acquired immune deficiency syndrome (AIDS), *Br. J. Ophthalmol.,* 67, 372, 1983.
627. Birx, D.L., Redfield, R.R., and Tosato, G., Defective regulation of Epstein-Barr virus infection in patients with acquired immunodeficiency syndrome (AIDS) or AIDS-related disorders, *N. Engl. J. Med.,* 314, 874, 1986.
628. Gendelman, H.E., Phelps, W., Feigenbaum, L., Ostrove, J.M., Adachi, A., Howley, P.M., Khoury, G., Ginsberg, H.S., and Martin, M.A., Trans-activation of the human immunodeficiency virus long terminal repeat sequence by DNA viruses, *Proc. Natl. Acad. Sci. U.S.A.,* 83, 9759, 1986.
629. Mosca, J.D., Bednarik, D.P., Raj, N.B.K., Rosen, C.A., Sodroski, J.G., Haseltine, W.A., Hayward, G.S., and Pitha, P.M., Activation of human immunodeficiency virus by herpesvirus infection: identification of a region within the long terminal repeat that responds to a trans-acting factor encoded by herpes simplex virus 1, *Proc. Natl. Acad. Sci. U.S.A.,* 84, 7408, 1987.
630. Kenney, S., Kamine, J., Markowitz, D., Fenrick, R., and Pagano, J., An Epstein-Barr virus immediate-early gene product trans-activates gene expression from the human immunodeficiency virus long terminal repeat, *Proc. Natl. Acad. Sci. U.S.A.,* 85, 1652, 1988.
631. Wong, G.H.W., Krowka, J.F., Stites, D.P., and Goeddel, D.V., *In vitro* anti-human immunodeficiency virus activities of tumor necrosis factor-alpha and interferon-gamma, *J. Immunol.,* 140, 120, 1988.
632. Hammer, S.M., Gillis, J.M., Groopman, J.E., and Rose, R.M., *In vitro* modification of human immunodeficiency virus infection by granulocyte-macrophage colony-stimulating factor and gamma interferon, *Proc. Natl. Acad. Sci. U.S.A.,* 83, 8734, 1986.
633. Böhnlein, E., Lowenthal, J.W., Siekevitz, M., Ballard, D.W., Franza, B.R., and Greene, W.C., The same inducible nuclear proteins regulates mitogen activation of both the interleukin-2 receptor-alpha gene and type 1 HIV, *Cell,* 53, 827, 1988.
634. Reuben, J.M., Hersh, E.M., Murray, J.L., Munn, C.G., Mehta, S.R., and Mansell, P.W.A., IL-2 production and response *in vitro* by the leukocytes of patients with acquired immune deficiency syndrome, *Lymphokine Res.,* 4, 103, 1985.
635. Kloster, B.E., John, P.A., Miller, L.E., Rubin, L.A., Nelson, D.L., Blair, D.C., and Tomar, R.H., Soluble interleukin 2 receptors are elevated in patients with AIDS or at risk of developing AIDS, *Clin. Immunol. Immunopathol.,* 45, 440, 1987.
636. Prince, H.E., Kleinman, S., and Williams, A.E., Soluble IL-2 receptor levels in serum from blood donors seropositive for HIV, *J. Immunol.,* 140, 1139, 1988.
637. Reddy, M.M. and Grieco, M.H., Elevated soluble interleukin-2 receptor levels in serum of human immunodeficiency virus infected populations, *AIDS Res. Hum. Retrovir.,* 4, 115, 1988.
638. Antonen, J. and Krohn, K., Interleukin 2 production in HTLV-III/LAV infection: evidence of defective antigen-induced, but normal mitogen-induced IL-2 production, *Clin. Exp. Immunol.,* 65, 489, 1986.
639. Guy, B., Kieny, M.P., Riviere, Y., Le Peuch, C., Dott, K., Girard, M., Montagnier, L., and Lecocq, J.-P., HIV F/3'*orf* encodes a phosphorylated GTP-binding protein resembling an oncogene product, *Nature,* 330, 266, 1987.
640. Delli Bovi, P., Donti, E., Knowles, D.M., II, Friedman-Kien, A., Luciw, P.A., Dina, D., Dalla-Favera, R., and Basilico, C., Presence of chromosomal abnormalities and lack or AIDS retrovirus DNA sequences in AIDS-associated Kaposi's sarcoma, *Cancer Res.,* 46, 6333, 1986.

641. Alonso, M.L., Richardson, M.E., Metroka, C.E., Mouradian, J.A., Koduru, P.R.K., Filippa, D.A., and Chaganti, R.S.K., Chromosome abnormalities in AIDS-associated lymphadenopathy, *Blood,* 69, 855, 1987.

642. Pelicci, P.-G., Knowles, D.M., II, Arlin, Z.A., Wieczorek, R., Luciw, P., Dina, D., Basilico, C., and Dalla-Favera, R., Multiple monoclonal B cell expansions and c-*myc* oncogene rearrangements in acquired immune deficiency syndrome-related lymphoproliferative disorders: implications for lymphomagenesis, *J. Exp. Med.,* 164, 2049, 1986.

643. Ablashi, D.V., Flagader, A., Markham, P.D., and Salahuddin, S.Z., Isolation of transforming Epstein-Barr virus from plasma of HTLV-III/LAV-infected patients, *Intervirology,* 27, 25, 1987.

644. Lo, S.-C. and Liotta, L.A., Vascular tumors produced by NIH/3T3 cells transfected with human AIDS Kaposi's sarcoma DNA, *Am. J. Pathol.,* 118, 7, 1985.

645. Fine, D. and Schochetman, G., Type D primate retroviruses: a review, *Cancer Res.,* 38, 3123, 1978.

646. Henrickson, R.V., Maul, D.H., Lerche, N.W., Osborn, K.G., Lowenstine, L.J., Prahalada, S., Sever, J.L., Madden, S.L., and Gardner, M.B., Clinical features of simian acquired immunodeficiency syndrome (SAIDS) in rhesus monkeys, *Lab. Anim. Sci.,* 34, 140, 1984.

647. Gardner, M.B. and Marx, P.A., Simian acquired immunodeficiency syndrome, *Adv. Viral Oncol.,* 5, 57, 1985.

648. King, N.W., Simian models of acquired immunodeficiency syndrome (AIDS): a review, *Vet. Pathol.,* 23, 345, 1986.

649. Marx, P.A. and Lowenstine, L.J., Mesenchymal neoplasms associated with type D retrovirus in macaques, *Cancer Surv.,* 6, 101, 1987.

650. Schneider, J. and Hunsmann, G., Simian lentiviruses — the SIV group, *AIDS,* 2, 1, 1988.

651. Fine, D.L., Landon, J.C., Pienta, R.J., Kubicek, M.T., Valerio, M.J., Loeb, W.F., and Chopra, H.C., Responses of infant rhesus monkeys to inoculation with Mason-Pfizer monkey virus materials, *J. Natl. Cancer Inst.,* 54, 651, 1975.

652. Daniel, M.D., King, N.W., Letvin, N.L., Hunt, R.D., Sehgal, P.K., and Desrosiers, R.C., A new type D retrovirus isolated from macaques with an immunodeficiency syndrome, *Science,* 223, 602, 1984.

653. Marx, P.A., Maul, D.H., Osborn, K.G., Lerche, N.W., Moody, P., Lowenstine, L.J., Hendrickson, R.V., Arthur, L.O., Gilden, R.V., Gravell, M., London, W.T., Wever, J.L., Levy, J.A., Munn, R.J., and Gardner, M.B., Simian AIDS: isolation of a type D retrovirus and transmission of the disease, *Science,* 223, 1083, 1984.

654. Heidecker, G., Lerche, N.W., Lowenstine, L.J., Lackner, A.A., Osborn, K.G., Gardner, M.B., and Marx, P.A., Induction of simian acquired immune deficiency syndrome (SAIDS) with a molecular clone of a type D SAIDS retrovirus, *J. Virol.,* 61, 3066, 1987.

655. Marx, P.A., Pedersen, N.C., Lerche, N.W., Osborn, K.G., Lowenstine, L.J., Lackner, A.A., Maul, D.H., Kwang, H.-S., Kluge, J.D., Zaiss, C.P., Sharpe, V., Spinner, A.P., Allison, A.C., and Gardner, M.B., Prevention of simian acquired immune deficiency syndrome with a formalin-inactivated type D retrovirus vaccine, *J. Virol.,* 60, 431, 1986.

656. Sanchez-Pescador, R., Power, M.D., Barr, P.J., Steimer, K.S., Stempien, M.M., Brown-Shimer, S.L., Gee, W.W., Renard, A., Randolph, A., Levy, J.A., Dina, D., and Luciw, P.A., Nucleotide sequence and expression of an AIDS-associated retrovirus (ARV-2), *Science,* 227, 484, 1985.

657. Thayer, R.M., Power, M.D., Bryant, M.L., Gardner, M.B., Barr, P.J., and Luciw, P.A., Sequence relationships to type D retroviruses which cause simian acquired immunodeficiency syndrome, *Virology,* 157, 317, 1987.

658. Bryant, M.L., Yamamoto, J., Luciw, P., Munn, R., Marx, P., Higgins, J., Pedersen, N., Levine, A., and Gardner, M.B., Molecular comparison of retroviruses associated with human and simian AIDS, *Hematol. Oncol.,* 3, 187, 1985.

659. Benveniste, R.E., Arthur, L.O., Tsai, C.-C., Sowder, R., Copeland, T.D., Henderson, L.E., and Oroszlan, S., Isolation of a lentivirus from a macaque with lymphoma: comparison with HTLV-III/LAV and other lentiviruses, *J. Virol.,* 60, 483, 1986.

660. Kanki, P.J., Alroy, J., and Essex, M., Isolation of T-lymphotropic retrovirus related to HTLV-III/LAV from wild-caught African green monkeys, *Science,* 230, 951, 1985.

661. Murphey-Corb, M., Martin, L.N., Rangan, S.R.S., Baskin, G.B., Gormus, B.J., Wolf, R.H., Andes, W.A., West, M., and Montelaro, R.C., Isolation of an HTLV-III-related retrovirus from macaques with simian AIDS and its possible origin in asymptomatic mangabeys, *Nature,* 321, 435, 1986.

662. Hirsch, V., Riedel, N., Kornfeld, H., Kanki, P.J., Essex, M., and Mullins, J.I., Cross-reactivity to human T-lymphotropic virus type III/lymphadenopathy-associated virus and molecular cloning of simian T-cell lymphotropic type III from African green monkeys, *Proc. Natl. Acad. Sci. U.S.A.,* 83, 9754, 1986.

663. Fukasawa, M., Miura, T., Hasegawa, A., Morikawa, S., Tsujimoto, H., Miki, K., Kitamura, T., and Hayami, M., Sequence of simian immunodeficiency virus from African green monkey, a new member of the HIV/SIV group, *Nature,* 333, 457, 1988.

664. Hirsch, V., Riedel, N., and Mullins, J.I., The genome organization of STLV-3 is similar to that of the AIDS virus except for a truncated transmembrane protein, *Cell,* 49, 307, 1987.

665. Kanki, P.J., West African human retroviruses related to STLV-III, *AIDS,* 1, 141, 1987.

666. Kestler, H.W., III, Li, Y., Naidu, Y.M., Butler, C.V., Ochs, M.F., Jaenel, G., King, N.W., Daniel, M.D., and Desrosiers, R.C., Comparison of simian immunodeficiency virus isolates, *Nature,* 331, 619, 1988.
667. Alter, H.J., Eichberg, J.W., Masur, H., Saxinger, W.C., Gallo, R., Macher, A.M., Lane, H.C., and Fauci, A.S., Transmission of HTLV-III infection from human plasma to chimpanzees: an animal model for AIDS, *Science,* 226, 549, 1984.
668. Saxinger, C., Alter, H.J., Eichberg, J.W., Fauci, A.S., Robey, W.G., and Gallo, R.C., Stages in the progression of HIV infection in chimpanzees, *AIDS Res. Hum. Retrovir.,* 3, 375, 1987.

Chapter 4

ENDOGENOUS PROVIRUSES

I. INTRODUCTION

Retroviruses are integrated as endogenous proviruses in the genome of most, if not all, vertebrate species, being vertically inherited as cellular genes through the germ line.[1] Endogenous proviruses are highly reiterated in the host cell genome. In the mouse, for example, they comprise up to 0.4% of the total genome and include approximately 50 type-C MuLV-related sequences, more than 900 intracisternal A particle (IAP) sequences, and other types of both defective and nondefective viral genome sequences. A process of DNA amplification, which would have occurred in a relatively recent evolutionary past, is apparently responsible for the multiplicity of endogenous retrovirus copies in mammalian species including rodents and primates.[2,3] Differences in endogenous retroviral sequences between closely related species may be attributed to the recent acquisition of such sequences by exogenous infection or to independent DNA deletion events that occurred during evolution of particular species. A family of essentially complete retroviral sequences present in the chimpanzee genome is absent in closely related species such as the human, the orangutan, and the gibbon.[4]

Amplification and dispersion of endogenous retroviral sequences in the mammalian genome may be linked events. Endogenous retroviral sequences are present even in avian species such as the Japanese quail that have been considered to be free of these viruses.[5] Endogenous retroviruses have been detected even in insects such as *Drosophila melanogaster* and *Ceratitis capitata*.[6,7] At least some of these proviral sequences are transcribed in normal cells. Although the molecular mechanisms involved in the control of expression of endogenous proviruses are not understood, differential expression of these viruses may be associated with development of malignant diseases, particularly with lymphomagenesis in mice and perhaps also in other animal species.[8]

The structure of endogenous viruses is highly conserved in evolution, especially at the 3'-terminal region and LTR,[9,10] which may indicate the biological importance of their polypeptide products. Endogenous proviruses may have entered the germ line by infecting early embryos of different animal species via retroviral particles. Structural similarities existing between exogenous viruses such as REV and endogenous viruses present in nonhuman primates indicate their physogenetic relationship.[11] Integration of endogenous proviruses frequently occurs in the vicinity of moderately repetitive cellular DNA sequences.[12]

The complex mechanisms involved in the regulation of endogenous provirus expression are little understood.[13] There is evidence that endogenous proviruses are involved in the processes of cell differentiation and in the normal developmental programs of specific tissues.[14,15] Some endogenous viral loci are tightly linked to loci coding for histocompatibility and differentiation antigens.[16,17] The specific structure of certain viral capsid proteins may play a critical role in the congenital transmission of endogenous, and perhaps also exogenous, retroviruses.[18] Infectious endogenous retroviruses can be recovered following transfection of recipient cells with cellular DNA containing proviral genomes.[19-22]

II. HUMAN ENDOGENOUS VIRUSES

The human genome contains sequences related to several types of retroviruses, including sequences related to type-A viruses,[23,24] type-B viruses such as MMTV,[25-28] and type-C viruses such as MuLV.[29-33] The sequences of human endogenous retroviruses are related to the genes *gag*, *pol*, and *env* of the respective rodent retroviruses, as well as LTR-related sequences, but they do not contain oncogenes. Some retroviral sequences may be absent from the genome of endogenous proviruses. There are two related families of human endogenous retroviral sequences: a family consisting of full-length (8.8 kb) proviral structures with typical LTRs, and a second family consisting of structures that contain only 4.1 kb of *gag-pol* sequences bounded by a tandem array of imperfect repeats 72 to 76 bp in length.[34] These endogenous retroviral sequences are widely dispersed throughout the human genome, which could be attributed to a process of amplification that occurred before the evolutionary divergence of humans and chimpanzees.[3]

Human genome contains about 50 copies of 9.2- to 9.5-kb endogenous viral sequences, termed HLM-2 or HERV-K, which have *env* gene sequences most closely related to type A (IAP) retroviruses, LTR sequences most homologous to type D viruses, and *pol* gene sequences related to each of these as well as to mammalian type B and avian type C viral genomes.[26,35,36] HLM-2/HERV-K *pol* gene is as much as 70% identical to MMTV *pol* gene. The MMTV-like HERV-K sequences are related to SINE elements and have been designated SINE-R.[28] SINE-R elements are present at 4000 to 5000 copies per haploid human genome.

In addition to MMTV- and MuLV-related endogenous proviruses, the human genome contains 800 to 1000 copies of a 5- to 6-kbp repetitive family of retroviral-like sequences which include LTR sequences of 415 bp without significant homology to LTRs of known retroviruses.[35,37] The new class of human retrovirus-like (RTVL) elements contains a poly-purine tract and a potential unique histidine tRNA primer binding site. The term RTVL-H (H representing histidine) has been proposed for designating the new family of human endogenous viruses.

Another family of human endogenous proviruses, termed HuERS, was isolated from a HeLa cell genomic library using the 3′-half fragment of proline tRNA as a hybridization probe.[38] This family is composed of three retrovirus-related sequences (HuERS-P1, -P2, and -P3) that include LTRs. Human and simian DNAs contain 10 to 40 copies of these elements, but they are apparently absent in mouse DNA.

A. FUNCTIONS OF HUMAN ENDOGENOUS PROVIRUSES

The normal functions of human endogenous viruses, and the regulatory signals controlling them, are not understood. At least some endogenous viruses are transcribed in normal human cells. mRNAs from endogenous retroviral sequences have been detected in human cells.[39] The transcripts vary in size, content, and quantity from tissue to tissue, being especially abundant in human placentas, but also detectable in human liver and spleen. The detected RNA species hybridize to sequences related to *env* and/or LTR. The possible physiological role of these RNAs is unknown. Some human LTRs may act as enhancers or promoters. Functional LTRs, if transposed or translocated into new positions, might play a role in neoplastic transformation or might act as mutagens to produce genetic disease.[34]

Tandem repeated sequences analogous to viral transcription enhancers are present in the human genome.[40] The human enhancer sequences are homologous to sequences present in some papovaviruses (SV40 and BKV) but, although sequences homologous to SV40 are present in multiple copies in the genome, there seems to be only one sequence homologous to BKV repeats. The functions of these enhancer sequences present in the human genome are also unclear.

B. CHROMOSOMAL LOCALIZATION OF HUMAN ENDOGENOUS PROVIRUSES

The chromosomal localization of human endogenous retroviruses is still poorly character-ized. An endogenous retroviral sequence, ERV1, has been assigned to human chromosome 18,[32] within the bands 18q22-q23.[41] Interestingly, translocations involving this chromosome are frequently found in a particular type of non-Hodgkin lymphoma.[42] ERV1 is found in human DNA in a single copy and is a defective provirus, containing a 3′ LTR but lacking a 5′ LTR. It contains *gag* and *pol* sequences related to MuLV and the baboon endogenous virus (BaEV).[30]

Another human endogenous virus, ERV3, consists also of a single copy and is located on chromosome 7.[43] Monosomy or partial deletion of human chromosome 7 is frequently observed in acute nonlymphocytic leukemia (ANLL). The protooncogene c-*erb*-B is located on the same chromosome but at a position (7p11-13) outside the usual site of breakage in ANLL (7q32-34). It remains to be determined whether ERV3 is located near this chromosomal breakpoint and whether it plays a role in the fragility of this site.[44] Although ERV3 retains the typical full-length gene order of retroviruses (5'LTR-*gag-pol-env*-3'LTR), it is apparently also a defective provirus due to the presence of terminator codons in the open reading frames of both its *gag* and *pol* gene sequences. ERV3 cannot function as an infectious virus but some of its genes may be capable of expression. The 5' and 3' LTRs of ERV3 resemble those of functional mammalian type-C retroviruses but have diverged from one another by 8.8%.[44] Infection of cultured human cells with BaEV frequently leads to an association of the viral DNA sequences with a specific genetic locus, *BEVI* (baboon endogenous viral infection), on human chromosome 6.[45] The *BEVI* locus would contain a short repeated DNA sequence with high affinity for the integration of BaEV in human cells. The physiologic role of the *BEVI* locus is unknown.

C. EXPRESSION OF ENDOGENOUS PROVIRUSES IN NORMAL HUMAN TISSUES

Endogenous proviruses may be expressed as either viral antigens or viral particles. The results of numerous studies indicate that both types of endogenous provirus expression are usually not found in most normal adult human tissues but can be detected in some particular tissues, especially in the placenta.

1. Viral Antigens

Antigens from type C or type D retroviruses are usually not present in normal adult human tissues.[46] An exception to this general rule is the placenta. A primate type-C retrovirus-related protein, called p30, was detected and immunologically characterized in 12 of 14 normal human placentas examined.[47,48] Protein p30 cross-reacts immunologically with the p30 antigen of the simian sarcoma-associated virus (SSAV)/gibbon ape lymphoma virus (GaLV) primate type C retrovirus group. Antibodies against p30 were detected in 7.7% of 1540 human cord-blood sera examined.[49] Expression of type C retroviral information is also observed in the placenta of nonhuman primates. Antigen related to the major internal structural protein p26 from rhesus monkey endogenous virus is expressed in rhesus placenta but not in fetal or adult tissues of the animal.[50] The p26 protein is expressed at higher levels on the external surface of the rhesus placenta, near decidua, than in the remainder of the placenta toward the amniotic surface. A monoclonal antibody specific for the p19 antigen of HTLV reacts with the syncytiotrophoblast cells of all human first-trimester placentas as well as with human choriocarcinoma cells.[51] Since HTLVs are infectious viruses the biological significance of the latter result is unknown.

2. Viral Particles

Viral particles from endogenous retroviruses are usually not visible by electron microscopy in adult human tissues, but such particles can be observed in up to 95% of fresh specimens of human placentas fixed immediately after delivery.[52] The particles observed in human placentas resemble type-D retroviruses.[53] A 75,000-mol wt polypeptide detected in syncytiotrophoblastic cells of human placentas by means of antibodies to a synthetic undecapeptide may correspond to expression of type-C endogenous retroviral sequences.[54] Using indirect immunofluorescence microscopy it was demonstrated that human cytotrophoblast of 6 to 10 weeks gestation contains MMTV-associated antigen, which is predominantly present in the periphery of the cells.[55] Retrovirus-like particles of endogenous origin have also been observed in normal human fetuses.[56] The latter particles contain reverse transcriptase and can be isolated from every human organ at certain stages of differentiation, which suggests a possible role in normal cell physiology. These retrovirus-like elements may be related to BaEV, and nucleotide sequences related to BaEV have been found in the normal human genome.[29] The mechanisms responsible for the emergence of viral particles in normal human placentas and fetuses and for the lack of such particles in adult human tissues are unknown. Particles similar to type C viruses were observed in 3 out of 16 oocytes from women treated with ovulation-inducing hormones.[57]

III. ENDOGENOUS RETROVIRUSES IN HUMAN TUMORS

The possible role of endogenous retroviruses in malignant diseases is not understood. Although endogenous viruses may not possess transforming capability, it is conceivable that they may have some role in the complex, multistage tumorigenic processes occurring in humans and other animals.

A. ENDOGENOUS TYPE-B RETROVIRUS EXPRESSION IN TUMORS

MMTV is a type B retrovirus that may be transmitted in mice either as an infectious agent or vertically, as an endogenous provirus, through the germ line. Antibodies to MMTV-related antigen can be detected in a relatively high proportion of women with breast cancer.[58] The proportion of women with breast cancer in whom circulating antibodies to MMTV-related antigen are detected may increase with advancing age of patients.[59] An antigen present in approximately half of human breast carcinomas is immunologically related to the envelope protein gp52 of MMTV.[60-63] The gp52 protein is usually not expressed on cell lines derived from human breast tumors or from the milk of normally lactating women.[64] Studies with a direct leukocyte migration inhibition test suggested that leukocytes from a proportion of breast cancer patients are presensitized to MMTV-related antigen.[65] Antibodies to MMTV-related antigens are present in 30% of patients with breast cancer but a similar increase is also found in patients with breast adenoma and benign fibrocystic breast disease.[66] Up to 70% of women in some human populations may have antibodies against MMTV-related antigens.[67] Although assays for these antigens are obviously not useful for the diagnosis of human breast cancer, it has been suggested that they could help to identify a small group of subjects with benign breast diseases associated with high risk for developing malignant breast tumors.[68]

MMTV-related sequences are present in the genome of human breast cancer cells but are also present in the genome of normal human breast cells as well as in human placenta.[27,69] These sequences are inherited through the germ line, and some of them are more than 80% homologous with regions of the MMTV genome. Sequences corresponding to *gag-pol* genes have the greatest homology, but sequences related to MMTV *env* and LTR are also present in the human genome. MMTV-like particles associated with the presence of reverse transcriptase activity were detected in the peripheral blood monocytes from 97% of breast cancer patients, in contrast to 11% of age- and sex-matched controls.[70] The possible role of the expression of MMTV-like viruses in human breast cancer is not known.

B. ENDOGENOUS TYPE-C RETROVIRUS EXPRESSION IN TUMORS

Virions morphologically identical to type-C retroviruses appear at low frequency in human tumor cells, including embryonal carcinoma cell lines established from human testicular tumors and teratocarcinoma cell lines.[71-73] Type C virus particles are usually not present in short term cultures of testicular tumors or choriocarcinoma. Retroviral particles are occasionally observed in primary human tumors, e.g., in metastatic melanomas.[74]

Endogenous retroviral sequences may be activated in human leukemia.[75] Antigens related to the core protein p30 of BaEV and/or SSV/SSAV have been detected in 35 to 80% of sera from patients with leukemia and lymphoma.[76,77] Lower positivity for p30 antigen was found in the sera of pregnant women (18%) and in normal controls (8%). Expression of type-C retrovirus-related sequences, including sequences with homology to MuLV, was found in human DNA, and polyadenylated RNAs transcribed from *env* and LTR type-C retrovirus-related sequences was detected in human colon tumors and colon carcinoma cell lines.[29,30,39,78] In most of the colon tumors examined, 3.6-kb LTR-related transcripts, which are prominent and abundant in the normal colon mucosa, were found to be strikingly increased, whereas LTR-*env*-related transcripts of 3.0 and 1.7 kb were increased to a variable degree in the tumors.[78] In addition, the primary tumors and tumor cell lines showed a high degree of variability in type-C endogenous provirus sequence expression as compared to the remarkably consistent pattern of expression exhibited by normal human colon mucosa specimens. The biological significance of such changes is unknown. Human lymphoma cell lines negative for EBV genome sequences express MuLV-related antigens after conversion with EBV.[79]

C. ENDOGENOUS TYPE-C RETROVIRUS EXPRESSION IN NONMALIGNANT DISEASES

Expression of endogenous retroviral sequences has been detected in human nonmalignant diseases. Immune complexes including antibodies against the p30 antigen of type C retroviruses have been detected in the kidney lesions occurring in patients with systemic lupus erythematosus (SLE).[80] Antibodies against MuLV *gag* proteins may be present detected in the sera of patients with autoimmune connective tissue disorders, including SLE and rheumatoid polyarthritis.[81] However, these findings do not necessarily implicate a causal relationship and the possible role of antiretrovirus antibodies in the etiology of human autoimmune diseases remains an open question. MuLV-related sequences are present in the murine major histocompatibility complex, which suggests the possibility that endogenous retroviruses may contribute to the generation of histocompatibility gene diversity.[17] It would be interesting to know if a similar situation also occurs with the human histocompatibility complex, HLA.

IV. REVERSE TRANSCRIPTASE ACTIVITY IN ANIMAL TISSUES

Reverse transcriptase and endonuclease activities are characteristically associated with retroviruses. Reverse transcriptase activity was first detected in the virions of the acute retrovirus RSV.[82,83] A similar or identical activity was found in the chronic retrovirus R-MuLV.[84,85] However, reverse transcriptase activity is not an exclusive property of retroviruses, since it is present in some DNA viruses such as the duck and human hepatitis B viruses.[86,87] Moreover, reverse transcriptase activity was detected in normal, uninfected cells.[88,89] An activity characteristic of reverse transcriptase, not serologically related to the DNA polymerase of ALV and AEV, was found in uninfected chicken embryos as well as in many other animal tissues.[90] Reverse transcriptase activity is frequently present in normal human placenta as well as in human ovarian follicular fluid.[57,91,92] Treatment of normal rat embryo fibroblasts with 5-iododeoxyuridine results in a transient appearance of reverse transcriptase activity.[93] This activity may be important in relation to several specialized functions of the genome even in higher animal species.

Enzymatic or immunologic activity for reverse transcriptase was detected in several types of tumor tissues, especially in human leukemias.[94-101] It has been suggested that quantitation of reverse transcriptase activity may be a useful parameter in the diagnosis of myeloproliferative disorders.[102] Abundant transcripts homologous to the mouse IAP *pol* gene, but not to the *gag* gene, were detected in both human colon adenocarcinoma and the surrounding mucosa.[24]

A glycoprotein with reverse transcriptase-like properties was detected in normal human blood and was found to be elevated in patients with different types of hematologic disorders, including leukemia.[103] Apparently, this glycoprotein is the product of endogenous retroviral information and would be associated with regulation of normal growth in hematopoietic cells. A component of this protein, p15E, possesses immunosuppressive properties, inhibiting the proliferative responses of a murine cytotoxic T-cell line as well as alloantigen-stimulated proliferation of murine and human lymphocytes.[104] p15E-related antigens are also present in murine and feline retroviruses as well as in the human retroviruses HTLV-I and HTLV-II.

A. ENDOGENOUS REVERSE TRANSCRIPTASE INHIBITORS

A specific inhibitor of reverse transcriptase has been detected in human placenta but its biological role has not been determined.[105,106] The inhibitor is a protein of 60,000 to 65,000 Da which is associated with retrovirus-like particles present in human placenta extracts and it is selective for mammalian retroviral reverse transcriptase since it does not substantially inhibit avian retrovirus polymerases α, β, and γ. Moreover, the inhibitor does not irreversibly inactivate the enzyme associated with the viral particles since upon its removal from these particles reverse transcriptase activity reappears.[105] Whether reverse transcriptase activities detected in human placentas and tumors by different laboratories are dependent on the same enzyme, and whether they are related to the presence of endogenous or exogenous retroviral genetic information in the respective tissues, have not yet been determined conclusively. Some of the difficulties encountered in detecting reverse transcriptase activity in human placental extracts may be eliminated by controlling conditions like the monovalent cation concentration and the protein/detergent ratio in the reaction mixture.[107]

B. ORIGIN OF REVERSE TRANSCRIPTASE IN ANIMAL TISSUES

The origin of reverse transcriptase activity present in normal or neoplastic animal tissues is not clear at all. The activity detected in noninfected animal tissues is generally believed to be due the expression of endogenous retroviruses in normal cells. Reverse transcriptase activity of rat liver is associated with endogenous retroviruses related to IAPs.[108] However, the exact origin of the activity present in normal tissues is difficult to define. Although it has been estimated that the human genome contains 30 to 40 copies of MMTV-related *pol* sequences, most or all of these sequences would be nonfunctional (i.e., would be pseudogenes) or would give origin to proteins without reverse transcriptase activity.[109] Genetic *pol* sequences are present in avian cells that lack endogenous retroviruses.[110] It is thus possible that at least some reverse transcriptase activity occurring in animal tissues depends not on retroviral genes but on a cellular gene. Such activity, corresponding to nonviral retroposons, would be related to the generation of genes, pseudogenes, and transposable genetic elements by the reverse flow of genetic information.[111]

V. ENDOGENOUS RETROVIRUSES IN NONHUMAN ANIMAL TISSUES

Endogenous retroviruses are universally present in mammalian species. Retroviruses described in rats are all endogenous; no horizontally transmitting retrovirus is known in rats.[112] Type C particles from endogenous retroviruses are observed in the placenta of normal rats.[113]

Endogenous and exogenous retroviruses, morphologically classified as types A, B, C, and D, have been detected in nonhuman primates.[114-117] The Mason-Pfizer monkey virus (MPMV), isolated from a spontaneous mammary tumor of a rhesus monkey, can proliferate in the lymph nodes of infant rhesus monkeys inoculated with the virus and is capable of productively infect human W138 fibroblasts *in vitro*.[118,119] Molecular hybridization studies demonstrated that a specific restriction fragment of DNA from the endogenous MMC-1 retrovirus isolated from rhesus monkeys is also contained in the gorilla and the chimpanzee but not in humans, gibbon apes, and orangutans.[120]

Computer-assisted comparison of the nucleotide sequences of endogenous retroviruses isolated from different monkey species has helped to delineate their structural relationships and the existence of separate subgroups of these viruses.[121] MuLV-related sequences were detected in the genome of the African green monkey.[122] The unintegrated and integrated BaEV genomes have been characterized and were analyzed thereafter with restriction enzymes. These genomes are heterogeneous and one of them was not defective as determined by transfection. Cocultivation of transformed human cells, but not normal human cells, with BaEV-producing human embryonic cells resulted in syncytium formation.[123] In contrast, three nonhuman primate type D retroviruses, namely, MMPV, the closely related langur virus PO-1-Lu, and the squirrel monkey retrovirus (SMRV), induced syncytia formation in normal human and nonhuman primate cells.[124] BaEV exhibits homology with an endogenous retrovirus of rhesus monkeys as well as with the GaLV and other retroviruses (SSV, FeLV, and several murine retroviruses).[125] GaLV is an infectious retrovirus whose genome has been cloned and studied by restriction endonuclease and DNA sequence analysis.[126] Antibodies against both endogenous and exogenous retroviruses are present in the sera of nonhuman primate species.[127]

Different types of endogenous and exogenous retroviruses have been identified in the domestic cat.[128,129] While the retrovirus RD-114 is only endogenous, FeLV is both an endogenous and exogenous, infectious virus. Multiple copies of RD-114 and FeLV are contained in the genome of the domestic cat and are expressed during embryogenesis in a partially tissue-specific fashion.[130]

Four types of retroviruses are contained as endogenous proviruses in the mouse genome: MuLVs, IAPs, MMTVs, and VL-30 sequences. The following discussion is mainly focused on type-C (MuLV) and type-B (MMTV) murine retroviruses.[131]

A. THE MOUSE LEUKEMIA RETROVIRUSES

A remarkable fraction (about 5%) of mouse chromosomal DNA consists of copies of endogenous proviruses. The proviral copies of MuLVs behave both as classical Mendelian genes and as mobile genetic elements.[132] These proviral genes are capable of reinsertion into the host genome, and this characteristic has resulted in genetic diversity among inbred and wild mice and produces similar variability in the somatic cells of individual mice. However, little is known about how or when these retroviral sequences entered the mouse genome or whether they benefit the host.

As implied by the name, mouse leukemia virus, the earliest isolates of these agents possessed leukemia-inducing activity, but later the term MuLV has been applied to all replication-competent and occasionally to replication-defective viruses that show some sequence homology to the original strains of MuLV.[8] MuLVs can be isolated from most inbred strains of mice as well as from feral mice populations, but in most cases the term MuLV is a misnomer because the great majority of naturally occurring MuLV strains are not leukemogenic. In fact, MuLVs range from strains possessing a leukemogenic potential to others that are not leukemogenic. No oncogenes are present in any of these strains.

1. Classification of Endogenous MuLVs

MuLVs, although related in general structure and nucleotide sequences to each other, are constituted by a collection of retroviruses with diverse patterns of host range and tissue tropisms.[133] The host range properties of MuLVs serve as a mean of classifying them into three families known as ecotropic, xenotropic, and amphotropic or polytropic.[8] Ecotropic MuLVs replicate in mouse cells but do not infect cells of other species. Xenotropic MuLVs grow on cells of species other than mouse but do not grow on mouse cells. This difference between ecotropic and xenotropic viruses is dictated by antigenic determinants contained in the viral envelope glycoprotein gp70, as demonstrated by means of artificial viral pseudotypes with an ecotropic genome contained in a xenotropic envelope and viceversa.[134] Amphotropic or polytropic MuLVs possess both ecotropic and xenotropic host ranges. Polytropic MuLVs arise stepwise by recombination of ecotropic MuLVs with endogenous retroviral sequences of mice and are implicated in the etiology of ecotropic MuLV-induced leukemias in several murine systems.[135]

2. Expression of Endogenous MuLVs

Expression of endogenous MuLV genomes in cells and tissues of different mouse strains differs both quantitatively and qualitatively from strain to strain.[8] High titers of endogenous ecotropic MuLV expression are observed in AKR mice, which is a prerequisite for the later development of thymic lymphoma. Blastocysts and egg cylinders from highly leukemogenic AKR mice contain budding and extracellularly located type C particles.[136] AKR mice express infectious ecotropic MuLVs at about 16 d of gestation and high titers of ecotropic MuLV antigens are found in all organs of newborn and young adult mice and persist throughout life.[137] In comparison, low leukemic mice strains such as BALB/c, C3H/He, and C57BL/6 express much lower levels of infectious MuLVs.[138] Mice from a variety of inbred strains produce IgG antibodies against MuLVs but it is not clear whether these antibodies are directed against endogenous or exogenous MuLVs or both.[139] Mitogenic stimulation of lymphocytes from different mouse strains is associated with expression of endogenous retrovirus transcripts.[140]

MuLVs are frequently expressed in certain types of murine tumors, including spontaneous lymphomas.[141] Endogenous viruses may be involved in radiation-induced leukemogenesis in mice. A virus called radiation murine leukemia virus (Rad-MuLV) was first isolated and was demonstrated to be capable of inducing a high incidence of lymphomas in C57 BL/6 (B6) mice.[142,143] A variant of this virus, designated D-Rad-MuLV, is weakly leukemogenic but is capable of inducing high-incidence lymphomas in mice exposed to a single dose of irradiation, whereas another variant, designated A-Rad-MuLV, which was spontaneously derived from a passaged line of D-Rad-MuLV, was capable of inducing high-incidence lymphomas in intact nonirradiated B6 mice.[144] The emergence of highly leukemogenic Rad-MuLV variants may involve activation of endogenous fibrotropic virus which is immunogenic in its natural host strain B6, followed by recombination of this virus with other retroviral genetic sequences, which would result in the generation of a suppressogenic and thymotropic, highly leukemogenic virus.[145] Immunization against retroviral antigens decreases the incidence of mouse thymic lymphomas.[146]

Endogenous MuLV-related sequences could be involved in the development of radiation-induced osteosarcomas in mice.[147] Mixed populations of endogenous viruses related to AKR MuLV are present in spontaneous and radiation-induced mouse bone tumors.[148] However, in spite of numerous studies performed for more than 20 years, many questions on this subject remain unanswered and the possible role of endogenous retroviruses in radiation-induced oncogenic processes remains controversial.[149] In a study on ^{90}Sr-induced osteosarcomas in CF1 mice, no proviruses were found to be integrated near the c-*myc* protooncogene and the results suggested that activated endogenous retrovirus may not be essential for the development of radiation-induced osteosarcomas in mice.[150]

Endogenous retrovirus-like sequences related to MuLVs, termed *TLev1* and *TLev2*, have been identified within the MHC *TL* locus of uninfected C57BL/10 mice.[151] It is not known whether *TLev* sequences play a role in the phenotypic expression of *TL* antigens but these sequences contain LTRs which are potential regions for regulation of the expression and replication of the viral genome. Normal thymocytes of C57BL/10 mice do not express *TL* antigens, while leukemic cells do express this antigen.

3. Induction of Type C Endogenous Retrovirus Expression

Ecotropic MuLV production can be induced from apparently virus-free mouse cells by treatment with halogenated pyrimidines (5-iododeoxyuridine and 5-bromodeoxyuridine).[152] In a similar manner, cultures of fetal diploid baboon fibroblasts treated with 5-bromodeoxyuridine synthesize protein antigenically related to the p28 protein product of BaEV *gag* gene.[153] Intramuscular injection of 5-bromodeoxyuridine into *Xiphophorus* fish bearing melanoma or lymphoma results in the induction of type B or type C particles in the tumors.[154] The mechanisms of this induction are unknown. Changes in the molecular mechanisms involved in the control of gene expression may be responsible for the induction of endogenous provirus expression. Treatment of synchronized K-MuSV-transformed BALB/c mouse cells with *n*-butyrate and cycloheximide promote expression of type C endogenous viruses.[155] The enhancing effect of *n*-

butyrate is limited to the G_1 phase of the cell cycle and correlates with a prolongation of G_1 and inhibition of DNA synthesis. It is known that *n*-butyrate treatment results in hyperacetylation of chromatin histones, which may induce changes in gene expression.

Endogenous proviruses contained in the chicken genome are expressed in form of viral particles with an associated reverse transcriptase activity after treatment of cultured embryo cells with metabolites of the chlorinated pesticide DDT and the antibacterial agent hexachlorophene.[156] The possible biological significance of the induction of endogenous retroviruses by chemical agents is not understood. Carcinogenic agents can induce qualitative and quantitative alterations in the expression of endogenous proviruses. Treatment of mouse cells (Eb lymphoma cells) with the alkylating agent MNNG results in retroviral gp70 molecules expressed at the cell surface.[157] The possible role of such mutagenized endogenous retroviral antigens in tumorigenic processes is unknown but their expression on the cell surface could be associated with marked changes in the immunogenicity of the tumor cells.

4. Mink Cell Focus-Inducing Viruses, Ecotropic Recombinant Virus, and Generation of MuLVs

A class of MuLVs isolated from spontaneous murine lymphomas is called mink cell focus (MCF)-inducing viruses because of the characteristic morphological changes induced by them in mink cells.[158] MCFs found in the highly leukemogenic AKR mouse strain are not endogenous viruses but are generated by multiple recombination events between ecotropic and nonecotropic virus progenitors.[159] Unlike the endogenous viruses contained in the genome of AKR mice, MCF viruses are highly leukemogenic.[160] Formation of MCF viruses may be a requisite for the high frequency induction of T-cell lymphomas in mice. Lymphomas occurring in recombinant inbred strain of mice derived by crossing the high leukemogenic AKR/J strain with the weakly lymphomatous strain DBA/2J were frequently associated with rearrangement of protooncogene loci including c-*myc*, *prt*-1, *pim*-1, *fis*-1, *Mlvi*-1, and *Mlvi*-2.[161] Some tumors contained rearrangement at two of these loci. Recombinant MCF proviruses were most commonly found to be integrated near c-*myc*.

MCF MuLV infect both mouse and xenogenic cells and may be constituted by *env* gene recombinants between the endogenous ecotropic AKR virus and endogenous xenotropic-related MuLV.[8] A diversity of MCF MuLV genomes have been recovered from mouse leukemic tissues and the susceptibility to infection by these viruses may critically depend on genetic factors. It seems likely that different types of MuLV proviruses can be amplified by cellular recombinational or correctional mechanisms involving cellular sequences showing only slight homology with MuLVs.[8]

The retroviral gene family of the mouse is subjected to a dynamic system of genetic recombination which results in generation of diverse types of MuLVs. During the development of thymic leukemias in AKR mice there is a period of recombination between the endogenous ecotropic and nonecotropic MuLVs as a leukemogenic MCF virus is generated that, beginning at 4 or 5 months, produces a massive infection of the major thymocyte population of immature T cells.[162] From this infection and the multiple virus chromosomal integrations, a monoclonal tumor develops containing many somatically acquired MCF proviruses. Although it is not known how the MCF proviruses induced the neoplastic transformation of thymocytes, there is evidence that factors which depend on a single dominant gene may determine the susceptibility of mice to leukemogenic recombinant retroviruses, permitting the infection of the thymocytes by these viruses.[163] Leukemia-resistant mice lack this gene.

Particular types of recombinant polytropic endogenous retroviruses may play a role during the induction of spontaneous nonthymic lymphomas in high-leukemia mice strains.[164] A novel group of MCF-related viruses, derived by inoculation of different mice strains with Friend or Moloney murine ecotropic viruses, was apparently generated by recombinational events between exogenous and endogenous retroviral sequences.[165,166]

The factors determining the apparent specificity of sequestration of endogenous provirus sequences in generation of MCF viruses and other recombinant viruses are not clear. It was observed that M-MuLV-derived MCF viruses are oncogenic, whereas F-MuLV-derived MCF viruses are not, which suggests that recombination with a particular *env* sequence may influence the oncogenicity of a recombinant virus.[165] However, the wild type FLV-A strain of F-MuLV is an infectious replication-competent virus that is fully pathogenic in the absence of virus components of endogenous origin.[167]

5. Role of MuLV-Related Endogenous Proviruses in Tumorigenic Processes

The role of MuLV-related endogenous viruses in the origin and/or development of either spontaneous or experimental mouse tumors is uncertain. No expression of endogenous type C viruses may be observed in spontaneous animal tumors, for example, in adrenal tumors occurring in aged NIH Swiss mice.[168] No evidence was obtained in favor of a possible participation of endogenous viruses in thymic lymphomas induced in RF/J mice by skin painting of MCA.[169] On the other hand, MuLV LTR sequences are expressed in murine squamous cell carcinomas of the skin induced by chemical carcinogens.[170] Treatment of mice with NMU can activate endogenous ecotropic MuLVs, but spontaneous activation of endogenous MuLVs occurs in older mice.[171] The combined action of suboptimal doses of NMU and activated endogenous MuLV genomes could result in a significantly high incidence of leukemias and solid tumors.[172]

The tumor promoter TPA decreases the induction of endogenous mouse retrovirus expression by bromodeoxyuridine and lipopolysaccharide.[173] Studies on the induction of type C endogenous retroviruses in mouse cells *in vitro* by caffeine or iododeoxyuridine in association with UV- or X-irradiation indicate that the mechanism of endogenous virus induction may be different in different cell types even when the same inducer agents are used.[174] Of 20 human tumors transplanted and passaged in nude mice, 1 was associated with a massive induction of endogenous ecotropic and xenotropic MuLVs in the host animal.[175] The human inducer tumor was an oat-cell lung carcinoma which possibly produced a specific hormone or factor with properties for inducing endogenous type C viruses.

The suspected carcinogenic agent 1,3-butadiene (a colorless gas used as a monomer in the production of synthetic or styrene-butadiene rubber) increases the expression of antigens from endogenous ecotropic viruses in hematopoietic tissues of B6C3F1 mice during the preleukemic phase of exposure to the agent.[176] An incidence of up to 60% of thymic lymphoma/leukemia is observed in B6C3F1 mice exposed to 1,3-butadiene. In contrast, the incidence of these tumors is much more lower (10%) in NIH Swiss mice that do not possess intact endogenous ecotropic retroviral sequences. These results suggest that expression of endogenous proviral sequences may be important for the development of certain tumors, at least in mice model systems. Emergence of type C retroviral particles may also be associated with tumorigenic processes induced by chemical carcinogens in hamsters.[177] However, the precise role of endogenous retroviruses in carcinogen-induced tumorigenic processes in general remains to be elucidated. Interestingly, expression of endogenous virus particles is associated not only with tumors induced by chemical carcinogens or radiation but also with foreign body tumorigenesis. Sarcomas induced in AKR mice by implanting plastic or glass coverslips are associated with the expression of type C particles.[178] IAPs are observed in sarcomas induced by similar procedures in other mouse strains.

B. INTRACISTERNAL A PARTICLES

Intracisternal A particles (IAPs) are constituted by a family of endogenous murine retroviral sequences whose transcripts are packaged in A particles in the cysternae of the endoplasmatic reticulum.[179-181] IAPs were first described as inclusion bodies in mouse mammary adenocarcinomas.[182] IAPs are noninfectious structures that may represent incomplete intracellular entities of MMTV since the particles are, at least in part, true precursors of the MMTV nucleoid, often incorporated into viruses budding at the cell surface.[183,184] The accumulation of IAPs observed in several normal and neoplastic mouse tissues may be explained by an inadequate maturation processing of virus precursor polypeptides and/or by disturbed virus budding.[185] The isolated IAPs contain a polyadenylated RNA molecule, a reverse transcriptase, and a *gag*-like 73-kDa protein.

1. IAP-Related Chromosomal DNA Sequences

DNA sequences related to the RNA sequences contained in IAPs are found widely distributed in rodent genomes and are designated IAP elements. Multiple IAP elements are found on all chromosomes of both mouse and hamster. IAP elements are reiterated to the extent of 1000 or more copies per haploid genome in *Mus musculus*.[2] In the hamster, more than one half of the IAP sequences are located in regions of noncentromeric constitutive heterochromatin and most of these sequences are apparently transcriptionally silent even in IAP-rich tumor cells, since extensive DNA methylation is observed at sites both within the IaP sequences and near their regulatory elements in the 5′ LTRs.[2] IAP-related genomic sequences are not exclusively found in rodent species but the presence of IAP-related gene products has been detected by serological methods in all mammalian species examined, whereas they are apparently absent in birds.[186] IAPs are consistently observed within cells of the inner cell mass of cat blastocysts.[187]

According to their size and genomic organization, IAPs are classified into types I and type II, and the latter into subtypes IIa, IIb, and IIc. The full size mouse type I IAP gene is 7.2 kbp in length but shorter IAP units have been detected containing deletion in various positions in addition to 350- to 450-bp LTR sequences. The majority of type II IAP clones isolated from a mouse genomic library contained highly repetitive DNA sequences in addition to moderately repetitive IAP elements.[188] The construction of cDNA clones and the sequentiation of IAP elements contained in the mouse genome has been reported.[189] The sequences contained in IAP elements resemble those of retroviral genomes and include *gag*-, *pol*-, and *env*-like regions which are highly conserved among the IAP elements of the species.

2. Expression of IAPs in Mouse Tissues

IAPs are observed in early embryos from numerous strains of mice.[136,190] IAPs are also found, although in small number, in the ovarian oocytes until they are released from the follicles; they are not observed in the later phase of maturation of the oocytes, nor in the fertilized eggs. Among normal mouse somatic tissues, IAP expression is highest in the thymus of young animals, where allelic forms of IAP elements may be expressed.[191] IAPs are present in normal epidermis of BALB/c mice and their number increase throughout polycyclic hydrocarbon-induced carcinogenesis produced with tobacco smoke condensate fractions.[192]

IAPs may be expressed in a variety of mouse tumors, including myelomas, leukemias, and a chemically induced mouse colon tumor.[193] IAP genes are transcriptionally active in mouse embryonal carcinoma cells.[194] In mouse myelomas there may be up to a 1000-fold increase in the abundance of IAP transcripts, which is mainly due to enhanced transcription of IAP sequences within the tumor cells.[195] The content of IAP transcripts in the cells of different transplanted tumors in mice may be 10- to 100-fold higher than in normal mice tissues.[196] The biological role of IAP expression in mouse embryos and tumors is unknown but this expression may be linked to the early G_1 phase of the cell cycle.[197]

Both IAPs and extracellular type C budding particles were detected in spontaneous BF murine osteosarcomas, their cultured cell lines, and the tumors induced by inoculation of these cultured cells into the original host mice.[198] Expression of IAPs and type C particles in tumors may depend, at least in part, on the particular mouse strain. In experiments with foreign body tumorigenesis, mice from the CBA/H and CBA/H-T6 strains (or their hybrids) expressed IAPs in the majority of the induced sarcomas, whereas mice of the highly leukemogenic AKR strain expressed immature type C particles in sarcomas induced by the same procedure.[178] The biological significance of the expression of IAPs or type C particles in natural and experimental mouse tumors is unknown.

3. Expression of IAP-Related Antigens in Human Tissues

IAPs represent intracellular entities related mainly to MMTV core constituents. Antibodies to IAPs are present in about one fourth of the sera obtained from both breast cancer patients and normal lactating women.[199,200] These antibodies recognize epitopes of p14, the nucleic acid-binding core protein of MMTV, which corresponds to the protein Ap14 of IAPs.[166]

The genome of the human endogenous retrovirus HERV-K10 is highly homologous to the Syrian hamster IAP genome. The putative protein product of the HERV-K10 *env* gene structurally resembles the MMTV *env* protein and it is possible that gp52-related antigen expressed in human breast cancer tissue is the *env* gene product of a potentially active HERV-K provirus.[26]

4. IAP-Induced Alteration of Differentiated Cellular Functions

IAP expression may be associated with altered regulatory mechanisms of certain differentiated cellular functions. The U3 region of IAP LTRs contains all the regulatory elements for bidirectional transcription in the LTRs. Many endogenous IAPs have the potential to be active and may stimulate the transcription of cellular genes in both the sense and antisense directions.[193] It is thus evident that the IAP genes may cause aberrant expression of flanking cellular genes, independent of the orientation of the IAP gene.

Glucose, which is the physiological stimulus of insulin secretion by the pancreatic β cells, may induce the transcription and translation of an IAP gene in the β cells.[201] The biological significance of this expression is unknown, but inbred strains of mice carrying the autosomal recessive obesity-diabetes mutation, "diabetes" (*db*), and expressing constitutively IAPs develop severe diabetes mellitus.[201] In contrast, mice strains unable to express IAPs in the β cells are resistant to diabetes. These results suggest a retroviral-related mechanism of the glucose-stressed β cells that can lead to the development of diabetes in genetically susceptible animals.

5. IAP-Induced Alteration of Protooncogenes

In some lymphomas induced in mice with pristane or mineral oil, the c-*mos* protooncogene may be rearranged and may contain an IAP LTR.[202-204] The rearranged c-*mos* genes are transcriptionally active and able to induce transformation in an NIH/3T3 DNA transfection assay. An IAP element has also been found to be inserted approximately 2 kb downstream of the exon 3 of c-*myc* in a murine plasmacytoma.[205] These findings suggest that endogenous IAPs may be a source of genetic variation in mice, representing transposon-like movable genetic elements, and that such elements may occasionally have a role in tumor origin and/or progression through activation of protooncogenes. However, IAP insertion near c-*mos* or c-*myc* is not associated with transcriptional activation of these genes in mouse plasmacytomas.[205] The possible role of IAP insertion in the origin of mouse lymphoid tumors is not understood, especially in relation to protooncogene activation.

6. IAP-Induced Alteration of other Cellular Genes

IAPs may also be involved in tumorigenic processes by their participation in activating nonprotooncogene cellular genes. For example, the myelomonocytic leukemic cell line WEHI-3B produces constitutively the hematopoietic growth factor interleukin 3 (IL-3) and this is due to insertion of an IAP with its 5′ LTR positioned close to the promoter region of the IL-3 gene.[206] Possibly, this alteration produces an autostimulatory effect in the WEHI-3B cells, thus contributing to the maintenance of a transformed phenotype in these cells.

7. Oncogene-Induced Alteration in IAP Expression

The products of several oncogenes or putative oncogenes (*myc* protein, p53 antigen, adenovirus E1A protein, and SV40 large T antigen) are able to enhance the activity of the 5′ LTR promoter transcribing the IAP genome.[207] Although the biological significance of this alteration is not clear, these results suggest that the activation of IAP expression may serve as an indicator of the activity of protooncogenes during both embryonic development and tumorigenic processes.

C. THE MOUSE MAMMARY TUMOR VIRUS

The mouse mammary tumor virus (MMTV) has been implicated, in association with genetic and hormonal factors, in the etiology of mouse mammary tumors.[208] MMTV may be acquired by either horizontal or milk-borne transmission infection in mice, but MMTV proviruses are present in the genome of all inbred strains of mice and are also found in many feral mice. Morphologically, extracellular mature MMTVs are classified as type B particles.[179,209] The structural characteristics of MMTV virions have been studied in detail.[210] Intracellular type A particles are also associated with MMTV expression. Both reverse transcriptase and its 70S RNA template are contained in MMTV particles.[211]

Proviral MMTV-related DNAs behave as cellular genes and are transmitted vertically, in a Mendelian fashion, through the germ line of the mouse. More than 20 MMTV-containing loci, designated *Mtv*, have been defined. These loci are very similar to each other but minor sequence polymorphisms between the endogenous MMTV copies can be detected by different methods and some copies may consist of incomplete proviral genes. A standardized nomenclature has been proposed for endogenous MMTVs.[212]

In the GR strain of mice, which is characterized by incidence of mammary tumors, a single genetic locus, *Mtv*-2, is involved in the control of complete MMTV particles expression. Only the MMTV copy contained in the *Mtv*-2 locus is totally homologous to the exogenous MMTV in GR mice, and the provirus located in the *Mtv*-2 locus would be transcriptionally active and responsible for the virus production.[213] The other *Mtv* loci contained in GR mice would be structurally heterogeneous. A glycoprotein of 130,000-mol wt (gp130) detected in the cytoplasm of mammary tumors occurring in GR mice appears to be translated from one of the *Mtv* loci contained in the GR mouse genome.[214] Protein gp130 is a polyprotein containing juxtaposed sequences translated from MMTV provirus genome and sequences of cellular origin. The biological significance of the gp130 polyprotein is unknown.

The preparation of DNA probes specific for cellular sequences flanking endogenous MMTV proviruses has permitted an unambiguous discrimination between the different units and to trace their patterns of segregation among a variety of inbred strains of mice.[215] The same probes also facilitated the assignment of MMTV proviruses to particular mouse chromosomes. For example, the loci designated *Mtv-17* and *Mtv-21* were assigned to mouse chromosomes 4 and 8, respectively. Integration of MMTV into mouse chromosomes is apparently nonrandom and endogenous MMTV sequences are preferentially localized in mouse DNA fractions ranging in GC content from 37 to 39%.[216]

1. Normal Functional Role of Endogenous MMTV Sequences

The possible normal functions of endogenous MMTV sequences have not been defined but its absence from some healthy feral mice indicates that the genetic information contained in this virus is probably dispensable for normal mouse development.[217-219] However, the existence of some normal function for these sequences is suggested by the fact that differential expression of endogenous MMTV genes is observed during development of the BALB/c mouse mammary gland.[220] Expression of endogenous MMTV sequences in BALB/c mice varies over the course of development of the mammary gland during pregnancy and lactation. Although all regions of the viral genome are expressed in these mice, both the level and temporal regulation of expression are different for LTR-, *env*-, and *gag-pol*-specific mRNAs.[220] However, LTR-specific mRNA is usually detected in much greater amounts than the other viral genome transcripts. The biological significance of this apparently noncoordinate regulation of MMTV expression, with differential expression from the different regions of the viral genome, is not understood.

2. Role of MMTV Proviruses in Carcinogenic Processes

The contribution of MMTV to mammary tumorigenesis in mouse strains that harbor the exogenous, milk-transmitted MMTV seems likely. A correlation exists between MMTV antigen expression in the milk (which reflects the animal's infection) and the risk of mammary tumor development.[221] However, factors other that virus infection are crucially involved in MMTV-associated mouse mammary tumorigenesis. Inoculation of purified exogenous MMTV into low-cancer-incidence mouse strains results in the appearance of mammary tumors in only a fraction of the animals.[222]

The possible role of endogenous MMTV sequences in mouse mammary tumorigenic processes still less well understood. A lack of correlation is frequently observed between the expression of endogenous MMTV genes and the occurrence of mammary tumors in different strains of mice.[223] The appearance of genetic cell variants may have an important role in mouse mammary tumorigenesis but the possible role of MMTV endogenous viruses in the origin of these variants is not clear. Acquisition of MMTV provirus copies does not seem to be an absolute requirement for the development of hormone- or carcinogen-induced mammary tumors in several mouse strains.[224] Induction of mouse mammary tumors by urethane is not accompanied by changes in MMTV or MuLV expression.[225] Loss of hormone dependence of mouse mammary tumors is not associated with extra MMTV DNA integrations.[226] Expression of MMTV-related antigens shows heterogeneity among different spontaneously arising mouse mammary tumors.[227,228] Treatment of cultured mouse mammary glands with potent chemical carcinogens (DMBA and FAA) results in their neoplastic transformation but this process is not associated with induction of endogenous MMTV expression.[229] Induction of mammary tumor in virgin female BALB/c or C3H mice by chemical carcinogens (DMBA or urethane), with or without prolonged hormonal stimulation, or induction with X-irradiation, is not clearly associated with increased levels of RNA or antigen from endogenous MMTV.[230,231] It is thus rather unlikely that endogenous MMTV expression is crucially required for spontaneous or experimentally induced mouse mammary tumorigenesis. In any case, it is clear that MMTV would at most be only one of several cooperating factors required to mediate the complete neoplastic transformation of mouse mammary cells.[232]

The endogenous MMTV provirus *Mtv*-2 is localized on mouse chromosome 18 and is associated with mammary carcinomas in virtually 100% of breeding females of the GR laboratory mouse strain.[233] The *Mtv*-2 endogenous provirus has been transferred from the inbred GR strain to a wild mouse line which is free of both endogenous and exogenous MMTVs.[234] The incidence of mammary tumors in the P through F2 generations of the new mouse line, designated WXG-2, was much more lower than would be expected in the parental GR strain. These results demonstrate that the natural resistance of wild animal populations to viral-induced tumorigenesis may not simply be a resistance to infection, but rather resistance at other levels of tumorigenesis.

Amplification and novel locations of endogenous MMTV genomes have been observed in mouse T-cell lymphomas.[235] MMTV transcripts of 2.2 kb containing LTR sequences are present in high amounts in certain mouse mammary tumors which arise spontaneously or are induced by hormonal or chemical carcinogens or both.[236] Such transcripts appear to include, in addition to proviral LTR sequences, sequences from either other parts of the MMTV genome or the mouse genome. The possible role of transcripts containing LTR sequences in the origin and/or maintenance of mouse mammary tumors remains undetermined. The fact that the appearance of *Mtv*-2 MMTV proviral sequences with a particular alteration is infrequent in T-cell leukemias of mouse strain GR and the observation that only certain LTR rearrangements are permitted in these leukemias and that each leukemia contains the same rearrangement, which appears at an early stage in the development of the disease, suggest that rearrangements of endogenous MMTV sequences may be implicated in some way in murine leukemogenesis.[237] Although each murine T-cell leukemia appears clonal with respect to extra MMTV provirus, since all extra MMTV proviruses of each leukemia contain the same rearrangement, the detected alterations are different for the different leukemias. Treatment of the carcinogen-induced mouse T-cell lymphoma cell line EL-4 with TPA results in induction of the synthesis of protein products of the LTR region of endogenous MMTV proviruses.[238]

Activation of specific cellular sequences, termed *int*-1, *int*-2, and *int*-3, by an enhancer effect of MMTV was discussed previously as a possible mechanism for the potential carcinogenic effects of MMTV. Mammary tumors in the GR mouse strain are associated with the expression of an endogenous MMTV provirus. The tumors progress from a hormone-dependent growth phase to autonomous, hormone-independent growth and a number of transplanted mammary tumors in the hormone-dependent phase are positive for proviral insertion at *int*-1, *int*-2, or both.[239] It is not known if *int* cellular sequences can be considered as protooncogenes or contain protooncogenes but the protein product of *int*-1 has no apparent homology to any known oncogene protein product.[240,241] The oncogenic potential of the *int*-1 gene on mammary cells is strongly suggested by the demonstration that infection of a mouse mammary epithelial cell line with a retrovirus vector carrying an intact coding sequence for *int*-1 protein produces several changes in morphology and growth control that are characteristic of neoplastic transformation.[242] Pregnancy-dependent MMTV provirus integration within *int*-2 occurs already at the earliest appearance of the mammary tumor and may therefore represent an important event in the multistage developmental processes of this type of neoplasia.[243] However, chemically induced tumors are pathogenically heterogeneous and some of these tumors may be independent of MMTV activation and *int* gene expression.[244]

D. VL-30 SEQUENCES

The mouse genome contains multiple 20 to 50 copies of closely related 5.2-kb DNA sequences, called virus-like 30 (VL-30) sequences.[245,246] These sequences normally express 30S RNA transcripts and have properties similar to those of retroviruses, including the presence of 400 bp-long terminal direct repeats. The biological significance of VL-30 sequences is unknown but they share some structural characteristics with eukaryotic transposons.

E. GENETIC AND NONGENETIC FACTORS CONTROLLING ENDOGENOUS PROVIRUS EXPRESSION

The expression of endogenous proviruses depends, at least in part, on their localization within chromosomes.[247] Genetic factors contribute to the regulation of provirus expression in several low leukemic strains of mice.[248] Regulation of endogenous MuLV expression occurs mainly at the transcriptional level.[249]

The *Fv-1* locus is prominent among the genes controlling the expression, replication, and spread of mouse mammary endogenous retroviruses.[250,251] Two major alleles of this gene, termed *Fv-1*^{n} and *Fv-1*^{b}, that occupy a single locus on mouse chromosome 4,[252] restrict infection by incompatible MuLVs which fall into *Fv-1* categories N-tropic or B-tropic, respectively. Another genetic locus, the *Gv-1* locus, is involved in a coordinate regulation of the expression of multiple endogenous murine retroviruses.[253] *Gv-1* acts by *trans* mechanisms through the production of an unknown diffusible factor, which is capable of regulating the expression of endogenous retroviruses in a tissue-specific manner. Endogenous MuLV proviruses are located at many different sites in the mouse genome and the viral genomes can be induced to be expressed with different efficiencies spontaneously *in vivo,* by chemicals *in vitro,* or by DNA transfection.[8]

Some mouse strains are genetically resistant to mammary tumorigenesis despite the fact that they release large amounts of MMTV in milk. While the resistance genes of most mouse strains inhibit both mammary tumorigenesis and MMTV expression, the II-TES strain of mice is unique in that it carries a recessive gene for mammary tumor resistance, which does not inhibit MMTV release, and two independent dominant mammary tumor promoting genes which are inhibited by the resistance gene.[254] The SL/Ni substrain of mice is highly polymorphic in the expression of endogenous ecotropic virus and this polymorphism among individuals is due to an epigenetic factor transmitted via milk from virus-free mothers to their offspring.[255] The maternal factor selectively restricts the expression of endogenous retroviruses.

1. Activity of LTRs from Endogenous Proviruses

The promoter activity of proviral LTRs may contribute to the level of expression of endogenous viruses. Markedly elevated expression of an endogenous retroviral LTR has been observed in a mouse colon tumor.[193] RNA molecules which hybridize to a cloned cDNA from this tumor are highly heterogeneous in size and are elevated more than 50-fold in the tumor as compared to the normal mouse colon. Some endogenous proviruses contain defects or changes in LTR and leader sequences, which may result in partial loss of promoter activity, this activity being lower than the "threshold" necessary for efficient cellular transformation.[256]

2. Amplification of Endogenous Provirus Sequences

In transplanted mouse T-cell lymphomas, MMTV replication may not be limited to a specific chromosome localization, but rather replication and reintegration of MMTV proviruses into different chromosomes is observed.[257] The newly integrated MMTV copies are produced by mechanisms which may generate a high degree of polymorphism as well as deletions in the viral DNA, which may result in high levels of truncated RNAs in the lymphoma cells. The possible role of these alterations in mouse lymphomagenesis is not known.

3. DNA Methylation and the Control of Endogenous Provirus Expression

DNA methylation may be important for the expression, or lack of expression, of proviral genomes.[258,259] All CpG sites in the germ line-transmitted M-MuLV proviral genome, as well as in the flanking DNA sequences, are highly methylated at day 12 of gestation.[260] At subsequent stages of development, specific CpG sites which are localized exclusively in the 5' and 3' enhancer regions of the LTRs become progressively demethylated. The extent of enhancer demethylation is tissue-specific and strongly affected by the chromosomal position of the respective proviral genome.[260] Silent retroviral genomes can be efficiently activated by treatment of mice or mice cells with 5-azacytidine, which induces altered patterns of DNA methylation.[261-263]

The methylation pattern of endogenous MMTV genes is tissue-specific and stably inherited.[264] Expression of MMTV proviruses in various mouse thymoma cell lines may correlate with methylation of the viral LTR.[265] MMTV proviruses are activated during mammary carcinogenesis, apparently through an alteration of their methylation patterns.[266] Specific demethylation of the viral loci is associated with the neoplastic phenotype, regardless of whether viral or chemical inducer agents are responsible for tumor formation.[267] Demethylation of the *Mtv*-6 MMTV locus was found in all mammary preneoplastic lesions (hyperplastic alveolar nodules) and tumors that were free from acquired proviruses in BALB/c mice. The chromosomal integration site may contribute to determine the tissue-specific methylation pattern of MMTV,[268] which would be involved in the control of MMTV transcriptional activity. However, endogenous MMTV genomes are hypomethylated not only in the mammary tumors but also in several nonmammary organs (testes, spleen, placenta, liver, lung), although they are sparingly transcribed or not transcribed at all in these organs.[268,269] Thus, a clear-cut correlation between MMTV hypomethylation and MMTV transcriptional activity is not apparent and additional factors must be involved in controlling this activity.

The mechanisms responsible for the regulation of endogenous proviruses (or other genetic elements) may not be the same in undifferentiated and differentiated cells. A cloned M-MuLV genome remained hypomethylated after transfection into undifferentiated teratocarcinoma cells, but its expression was suppressed in the undifferentiated cells.[270] When these cells were induced to differentiate into epithelial tissues, the pattern of DNA methylation of the viral genome remained unchanged but spontaneous M-MuLV expression was detected in the differentiated cells.

4. Hormonal Control of Endogenous Provirus Expression

Expression of endogenous proviruses depends, at least in part, on hormone-regulated mechanisms. Estrogen treatment induces the expression of type C retroviruses in the uteri of either sexually immature or ovariectomized mice.[271] Expression of MMTV has been studied extensively. Several hormones, especially steroids, but also insulin and growth hormone, contribute to the regulation of MMTV expression.[4,272-275] Expression of the MMTV-homologous human endogenous retrovirus HERV-K in the human breast cancer cell line T47D is stimulated by progesterone after pretreatment with estradiol but is not affected in the presence of either estradiol or progesterone alone.[276]

Glucocorticoids, as well as other steroid hormones, can affect transcriptional processes in genes responsive to the hormone by interacting with DNA sequences that may be located at relatively far distant sites.[247] The sequence that is minimally required for specific interaction of the glucocorticoid receptor with its DNA-binding site is represented by a partially symmetric sequence of 15 bp. The progesterone receptor interacts with the same sequence and the estradiol receptor recognizes a strongly related but distinct element. In the intact cell, but not *in vitro,* the hormone is required for the interaction of the receptor with the specific regulatory DNA sequence. The regulatory signals recognized by glucocorticoids in endogenous virus sequences are located within a restricted segment of the LTR sequences of the viral genome, the hormone regulatory element (HRE), or glucocorticoid regulatory element (GRE), and the regulation seems to occur at the level of the initiation of transcription.[278-283] The glucocorticoid-receptor complex binds specifically to a 340 bp-restriction fragment of MMTV LTR. Two strong glucocorticoid-receptor complex binding sites have been found between nucleotide positions -72 and -192 with respect to the LTR RNA initiation site.[281] Only glucocorticoids, but also progestins and androgens, can induce the transcription of the MMTV LTR promoter.[284] As in the case of the glucocorticoid-induced stimulation of transcription, a particular DNA sequence element mediates the progestin and androgen responsiveness or MMTV LTR transcription. These results suggest the existence of some common structural features of steroid hormone receptors which are capable of recognizing and binding to HRE. However, in contrast to glucocorticoids, progestins, and androgens, estradiol does not induce transcription at the MMTV LTR promoter, which indicates a lesser degree of homology between the estradiol receptor and other steroid hormone receptors. An estrogen response element is apparently not contained within the MMTV LTR.[285]

Altered chromatin conformation reflected in specific sites of DNase I hypersensitivity are associated with the hormone-induced transcriptional activation of the proviral genome.[286] Alteration in ADP-ribosylation of proteins could be important in the glucocorticoid-induced chromatin changes and it has been suggested that ADP-ribose may serve as a negative regulator of certain genes.[287]

The hormonal regulation of endogenous or exogenous MMTV proviruses does not follow, however, simple, clear rules. The presence of multiple glucocorticoid response element sequences, acting as transcriptional enhancers in relatively independent position with respect to the MMTV promoter, can differentially activate the promoter in an additive fashion.[288] The exact role of the glucocorticoid hormone in the process of activation of this specific cellular receptor is not understood. The steroid ligand is apparently not an absolute requirement for generating the conformation of the glucocorticoid receptor that allows its interaction with the MMTV HRE *in vitro*.[289] Two proteins (NF-1 and F-i), present in crude nuclear extracts, would interact with the steroid hormone-activated virus promoter for loading the system responsible for the transcriptional activation of MMTV sequences.[290]

The ovarian hormones 17 β-estradiol and progesterone can modify the proliferative response of the mouse mammary gland to MMTV infection.[291] Many other endogenous and/or exogenous factors may be involved in the regulatory phenomena occurring in the mouse mammary gland. Expression of either a v-*mos* oncogene or an activated human c-H-*ras* protooncogene by *in vitro* recombination with the MMTV LTR interferes with the mechanism of glucocorticoid-induced MMTV transcription.[292]

A correlation between induced endogenous virus products and neoplastic changes in mice during hormonal mammary carcinogenesis has not been established.[293] Different variants of MMTV may have different properties in relation to mammary gland tumorigenesis. For example, the MMTV variant RIII has low tumorigenic action and, on the contrary, may induce lobuloalveolar differentiation, whereas the variant C3H of the same virus shows low differentiative activity and high tumorigenic activity.[294] The molecular mechanisms related to such differential effects remain undetermined but possible explanations include different sites of virus integration in the host genome and/or different sensitivity of the infected mammary cells to hormones. Additional studies are required for a better characterization of the role of endogenous and exogenous MMTV, in conjunction with genetic and hormonal factors, in mouse mammary tumorigenesis.

5. Immunologic Factors

An important question about endogenous retroviruses is whether they can be activated by infectious and immunologic processes. Although activation of endogenous viruses can be induced by different chemical, physical, hormonal, mitogenic, allogeneic, and viral stimuli *in vitro,* or may even occur in an apparently spontaneous fashion, the factors involved in activation of endogenous viruses *in vivo* remain little known. Immunologic changes or stimuli may be, in principle, involved in this activation. Inoculation of fetal bovine serum of horse serum plus Freund's complete adjuvant into baboons resulted in activation of humoral immune response against the endogenous virus of this primate, BaEV, and the glycoprotein gp71 of the same virus.[295] These results suggest *in vivo* activation of BaEV expression by an immune response to nonviral antigens. A possible association between autoimmunity and neoplasia in relation to activation of type C endogenous retroviruses has been discussed.[296] A general conclusion on this subject cannot be reached on the basis of the available evidence.

VI. SUMMARY

Sequences related to different retroviruses are present in the mammalian genome, being inherited through the germ line, and some of these sequences are expressed as RNA and protein products. The ubiquituous presence of these viral sequences suggests that they are related to some essential cellular functions. However, these functions remain to be defined. The possible role of endogenous provirus expression in cell differentiation and proliferation as well as in tumorigenic processes remains enigmatic.

REFERENCES

1. Jaenisch, R., Endogenous retroviruses, *Cell*, 32, 5, 1983.
2. Kuff, E.L., Fewell, J.E., Lueders, K.K., DiPaolo, J.A., Amsbaugh, S.C., and Popescu, N.C., Chromosome distribution of intracisternal A-particle sequences in the Syrian hamster and mouse, *Chromosoma (Berlin)*, 83, 213, 1986.
3. Steele, P.E., Martin, M.A., Rabson, A.B., Bryan, T., and O'Brien, S.J., Amplification and chromosomal dispersion of human endogenous retroviral sequences, *J. Virol.*, 59, 545, 1986.
4. Bonner, T.I., Birkenmeier, E.H., Gonda, M.A., Mark, G.E., Searfoss, G.H., and Todaro, G.J., Molecular cloning of a family of retroviral sequences found in chimpanzee but not human DNA, *J. Virol.*, 43, 914, 1982.
5. Chambers, J.A., Cywinski, A., Chen, P.-J., and Taylor, J.M., Characterization of Rous sarcoma virus-related sequences in the Japanese quail, *J. Virol.*, 59, 354, 1986.
6. Plus, N., Further studies on the origin of the endogenous viruses of *Drosophila melanogaster* cell lines, in *Invertebrate Systems In Vitro*, Kustak, E., Maramorosch, K., and Dübendorfer, A., Eds., Elsevier, Amsterdam, 1980, 435.
7. Plus, N., Veyrunes, J.C., and Cavalloro, R., Endogenous viruses of *Ceratitis capitata* Wied. "J.R.C. Ispra" strain, and of *C. capitata* permanent cell lines, *Ann. Virol. (Paris)*, 132E, 91, 1981.
8. Risser, R., Horowitz, J.M., and McCubrey, J., Endogenous mouse leukemia viruses, *Annu. Rev. Genet.*, 17, 85, 1983.
9. Kominami, R., Tomita, Y., Connors, E.C., and Hatanaka, M., Conserved sequence related to the 3'-terminal region of retrovirus RNAs in normal cellular DNAs, *J. Virol.*, 34, 684, 1980.
10. Devare, S.G., Reddy, E.P., Law, J.D., and Aaronson, S.A., Nucleotide sequence analysis of the long terminal repeat of integrated simian sarcoma virus: evolutionary relationship with other mammalian retroviral long terminal repeats, *J. Virol.*, 42, 1108, 1982.
11. Rice, N.R., Bonner, T.I., and Gilden, R.V., Nucleic acid homology between avian and mammalian type C viruses: relatedness of reticuloendotheliosis virus cDNA to cloned proviral DNA of the endogenous colobus virus CPC-1, *Virology*, 114, 286, 1981.
12. Evans, R.M., Baluda, M.A., and Shoyab, M., Differences between the integration of avian myeloblastosis virus DNA in leukemic cells and of endogenous viral DNA in normal chicken cells, *Proc. Natl. Acad. Sci. U.S.A.*, 71, 3152, 1974.
13. Weinberg, R.A. and Steffen, D.L., Regulation of expression of the integrated retrovirus genome, *J. Gen. Virol.*, 54, 1, 1981.
14. Liebermann, D., Hoffman-Liebermann, B., and Sachs, L., Regulation of endogenous type C virus expression during normal myeloid cell differentiation: evidence for a role in promoting myeloid cell proliferation and differentiation, *Virology*, 107, 121, 1980.
15. Rasheed, S., Role of endogenous cat retrovirus in cell differentiation, *Proc. Natl. Acad. Sci. U.S.A.*, 79, 7371, 1982.
16. Meruelo, D., Rossomando, A., Offer, M., Buxbaum, M., and Pellicer, A., Association of endogenous viral loci with genes encoding histocompatibility and lymphocyte differentiation antigens, *Proc. Natl. Acad. Sci. U.S.A.*, 80, 5032, 1983.
17. Meruelo, D., Kornreich, R., Rossomando, A., Pampeno, C., Mellor, A.L., Weiss, E.H., Flavell, R.A., and Pellicer, A., Murine leukemia virus sequences are encoded in the murine major histocompatibility complex, *Proc. Natl. Acad. Sci. U.S.A.*, 81, 1804, 1984.
18. Robinson, H.L. and Eisenman, R.N., New findings on the congenital transmission of avian leukosis viruses, *Science*, 225, 417, 1984.
19. Cooper, G.M. and Temin, H.M., Lack of infectivity of the endogenous avian leukosis virus-related genes in the DNA of uninfected chicken cells, *J. Virol.*, 17, 422, 1976.
20. Lowy, D.R., Infectious murine leukemia virus from DNA of virus-negative AKR mouse embryo cells, *Proc. Natl. Acad. Sci. U.S.A.*, 75, 5539, 1978.
21. Copeland, N.G. and Cooper, G.M., Transfection by exogenous and endogenous murine retrovirus DNAs, *Cell*, 16, 347, 1979.
22. McCubrey J. and Risser, R., Activation of nonexpressed endogenous ecotropic murine leukemia virus by transfection of genomic DNA into embryo cells, *J. Virol.*, 45, 950, 1983.
23. Ono, M., Molecular cloning and long terminal repeat sequences of human endogenous retrovirus genes related to types A and B retrovirus genes, *J. Virol.*, 58, 937, 1986.
24. Moshier, J.A., Luk, G.D., and Huang, R.C.C., mRNA from human colon tumor and mucosa related to the *pol* gene of an endogenous A-type retrovirus, *Biochem. Biophys. Res. Commun.*, 139, 1071, 1986.
25. Callahan, R., Drohan, W., Tronick, S., and Schlom, J., Detection of human DNA sequences related to the mouse mammary tumor virus genome, *Proc. Natl. Acad. Sci. U.S.A.*, 79, 5503, 1982.
26. Ono, M., Yasunaga, T., Miyata, T., and Ushikubo, H., Nucleotide sequence of human endogenous retrovirus genome related to the mouse mammary tumor virus genome, *J. Virol.*, 60, 589, 1986.

27. May, F.E.B. and Westley, B.R., Structure of a human retroviral sequence related to mouse mammary tumor virus, *J. Virol.*, 60, 743, 1986.

28. Ono, M., Kawakami, M., and Takezawa, T., A novel human nonviral retroposon derived from an endogenous retrovirus, *Nucleic Acids Res.*, 15, 8725, 1987.

29. Martin, M.A., Bryan, T., Rasheed, S., and Khan, A.S., Identification and cloning of endogenous retroviral sequences present in human DNA, *Proc. Natl. Acad. Sci. U.S.A.*, 78, 4892, 1981.

30. Bonner, T.I., O'Connell, C., and Cohen, M., Cloned endogenous retroviral sequences from human DNA, *Proc. Natl. Acad. Sci. U.S.A.*, 79, 4709, 1982.

31. Repaske R., O'Neill, R.R., Steele, P.E., and Martin, M.A., Characterization and partial nucleotide sequence of endogenous type C retrovirus segments in human chromosomal DNA, *Proc. Natl. Acad. Sci. U.S.A.*, 80, 678, 1983.

32. O'Brien, S.J., Bonner, T.I., Cohen, M., O'Connell, C., and Nash, W.G., Mapping of an endogenous retroviral sequence to human chromosome 18, *Nature*, 303, 77, 1983.

33. Repaske, R., Nucleotide sequence of a full-length human endogenous retroviral segment, *J. Virol*, 54, 764, 1985.

34. Steele, P.E., Rabson, A.B., Bryan, T., and Martin, M.A., Distinctive termini characterize two families of human endogenous retroviral sequences, *Science*, 225, 943, 1984.

35. Callahan, R., Chiu, I.-M., Wong, J.F.H., Tronick, S.R., Roe, B.A., Aaronson, S.A., and Schlom, J., A new class of endogenous human retroviral genomes, *Science*, 228, 1208, 1985.

36. Horn, T.M., Huebner, K., Croce, C., and Callahan, R., Chromosomal locations of members of a family of novel endogenous human retroviral genomes, *J. Virol.*, 58, 955, 1986.

37. Mager, D.L. and Henthorn, P.S., Identification of a retrovirus-like repetitive element in human DNA, *Proc. Natl. Acad. Sci. U.S.A.*, 81, 7510, 1984.

38. Harada, F., Tsukada, N., and Kato, N., Isolation of three kinds of human endogenous retrovirus-like sequences using tRNA[Pro] as a probe, *Nucleic Acids Res.*, 15, 9153, 1987.

39. Rabson, A.B., Steele, P.E., Garon, C.F., and Martin, M.A., mRNA transcripts related to full-length endogenous retroviral DNA in human cells, *Nature*, 306, 604, 1983.

40. Rosenthal, N., Kress, M., Gruss, P., and Khoury, G., BK viral enhancer element and a human cellular homolog, *Science*, 222, 749, 1983.

41. Renan, M.J. and Reeves, B.R., Chromosomal localization of human endogenous retroviral element ERV1 to 18q22-q23 by *in situ* hybridization, *Cytogenet. Cell Genet.*, 44, 167, 1987.

42. Yunis, J.J., Oken, M.M., Kaplan, M.E., Ensrud, K.M., Howe, R.R., and Theologides, A., Distinctive chromosomal abnormalities in histologic subtypes of non-Hodgkin's lymphomas, *N. Engl. J. Med.*, 307, 1231, 1982.

43. O'Connell, C., O'Brien, S., Nash, W.G., and Cohen, M., ERV3, a full length human endogenous provirus: chromosomal localization and evolutionary relationship, *Virology*, 138, 225, 1984.

44. O'Connell, C.D. and Cohen, M., The long terminal repeat sequences of a novel human endogenous retrovirus, *Science*, 226, 1204, 1984.

45. Cohen, J.C. and Murphey-Corb, M., Targeted integration of baboon endogenous virus in the *BEVI* locus on human chromosome 6, *Nature*, 301, 129, 1983.

46. Micheel, B., Wunderlich, V., and Hertling, I., Search for retrovirus expression in men — failure to demonstrate retrovirus-specific antigens in normal and malignant tissue, *Arch. Geschwulstforsch.*, 52, 169, 1982.

47. Maeda, S., Mellors, R.C., Mellors, J.W., Jerabek, L.B., and Zervoudakis, I.A., Immunohistologic detection of antigen related to primate type C retrovirus p30 in normal human placentas, *Am. J. Pathol.*, 112, 347, 1983.

48. Jerabek, L.B., Mellors, R.C., Elkon, K.B., and Mellors, J.W., Detection and immunochemical characterization of a primate type C retrovirus-related p30 protein in normal human placentas, *Proc. Natl. Acad. Sci. U.S.A.*, 81, 6501, 1984.

49. Suni, J., Wahlström, T., and Vaheri, A., Retrovirus p30-related antigen in human syncytiotrophoblasts and IgG antibodies in cord-blood sera, *Int. J. Cancer*, 28, 559, 1981.

50. Stromberg, K. and Huot, R.I., Preferential expression of endogenous type C viral antigen in rhesus placenta during ontogenesis, *Virology*, 112, 365, 1981.

51. Suni, J., Narvanen, A., Wahlström, T., Lehtovirta, P., and Vaheri, A., Monoclonal antibody to human T-cell leukemia virus p19 defines polypeptide antigen in human choriocarcinoma cells and syncytiotrophoblasts of first-trimester placentas, *Int. J. Cancer*, 33, 293, 1984.

52. Ueno, H., Imamura, M., and Kikuchi, K., Frequency and antigenicity of type C retrovirus-like particles in human placentas, *Virchows Arch. Pathol. Anat.*, 400, 31, 1983.

53. Dirksen, E.R. and Levy, J.A., Virus-like particles in placentas from normal individuals and patients with systemic lupus erythematosus, *J. Natl. Cancer Inst.*, 59, 1187, 1977.

54. Suni, J., Närvänen, A., Wahlström, T., Aho, M., Pakkanen, R., Vaheri, A., Copeland, T., Cohen, M., and Oroszlan, S., Human placental syncytiotrophoblastic M_r 75,000 polypeptide defined by antibodies to a synthetic peptide based on a cloned human endogenous retroviral DNA sequence, *Proc. Natl. Acad. Sci. U.S.A.*, 81, 6197, 1984.

55. Klavins, J.V., Shapiro, S.H., Wessely, Z., and Berkman, J.I., RNA virus associated antigen in human placenta, *Ann. Clin. Lab. Sci.,* 10, 137, 1980.

56. Mondal, H. and Hofschneider, P.H., Isolation and characterization of retrovirus-like elements from normal human fetuses, *Int. J. Cancer,* 30, 281, 1982.

57. Larsson, E., Nilsson, B.O., Sundström, P., and Widéhn, S., Morphological and microbiological signs of endogenous C-virus in human oocytes, *Int. J. Cancer,* 28, 551, 1981.

58. Witkin, S.S., Sarkar, N.H., Kinne, D.W., Good, R.A., and Day, N.K., Antibodies reactive with the mouse mammary tumor virus in sera of breast cancer patients, *Int. J. Cancer,* 25, 271, 1980.

59. Tomana, M., Niedermeier, W., and Mukherjee, D., Antibodies to MMTV-related antigen in breast cancer patients of different ages, *Cancer Immunol. Immunother.,* 11, 59, 1981.

60. Mesa-Tejada, R., Keydar, I., Ramanarayanan, M., Ohta, T., Fenoglio, C., and Spiegelman, S., Detection in human breast carcinomas of an antigen immunologically related to a group-specific antigen of mouse mammary tumor virus, *Proc. Natl. Acad. Sci. U.S.A.,* 75, 1524, 1978.

61. Mesa-Tejada, R., Oster, M.W., Fenoglio, C.M., Madigson, J., and Spiegelman, S., Diagnosis of primary breast carcinoma through immunohistochemical detection of antigen related to mouse mammary tumor virus in metastatic lesions: a report of two cases, *Cancer,* 49, 261, 1982.

62. Keydar, I., Selzer, G., Chaitchik, S., Hareuveni, M., Karby, S., and Hizi, A., A viral antigen as a marker for the prognosis of human breast cancer, *Eur. J. Cancer Clin. Oncol.,* 18, 1321, 1982.

63. Keydar, I., Ohno, T., Nayak, R., Sweet, R., Simoni, F., Weiss, F., Karby, S., Mesa-Tejada, R., and Spiegelman, S., Properties of retrovirus-like particles produced by a human breast carcinoma cell line: immunological relationship with mouse mammary tumor virus proteins, *Proc. Natl. Acad. Sci. U.S.A.,* 81, 4188, 1984.

64. Callis, A.H. and Ritzi, E.M., Protein A assay for mouse mammary tumor virus gp52 determinants on murine and human mammary tumor cells, *Virology,* 111, 656, 1981.

65. Fukuda, M., Wanebo, H.J., Tsuel, L., Ashikari, R., and Sarkar, N.H., Leukocyte migration inhibition among breast cancer patients in response to various oncogenic viruses, *J. Natl. Cancer Inst.,* 64, 431, 1980.

66. Zotter, S., Grossmann, H., Francois, C., Kozma, S., Hainaut, P., Calberg-Bacq, C.-M., and Osterrieth, P.M., Among the human antibodies reacting with intracytoplasmic A particles of mouse mammary tumor virus, some react with MMTV p14, the nucleic acid-binding protein, and others with MMTV p28, the main core protein, *Int. J. Cancer,* 32, 27, 1983.

67. Levine, P.H., Mesa-Tejada, R., Keydar, I., Tabbane, F., Spiegelman, S., and Mourali, N., Increased incidence of mouse mammary tumor virus-related antigen in Tunisian patients with breast cancer, *Int. J. Cancer,* 33, 305, 1984.

68. Cannon, G.B., Barsky, S.H., Alford, T.C., Jerome, L.F., Tinley, V., McCoy, J.L., and Dean, J.H., Cell-mediated immunity to mouse mammary tumor virus antigens by patients with hyperplastic benign breast disease, *J. Natl. Cancer Inst.,* 68, 935, 1982.

69. May, F.E.B., Westley, B.R., and Rochefort, H., Mouse mammary tumour virus related sequences are present in human DNA, *Nucleic Acids Res.,* 11, 4127, 1983.

70. Al-Sumidaie, A.M., Leinster, S.J., Hart, C.A., Green, C.D., and McCarthy, K., Particles with properties of retroviruses in monocytes from patients with breast cancer, *Lancet,* 1, 5, 1988.

71. Harzmann, R., Löwer, J., Löwer, R., Bichler, K.-H., and Kurth, R., Synthesis of retrovirus-like particles in testicular teratocarcinomas, *J. Urol.,* 128, 1055, 1982.

72. Bronson, D.L., Saxinger, W.C., Ritz, D.M., and Fraley, E.E., Production of virions with retrovirus morphology by human embryonal carcinoma cells *in vitro, J. Gen. Virol.,* 65, 1043, 1984.

73. Löwer, R., Löwer, J., Frank, H., Harzmann, R., and Kurth, R., Human teratocarcinomas cultured *in vitro* produce unique retrovirus-like viruses, *J. Gen. Virol.,* 65, 887, 1984.

74. Birkmayer, G.D., Balda, B.-R., Miller, F., and Braun-Falco, O., Virus-like particles in metastases of human malignant melanoma, *Naturwissenschaften,* 59, 369, 1972.

75. McClain, K. and Wilkowski, C., Activation of endogenous retroviral sequences in human leukemia, *Biochem. Biophys. Res. Commun.,* 133, 945, 1985.

76. Hehlmann, R., Schetters, H., Erfle, V., and Leib-Mosch, C., Detection and biochemical characterization of antigens in human leukemic sera that cross-react with primate C-type viral proteins (M_r 30,000), *Cancer Res.,* 43, 392, 1983.

77. Maeda, S., Yonezawa, K., Yoshizaki, H., Mori, M., Kobayashi, T., Akahonai, Y., Yachi, A., and Mellors, R.C., Leukemia serum reactive with retrovirus-related antigen in normal human placenta, *Int. J. Cancer,* 38, 309, 1986.

78. Gattoni-Celli, S., Kirsch, K., Kalled, S., and Isselbacher, K.J., Expression of type C-related endogenous retroviral sequences in human colon tumors and colon cancer cell lines, *Proc. Natl. Acad. Sci. U.S.A.,* 83, 6127, 1986.

79. Lasky, R.D. and Troy, F.A., Possible DNA-RNA tumor virus interaction in human lymphomas: expression of retroviral proteins in Ramos lymphoma lines is enhanced after conversion with Epstein-Barr virus, *Proc. Natl. Acad. Sci. U.S.A.,* 81, 33, 1984.

80. Reynolds, J.T. and Panem, S., Characterization of antibody to C-type virus antigens isolated from immune complexes in kidneys of patients with systemic lupus erythematosus, *Lab. Invest.,* 44, 410, 1981.

81. Rucheton, M., Graafland, H., Fanton, H., Ursule, L., Ferrier, P., and Larsen, C.J., Presence of circulating antibodies against *gag*-gene MuLV proteins in patients with autoimmune connective tissue disorders, *Virology,* 144, 468, 1985.

82. Temin, H.M. and Mizutani, S., RNA-dependent DNA-polymerase in virions of Rous sarcoma virus, *Nature,* 226, 1211, 1970.

83. Mizutani, S., Boettiger, D., and Temin, H.M., A DNA-dependent DNA polymerase and a DNA endonuclease in virions of Rous sarcoma virus, *Nature,* 228, 424, 1970.

84. Baltimore, D., An RNA-dependent DNA polymerase in virions of RNA tumor viruses, *Nature,* 226, 1209, 1970.

85. Baltimore, D., RNA-dependent synthesis of DNA by virions of mouse leukemia virus, *Cold Spring Harbor Symp. Quant. Biol.,* 35, 843, 1970.

86. Summers, J. and Mason, W.S., Replication of the genome of a hepatitis B-like virus by reverse transcription of an RNA intermediate, *Cell,* 29, 403, 1982.

87. Miller, R.H., Close evolutionary relatedness of the hepatitis B virus and murine leukemia virus polymerase gene sequences, *Virology,* 164, 147, 1988.

88. Coffin, J.M. and Temin, H.M., Ribonuclease-sensitive deoxyribonucleic acid polymerase activity in uninfected rat cells and rat cells infected with Rous sarcoma virus, *J. Virol.,* 8, 630, 1971.

89. Temin, H.M., RNA-directed DNA polymerase systems: not necessarily transforming Rous viruses, *J. Natl. Cancer Inst.,* 48, 1181, 1972.

90. Kang, C.-Y. and Temin, H.M., Endogenous RNA-directed DNA polymerase activity in uninfected chicken embryos, *Proc. Natl. Acad. Sci. U.S.A.,* 69, 1550, 1972.

91. Nelson, J., Leong, J.-A., Levy, J.A., Normal human placentas contain RNA-directed DNA polymerase activity like that in viruses, *Proc. Natl. Acad. Sci. U.S.A.,* 75, 6263, 1978.

92. Vogel, A. and Chandra, P., Evidence for two forms of reverse transcriptase in human placenta of a patient with breast cancer, *Biochem. J.,* 197, 553, 1981.

93. Verwoerd, D.W. and Sarma, P.S., Induction of type C virus-related functions in nomral rat embryo fibroblasts by treatment with 5-iododeoxyuridine, *Int. J. Cancer,* 12, 551, 1973.

94. Gallo, R.C., Yang, S.S., and Ting, R.C., RNA-dependent DNA polymerase of human acute leukaemic cells, *Nature,* 228, 927, 1970.

95. Reid, T.W. and Albert, D.M., RNA-dependent DNA-polymerase activity in human tumors, *Biochem. Biophys. Res. Commun.,* 46, 383, 1972.

96. Sarngadharan, M.G., Sarin, P.S., Reitz, M.S., and Gallo, R.C., Reverse transcriptase activity of human acute leukemic cells: purification of the enzyme, response to AMV 70S RNA and characterization of the DNA product, *Nature,* 240, 67, 1972.

97. Wittkin, S.S., Ohno, T., and Spiegelman, S., Purification of RNA-instructed DNA polymerase from human leukemic spleen, *Proc. Natl. Acad. Sci. U.S.A.,* 72, 4133, 1975.

98. Jacquemin, P.C., Antibodies against feline and gibbon ape reverse transcriptase on surface of spleen cells in human myelogenous leukemia, *Eur. J. Cancer Clin. Oncol.,* 17, 1283, 1981.

99. Weiss, G.B., Carr, B.K., and Hannigan, E.V., Template specificities of a RNA-directed DNA polymerase from a human homologous mixed mesodermal sarcoma, *Oncology,* 40, 293, 1983.

100. Chandra, P., Immunological characterization of reverse transcriptase from human tumor tissues, *Surv. Immunol. Res.,* 2, 170, 1983.

101. Weiss, G.B., Carr, B.K., and Rae-Venter-Huff, B., RNA-directed DNA polymerase activity in human breast cancer biopsy specimens: relation to estrogen receptor protein, *Oncology,* 41, 257, 1984.

102. Strayer, D.R., Brodsky, I., Caranfa, M.J., and Gillespie, D.H., Quantitation of RNA-dependent platelet DNA polymerase in patients with myeloproliferative disorders, *Br. J. Haematol.,* 50, 521, 1982.

103. Jacquemin, P.C., Strijckmans, P., and Thiry, L., Study of the expression of a glycoprotein of retroviral origin in the plasma of patients with hematologic disorders and in the plasma of normal individuals, *Blood,* 64, 832, 1984.

104. Cianciolo, G.J., Copeland, T.D., Oroszlan, S., and Snyderman, R., Inhibition of lymphocyte proliferation by a synthetic peptide homologous to retroviral envelope proteins, *Science,* 230, 453, 1985.

105. Nelson, J., Levy, J.A., and Leong, J.C., Human placentas contain a specific inhibitor of DNA polymerase, *Proc. Natl. Acad. Sci. U.S.A.,* 78, 1670, 1981.

106. Leong, J.C., Wood, S.O., Lyford, A.O., and Levy, J.A., Purification of a specific inhibitor of reverse transcriptase from human placenta, *Int. J. Cancer,* 33, 435, 1984.

107. Leong, J.C., Nelson, J.A., and Levy, J.A., Optimal conditions for detection of reverse transcriptase activity in human placentas, *Biochim. Biophys. Acta,* 782, 441, 1984.

108. Salganik, R.I., Tomsons, V.P., Pyrinova, G.B., Korokhov, N.P., Kiseleva, E.V., and Khristolyubova, N.B., Reverse transcriptase of rat liver associated with the endogenous retrovirus related to the mouse intracisternal A-particle, *Biochem. Biophys. Res. Commun.,* 131, 492, 1985.

109. Deen, K.C. and Sweet, R.W., Murine mammary tumor virus *pol*-related sequences in human DNA: characterization and sequence comparison with the complete murine mammary tumor virus *pol* gene, *J. Virol.*, 57, 422, 1986.
110. Dunwiddie, C. and Faras, A.J., Presence of retrovirus reverse transcriptase-related gene sequences in avian cells lacking endogenous avian leukosis viruses, *Proc. Natl. Acad. Sci. U.S.A.*, 82, 5097, 1985.
111. Weiner, A.M., Deininger, P.L., and Efstratiadis, A., Nonviral retroposons: genes, pseudogenes, and transposable elements generated by the reverse flow of genetic information, *Annu. Rev. Biochem.*, 55, 631, 1986.
112. Rasheed, S., Retroviruses and oncogenes in rats, in *Retroviruses and Human Pathology*, Gallo, R.C., Stehelin, D., and Varnier, O.E., Eds., Humana Press, Clifton, NJ, 1985, 153.
113. Gross, L., Schidlovsky, G., Feldman, D., Dreyfuss, Y., and Moore, L.A., C-type virus particles in placenta of normal healthy Sprague-Dawley rats, *Proc. Natl. Acad. Sci. U.S.A.*, 72, 3240, 1975.
114. Fine, D. and Schochetman, G., Type D primate retroviruses: a review, *Cancer Res.*, 38, 3123, 1978.
115. Nooter K. and Bentvelzen, P., Primate type-C oncoviruses, *Biochim. Biophys. Acta*, 605, 461, 1980.
116. Gardner, M.B. and Marx, P.A., Simian acquired immunodeficiency syndrome, *Adv. Viral Oncol.*, 5, 57, 1985.
117. Marx, P.A. and Lowenstine, L.J., Mesenchymal neoplasms associated with type D retroviruses in macaques, *Cancer Surv.*, 6, 101, 1987.
118. Nowinski, R.C., Edynak, E., and Sarkar, N.H., Serological and structural properties of Mason-Pfizer monkey virus isolated from the mammary tumor of a rhesus monkey, *Proc. Natl. Acad. Sci. U.S.A.*, 68, 1608, 1971.
119. Fine, D.L., Kingsbury, E.W., Valerio, M.G., Kubicek, M.T., Landon, J.C., and Chopra, H.C., Simian tumour virus proliferation in inoculated *Macaca mulatta*, *Nature New Biol.*, 238, 191, 1972.
120. Tainsky, M.A., Analysis of the virogenes related to the rhesus monkey endogenous type C retrovirus in monkeys and apes, *J. Virol.*, 37, 922, 1981.
121. Lovinger, G.G., Mark, G., Todaro, G.J., and Schochetman, G., 5′-Terminal nucleotide noncoding sequences of retroviruses: relatedness of two old world primate type C viruses and avian spleen necrosis virus, *J. Virol.*, 39, 238, 1981.
122. Martin, M.A., Bryan, T., McCutchan, T.F., and Chan, H.W., Detection and cloning of murine leukemia virus-related sequences from African green monkey liver DNA, *J. Virol.*, 39, 835, 1981.
123. Tanaka, T., Ogura, H., Ocho, M., Namba, M., Omura, S., and Oda, T., Syncytium formation induced by baboon endogenous virus in several transformed human cell lines, *Virology*, 108, 230, 1981.
124. Chatterjee, S. and Hunter, E., Fusion of normal primate cells: a common biological property of the D-type retroviruses, *Virology*, 1907, 100, 1980.
125. Cohen, M., Rice, N., Stephens, R., and O'Connell, C., DNA sequence relationship of the baboon endogenous virus genome to the genomes of other type C and type D retroviruses, *J. Virol.*, 41, 801, 1982.
126. Scott, M.L., McKereghan, K., Kaplan, H.S., and Fry, K.E., Molecular cloning and partial characterization of unintegrated linear DNA from gibbon ape leukemia virus, *Proc. Natl. Acad. Sci. U.S.A.*, 78, 4213, 1981.
127. Fine, D.L. and Arthur, L.O., Expression of natural antibodies against endogenous and horizontally transmitted macaque retroviruses in captive primates, *Virology*, 112, 49, 1981.
128. O'Brien, S.J., Reeves, R.H., Simonson, J.M., Eichelberger, M.A., and Nash, W.G., Parallels of genomic organization and of endogenous retrovirus organization in cat and man, *Dev. Genet.*, 4, 341, 1984.
129. Hardy, W.D., Jr., Feline retroviruses, *Adv. Viral Oncol.*, 5, 1, 1985.
130. Niman, H.L., Akhavi, M., Gardner, M.B., Stephenson, J.R., and Roy-Burman, P., Differential expression of two distinct endogenous virus genomes in developing tissues of the domestic cat, *J. Natl. Cancer Inst.*, 64, 587, 1980.
131. Kozak, C.A., Retroviruses as chromosomal genes in the mouse, *Adv. Cancer Res.*, 44, 295, 1985.
132. Kozak, C. and Silver, J., The transmission and activation of endogenous mouse retroviral genomes, *Trends Genet.*, 1, 331, 1985.
133. Rowe, W.P., Leukemia virus genomes in the chromosomal DNA of the mouse, *Harvey Lect.*, 1978: 173, 1978.
134. Ishimoto, A., Hartley, J.W., and Rowe, W.P., Detection and quantitation of phenotypically mixed viruses: mixing of ecotropic and xenotropic murine leukemia viruses, *Virology*, 81, 263, 1977.
135. Evans, L.H. and Malik, F.G., Class II polytropic murine leukemia viruses (MuLVs) of AKR/J mice: possible role in the generation of class I oncogenic polytropic MuLVs, *J. Virol.*, 61, 1882, 1987.
136. Biczysko, W., Pienkowski, M., Solter, D., and Koprowski, H., Virus particles in early mouse embryos, *J. Natl. Cancer Inst.*, 51, 1041, 1973.
137. Rowe, W.P. and Pincus, T., Quantitative studies of naturally occurring murine leukemia virus infection of AKR mice, *J. Exp. Med.*, 135, 429, 1972.
138. McCubrey, J. and Risser, R., Genetic interaction in the spontaneous production of endogenous murine leukemia virus in low leukemic mouse strains, *J. Exp. Med.*, 156, 337, 1982.
139. Nowinski, R.C. and Kaehler, S.L., Antibody to leukemia virus: widespread occurrence in inbred mice, *Science*, 185, 869, 1974.
140. DeLamarter, J.F., Monckton, R.P., and Moroni, C., Transcriptional control of endogenous virus genes in murine lymphocytes, *J. Gen. Virol.*, 52, 371, 1981.

141. Gardner, M.B., Henderson, B.E., Rongey, R.W., Estes, J.D., and Huebner, R.J., Spontaneous tumors of aging wild house mice. Incidence, pathology, and C-type virus expression, *J. Natl. Cancer Inst.,* 50, 719, 1973.

142. Lieberman, M. and Kaplan, H.S., Leukemogenic activity of filtrates from radiation induced lymphoid tumors in mice, *Science,* 130, 387, 1959.

143. Declève, A., Lieberman, M., Ihle, J.N., and Kaplan, H.S., Biological and serological characterization of radiation leukemia virus, *Proc. Natl. Acad. Sci. U.S.A.,* 73, 4675, 1976.

144. Haran-Ghera, N., Ben-Yaakov, M., and Peled, A., Immunologic characteristics in relation to high and low leukemogenic activity of radiation leukemia virus variants, *J. Immunol.,* 118, 600, 1977.

145. Ben David, Y., Kotler, M., and Yefenof, E., A highly leukemogenic radiation leukemia virus isolate is a thymotropic, immunosuppressive retrovirus with a unique RNA structure, *Int. J. Cancer,* 39, 492, 1987.

146. Ferrer, J.F., Lieberman, M., and Kaplan, H.S., Protection against radiation leukemogenesis by repeated injections of immune and nonimmune sera, *Cancer Res.,* 33, 1339, 1973.

147. Erfle, V., Schmidt, J., Strauss, G.P., Hehlmann, R., and Luz, A., Activation and biological properties of endogenous retroviruses in radiation osteosarcomagenesis, *Leukemia Res.,* 10, 905, 1986.

148. Pedersen, F.S. and Etzerodt, M., Structure of endogenous retroviruses expressed in radiation-induced and spontaneous murine bone tumours, *Leukemia Res.,* 10, 923, 1986.

149. Janowski, M. and Boniver, J., Radiation-induced lymphomas and leukemias, *Leukemia Res.,* 10, 875, 1986.

150. Van der Rauwelaert, E., Maisin, J.R., and Merregaert, J., Provirus integration and *myc* amplification in ^{90}Sr induced osteosarcomas of CF1 mice, *Oncogene,* 2, 215, 1988.

151. Pampeno, C.L. and Meruelo, D., Isolation of a retroviruslike sequence from the *TL* locus of the C57BL/10 murine major histocompatibility complex, *J. Virol.,* 58, 296, 1986.

152. Lowy, D.R., Rowe, W.P., Teich, N., and Hartley, J.W., Murine leukemia virus: high frequency activation *in vitro* by 5-iododeoxyuridine and 5-bromodeoxyuridine, *Science,* 174, 155, 1971.

153. Lavelle, G., Kennel, S.J., and Foote, L.J., Endogenous type C viral expression in cultures of fetal diploid baboon cells treated with 5'-bromodeoxyuridine, *Virology,* 110, 427, 1981.

154. Jollinger, G., Schwab, M., and Anders, F., Virus-like particles induced by bromodeoxyuridine in melanoma and neuroblastoma of *Xiphophorus, J. Cancer Res. Clin. Oncol.,* 95, 239, 1979.

155. Long, C.W., Suk, W.A., Snead, R.M., and Christensen, W.L., Cell cycle-specific enhancement of type C virus activation by sodium *n*-butyrate, *Cancer Res.,* 40, 3886, 1980.

156. Pearson, M.N., Beaudreau, G.S., and Deeney, A.O'C., Induction of endogenous viral gene expression by halogenated hydrocarbons, *Carcinogenesis,* 2, 489, 1981.

157. Altevogt, P. and Apt, D., High-frequency generation of altered M_r 70,000 *env* glycoprotein in *N*-methyl-*N'*-nitro-*N*-nitrosoguanidine-treated murine tumor cells, *Cancer Res.,* 48, 1137, 1988.

158. Hartley, J.W., Wolford, N.K., Old, L.J., and Rowe, W.P., A new class of murine leukemia virus associated with development of spontaneous lymphomas, *Proc. Natl. Acad. Sci. U.S.A.,* 74, 789, 1977.

159. Quint, W., Boelens, W., van Wezenbeek, P., Cuypers, T., Maandag, E.R., Selten, G., and Berns, A., Generation of AKR mink cell focus-forming viruses: a conserved single copy xenotropic-like provirus provides recombinant long terminal repeat sequences, *J. Virol.,* 50, 432, 1984.

160. Holland, C.A., Hartley, J.W., Rowe, W.P., and Hopkins, N., At least four viral genes contribute to the leukemogenicity of murine retrovirus MCF 247 in AKR mice, *J. Virol.,* 53, 158, 1985.

161. Mucenski, M.L., Gilbert, D.J., Taylor, B.A., Jenkins, N.A., and Copeland, N.G., Common sites of viral integration in lymphomas arising in AKXD recombinant inbred mouse strains, *Oncogene Res.,* 2, 33, 1987.

162. Herr, W. and Gilbert, W., Free and integrated recombinant murine leukemia virus DNAs appear in preleukemic thymuses of AKR/J mice, *J. Virol.,* 50, 155, 1984.

163. Schwartz, R.S. and Khiroya, R.H., A single dominant gene determines susceptibility to a leukaemogenic recombinant retrovirus, *Nature,* 292, 245, 1981.

164. Thomas, C.Y., Boykin, B.J., Famulari, N.G., and Coppola, M.A., Association of recombinant murine leukemia viruses of the class II genotype with spontaneous lymphomas in CWD mice, *J. Virol.,* 58, 314, 1986.

165. Evans, J.H. and Cloyd, M.W., Friend and Moloney murine leukemia viruses specifically recombine with different endogenous retroviral sequences to generate mink cell focus-forming viruses, *Proc. Natl. Acad. Sci. U.S.A.,* 82, 459, 1985.

166. Cloyd, M.W. and Chattopadhyay, S.K., A new class of retrovirus present in many murine leukemia systems, *Virology,* 151, 31, 1986.

167. Brown, E.H., Zajac-Kaye, M., Pogo, B.G.-T., and Friend, C., Rat cells infected with anemia-inducing Friend leukemia virus contain integrated replication-competent but not defective proviral genomes, *Proc. Natl. Acad. Sci. U.S.A.,* 82, 5925, 1985.

168. Strickland, J.E., Saviolakis, G.A., Weislow, O.S., Allen, P.T., Hellman, A., and Fowler, A.K., Spontaneous adrenal tumors in the aged, ovariectomized NIH Swiss mouse without enhanced retrovirus expression, *Cancer Res.,* 40, 3570, 1980.

169. Goodenow M.M. and Lilly, F., Expression of differentiation and murine leukemia virus antigens on cells of primary tumors and cell lines derived from chemically induced lymphomas of RF/J mice, *Proc. Natl. Acad. Sci. U.S.A.,* 81, 7612, 1984.

170. Housey, G.M., Kirschmeier, P., Garte, S.J., Burns, F., Troll, W., and Weinstein, I.B., Expression of long terminal repeat (LTR) sequences in carcinogen-induced murine skin carcinomas, *Biochem. Biophys. Res. Commun.*, 127, 391, 1985.

171. Pintér, A. and Börzsönyi, M., RNA oncovirus expression in *N*-methyl-*N*-nitrosourea-induced lymphomas in mice, *Int. J. Cancer*, 28, 219, 1981.

172. Fey, F., Ehm, I., Drescher, B., Rentz, E., and Seidel, G., Demonstration of a syncarcinogenic effect of endogenous MuLV, reduced from MNU-induced leukemias, and suboptimal MNU doses in mice, *Neoplasma*, 28, 265, 1981.

173. Lipp, M., Scherer, B., Lips, G., Brandner, G., and Hunsmann, G., Diverse effects: augmentation, inhibition, and non-efficacy of 12-*O*-tetradecanoylphorbol-13-acetate (TPA) on retrovirus expression *in vivo* and *in vitro*, *Carcinogenesis*, 3, 261, 1982.

174. Niwa, O. and Sugahara, T., Effect of caffeine on induction of endogenous type C virus in mouse cells *in vitro*, *Cancer Res.*, 41, 3253, 1981.

175. Gautsch, J.W., Knowles, A.F., Jensen, F.C., and Kaplan, N.O., Highly efficient induction of type C retroviruses by a human tumor in athymic mice, *Proc. Natl. Acad. Sci. U.S.A.*, 77, 2247, 1980.

176. Irons, R.D., Stillman, W.S., and Cloyd, M.W., Selective activation of endogenous ecotropic retrovirus in hematopoietic tissues of B6C3F1 mice during the preleukemic phase of 1,3-butadiene exposure, *Virology*, 161, 457, 1987.

177. Freeman, A.E., Kelloff, G.J., Gilden, R.V., Lane, W.T., Swain, A.P., and Huebner, R.J., Activation and isolation of hamster-specific C-type RNA viruses from tumors induced by cell cultures transformed by chemical carcinogens, *Proc. Natl. Acad. Sci. U.S.A.*, 68, 2386, 1971.

178. Johnson, K.H., Ghobrial, H.K.G., Buoen, L.C., Brand, I., and Brand, K.G., Nonfibroblastic origin of foreign body sarcomas implicated by histological and electron microscopic studies, *Cancer Res.*, 33, 3139, 1973.

179. Bernhard, W., The detection and study of tumor viruses with the electron microscope, *Cancer Res.*, 20, 712, 1960.

180. Kelly, F. and Condamine, H., Tumor viruses and early mouse embryos, *Biochim. Biophys. Acta*, 651, 105, 1982.

181. Pikó, L., Hammons, M.D., and Taylor, K.D., Amounts, synthesis, and some properties of intracisternal A particle-related RNA in early mouse embryos, *Proc. Natl. Acad. Sci. U.S.A.*, 81, 488, 1984.

182. Guérin, M., Corps d'inclusion dans les adenocarcinomes mammaires de la souris, *Bull. Cancer (Paris)*, 42, 14, 1955.

183. Zotter, S. and Müller, M., Natural antibody in mammary tumor virus-infected mice that reacts with intracytoplasmic A particles of mouse mammary tumors, *J. Natl. Cancer Inst.*, 58, 967, 1977.

184. Sarkar, N.H. and Whittington, E.S., Identification of the structural proteins of the murine mammary tumor virus that are serologically related to the antigens of intracytoplasmic type-A particles, *Virology*, 81, 91, 1977.

185. Nusse, R., van der Ploeg, L., van Duijn, L., Michalides, R., and Hilgers, J., Impaired maturation of mouse mammary tumor virus precursor polypeptides in lymphoid leukemia cells, producing intracytoplasmic A particles and no extracellular B-type virus, *J. Virol.*, 32, 251, 1979.

186. Zotter, S., Widespread occurrence in mammals of antibodies reactive to intracytoplasmic A particles of the mouse mammary tumor virus, *Arch. Geschwulstforsch.*, 53, 315, 1983.

187. Bowen, R.A., Expression of virus-like particles in feline preimplantation embryos, *J. Natl. Cancer Inst.*, 65, 1320, 1980.

188. Lueders, K.K., Specific association between type-II intracisternal A-particle elements and other repetitive sequences in the mouse genome, *Gene*, 52, 139, 1987.

189. Aota, S., Gojobori, T., Shigesada, K., Ozeki, H., and Ikemura, T., Nucleotide sequence and molecular evolution of mouse retrovirus-like IAP elements, *Gene*, 56, 1, 1987.

190. Chase, D.G. and Pikó, L., Expression of A- and C-type particles in early mouse embryos, *J. Natl. Cancer Inst.*, 51, 1971, 1973.

191. Grossman, Z., Mietz, J.A., and Kuff, E.L., Nearly identical members of the heterogeneous IAP gene family are expressed in thymus of different mouse strains, *Nucleic Acids Res.*, 15, 3823, 1987.

192. Bibby, M.C. and Smith, G.M., C-type and intracisternal A-type virus particles during epidermal carcinogenesis by tobacco smoke condensate in BALB/c mice, *Br. J. Cancer*, 35, 743, 1977.

193. Augenlicht, L.H., Kobrin, D., Pavlovec, A., and Royston, M.E., Elevated expression of an endogenous retroviral long terminal repeat in a mouse colon tumor, *J. Biol. Chem.*, 259, 1842, 1984.

194. Christy, R.J. and Huang, R.C.C., Functional analysis of the long terminal repeats of intracisternal A-particle genes: sequences within the U3 region determine both the efficiency and direction of promoter activity, *Mol. Cell. Biol.*, 8, 1093, 1988.

195. Lueders, K.K., Segal, S., and Kuff, E.L., RNA sequences specifically associated with mouse intracisternal A-particles, *Cell*, 11, 83, 1977.

196. Grigoryan, M.S., Kramerov, D.A., Tulchinsky, E.M., Revasova, E.S., and Lukanidin, E.M., Activation of putative transposition intermediate in tumor cells, *EMBO J.*, 4, 2209, 1985.

197. Augenlicht, L.H. and Halsey, H., Expression of a mouse long terminal repeat is cell cycle-linked, *Proc. Natl. Acad. Sci. U.S.A.,* 82, 1946, 1985.

198. Nakata, Y., Ochi, T., Kurisaki, E., Okano, H., Hamada, H., Amitani, K., Tanabe, S., Ono, K., and Sakamoto, Y., Identification of type A and type C virus particles in BF murine osteosarcoma, *Cancer Res.,* 40, 127, 1980.

199. Müller, M., Zotter, S., and Kemmer, C., Specificity of human antibodies to intracytoplasmic type-A particles of the murine mammary tumor virus, *J. Natl. Cancer Inst.,* 56, 295, 1976.

200. Zotter, S., Grossmann, H., Johannsen, B.A., and Pilz, C., Is there any diagnostic relevance of human antibodies which react with the mouse mammary tumor virus (MuMTV)?, *Arch. Geschwulstforsch.,* 51, 338, 1981.

201. Leiter, E.H., Fewell, J.W., and Kuff, E.L., Glucose induces intracisternal type A retroviral gene transcription and translation in pancreatic beta cells, *J. Exp. Med.,* 163, 87, 1986.

202. Kuff, E.L., Feenstra, A., Lueders, K., Rechavi, G., Givol, D., and Canaani, E., Homology between an endogenous viral LTR and sequences inserted in an activated cellular oncogene, *Nature,* 302, 547, 1983.

203. Gattoni-Celli, S., Hsiao, W-L.W., and Weinstein, I.B., Rearranged c-*mos* locus in a MOPC 21 murine myeloma cell line and its persistence in hybridomas, *Nature,* 306, 795, 1983.

204. Cohen, J.B., Unger, T., Rechavi, G., Canaani, E., and Givol, D., Rearrangement of the oncogene c-*mos* in mouse myeloma NSI and hybridomas, *Nature,* 306, 797, 1983.

205. Greenberg, R., Hawley, R., and Marcu, K.B., Acquisition of an intracisternal A-particle element by a translocated c-*myc* gene in a murine plasma cell tumor, *Mol. Cell. Biol.,* 5, 3625, 1985.

206. Ymer, S., Tucker, W.Q.J., Sanderson, C.J., Hapel, A.J., Campbell, H.D., and Young, I.G., Constitutive synthesis of interleukin-3 by leukaemia cell line WEHI-3B is due to retroviral insertion near the gene, *Nature,* 317, 255, 1985.

207. Luria, S. and Horowitz, M., The long terminal repeat of the intracisternal A particle as a target for transactivation by oncogene products, *J. Virol.,* 57, 998, 1986.

208. Ponta, H., Günzburg, W.H., Salmons, B., Groner, B., and Herrlich, P., Mouse mammary tumour virus: a proviral gene contributes to the understanding of eukaryotic gene expression and mammary tumorigenesis, *J. Gen. Virol.,* 66, 931, 1985.

209. Dalton, A.J., RNA tumor viruses — terminology and ultrastructural aspects of virion morphology and replication, *J. Natl. Cancer Inst.,* 49, 323, 1972.

210. Sarkar, N.H. and Moore, D.H., Surface structure of mouse mammary tumor virus, *Virology,* 61, 38, 1974.

211. Gulati, S.C., Axel, R., and Spiegelman, S., Detection of RNA-instructed DNA polymerase and high molecular weight RNA in malignant tissue, *Proc. Natl. Acad. Sci. U.S.A.,* 69, 2020, 1972.

212. Kozak, C., Peters, G., Pauley, R., Morris, V., Michalides, R., Dudley, J., Green, M., Davisson, M., Prakash, O., Vaidya, A., Hilgers, J., Verstraeten, A., Hynes, N., Diggelmann, H., Peterson, D., Cohen, J.C., Dickson, C., Sarkar, N., Nusse, R., Varmus, H., and Callahan, R., A standardized nomenclature for endogenous mouse mammary tumor viruses, *J. Virol.,* 61, 1651, 1987.

213. Herrlich, P., Hynes, N.E., Ponta, H., Rahmsdorf, U., Kennedy, N., and Groner, B., The endogenous proviral mouse mammary tumor virus genes of the GR mouse are not identical and only one corresponds to the exogenous virus, *Nucleic Acids Res.,* 9, 4981, 1981.

214. Anderson, S.J. and Naso, R.B., A unique glycoprotein containing GR-mouse mammary tumor virus peptides and additional peptides unrelated to viral structural proteins, *Cell,* 21, 837, 1980.

215. Peters, G., Placzek, M., Brookes, S., Kozak, C., Smith, R., and Dickson, C., Characterization, chromosome assignment, and segregation analysis of endogenous proviral units of mouse mammary tumor virus, *J. Virol.,* 59, 535, 1986.

216. Salinas, J., Zerial, M., Filipski, J., Crepin, M., and Bernardi, G., Nonrandom distribution of MMTV proviral sequences in the mouse genome, *Nucleic Acids Res.,* 15, 3009, 1987.

217. Cohen, J.C. and Varmus, H.E., Endogenous mammary tumour virus DNA varies among wild mice and segregates during inbreeding, *Nature,* 278, 418, 1979.

218. Cohen, J.D., Traina, V.L., Breznik, T., and Gardner, M.B., Development of a mouse mammary tumor virus-negative strain: a new system for the study of mammary carcinogenesis, *J. Virol.,* 4, 882, 1982.

219. Callahan, R., Drohan, W., Gallahan, D., D'Hoostelaere, L., and Potter, M., Novel class of mouse mammary tumor virus-related DNA sequences found in all species of *Mus,* including mice lacking the virus proviral genome, *Proc. Natl. Acad. Sci. U.S.A.,* 79, 4113, 1982.

220. Knepper, J.E., Medina, D., and Butel, J.S., Differential expression of endogenous mouse mammary tumor virus genes during development of the BALB/c mammary gland, *J. Virol.,* 51, 518, 1986.

221. Altrock, B.W. and Cardiff, R.D., Mouse mammary tumor virus infections: viral expression and tumor risk, *J. Natl. Cancer Inst.,* 63, 1075, 1979.

222. Moore, D.H., Holben, J.A., and Charney, J., Biologic characteristics of some mouse mammary tumor viruses, *J. Natl. Cancer Inst.,* 57, 889, 1976.

223. Lasfargues, E.Y. and Lasfargues, J.C., Possible role of genetic cell variants in the viral induction of mouse mammary tumors, *In Vitro,* 17, 805, 1981.

224. Michalides, R., Wagenaar, E., Groner, B., and Hynes, N.E., Mammary tumor virus proviral DNA in normal murine tissue and non-virally induced mammary tumors, *J. Virol.,* 39, 367, 1981.

225. Imai, S., Morimoto, J., Tsubura, Y., and Hilgers, J., Mammary tumor induction in inbred mouse strains with urethane is not accompanied by changes in the expression of B- and C-type retroviral structure proteins, *Int. J. Cancer*, 30, 101, 1982.

226. Sluyser, M., Moncharmont, B., Ramp, G., de Goeij, C.C.J., and Evers, S.G., Hormonal regulation of mouse mammary tumor growth, *J. Steroid Biochem.*, 27, 209, 1987.

227. Gardner, M.B., Lund, J.K., and Cardiff, R.D., Prevalence and distribution of murine mammary tumor virus antigen detectable by immunocytochemistry in spontaneous breast tumors of wild mice, *J. Natl. Cancer Inst.*, 64, 1251, 1980.

228. Hager, J.C. and Heppner, G.H., Heterogeneity of expression and induction of mouse mammary tumor virus antigens in mouse mammary tumors, *Cancer Res.*, 42, 4325, 1982.

229. Tonelli, Q.J., Long, C.A., Vaidya, A.B., and Sorof, S., Lack of induction of murine mammary tumor virus expression in cultured mammary glands treated with chemical carcinogens, *Int. J. Cancer*, 27, 811, 1981.

230. Butel, J.S., Dusing-Swartz, S., Socher, S.H., and Medina, D., Partial expression of endogenous mouse mammary tumor virus in mammary tumors induced in BALB/c mice by chemical, hormonal, and physical agents, *J. Virol.*, 38, 571, 1981.

231. Smith, G.H., Teramoto, Y.A., and Medina, D., Hormones, chemicals and proviral gene expression as contributing factors during mammary carcinogensis in C3H/StWi mice, *Int. J. Cancer*, 81, 1981.

232. Slagle, B.L., Medina, D., and Butel, J.S., Mammary cancer stages in BALB/cV mice: mouse mammary tumor virus expression and virus-host interactions, *J. Natl. Cancer Inst.*, 79, 323, 1987.

233. Michalides, R., Verstraeten, R., Shen, F.W., and Hilgers, J., Characterization and chromosomal distribution of endogenous mouse mammary tumor viruses of European mouse strains STS/A and GR/A, *Virology*, 142, 278, 1985.

234. Morris, D.W., Young, L.J.T., Gardner, M.B., and Cardiff, R.D., Transfer, by selective breeding, of the pathogenic *Mtv-2* endogenous provirus from the GR strain of a wild mouse line free of endogenous and exogenous mouse mammary tumor virus, *J. Virol.*, 58, 247, 1986.

235. Dudley, J. and Risser, R., Amplification and novel locations of endogenous mouse mammary tumor virus genomes in mouse T-cell lymphomas, *J. Virol.*, 49, 92, 1984.

236. Graham, D.E., Medina, D., and Smith, G.H., Increased concentration of an indigenous proviral mouse mammary tumor virus long terminal repeat-containing transcript is associated with neoplastic transformation of mammary epithelium in C3H/Sm mice, *J. Virol.*, 49, 819, 1984.

237. Michalides, R. and Wagenaar, E., Site-specific rearrangements in the long terminal repeat of extra mouse mammary tumor proviruses in murine T-cell leukemias, *Virology*, 154, 76, 1986.

238. Racevskis, J., Expression of the protein product of the mouse mammary tumor virus long terminal repeat gene in phorbol ester-treated mouse T-cell-leukemia cells, *J. Virol.*, 58, 441, 1986.

239. Mester, J, Wagenaar, E., Sluyser, M., and Nusse, R., Activation of *int*-1 and *int*-2 mammary oncogenes in hormone-dependent and -independent mammary tumors of GR mice, *J. Virol.*, 61, 1073, 1987.

240. Nusse, R., van Ooyen, A., Cox, D., Fung, Y.K.T., and Varmus, H., Mode of proviral activation of a putative mammary oncogene (*int*-1) on mouse chromosome 15, *Nature*, 307, 131, 1984.

241. van Ooyen, A. and Nusse, R., Structure and nucleotide sequence of the putative mammary oncogene *int*-1: proviral insertions leave the protein encoding domain intact, *Cell*, 39, 233, 1984.

242. Brown, A.M.C., Wildin, R.S., Prendergast, T.J., and Varmus, H.E., A retrovirus vector expressing the putative mammary oncogene *int*-1 causes partial transformation of a mammary epithelial cell line, *Cell*, 46, 1001, 1986.

243. Peters, G., Lee, A.E., and Dickson, C., Activation of cellular gene by mouse mammary tumour virus may occur early in mammary tumour development, *Nature*, 309, 273, 1984.

244. Knepper, J.E., Medina, D., and Butel, J.S., Activation of endogenous MMTV proviruses in murine mammary cancer induced by chemical carcinogen, *Int. J. Cancer*, 40, 414, 1987.

245. Keshet, E., Shaul, Y., Kaminchik, J., and Aviv, H., Heterogeneity of "virus-like" genes encoding retrovirus-associated 30S RNA and their organization within the mouse genome, *Cell*, 20, 431, 1980.

246. Keshet, E. and Shaul, Y., Terminal direct repeats in a retrovirus-like repeated mouse gene family, *Nature*, 289, 83, 1981.

247. Jähner, D. and Jaenisch, R., Integration of Moloney leukaemia virus into the germ line of mice: correlation between site of integration and virus activation, *Nature*, 287, 456, 1980.

248. McCubrey, J. and Risser, R., Genetic interactions in induction of endogenous murine leukemia virus from low leukemic mice, *Cell*, 28, 881, 1982.

249. Thomson, J.A., Laipis, P.J., Stein, G.S., Stein, J.L., Lander, M.R., and Chattopadhyay, S.K., Regulation of endogenous type C viruses: evidence for transcriptional control of AKR viral expression, *Virology*, 101, 529, 1980.

250. Lilly, F., Fv-2: identification and localization of a second gene governing the spleen focus response to Friend leukemia virus in mice, *J. Natl. Cancer Inst.*, 45, 163, 1970.

251. Pincus, T., Hartley, J.W., and Rowe, W.P., A major genetic locus affecting resistance to infection with murine leukemia viruses. I. Tissue culture studies of naturally occurring viruses, *J. Exp. Med.*, 133, 1219, 1971.

252. Rowe, W.P. and Sato, H., Genetic mapping of the Fv-1 locus on the mouse, *Science*, 18, 640, 1973.

253. Levy D.E., Lerner, R.A., and Wilson, M.C., The Gv-1 locus coordinately regulates the expression of multiple endogenous murine retroviruses, *Cell,* 41, 289, 1985.

254. Aoyama, A., Nagayoshi, S., Saga, S., Malavasi-Yamashiro, J., Yokoi, T., Takenaka, T., Miyaishi, O., Lu, J., Imai, M., Tomita, T., and Hoshino, M., Genetic resistance to mammary tumorigenesis in a mouse strain with high murine mammary tumor virus expression, *Cancer Lett.,* 36, 119, 1987.

255. Hsiai, H., Buma, Y.O., Ikeda, H., Moriwaki, K., and Nishizuka, Y., Epigenetic control of endogenous ecotropic virus expression in SL/Ni mice, *J. Natl. Cancer Inst.,* 79, 781, 1987.

256. Cullen, B.R., Skalka, A.M., and Ju, G., Endogenous avian retroviruses contain deficient promoter and leader sequences, *Proc. Natl. Acad. Sci. U.S.A.,* 80, 2946, 1983.

257. Dudley, J.P., Arfsten, A., Hsu, C.-L.L., Kozak, C., and Risser, R., Molecular cloning and characterization of mouse mammary tumor proviruses from a T-cell lymphoma, *J. Virol.,* 57, 385, 1986.

258. Stuhlmann, H., Jahner, D., and Jaenisch, R., Infectivity and methylation of retroviral genomes is correlated with expression in the animal, *Cell,* 26, 221, 1981.

259. Harbers, K., Schnieke, A., Stuhlmann, H., Jahner, D., and Jaenisch, R., DNA methylation and gene expression: endogenous retroviral genomes becomes infectious after molecular cloning, *Proc. Natl. Acad. Sci. U.S.A.,* 78, 7609, 1981.

260. Jähner, D. and Jaenisch, R., Chromosomal position and specific demethylation in enhancer sequences of germ line-transmitted retroviral genomes during mouse development, *Mol. Cell. Biol.,* 5, 2212, 1985.

261. Niwa, O. and Sugahara, T., 5-Azacytidine induction of mouse endogenous type C virus and suppression of DNA methylation, *Proc. Natl. Acad. Sci. U.S.A.,* 78, 6290, 1981.

262. Jaenisch, R., Schnieke, A., and Harbers, K., Treatment of mice with 5-azacytidine efficiently activates silent retroviral genomes in different tissues, *Proc. Natl. Acad. Sci. U.S.A.,* 82, 1451, 1985.

263. Hsiao, W.-L.W., Gattoni-Celli, S., and Weinstein, I.B., Effects of 5-azacytidine on expression of endogenous retrovirus-related sequences in C3H 10T1/2 cells, *J. Virol.,* 57, 1119, 1986.

264. Gunzburg, W.H., Hynes, N.E., and Groner, B., The methylation pattern of endogenous mouse mammary tumor virus proviral genes is tissue specific and stably inherited, *Virology,* 138, 212, 1984.

265. Mermod, J.-J., Bourgeois, S., Defer, N., and Crépin, M., Demethylation and expression of murine mammary tumor proviruses in mouse thymoma cell lines, *Proc. Natl. Acad. Sci. U.S.A.,* 80, 110, 1983.

266. Breznik, T. and Cohen, J.C., Altered methylation of endogenous viral promoter sequences during mammary carcinogenesis, *Nature,* 295, 255, 1982.

267. Gama-Sosa, M.A., Breznik, T., Butel, J.S., Medina, D., and Cohen, J.C., Mammary preneoplasia and tumorigenesis in the BALB/c mouse: structure and modification of mouse mammary tumor virus DNA sequences, *Virus Res.,* 7, 1, 1987.

268. Gunzburg, W.H. and Groner, B., The chromosomal integration site determines the tissue-specific methylation of mouse mammary tumour virus proviral genes, *EMBO J.,* 3, 1129, 1984.

269. Hu, W.-S., Fanning, T.G., and Cardiff, R.D., Mouse mammary tumor virus: specific methylation patterns of proviral DNA in normal mouse tissues, *J. Virol.,* 49, 66, 1984.

270. Niwa, O., Suppression of the hypomethylated Moloney leukemia virus genome in undifferentiated teratocarcinoma cells and inefficiency of transformation by a bacterial gene under control of the long terminal repeat, *Mol. Cell. Biol.,* 5, 2325, 1985.

271. Fowler, A.K., Reed, C.D., Todaro, G.J., and Hellman, A., Activation of C-type RNA virus markers in mouse uterine tissue, *Proc. Natl. Acad. Sci. U.S.A.,* 69, 2254, 1972.

272. Parks, W.P., Scolnick, E.M., and Kozikowski, E.H., Dexamethasone stimulation of murine mammary tumor virus expression: a tissue culture source of the virus, *Science,* 184, 158, 1974.

273. Sluyser, M., Verstraeten, R.A., and Van Nie, R., Effect of hormones on the expression of proviral genes Mtv-2 and Mtv-3 in mouse mammary gland, *Int. J. Cancer,* 31, 217, 1983.

274. Groner, B., Ponta, H., Beato, M., and Hynes, N.E., The proviral DNA of mouse mammary tumor virus: its use in the study of the molecular details of steroid hormone action, *Mol. Cell. Endocrinol.,* 32, 101, 1983.

275. Ringold, G.M., Regulation of mouse mammary tumor virus gene expression by glucocorticoid hormones, *Curr. Top. Microbiol. Immunol.,* 106, 79, 1983.

276. Ono, M., Kawakami, M., and Ushikubo, H., Stimulation of expression of the human endogenous retrovirus genome by female steroid hormones in human breast cancer cell line T47D, *J. Virol.,* 61, 2059, 1987.

277. Schütz, G., Control of gene expression by steroid hormones, *Biol. Chem. Hoppe-Seyler,* 369, 77, 1988.

278. Groner, B., Hynes, N.E., Rahmsdorf, U., and Ponta, H., Transcription initiation of transfected mouse mammary tumor virus LTR DNA is regulated by glucocorticoid hormones, *Nucleic Acids Res.,* 11, 4713, 1983.

279. Groner, B., Kennedy, N., Skroch, P., Hynes, N.E., and Ponta, H., DNA sequences involved in the regulation of gene expression by glucocorticoid hormones, *Biochim. Biophys. Acta,* 781, 1, 1984.

280. Firzlaff, J.M. and Diggelmann, H., Dexamethasone increases the number of RNA polymerase II molecules transcribing integrated mouse mammary tumor virus DNA and flanking mouse sequences, *Mol. Cell. Biol.,* 4, 1057, 1984.

281. Scheidereit, C. and Beato, M., Contacts between hormone receptor and DNA double helix within a glucocorticoid regulatory element of mouse mammary tumor virus, *Proc. Natl. Acad. Sci. U.S.A.,* 81, 3029, 1984.

282. Lee, F., Hall, C.V., Ringold, G.M., Dobson, D.E., Luh, J., and Jacob, P.E., Functional analysis of the steroid hormone control region of mouse mammary tumor virus, *Nucleic Acids Res.,* 12, 4191, 1984.

283. Beato, M., Arnemann, J., Chalepakis, G., Slater, E., and Willmann, T., Gene regulation by steroid hormones, *J. Steroid Biochem.,* 27, 9, 1987.

284. Cato, A.C.B., Henderson, D., and Ponta, H., The hormone response element of the mouse mammary tumour virus DNA mediates the progestin and androgen induction of transcription in the proviral long terminal repeat region, *EMBO J.,* 6, 363, 1987.

285. Otten, A.D., Sanders, M.M., and McKnight, G.S., The MMTV LTR promoter is induced by progesterone and dihydrotestosterone but not by estrogen, *Mol. Endocrinol.,* 2, 143, 1988.

286. Peterson, D.O., Alterations in chromatin structure associated with glucocorticoid-induced expression of endogenous mouse mammary tumor virus genes, *Mol. Cell. Biol.,* 5, 1104, 1985.

287. Johnson, G.S. and Ralhan, R., Glucocorticoid agonists as well as antagonists are effective inducers of mouse mammary tumor virus RNA in mouse mammary tumor cells treated with inhibitors of ADP-ribosylation, *J. Cell. Physiol.,* 129, 36, 1986.

288. Toohey, M.G., Morley, K.L., and Peterson, D.O., Multiple hormone-induced enhancers as mediators of differential transcription, *Mol. Cell. Biol.,* 6, 4526, 1986.

289. Willmann T. and Beato, M., Steroid-free glucocorticoid receptor binds specifically to mouse mammary tumour virus DNA, *Nature,* 324, 688, 1986.

290. Cordingley, M.G., Riegel, A.T., and Hager, G.L., Steroid-dependent interaction of transcription factors with the inducible promoter of mouse mammary tumor virus *in vivo, Cell,* 48, 261, 1987.

291. Lee, A.E., Proliferative responses of mouse mammary glands to 17β-estradiol and progesterone and modification by mouse mammary tumor virus, *J. Natl. Cancer Inst.,* 71, 1265, 1983.

292. Jaggi, R., Salmons, B., Muellener, D., and Groner, B., The v-*mos* and H-*ras* oncogene expression represses glucocorticoid hormone-dependent transcription from the mouse mammary tumor virus LTR, *EMBO J.,* 5, 2609, 1986.

293. McGrath, C.M., Prass, W.A., Maloney, T.M., and Jones, R.F., Induction of endogenous mammary tumor virus expression during hormonal induction of mammary adenoacanthomas and carcinomas of BALB/c female mice, *J. Natl. Cancer Inst.,* 67, 841, 1981.

294. Squartini, F., Basolo, F., and Bistocchi, M., Lobuloalveolar differentiation and tumorigenesis: two separate activities of mouse mammary tumor virus, *Cancer Res.,* 43, 1983.

295. Eichberg, J.W., Kalter, S.S., Heberling, R.L., Lawlor, D.A., Morrison, J.D., Bandyopadhyay, A.K., Levy, C.-C., Yoshinoya, S., and Pope, R.M., *In vivo* activation of baboon endogenous virus, *Proc. Soc. Exp. Biol. Med.,* 166, 271, 1981.

296. Levy, J.A., Autoimmunity and neoplasia: the possible role of C-type viruses, *Am. J. Clin. Pathol.,* 62, 258, 1974.

Chapter 5

DNA VIRUSES

I. INTRODUCTION

DNA viruses with pathogenetic potential are widely distributed in nature, infecting a diversity of animal species. Evidence, derived mainly from epidemiological studies, is suggestive for a possible role of some DNA viruses in the etiology of malignant diseases occurring spontaneously in humans and other animals.[1-3] DNA viruses with suspected oncogenic potential include some types of herpesviruses and papillomaviruses as well as the hepatitis B virus. Unfortunately, epidemiological methods alone cannot serve to demonstrate, or to discard, etiological associations, and the mechanisms possibly involved in these associations remain poorly understood.

DNA viruses associated with some common human cancers are not novel, rare viruses, but are well-known, ubiquitous viruses. The higher incidence of these viruses in tumor cells does not necessarily implicate an etiological relationship. A possible interpretation is that tumor cells are more susceptible to viral infection than normal cells and/or that such ubiquitous viruses may find in the tumor cells a more appropriate environment for their replication. This possibility is reinforced by the results obtained, for example, with the replication of herpesviruses, *in vitro* and *in vivo*, in leukemic lymphoid cells.[4,5] However, a consistent association between particular subtypes of DNA viruses and specific types of tumors would lend support to the hypothesis of a causal relationship between the virus and the tumor.

Host factors, including genetic, hormonal, and immunologic conditions, are of great importance in determining the final result of infections by DNA viruses with oncogenic potential. In general, human cells are more resistant than murine cells to virus-induced oncogenic transformation. DNA viruses could evoke malignancies in individuals with inherited or acquired defects in certain immunological responses, i.e., with impaired immune surveillance.[6,7] Several types of malignant neoplasms occur with increased frequency in immune deficient patients, and without an adequate immune defense system some common viruses may induce uncontrolled proliferation in target cells. The complexity of the etiopathogenetic mechanisms involved in malignant diseases associated with infection by DNA viruses is exemplified by Marek's disease occurring in fowls.[8]

The oncogenic potential of certain DNA viruses, especially those with small genomes, like polyoma virus and SV40, may be related to specific sequences or transforming genes, which could be considered as oncogenic since they would be necessary for the initiation and maintenance of a transformed phenotype in the virus-infected cells. In particular, it is interesting to look for the possible presence of sequences with homology to cellular sequences,[9] including oncogene-related sequences, in the genome of DNA viruses. In fact, there is evidence that the human and murine genomes contain sequences homologous to sequences present in the genomes of certain DNA viruses, including Epstein-Barr virus (EBV), herpes simplex virus (HSV), human cytomegalovirus (HCMV), and human adenovirus types 2, 3 and 12, because cytoplasmic RNA prepared from normal and malignant human cells hybridize to specific genomic regions of these viruses but not to papovavirus DNA.[10-12] The detected viral sequences are apparently homologous to conserved repetitive sequences of higher organisms.

DNA viruses with little oncogenic potential, or without a recognized oncogenic potential, may also show intriguing homologies with cellular DNA sequences. The vaccinia virus, which is a cytolytic poxvirus, encodes a polypeptide, the vaccinia virus growth factor (VVGF), which exhibits structural homology with the growth factors EGF and TGF-α.[13-15] VVGF is secreted into the medium of vaccinia virus-infected cells, is recognized by antibodies to mouse EGF, and is capable of binding to the cellular EGF receptor, inducing its autophosphorylation.[16] Another poxvirus, the Shope fibroma virus (SFV), also encodes a gene product which shows significant homology with both EGF and TGF-α.[17] These findings suggest that some nononcogenic DNA viruses, such as the vaccinia virus and SFV, can acquire, in a manner similar to that of acute transforming retroviruses, cellular DNA sequences related to growth factors, which may confer some advantage for inducing growth in cells infected by the virus.

The following discussion is mainly focused on the molecular events which would be involved in malignant transformation associated with DNA viruses and the possible relation between the genes of DNA viruses and specific cellular genes, especially protooncogenes, both at the nucleic acid and protein levels. Among the possibilities to be considered *a priori* are (1) derangement of cellular oncogene functions by the presence of unintegrated or integrated DNA viruses within the cell, (2) production of oncogene-like proteins by oncogenic DNA viruses, and (3) interaction between DNA viruses protein products and specific protooncogene protein products.

II. EPSTEIN-BARR VIRUS

The Epstein-Barr virus (EBV) is an ubiquitous pathogen that has been implicated as an environmental agent contributing to the origin of a number of human malignant and nonmalignant diseases but that can also produce asymptomatic infection.[18-20] In general, EBV is associated with a wide spectrum of lymphoproliferative disorders ranging from benign polyclonal B cell hyperplasias, without cytogenetic abnormalities and resembling infectious mononucleosis, to more classic monoclonal malignant lymphomas with clonal chromosome abnormalities.[21] These associations do not necessarily implicate, by themselves, a causal relationship. However, EBV is capable of inducing immortalization of human B cells and it could act as a cofactor in the development of certain human tumors.

EBV has been recognized as the etiologic agent of infectious mononucleosis, a benign polyclonal B cell proliferation. Several types of human tumors, especially African Burkitt's lymphoma and nasopharyngeal carcinoma, have been found to be frequently associated with EBV infection.[1,22,23] However, only a minority of Burkitt's lymphomas reported from non-African countries are associated with EBV. In one study of human nasopharyngeal carcinoma all of the normal nasopharyngeal biopsies examined as control samples expressed EBV-specific RNA transcripts.[24] It is thus difficult to attribute the malignant transformation of nasopharyngeal epithelial cells to the sole presence of EBV. Although a variety of wild-type EBV strains may exist,[25] there is no clear evidence that particular EBV strains are more frequently associated with human neoplastic or nonneoplastic diseases. In any case, definitive proof for a causal relationship between EBV infection and Burkitt's lymphoma or nasopharyngeal carcinoma is still lacking. Recently, EBV genomes were detected in the tumor cells of three patients with T-cell lymphomas.[26]

A. STRUCTURE OF EBV

EBV is a double-stranded DNA herpesvirus with a large genome of approximately 172 kb.[27] The DNA of EBV virions is methylated to a very large extent, approaching 15% in the HR-1 strain.[28] The genome is linear in the virus particle but exists as a circular episome inside the nucleus of the infected cell. The circularization is mediated by means of multiple direct terminal repeats about 0.5 kb long, which become joined in the circular form. The genome is further divided into a short (U_s) and a long (U_L) unique region by direct sequence repeats of approximately 3 kb.[27] The EBV genome encompasses 84 major ORFs but the total number of proteins expressed from the genome is unknown. Some ORFs could be spliced together, tending to reduce the total number of proteins expressed by the virus, while alternate splicing patterns would increase the number of proteins.[27] Some proteins would correspond to the major antigens of the virus, including an early antigen (EA), an EBV-associated nuclear antigen (EBNA), a membrane antigen (MA), and the capsid antigen (VCA).

B. MECHANISMS OF EBV-INDUCED TRANSFORMATION

EBV infects specifically human B-lymphocytes and this process depends on its interaction with the specific cell membrane protein CR2, and can be blocked by calmodulin antagonists.[29] Tumor necrosis factor α (TNF-α) selectively inhibits the stimulation of human B cells by EBV, including proliferation and Ig secretion.[30] The mechanism of this inhibition is not understood but the presence of macrophages in the B cell population is required for the inhibition to occur.

EBV-infected lymphocytes, whether derived from an *in vitro* infection or from EBV-infected individuals, contain multiple copies of the EBV genome, most of them in form of closed circular episomal DNA. Infection of human B lymphocytes with EBV may result in immortalization of these cells as reflected by an acquired ability to proliferate indefinitely in cell culture. Since immortalization is only one of the components of the malignant phenotype, these cells, although frequently called transformed cells, cannot be considered as true malignant cells.

1. EBV Genes Involved in Cellular Transformation

The expression of the EBV genome in latently infected cells is highly restricted but these cells transcribe mRNAs from at least three regions of the genome and contain some viral antigens, especially EBNA. At least four different EBNA nuclear proteins have been identified. Human sera with antibodies to EBNA react with a 62,000-Da (62K) protein present in both EBV genome-positive and EBV genome-negative human cell lines.[31] Although analysis with protease degradation indicates that EBNA and the 62K protein are not identical, they may contain a similar epitope. Thus, EBNA may contain sequences of cellular origin. Artificial introduction of EBV DNA fragments containing the EBNA encoding gene into normal human lymphocytes results in EBNA expression at levels comparable to those seen during the natural transforming infection by EBV, but the transfected lymphocytes do not proliferate and no immortalization is observed.[32] It is thus apparent that, although EBNA may be necessary for cellular immortalization by EBV, it alone is not sufficient, and EBNA cannot be considered as an oncogene product.

A cell membrane protein, termed LMP, is expressed in latent EBV infection and is likely to be an important mediator of EBV-induced cell proliferation.[33] Moreover, production of this protein in Rat-1 cells results in their conversion to a fully transformed phenotype. LMP is localized to patches at the cell periphery and is also associated with the cytoskeletal protein vimentin in EBV-infected lymphocytes. Although the role of LMP-vimentin association in EBV-induced transformation is unknown, the vimentin action is abnormal in EBV-transformed lymphocytes and EBV-infected tumor cells.

Tumor initiators and promoters such as phorbol diester (TPA) may enhance EBV replication in cultures of human lymphoblastoid cells.[34] The expression of a gene, or genes, located in a specific region of the EBV genome is required for the initiation of EBV replication, whereas expression of genes located in other regions of the viral genome are important for the establishment of lymphocyte immortalization.[35] A specific region of the EBV genome (the 0.26 to 0.36 region) is necessary for the initiation of EBV-induced cellular transformation but may be dispensable for the maintenance of a transformed phenotype.[36] EBV is the only known mitogen for human B lymphocytes which acts independently of factors produced by accessory cells, including cytokines produced by T-cells. Following EBV-induced transformation, B lymphoblasts release a soluble factor which mimics the B cell stimulatory products of mitogen-conditioned T lymphocytes and, apparently, the virally transformed cells utilize this activity to sustain their own growth.[37]

Mouse and human DNA contain repeat arrays related to an EBV repeat, IR3.[38] These repeats are not dispersed copies of a single sequence, but instead are a family of related sequences characterized by a high frequency of GGA triplets. The significance of the homology between repeats contained in EBV and the mammalian genome is not understood. It not is known if these homologous repeats may have a role in EBV-induced transformation.

The mechanisms involved in immortalization of human B lymphocytes by EBV, as well as those related to the putative oncogenic ability of this virus, remain uncharacterized.[39] Although usually only human mature B lymphocytes expressing specific viral receptors can be infected and immortalized by EBV, two immortalized human T lymphoblastoid cell lines have been established by transfecting cord blood lymphocytes with purified EBV DNA enclosed in fusogenic Sendai virus envelopes.[40] These cells are immortalized and do not require the specific growth factor IL-2 for growth, but they contain incomplete EBV genomes and do not express the EBNA antigen.

The study of EBV deletion mutants with nontransforming ability indicates that a particular region(s) of the EBV genome is required for the initiation of EBV-induced transformation of susceptible cells.[41] Inactivation studies indicate that only one fourth of the EBV genome is required for the initiation and maintenance of lymphocyte transformation.[42] Spontaneously defective EBVs that have undergone rearrangements may be unable to induce transformation of cord blood lymphocytes.[43] However, an oncogene is apparently not contained in the EBV genome and a transforming protein product of the EBV genome has not been identified. Normal human B lymphocytes can be immortalized by EBV infection but the resulting cells lack tumorigenic properties in nude mice.[44,45]

The entire EBV genome is integrated into Burkitt's tumor cell DNA at the terminal repeat sequences of the virus.[46] The EBV genomes carried in Burkitt's lymphoma cells and nonmalignant lymphoblastoid cells from the same patients are identical and it is unlikely that specific types or variants of EBV are associated with malignant disease.[46,47] Two types of EBV, termed A and B, have been identified and these types show different prevalence in geographical areas of the world, but it is not known if they are preferentially involved in particular types of diseases, especially in Burkitt's lymphomas.[48] There is some evidence that EBV strain-related variation may determine variations in the immune response to EBV infection and may affect the outcome of the infection.[49]

Certain fragments of EBV DNA may confer the property of unlimited growth on monkey epithelial cells in culture but these cells fail to produce tumors in whole animal (nude mice) experiments.[50] It may be concluded that EBV does not contain transforming sequences (oncogenes) and that it lacks *per se* the ability to induce malignant transformation of cells. EBV would thus require the action of additional factors, which may include chemical carcinogens or other viruses, for inducing neoplastic transformation.

2. Cooperation with Growth Factors

Production of an autocrine growth factor(s) is a possible mechanism for EBV-induced immortalization of human B cells. A soluble factor, termed BLAST-2, purified to homogeneity from EBV-immortalized B lymphocytes, may have a role as an autocrine growth factor for these cells and may also act as a comitogen for thymocytes.[51] BLAST-2 has properties similar to those of IL-1.

Specific cellular growth factors could cooperate with EBV-coded proteins for the proliferation and/or immortalization of EBV infected cells. EBV infection of B lymphocytes could mediate a switch in responsiveness to growth factors such as TGF-β.[52] While growth of normal human B lymphocytes is inhibited by TGF-β, the growth of EBV-infected normal cells as well as EBV-positive Burkitt's lymphoma cell lines is slightly stimulated. Irradiated EBV, which retains its capacity to bind to the CR2 receptor protein on the cell surface but loses its ability to function as a B cell activator, can synergize with the specific growth factor, BCGF, to stimulate B-cell division.[53] A monocyte-derived growth factor that promotes the growth of EBV-infected cells was recognized as a 16-kDa protein which is identical to the interleukin BSF-2/IFN-β_2/IL-6.[54] It seems thus clear that both autocrine and paracrine factors are involved in stimulating the proliferation of EBV-infected lymphocytes.

3. Cooperation with other Viruses and with Chemical Agents

Cooperation between EBV and other viruses could result in the immortalization and/or malignant transformation of cells. Lymphomas are observed in a number of AIDS patients and it has been suggested that HIV or HIV-related viruses may contribute as additional cofactors to the pathogenesis of both African and AIDS-associated EBV-positive lymphomas.[55] Elevated levels of antibodies for both HIV- and EBV-related antigens are found in AIDS patients.[56] An EBV immediate-early gene product, *Bam*HI *MLF1*, can activate the expression of a heterologous gene linked to the HIV promoter.[57] A molecular interaction between EBV and HIV may be biologically significant in patients with coinfection of B lymphocytes by EBV and HIV viruses.

Chemical promoters or carcinogens could also act as cofactors in carcinogenic processes associated with EBV infection. Transformation of normal human epithelial cells by EBV *in vitro* is dependent on the presence of phorbol esters.[58] Epidemiological studies in southern regions of China, where nasopharyngeal carcinoma is prevalent, suggest the possible participation of tumor promoters from plant (*Croton tiglium*) origin in the development of the tumor.[59]

4. Protooncogene Expression in EBV-Infected Cells

Protooncogene expression has been studied in isogenic, EBV-positive and EBV-negative Burkitt's lymphoma cell lines.[60] The level of expression of c-*myc*, c-H-*ras,* and c-B-*lym* was elevated but not different in the two types of cell lines, thus suggesting that the growth properties of these cell lines do not depend on the induction of protooncogenes. In addition, the karyotypic analysis of these cells demonstrated that the pairs of chromosomes 8 and 14 were normal and the human lymphoma cells (BJAB cells) did not present the characteristic t(8;14) translocation observed in other Burkitt's lymphoma cells. However, in an EBV-negative Burkitt's lymphoma cell line (BJAB), *in vitro* infection with EBV was associated with deregulation and amplification of the c-*myc* protooncogene.[61] Loss of the virus was associated with reversion of the altered pattern of c-*myc* expression but not with reversion of the amplification event, which indicates that this amplification was not responsible for the deregulation of c-*myc* gene expression. Infection of EBV-negative BJAB cells with EBV results in the expression of higher levels of c-*myc* transcripts.[62] However, it is not known whether the altered expression of c-*myc* is the consequence rather than the cause of altered growth in the EBV-positive BJAB cell line. No characteristic chromosome abnormalities similar to those considered important in protooncogene activation in human lymphomas are found in lymphomas induced in tamarin monkeys by EBV inoculation.[63] Moreover, different lymphomas in the same tamarin arise from different clones.

Transcripts of the human c-*fgr* protooncogene are present in Burkitt's lymphoma cell lines naturally infected with EBV, but not in EBV-negative Burkitt's lymphoma cells.[64] Normal umbilical cord or peripheral blood lymphocyte lines established *in vitro* by EBV infection also contain detectable levels of c-*fgr* mRNA and a 50-fold increase of the steady-state c-*fgr* mRNA concentration is observed when uninfected Burkitt's lymphoma cell lines are deliberately infected with EBV.[64] Relatively high levels of c-*fgr* transcripts are present in the human leukemia cell line IM-9, which was derived from a lymphocyte cell established by EBV infection.[65] However, increased concentrations of c-*fgr* mRNA alone are not sufficient to induce malignant transformation of normal human lymphocytes or even to immortalize them as continuous cell lines. Moreover, there is no evidence that EBV-induced lymphocyte immortalization involves the c-*fgr* gene or any other protooncogene.

C. CONCLUSION

In conclusion, there are no strong arguments for considering EBV as a true oncogenic virus and there is no definitive proof for a crucial etiologic role of EBV in human tumors. However, EBV is a potent lymphoproliferation-inducing agent involved in the etiology of the benign disease, infectious mononucleosis, and it seems plausible that in certain geographical areas EBV may act as a cofactor related to the development of malignant diseases such as Burkitt's lymphomas and nasopharyngeal carcinomas. In any case, the mechanisms involved in EBV-induced cellular immortalization and/or transformation have not been characterized as yet.

III. HUMAN CYTOMEGALOVIRUS

Cytomegaloviruses (CMVs) are members of the family of herpesviruses. Human cytomegalovirus (HCMV) is an ubiquitous agent that can produce either asymptomatic infection or a wide variety of clinical manifestations, including congenital abnormalities, intrauterine fetal death, mental retardation, mononucleosis, and interstitial pneumonia in organ transplant and immune deficient patients.[66,67] Although experimental observations indicate a definite potential for oncogenicity of HCMV, the possible causal role of this virus in human cancer remains disputable,[68] the main obstacle in epidemiological studies being the ubiquitous distribution of HCMV. This virus has been suggested as a possible infectious agent related to the development of AIDS and Kaposi's sarcoma,[69-71] but definitive proof in favor of this association is still lacking.

A. STRUCTURE OF HCMV
HCMV is a double-stranded DNA herpesvirus with a very large genome composed of 230 to 240 kbp and with an approximate mol wt of 150 to 160×10^6. Strain variations of HCMV can be detected by means of restriction endonucleases. HCMV genome codes for more than 50 polypeptides with MWs ranging from 10 to 200 kDa. High antigenic heterogeneity has been detected in HCMV.

B. MECHANISMS OF HCMV-INDUCED TRANSFORMATION
Specific sequences of the HCMV genome are responsible for the transforming ability of the virus.[72] A gene fragment coding for a major structural glycoprotein of the virus, gp64, which is a 64-kDa late antigen, has been cloned and physically mapped.[73] The coding sequences of HCMV gp64 correspond to an area of the viral genome with no homology to cellular genes. However, the HCMV H301 gene encodes a glycoprotein with an amino acid sequence similar to that of MHC class I antigens of higher eukaryotes, which may be responsible for the observed β_2-microglobulin-binding properties of HCMV.[74] β_2-Microglobulin is a protein normally associated with class I MHC antigens, which are essential for self/non-self recognition in the immune response.

HCMV has no nucleotide sequences with homology to the oncogenes like c-*myc*,[75] but may have sequences with homology to HSV-2.[76] A viral fragment containing the latter sequences is able to induce rapid transformation in the NIH/3T3 DNA transfection assay.

Activation of endogenous proviruses is a possible mechanism for transformation induced by DNA viruses, but there is little evidence in favor of this possibility. Induction of a xenotropic type C endogenous virus has been observed in K-MuSV-transformed nonproducer BALB/c 3T3 cells when treated with UV-irradiated mouse cytomegalovirus (MCMV).[77]

C. CONCLUSION
An etiological role of CMVs in nonexperimental animal tumors is still unproven. Although DNA sequences that hybridize to HCMV have been detected in some human tumors, e.g., in cervical neoplastic tissue,[78] there is no firm evidence for a role of HCMV in human cancer. CMVs have been isolated in cell cultures derived from biopsy specimens with EBV-associated nasopharyngeal carcinoma.[79] A possible etiological role of HCMV in Kaposi's sarcoma, associated or not with HIV infection, is still unsettled.[80] Most probably, CMVs found in these tumors are only passenger viruses. Since CMVs are ubiquitous agents, it is conceivable that CMVs may simply find a more appropriate milieu for replication in malignant cells than in normal cells, which would explain their more frequent prevalence in tumors.[4,5] The same consideration could also be valid for at least other herpesviruses as well.

IV. HERPES SIMPLEX VIRUSES

Herpes simplex viruses (HSVs) are members of the Herpesviridae family, which is a very complex one.[81] The members of this family are widely distributed among vertebrate species and have been found to be associated with both neoplastic and nonneoplastic diseases. However, it has been difficult to prove the etiological relationship of this association. A renal adenocarcinoma of the leopard frog (*Rana pipiens*), the Lucké's tumor, has been studied in detail and is most probably associated etiologically with a herpesvirus.[82-84]

HSVs are ubiquituous infectious agents in human populations.[85] Herpes simplex virus type 2 (HSV-2) has been suggested to be involved in the etiology of carcinoma of the human uterine cervix but definitive proof of a causal association is still lacking.[3] Recent epidemiological evidence points against this association.[86] Cervical cancer, as cancers in general, are the result of a complex multistage process and, most probably, multiple factors are involved in its etiology and pathogenesis.[87] The development of effective vaccines against HSV-1 and HSV-2 by recombinant DNA technology, as reported recently,[88] may contribute to a better understanding of the possible role of these viruses in human neoplastic diseases.

A. STRUCTURE OF HSVs

As other herpesviruses, HSVs are large, enveloped viruses approximately 150 nm in size which contain a genome constituted by double-stranded DNA with a total size of about 160 kbp. Some defined portions of this genome may be associated with the oncogenic potential of HSVs. Human DNA contains sequences with homology to a specific restriction fragment of HSV-1.[89] The fragment, termed *Bam*HI-Z, is represented in 10 to 60 copies per human haploid genome and contains a 0.29-kb segment which is responsible for the homology. The biological significance of this homology is unclear but it could be related to host-viral interaction and host DNA rearrangement.

B. MECHANISMS OF HSV-INDUCED TRANSFORMATION

The mechanisms involved in transformation associated with HSV infection have not been elucidated, but small fragments of HSV DNA with no apparent ability to specify a viral polypeptide may have transforming capability. This capability is contained in insertion sequence (IS)-like structures.[90] After integration, such structures could induce alterations in regulatory functions of the host genome, including the possibility of activation of protooncogenes or the production of a more general alteration in genomic functions through a mutagen-like mechanism. The immediate-early enhancer element of HSV-1 can replace a regulatory region of the c-H-*ras*-1 protooncogene required for transformation.[91]

1. HSV-2 Genes Involved in Cellular Transformation

Multistage transformation may be induced by defined fragments of HSV-2 and some particular regions of the HSV-2 genome that may be responsible for the oncogenic properties of HSV-2 in defined experimental conditions have been identified.[92,93] The transformation-associated fragment corresponds to the *Bam*HI fragment E (map position 0.533-0.583) of HSV-2 DNA, which encodes for 140-kDa ribonucleotide reductase. This enzyme catalyzes the first step in DNA synthesis by direct reduction of all four ribonucleotides to the corresponding deoxyribonucleotides. The cloned fragment of HSV-2 is able to transform established Rat-2 cells but, unlike *ras* oncogene-induced transformation, the HSV-2 DNA fragment induces transformation at low efficiency and after a relatively long latency period, which suggests that the activation of particular cellular genes, perhaps of protooncogenes, is involved in such transformation.[94] Moreover, DNA sequences homologous to HSV-2 *Bam*HI fragment E are present in normal Rat-2 cells DNA, and these sequences may be amplified in association with transformation induced in the same cells by the HSV-2 fragment.

Similarly derived HSV-2 sequences, termed mtr-II (map position 0.585-0.601), are capable of inducing morphological transformation of rat 3Y1 cell lines upon cloning and transfection.[95] Moreover, the HSV-2 mtr-II region may affect transformation by rearranging cellular sequences that exhibit homology with HSV-2 sequences, termed mtr-III, contained between 0.53 and 0.58 map units of the HSV-2 genome, i.e., the same sequences contained in *Bam*HI fragment E of the virus genome.

From ten human genital invasive squamous cell carcinomas and five genital premalignant lesions analyzed for the presence of HSV-2 DNA sequences, two vulvar tumors and two vulvar dysplastic tissues were found to contain DNA sequences homologous to the *Bgl*II O fragment (coordinates 0.38 to 0.42) and the *Bgl*II N fragment (coordinates 0.58 to 0.63) of HSV DNA.[96] These two fragments overlap the subsets of HSV-1 and HSV-2 DNA sequences, respectively, shown previously to transform cells in culture. Moreover, in each of the two positive vulvar tumors, the *Bgl*II N and *Bgl*II O sequences appeared to be linked, whereas in the standard HSV-2 genome the two fragments are separated by approximately 26 kb. This finding suggest that the two set of viral DNA sequences may have rearranged prior to or following the association of the HSV DNA with the tumor cells.[96] The possible role, if any, of this rearrangement in the tumorigenic process is unknown.

2. Expression of Cellular Genes in HSV-2-Infected Cells

The possible role of the expression of cellular genes, including protooncogenes, in the potential oncogenic properties of HSV-2 is not clear. Cellular proteins expressed in HSV-transformed cells also accumulate during HSV infection.[97] Infection of cultured human and hamster cells with HSV-1 results in the transcriptional activation of a small number of cellular genes.[98] Although the majority of these cellular genes depends on viral protein synthesis for their induction, a small minority does not require this synthesis and are induced by events occurring early upon binding of the virion to the cell surface and its entry into the cell. The physiological significance of HSV-induced proteins is unknown.

Infection of either human diploid cell strains or mouse heteroploid cell lines with HSV-2, but not with HSV-1, results in a rapid and transient induction of c-*fos* protooncogene expression.[99] Virus-specific protein synthesis is an absolute requirement for the production of HSV-2-induced c-*fos* mRNA and it seems likely that one of the several HSV-2 immediate early functions is responsible for the transcriptional activation of the c-*fos* gene.

3. Interaction of HSV with Chemical Carcinogens

Interaction with chemical carcinogens may be important for HSV-associated transformation. Different carcinogens and procarcinogens enhance the morphological transformation of 3T3 Swiss mouse cells by HSV-2.[100] Presumably, chemical carcinogens enhance the oncogenic potential of HSVs and other DNA viruses by causing structural alterations in the host cell genome, including point mutations, DNA strand breaks, and chromosome aberrations. Such changes could involve protooncogenes.

4. Oncogenic Potential of *Herpesvirus saimiri*

Herpesvirus saimiri is a virus closely related to human HSVs. This virus naturally infects squirrel monkeys (*Saimiri sciureus*) without producing signs of disease, but the experimental infection of other New World primates results in the induction of malignant T-cell lymphoma. A region of the viral genome not required for replication is required for oncogenicity of *H. saimiri* in owl monkeys (*Aotus trivirgatus*).[101,102] The protein product of this oncogenic viral region has not been identified.

5. Marek's Disease of Chickens

Marek's disease is a naturally occurring lymphoproliferative disease of chickens caused by a herpesvirus, the Marek's disease virus (MDV).[8,103] Three serotypes of MDV have been characterized: serotype 1 or oncogenic MDV, serotype 2 or nononcogenic MDV, and serotype 3 or herpesvirus of turkeys (HVT). The sequential events of Marek's disease caused in chickens by serotype 1 MDV can be divided in three phases: early cytolytic infection accompanied by temporary immunosuppression, latent infection, and the final phase of secondary cytolytic infection with permanent immunosuppression and tumor development. However, the third phase may never develop, depending on the oncogenic potential of the viral strain and host factors such as genetic resistance, presence of maternal antibodies, age at infection, and immunosuppression by other agents. The lymphoid tumors induced by MDV can develop in visceral organs, nerves, muscles, and skin but the exact target cell as well as the mechanisms of MDV-induced transformation remain poorly defined.

6. Conclusion

Although HSVs have defined oncogenic potential under specific experimental conditions, the possible role of these viruses in natural carcinogenic processes occurring in humans and other animals is still under discussion. The mechanisms involved in HSV-induced neoplastic transformation are not known but HSV are capable of inducing alterations in genome expression of the infected cells.

V. HUMAN B-LYMPHOTROPIC VIRUS

A novel herpesvirus, called human B-lymphotropic virus (HBLV), has been isolated recently from the peripheral blood leukocytes of six individuals with diverse lymphoproliferative disorders, including two AIDS patients.[104] HBLV was detected in 3 of 82 human B-cell lymphomas of different histologic types.[105] The virus is apparently not usually present in normal individuals (it was found to be present in only 4 of 220 randomly selected healthy donors) or in patients with AIDS (it was absent in 12 additional AIDS patients). HBLV infects selectively human B cells, converting them into large, refractile mono- or binucleated cells with nuclear and cytoplasmic inclusion bodies. HBLV is morphologically similar to viruses of the herpesvirus family but is readily distinguishable from the known human and nonhuman primate herpesviruses by host range, *in vitro* biological effects, and antigenic features.[104] HBLV contains a 110-kb double-stranded DNA genome.[106]

VI. HEPATITIS B VIRUS

Hepatitis B virus (HBV) is the main etiological agent of human viral hepatitis, a worldwide distributed infectious disease. There are about 200 million HBV carriers throughout the world, many of them asymptomatic, but the hepatitis induced by this infectious agent may progress to chronic liver disease, including cirrhosis and, probably, primary liver cancer.[107-114] A striking association exists in children between chronic HBV infection and the development of liver cirrhosis and hepatocellular carcinoma. Hepatitis B surface antigen (HBsAg) was detected in the liver and/or serum of 100% of 42 Taiwanese children by immunocytochemical techniques and/ or radioimmunoassay.[115] HBV infection in children may occur from familial carriers of the virus, especially from carrier mothers. However, studies performed in certain human populations, like Greenland Eskimos, indicate that infection with HBV alone does not necessarily enhance the risk for primary hepatocellular carcinoma.[116] Eskimos do not have a high incidence of PHC despite a high prevalence of antibodies against HBV (HBsAg), which suggests that other carcinogenic factors in their environment may be absent or that protective factors are present. Seroepidemiological studies performed in China also indicate wide variation in the association between HBV infection and the incidence of hepatocellular carcinoma; in some regions of the country, only half of the tumor cases are positive for HBV DNA.[117] The results of these and other studies strongly suggest that etiologic factors in addition to HBV infection are required for hepatocellular carcinoma to develop and that in some cases HBV is not involved at all in the etiology of the tumor. Hepatocarcinogenic substances such as aflatoxin B_1 are suspected to be involved in the etiology of human hepatocellular carcinoma in Asia and Africa,[118] but definitive proof of this association does not exist as yet.

A. STRUCTURE AND INTEGRATION OF THE HBV GENOME

The HBV genome is composed of approximately 3200 bp of partially single-stranded DNA and the complete nucleotide sequences of two different HBV subtypes have been determined after cloning in molecular vectors.[119] DNA replication of HBV and HBV-like viruses such as the duck hepatitis B virus occurs through an RNA intermediate by reverse transcription in a way similar to that of retroviruses.[120] Moreover, reverse transcriptase activity is present in the viral particles and nucleotide sequence studies gave evidence for a common evolutionary origin of HBV and retroviruses.[121,122] Putative reverse transcriptase intermediates of HBV have been detected by serological screening in primary human liver carcinomas.[123] However, no onco-gene-like sequences have been identified in the HBV genome.

In human hepatocellular carcinoma, HBV DNA may exist either in an unintegrated, episomal state or may be integrated in the chromosomes of the liver cells. Integration of HBV DNA into the genome of HBV-positive human hepatocarcinoma cells may occur by a mechanism in which minus-strand replicative intermediates synthesized by reverse transcription of the pregenomic RNA template of the virus are inserted into host cell chromosomal DNA in the presence of defective nucleocapsid synthesis.[124] In HbsAg-positive human hepatocellular carcinoma, study of the integration site of HBV DNA into host cell genome indicates that most of these tumors, including metastatic tumors, are clonal in origin.[125] Expression of HBV antigen genes in patients with hepatocellular carcinoma does not depend only on the state of HBV DNA methylation, but would require additional factors such as gene rearrangements.[126]

Various molecular forms of HBV DNA have been detected not only in hepatocellular carcinoma but also in Kaposi's sarcoma.[127] At least in some cases of hepatocellular carcinoma, neither deletion nor rearrangement is detected in the cellular DNA-flanking sequences following integration of the HBV genome, except for generation of short direct repeats at the virus-cell junction.[128] Despite their origin from a common HBV subtype, fragments cloned from the integrated HBV virus show an unexpected degree of sequence divergence.[129] Furthermore, unlike the retroviruses, the HBV DNA is highly fragmented in the integrated state and the HBsAg gene coding for the surface antigen may be the only intact gene present in the integrated HBV fragments.

B. MECHANISMS OF HBV-INDUCED TRANSFORMATION

DNA sequences responsible for the putative oncogenic potential of HBV have not been characterized. The glucocorticoid derivative dexamethasone stimulates HBV expression in some human hepatocellular carcinoma cell lines, and a glucocorticoid-responsive enhancer element has been identified in a particular fragment of the HBV genome that has been cloned in molecular vectors.[130] The possible role of glucocorticoid hormones in human liver carcino-genesis is not understood. A biological system where HBV mRNAs and proteins are expressed would contribute to a better understanding of the viral genome function and the characterization of the biochemical and physiological properties of HBV protein products.[131]

1. HBV-Induced Chromosome Alterations

Certain types of chromosome alterations are closely related to cancer origin and/or development. A possible mechanism for HBV-induced oncogenic transformation is chromosome deletion including some critical regulatory DNA region. Deletion of chromosome 11 at region 11p13-p14 has been detected in the tumor cells of a human hepatocellular carcinoma.[132] The deletion was produced as a consequence of HBV integration at this site and left only a single copy of the remaining normal allele. A deletion at the same chromosome location has been observed in the tumor cells of Wilms' tumor.[133,134]

A human hepatoma cell line (huH2-2) contains a single copy of the 1895-bp subgenomic region of HBV DNA integrated into the human chromosomal DNA and flanked by 12 bp directly repeating cellular DNA sequences but without causing deletion or rearrangement in the cellular flanking DNA sequences.[128] In another human hepatocellular carcinoma, linear HBV DNA integration was localized at a site involved in translocation between chromosomes 17 and 18 associated with deletion of a DNA segment of at least 1.3 kb at the translocation site.[135]

2. Protooncogene Expression in HBV-Infected Cells

Another possible mechanism of HBV-induced transformation would consist in insertional or noninsertional activation of protooncogenes but no evidence in favor of this possibility was obtained in DNA hybridization experiments with a human hepatoma-derived cell line in which several protooncogenes (c-*myc*, c-K-*ras*, c-H-*ras*, c-*mos*, c-*abl*, c-*bas*, c-*sis*, and c-*fps*) were examined for the presence of HBV DNA at cloned cellular flanking DNA in the sites of virus insertion.[136] Apparently, HBV DNA integrates randomly into the host cell genome. However, HBV DNA integration in a sequence homologous to v-*erb*-A and steroid receptor genes has been observed in a human hepatocellular carcinoma.[137] DNA from the human hepatoma cell line HCC-M, which has HBV DNA in integrated form, has an ability to transform NIH/3T3 cells in the DNA transfection assay.[138] The transforming gene(s) activated in this cell line, as well as the mechanism(s) of their activation, were not characterized.

C. WOODCHUCK HEPATITIS VIRUS

Woodchucks chronically infected with woodchuck hepatitis virus (WHV) may eventually develop hepatocellular carcinoma. WHV sequences integrated into the DNA of tumor cells are extensively rearranged and contain only parts of the viral genome.[139] WHV-associated hepatocellular carcinomas of woodchucks were screened for activation of protooncogenes including c-*abl*, c-*erb*-A, c-*erb*-B, c-*ets*, c-*fes*, c-*fms*, c-*myb*, c-*mos*, c-*raf*, c-H-*ras*, c-K-*ras*, N-*ras*, c-*sis*, and c-*src*.[140] The only protooncogene detected with an altered expression was c-*myc* in three out of nine carcinomas. These 3 tumors exhibited a 5- to 50-fold higher level of c-*myc* transcripts in comparison to the adjacent liver tissues, and the size of c-*myc* transcripts varied between 2.0 and 5.6 kb. Studies at the DNA level demonstrated rearrangement of the c-*myc* locus in these three tumors, and one of the tumors showed truncation of the c-*myc* gene and joining to a cellular DNA sequence of unknown function. WHV DNA was not found to be integrated near the c-*myc* coding exons, excluding insertional mutagenesis as an activating mechanism of c-*myc* expression.

D. CONCLUSION

The structural organization of the HBV genome suggests that it may share a common ancestor with retroviruses. Epidemiological studies performed in human populations living in different geographical areas indicate the frequent existence of a significant correlation between HBV infection and hepatocellular carcinoma. HBV could act as a cofactor in human liver carcinogenesis but an essential, indispensable role of HBV in the origin of PHC is unlikely. Definitive proof for the oncogenic potential of HBV under natural conditions is still lacking, and the molecular mechanisms possibly involved in HBV-induced oncogenicity have not been identified.

VII. ADENOVIRUSES

Adenoviruses are particularly interesting viruses because they afforded the first examples of human viruses capable of transforming cells *in vitro* and inducing tumors in experimental animals.[141-145] Moreover, certain adenoviruses may be capable of inducing tumors such as subcutaneous polymorphic sarcomas in the offspring of animals (Syrian golden hamsters) after inoculation of the mothers during gestation,[146] which may represent the first example of transplacental experimental tumor induction by potentially oncogenic viruses.

There are several different serotypes of human adenoviruses and although not all of them are able to induce tumors in rodents following injection, almost all are able to transform cells in culture. Based on the oncogenic potential for newborn hamsters, human adenoviruses have been classified into three groups: the highly oncogenic group A (Ad12, Ad18, and Ad31), the weakly oncogenic group B (Ad3, Ad7, Ad11, Ad14, Ad16, and Ad21), and the nononcogenic group C (Ad1, Ad2, Ad5, and Ad6).[147] This classification has some inconveniences. Although Ad5 is a member of the non-oncogenic group of adenoviruses, it is 10 to 50 times more efficient than oncogenic Ad12 in transforming rodent cells *in vitro*.[148] In addition, a group D of human adenoviruses has been defined, comprising 18 different types of the 41 identified human adenoviruses. Members of group D Ads have been shown to produce benign mammary tumors at almost 100% incidence when inoculated into female rats and some of these tumors can subsequently progress to malignancy.[149] A human adenovirus of group D, Ad9, induces efficient transformation of a rat embryo fibroblast cell line.[150]

Primary cultures of adult rat hepatocytes can be transformed by infection with Ad5 or transfection with Ad5 DNA, but the transformed cells are not tumorigenic when inoculated into neonatal syngeneic rats.[151] Some of these Ad5-transformed rat liver cells retain differentiated functions such as the capacity to secrete albumin, transferrin, hemopexin, and other plasma proteins. Retinoblastomas have been induced in baboons by intraocular inoculation of Ad12.[152] However, there is no evidence that Ad12 plays any role in human retinoblastoma.[153] In general, there is no firm evidence that adenoviruses are involved in the etiology of human cancer. However, the molecular mechanisms of experimental adenovirus-induced neoplastic transformation may contribute to a better knowledge of the complex processes associated with the malignant transformation of cells.

A. STRUCTURE AND REPLICATION OF ADENOVIRUSES

The genome of the best characterized adenovirus, adenovirus type 5 (Ad5), consists of a linear duplex of DNA, 36,000 bp in length, encoding 30 to 40 proteins involved in virus replication. The adenovirus genome is transcribed in both the leftward and rightward directions and contains inverted terminal repeat sequences (ITRs), 103 bp in length, and a terminal protein covalently attached to the 5′ nucleotide of each strand through a phosphodiester linkage. The adenovirus genes, which are of major importance in malignant transformation of cells in culture and in experimental induction of tumors *in vivo,* are those contained within the left approximately 12%, early region 1 (E1), of the viral genome. These sequences are the only ones which are consistently retained and expressed in transformed cells and the only ones which are both necessary and sufficient for DNA-mediated transformation.[143] Adenovirus region E1 contains two independently promoted transcriptional units, E1A and E1B, and different mRNAs are expressed from each one of these units: 9S, 12S, and 13S mRNA species from E1A, and 13S and 22S mRNA species from E1B.[154-158] Plasmid constructs carrying E1A nucleotide sequences can induce DNA synthesis in growth-arrested NIH/3T3 fibroblasts when they express either 12S or 13S mRNA, but not when they express only 9S mRNA.[159] Expression of adenovirus early promoters depends, at least in part, on the action of specific cellular proteins.[160] The 19-kDa E1B gene protein product can activate all the adenovirus early promoters as well as the promoter of the cellular HSP-70 gene, but not the adenovirus late promoters.[161]

Replication of the adenovirus genome can be initiated at either terminus and depends on the presence of specific nucleotide sequence domains within the terminal region of the viral DNA. Both virus- and cell-encoded proteins are required for initiation of adenovirus replication *in vitro*, which depends on the specific interaction of multiple proteins with the viral origin of DNA replication.[162]

B. MECHANISMS OF ADENOVIRUS-INDUCED TRANSFORMATION

Many efforts have been dedicated to elucidate the mechanisms involved in adenovirus-induced malignant transformation.[148,154-156] Comparison of nucleotide sequences at a number of sites for recombination between adenovirus and cellular DNA have not provided evidence that adenovirus DNA insertion occurs at unique, highly specific cellular DNA sequences.[163] Recent evidence indicates that at least some of the cellular DNA sequences at sites of insertion of adenovirus DNA are transcriptionally active and that this activity may be a necessary, but not sufficient, precondition for the insertion of adenovirus DNA.[164] An Ad12 genome was found to be inserted in the vicinity of an IAP in the cells of a Syrian hamster tumor induced by the adenovirus.[165] Chemical carcinogens that induce DNA lesions may enhance the transforming capacity of adenoviruses.[166] This result and other similar results obtained with other DNA viruses suggest that interactions between the viruses and chemical carcinogenic agents may be relevant to the etiology of tumors occurring in animal species, possibly including the human species.

1. Transformation-Related Adenovirus-Encoded Proteins

Expression of discrete adenovirus functions is required for adenovirus-induced neoplastic transformation of cells. The protein products of at least some adenovirus RNA species are critically involved in the molecular mechanisms leading to adenovirus-induced oncogenic transformation, as can be defined from results obtained with different virus mutants.[167,168] Although no oncogenes are apparently contained in the adenovirus genome, some adenovirus-encoded proteins could act through cellular metabolic pathways similar or identical to that used by oncogene protein products or could produce derangement in endogenous protooncogene functions.

The two related proteins encoded by the E1A region of the Ad2 genome are required for transformation.[168] Cells containing only the E1A region are immortal but lack many of the properties of fully transformed cells, including tumorigenicity, and the 5' half of E1B is required for complete transformation. Vectors expressing the 12S sequences from the E1A region of Ad5 have higher immortalizing capacity than those expressing 13S sequences and can induce proliferation and immortalization of epithelial cells in rat kidney, liver, heart, pancreas, and thyroid primary cultures.[169] The 12S E1A protein expressed at moderated levels by these vectors does not transform cells to a tumorigenic phenotype nor allow them to grow in soft agar. However, constructed plasmids expressing very high levels of E1A gene proteins alone are able to induce in some cellular systems many of the attributes of morphological transformation that have been assigned to E1B proteins.[170] The Ad5 E1A region is capable of inducing mouse NIH/3T3 fibroblasts to acquire several properties of transformed cells, including anchorage-independent growth, a lowered serum requirement, and a tumorigenic phenotype without significant morphological alteration.[171]

The cloned E1 region of Ad12 can transform human embryo retinoblasts which, upon inoculation into athymic mice, form tumors resembling poorly differentiated retinoblasto-mas.[172] Cooperation between E1A and E1B regions of the virus genome is usually required for the induction of a fully transformed phenotype. The human Ad5 E1A region is capable of inducing immortalization of primary cultures of BRK cells but requires the presence of E1B region for complete oncogenic transformation. One of the effects of the E1B region in the transformation process is the activation of E1A expression by a *cis* effect that enhances transcription initiation.[173] This activation is mainly observed when E1A and E1B regions of the viral genome are integrated simultaneously into the cellular genome and is only minimal when these regions are integrated separately, which strongly suggests that a close physical linkage of E1A and E1B regions is essential for the enhancing effect. It is thus possible that the major function of E1B in cell transformation is the activation of E1A expression. However, the possibility that a viral protein product is involved in activation of E1A transcription is suggested by the fact that a product of a herpesvirus (the pseudorabies virus) can activate the transcription of adenovirus E1A region even more efficiently than would do the putative adenovirus gene product.[174]

The larger 13S mRNA from Ad2 and Ad5 E1A region encodes a protein of 289 amino acids, while the smaller 12S mRNA encodes a 243-amino acid protein, which differs from the 13S mRNA-encoded product by the internal deletion of 46 amino acid residues.[175] The purified 13S and 12S mRNA-encoded proteins are able to induce cellular DNA synthesis when introduced by microinjection, either individually or in combination, into quiescent, G_0-arrested mammalian cells from immortalized cell lines.[176] Studies with deletion mutants showed that the 85 amino acids of the amino-terminal region common to both the proteins coded by the 12S and 13S mRNAs of E1A region of the virus may be sufficient for the induction of synthesis of proliferating nuclear antigen and the stimulation of DNA synthesis in BRK cells.[177] A second domain also common to the amino-terminal exon of both of these proteins is required for the induction of mitosis and stimulation of proliferation of primary BRK cells.

The 243-amino acid protein from region E1A of Ad2, encoded by 12S mRNA, is required for full transformation of rat embryo cells.[178] Mutants of Ad5 that contain defects in the gene encoding the E1A 289-amino acid polypeptide encoded by 13S mRNA, but producing a wild-type 12S mRNA-encoded 243-amino acid protein, are capable of inducing tumors in nude mice as well as in immunocompetent syngeneic Fischer rats.[179] In contrast, cells expressing Ad5 wild-type 289-amino acid protein are unable to induce tumors in either nude mice or syngeneic rats. Adenovirus mutants carrying an identical 69-bp deletion in the first exon of E1A are fully competent for replication and growth in their normal hosts and have a host range extended to include the Vero cell line of African green monkey origin but are almost totally defective with regard to neoplastic transformation.[180]

The capacity of Ad12 to transform primary baby rat kidney (BRK) cells *in vitro* resides also in the left-terminal part of the viral DNA, which encodes several types of proteins.[181] Expression of one of these proteins, a 60-kDa protein encoded by the E1 region of the viral genome, is required for oncogenicity in nude mice, but not for morphological transformation of the cultured cells. A cDNA clone corresponding to the E1A 12S gene has been recombined with viruses and such viruses induce immortalization in BRK cells at a very high efficiency, although the immortalized foci are not fully transformed.[182] It is thus apparent that functions additional to those encoded by E1A genes are necessary for the transformation of cultured primary cells. Such functions may be supplied by particular types of oncogene proteins or growth factors.

2. Complementation of Adenovirus Proteins and Oncogene Products for the Induction of Neoplastic Transformation

Protein products from the E1 region of adenoviruses may complement the action of oncogenes to induce neoplastic transformation. The T24/EJ mutant human c-H-*ras* protooncogene is unable to transform BRK cells but this oncogene can be complemented by the Ad2 E1A gene to produce full transformation and tumorigenicity.[183] Plasmids expressing partial adenovirus E1A coding sequences may enable T24/EJ c-H-*ras* and polyoma virus *pmt* genes to transform cultured primary BRK cells.[184] This transformation requires the complementation of functions specified by different domains of E1A products, suggesting that transformation induced by adenoviruses in cooperation with *ras* oncogenes is a process that involves at least three steps.[185] Different activities of Ad5 and Ad12 E1A regions may be involved in transformation with the T24/EJ c-H-*ras* gene.[186] In spite of the fact that Ad5 is less oncogenic than Ad12, the Ad5 E1A plus *ras*-transformed cells are highly oncogenic, whereas the Ad12 E1A plus *ras*-transformed cells are weakly oncogenic with respect to both their behavior *in vitro* and their tumorigenic properties. The reason for this difference could not be identified in these studies but no differences were detected in the levels of expression of Ad E1A regions of T24/EJ c-H-*ras* gene in the two cell types.

The DNAs of human adenoviruses Ad2 and Ad5 hybridize to genomic DNAs from human and chicken tissue.[187] The hybridization of human and adenoviral DNA has specificity, as only certain regions of viral DNA hybridize, and it is contained within short regions (around 200 bp) of viral DNA, occurring to regions which are known to be transcription units. Interestingly, adenovirus E1A region can substitute for the *myc* oncogene in DNA transfection/transformation assays.[183] Moreover, Ad2 E1A can provide functions required by polyoma virus middle-T antigen and T24 c-H-*ras*-1 genes for transforming BRK cells. In contradiction to a previous conclusion,[188] no significant structural homology exists between the c-*myc* protooncogene protein product and adenovirus E1A proteins.[189,190] In E1A-transformed NIH/3T3 cells the endogenous c-*myc* gene is expressed at high levels, which suggest its possible participation in the expression of a transformed phenotype in these cells.[171]

3. Regulation of Cellular Functions by Adenovirus-Encoded Proteins

E1A proteins are involved in regulating the expression of certain host cell genomic functions, including DNA synthesis.[176] The carboxyl-terminus of E1A contains sequences essential for rapid and efficient nuclear localization of the adenovirus-encoded protein.[191] The mechanisms responsible for the nuclear localization and retention of E1A proteins are not understood but there is evidence that particular portions of the E1A proteins amino acid sequence, including a pentapeptide signal sequence from the extreme carboxyl terminus, are involved in these phenomena.[192] Interestingly, the attachment of this signal to a heterologous protein (*Escherichia coli* galactokinase) rapidly directs it into the nucleus. Apparently, the signal pentapeptide is capable of enhancing the rate of nuclear entry of proteins. The molecular and cellular events involved in the rapid translocation of cytoplasmic proteins possessing specific signal oligopeptides into the nucleus remains to be elucidated. In addition to favoring the entry of proteins into the nucleus, the same or other signal oligopeptides contained in nuclear proteins may be involved in their subsequent nuclear retention, perhaps by specific interactions with certain nuclear components.

Both the 289- and the 243-amino acid Ad2 E1A proteins are localized predominantly in the nucleus and a fraction of the 289-amino acid proteins is associated with the nuclear matrix.[193] By means of monoclonal antibodies to the protein products of human Ad12 it has been demonstrated that a putative transforming 58-kDa phosphoprotein encoded by the virus is localized in the nucleus of the infected cells, which suggests a possible role of this protein in regulation of gene expression.[194] A factor encoded by adenovirus E1A region has properties in common with a transcription factor which may be involved in the differentiation of murine embryonal carcinoma stem cells.[195] The immortalizing and transforming properties of E1A proteins on primary BRK cells could be exerted through the production of a growth factor whose synthesis would depend on some function residing within amino acid residues located on the amino-terminal region of the E1A proteins.[196] The putative growth factor would have specificity for epithelial tissues, but it has not been identified as yet.

The role of adenovirus-encoded nuclear proteins in the regulation of host genomic functions related to the expression of a transformed phenotype is not clear. The construction and genetic analysis of E1A mutations has indicated that the transforming function of E1A can be dissociated from its transcriptional regulatory functions.[197] More than half of the E1A proteins not released into the soluble fraction in adenovirus-infected and -transformed human cells are associated with the cytoskeleton and only small quantities of the E1A proteins are found in the nuclear fraction, including the chromatin and the nuclear matrix.[198] Thus, the possible role of adenovirus proteins in the regulation of nuclear functions remains uncharacterized. Cellular gene expression may also be regulated in adenovirus-transformed cells at the level of posttranscriptional mechanisms.[199]

4. Association of Adenovirus-Encoded Proteins with the p53 Cellular Antigen

In rat cell lines transformed by Ad5, but not by Ad12, the 55-kDa protein encoded by the E1B region of the virus forms a complex with the cellular antigen p53.[200] The stability of p53 in both Ad5- and Ad12-transformed cells is increased relative to that in primary cells and this stability appears to correlate with morphological transformation.

5. The *cyt* Gene

A gene of Ad2 and Ad5, termed *cyt*, is responsible for the transforming properties of these adenoviruses in rat 3Y1 cells.[201,202] The gene *cyt* encodes a 19,000-mol wt (19K) polypeptide whose amino acid sequence has been determined and it has been postulated that this gene may be considered as an oncogene. The cyt⁺ locus is an allele of the lp⁺ locus which maps within the 19K tumor antigen and the *cyt* phenotype may be the result of mutations in specific domains of the 19K tumor antigen. The majority of 59 *cyt* mutants examined are transformation defective whereas *cyt⁺* revertants and *cyt⁺* intragenic recombinants can recover fully the transforming ability. However, the function of the *cyt* protein product is unknown.

6. Expression of Cellular Genes in Adenovirus-Transformed Cells

Adenoviruses may either induce or inhibit the expression of cellular genes. Ad2 activates cell cycle-dependent genes that are a subset of those activated by serum.[203] Deregulation of the serum-induced expression of c-*myc*, but not c-K-*ras* or p53 genes, is observed during the cell cycle in adenovirus-transformed mouse cell lines.[204] One of the adenovirus- and serum-activated genes is the gene that encodes the major heat shock protein, HSP70.[205] The levels of expression of different cellular genes may be differentially modulated in Ad12-infected cells and Ad12-transformed human cells.[206] Whereas the level of expression of HSP70, β-tubulin, and p53 antigen are unchanged following Ad12 infection of human embryo kidney (HEK) cells, thymidine kinase activity shows a marked increase in the infected cells. In cell lines transformed with either Ad12 or Ad5 E1 DNA, HSP70 and β-tubulin levels are greatly increased, but p53 is only expressed at high levels in Ad12-transformed lines expressing both E1A and E1B proteins.[206] HSP70 gene expression is induced in HeLa cells by Ad5 infection even in the absence of exogenous growth factors.[207] The 13S product of Ad5 E1A region is the specific *trans*-activator of the HSP70 gene in Ad5-infected cells.

Adenoviruses may not stimulate but repress the expression of particular cellular genes. The complete myogenic program of cultured rodent myoblasts can be blocked by the introduction of constitutively expressing Ad5 E1A genes, which is due to the inhibition of the transcriptional activity of muscle-specific genes.[208] In particular, the promoter-inducing activities of well-defined elements that are required for the muscle-specific expression of two sarcomeric α-actins, and which normally bind cellular *trans*-acting factors, become targets for E1A-induced suppression. The construction of an extensive series of mutations within the E1A gene have given new insights about the importance of gene repression in adenovirus-induced transformation.[209] The results obtained with these mutants strongly suggest that it is transcriptional repression rather than transcriptional activation that is important for transformation. The cellular gene(s) whose repression is directly associated with adenovirus-induced transformation remains uncharacterized but it could hypothetically correspond to some tumor suppressor genes (antioncogenes).

There are differences between the cellular proteins of nontumorigenic Ad5- and tumorigenic Ad12-transformed mouse cells.[210] From these studies it may be concluded that different adenoviruses may elicit different responses in different host cell types and that vast differences in the levels of expression of different genes may exist between viral infection and viral transformation.[206] However, the cellular genes specifically involved in the expression of adenovirus-induced neoplastic transformation have not been identified. It is also not known whether these genes are protooncogenes or other class of cellular genes. Moreover, not only nuclear genes but also mitochondrial genes can be activated by adenovirus E1A products. Increased levels of the mitochondrial mRNA encoding subunit II of cytochrome oxidase have been found in rat fibroblast cells immortalized by transfer of E1A DNA.[211] Similar changes in the expression of this mitochondrial gene are observed after transfer of polyoma virus *plt* gene or a rearranged c-*myc* protooncogene.

The mechanisms responsible for adenovirus-induced activation or repression of cellular genes are not understood. Progression of Ad5-transformed cells is associated with altered patterns of DNA methylation and may be reversed by treatment with the demethylating agent, 5-azacytidine.[212] There is evidence that Ad12 DNA is preferentially integrated into particular chromosomes after infection of human cells with the virus,[213] but the biological significance of this difference is not understood.

Protein kinase activity is associated with purified human adenoviruses.[214] The activity of the viral enzyme is regulated by divalent cations,[215] but the possible role of this kinase in the regulation of host genome functions has not been established. The enzyme is probably involved at some early stage of the viral infection.

7. Influence of Hormones and Growth Factors

Hormones and growth factors may exert remarkable modulatory effects on adenovirus-induced transformation. Both enhancing and inhibiting effects can be observed, according to the agent and the type of cell. Treatment of primary hamster embryo cells with glucocorticoids *in vitro* results in a significant increase in the number of Ad12-induced foci of transformed cells.[216] In contrast, marked inhibition of transformation in this system is produced when the cells are treated with estrogen, progesterone, or aldosterone. The mechanisms of enhancement and inhibition of adenovirus-induced transformation by steroid hormones are unknown. Cells transformed by vector plasmids carrying the Ad5 E1A gene become largely independent of the exogenous supply of growth factors.[217] Reversion to anchorage-dependent growth, flat morphology, and nontumorigenicity of rat brain cells infected with Ad2 is accompanied by increased expression of EGF receptors on the cell surface and decreased production of TGF-α.[218]

Infection of REF cells with a specific host-range mutant (H5hr1) results in cold-sensitive (*cs*) expression of both the initiation and maintenance of the the transformed phenotype.[219] Studies using this *cs* mutant showed that Ad5-induced transformation results in the loss of inducibility of the Na$^+$/K$^+$-ATPase by thyroid hormone and decreased binding of radiolabeled EGF.[220] In general, it is not known whether the complex changes in the responses of adenovirus-transformed cells to hormones and growth factors are causally associated with the process of neoplastic transformation or are rather the consequence of this process.

8. Dependence of Adenovirus-Induced Tumorigenicity on the Immune Status of the Host

Expression of the adenovirus E1A protein alone is sufficient to cause increased susceptibility to lysis by NK cells and activated macrophages in the absence of detectable cell surface expression of viral transplantation antigens.[221] The E1A products can be detected in the cell nucleus and the cytoplasm of the adenovirus-transformed cells but are apparently not present on the cell membrane.

A lack of expression of MHC class I antigens would allow the tumor cells to escape immune surveillance from the host and could contribute to the growth of tumor cells *in vivo*. Mouse cells transformed by the highly oncogenic adenovirus strain Ad12 express reduced levels of class I antigens on their surface, in contrast to the nononcogenic Ad5 strain of the same virus which do not produce such an alteration.[222] Proteins of Ad-12 E1A gene, in the absence of the E1B gene, may repress the expression of class I HLA antigens (HLA-B, -B, and -C) in transformed human cells.[223] These results suggest that Ad12 E1A proteins repress MHC class I gene expression by similar mechanisms in both rodent and human transformed cells. Interestingly, transfection of a functional class I gene into highly tumorigenic Ad12-transformed cell line that express no detectable MHC class I surface antigens results in its complete loss of oncogenicity.[224]

Moreover, cells transfected with an MHC class I gene (the K gene) can immunize animals against the parental Ad12-induced tumor not expressing any class I antigen.[225] However, according to results from other studies, there is no correlation between the tumorigenicity in immunocompetent syngeneic adult rodents of Ad2- and Ad5-transformed hamster and mouse cells and the level of class I MHC antigens expressed on the surfaces of these cells.[226] Thus, the expression of different levels of class I MHC proteins could not explain the differences in the oncogenicity between nononcogenic and highly oncogenic human adenovirus types.

Ad2 infection of lymphoid cells (MPC11 plasmacytoma cells) may result in an inhibition of transcription of the Ig γ-2b heavy chain gene.[227] This inhibition is due to repression of the activity of the gene enhancer by the Ad2 E1A products. The possible biological significance of this inhibition is unknown but Ad2 is commonly found in a latent state in human lymphoid tissues, especially adenoids and tonsils.

9. Induction of Cell Differentiation by Adenoviruses

Plasmids encoding Ad5 E1A gene products can induce differentiation of F9 teratocarcinoma stem cells.[228] The morphological changes and the acquisition of differentiation-specific proteins induced by Ad5 E1A-carrying plasmids are similar to those induced by retinoic acid or the c-*fos* protooncogene.[229] The molecular mechanisms of Ad5 E1A-induced differentiation are unknown but they may depend on the induction and/or repression of cellular genes.

C. CONCLUSION

Although it is unlikely that adenoviruses play any role in the etiology of human cancer, the study of these viruses may lend interesting results for understanding the molecular mechanisms involved in the oncogenic potential of DNA viruses in general. Neoplastic transformation of normal cells by adenoviruses depends on the products of two early viral genes, E1A and E1B, which have been considered as oncogenes but are functionally not identical to the oncogenes contained in the genome of acute retroviruses. The function of E1A- and E1B-encoded proteins are little understood. These proteins are associated with the nucleus and the cytoplasm but are not present in the cell membrane. The molecular mechanisms of adenovirus-induced neoplastic transformation are unknown but E1A has been considered as an oncogene-like gene and there is evidence that the E1A product is capable of inducing transformation by a mechanism involving the repression of a cellular enhancer, rather than by transcriptional activation of cellular protooncogenes or other genes.[209] The gene whose expression is repressed by the E1A product in adenovirus-transformed cells has not been identified but it could correspond to a tumor-suppressor gene (antioncogene).

VIII. PAPILLOMAVIRUSES

Papillomaviruses are members of the papovavirus group (which include also polyoma virus and SV40) and have been etiologically related to the appearance of benign epithelial cell proliferative processes of animals and man, including papillomas and warts, which may eventually undergo malignant conversion under particular genetic and/or environmental conditions.[230-239] Most papillomaviruses of either human (HPVs) or bovine (BPVs) origin are strictly epitheliotropic, infecting basal epidermal cells. However, two classes of BPVs have been described: subgroup A BPVs infect both fibroblasts and keratinocytes, whereas subgroup B BPVs infect only epithelial cells.[240] The study of papillomaviruses has been hampered by the lack of a cellular culture system suitable for virus propagation. In spite of this difficulty, these viruses have been studied by molecular cloning, reassociation kinetics of genomic sequences and serological procedures, which has permitted the identification of up to 42 different types of HPVs and 6 types of BPVs have been described.[241] Importantly, the molecular heterogeneity of papillomaviruses appears to underlie their different cytopathological effects; some particular types are more frequently associated with malignant lesion than other types. The strongest association is observed between HPV-16 and HPV-18 infection and cancers of the genital region, especially cervical cancer, but also cancers of the vulva, the vagina, and the penis as well as oral cancers. HPV-39 may also be associated with human cervical cancer.[242]

A. STRUCTURE AND EXPRESSION OF PAPILLOMAVIRUSES

The papillomavirus genomes are constituted by double-stranded circular molecules containing approximately 8000 bp. In spite of their extreme heterogeneity, all types of papillomaviruses show the same overall genomic organization and the large or conserved ORFs are found at similar positions on a single strand of the viral DNA duplex, the other DNA strand being apparently noncoding.[234] Different molecular species of BPV mRNAs may be generated by differential posttranscriptional splicing processes.

Comparison of BPV-1-transformed mouse fibroblasts, which may be regarded as benign cells, with human cervical carcinoma-derived cell lines (HeLa and C4-I cells) demonstrates differences in regulation of the viral genome transcription.[243] Whereas inhibition of protein synthesis by cycloheximide results in an increased level of BPV-1 transcription in fibroblasts by about one order of magnitude, transcription of the HPV-16 and HPV-18 in cervical carcinoma cells is not affected by cycloheximide treatment in carcinoma-derived cell lines. These results may reflect differential control mechanisms of individual virus and/or cell types. Although changed physiology of the cancer cell could account for the inability to control viral gene expression, it is attractive to consider the possibility that the loss of down-regulation of viral transcription could play a role in malignant conversion.

HPV-16 contains a DNA sequence element with a large degree of homology to a palindromic sequence which is the consensus sequence of glucocorticoid responsive elements of known genes regulated by this steroid hormone.[244] The glucocorticoid receptor protein binds to this HPV-16 sequence *in vitro* and stimulates transcription from a promoter linked in *cis* but the biological relevance of these observations in relation to the oncogenic potential of HPV-16 is unclear.

B. PAPILLOMAVIRUSES AND HUMAN CANCER

HPVs appear to act as cofactors in the etiology of human genital and laryngeal cancers.[232-239,245,246] Specific HPV types would have an enhanced oncogenic potential and are associated more frequently with human cancer.[247,248] HPV-16 was found to be associated with vulvar cancer, as demonstrated by *in situ* hybridization using specific viral DNA probes.[249] HPV-18 genome was found to be integrated into the genome of cell lines derived from carcinomas of the human uterine cervix (HeLa and 756 cells).[250] However, HPV DNA sequences usually occur in an episomal form in tumors of the human uterine cervix. Some cell lines, as well as cells from human cervical carcinoma biopsies, contain polyadenylated RNA transcripts derived from HPV-16 and HPV-18 sequences.

The study of cervical biopsy specimens from different geographical areas (U.S., Brazil, and Peru) suggests that, while HPV-6 and HPV-11 appear to have very little oncogenic association and HPV-31 has a low oncogenic association, HPV-16 and HPV-18 have high oncogenic association.[248] Infection with HPV-16 or HPV-18 would result in an epithelial proliferation with a strong likelihood of developing into an invasive cervical squamous carcinoma or adenocarcinoma. HPV-16 and HPV-18 have been detected in neoplastic lesions of the human female genital tract, including cervical intraepithelial and invasive lesions, as well as vulvar intraepithelial neoplasias and invasive carcinomas.[251-256] Between 17 and 91% of human cervical tumors are positive for the presence of HPV-16 or HPV-18 DNA, depending on differences in geographical distribution. A problem in the interpretation of these epidemiological studies is that a high prevalence of positivity for HPV infection is found in control women from the same populations; in some geographical areas, e.g., in Latin America, more than half of the women are infected with either HPV-16 or HPV-18.[257] Mild displastic (grade I) cervical lesions are usually free of HPV-16 sequences but a minor proportion (23%) of these lesions may be positive for HPV-18 sequences.[254] More advanced cervical neoplastic lesions (grades II and III) are more frequently positive (23 to 50%) for HPV-16 but the proportion of positivity for HPV-18 remains about the same (20 to 26%).[254] However, these distributions can be different in different human populations and different geographical areas. In some areas the association between invasive carcinoma of the cervix and HPV is rather low.[258] The results of a comparative epidemiological study on the incidence of cervical cancer and HPV-16/HPV-18 infection in two distinct geographical regions (Denmark and Greenland) did not lend support to the hypothesis that HPV-16/HPV-18 are causal determinants of cervical cancer incidence.[259] In a recent critical review on the state of the evidence about the possible role of HPVs in human cervical cancer, it was concluded that "while experimental data suggest an oncogenic potential for HPV, the epidemiological evidence implicating it as a cause of cervical neoplasia is rather limited", and that "no epidemiological study has convincingly demonstrated that HPV causes cervical cancer."[239]

In conclusion, although certain types of HPVs could be involved in the etiology of human cervical cancer, factors other than HPV infection are most probably responsible for the development of human cervical carcinomas, at least in certain geographical areas. In cattle living in the Scottish Western Highlands, bovine papilloma virus type 4 (BPV-4) is the causative agent of benign papillomas of the alimentary canal, which can become the focus for the development of carcinomas in animals feeding on the bracken fern.[237]

C. MECHANISMS OF PAPILLOMAVIRUS-INDUCED TRANSFORMATION

The mechanisms of papillomavirus-induced transformation are little understood. HPV-16 can induce immortalization upon transfection into human foreskin keratinocytes.[260] The immortalized keratinocytes exhibit karyotypic abnormalities with tendency to near triploidy and the presence of a marker isochromosome 21. Studies on transformation of established murine fibroblast cell lines (NIH/3T3 and 3Y1) with cloned HPV-16 DNA suggest that at least two sequential events may be required for the expression of morphological transformation and that the secondary changes occurring in the growth properties of the transfected cells are due to some cellular alterations.[261]

Integration and persistence of BPV DNA is apparently not required for the maintenance or progression of the state of cell transformation in cattle.[262,263] BPVs may induce cell transformation by executing one or more early events, and once the transformed phenotype is attained viral functions may no longer be required.[264] In contrast, HPV DNA may persist in human tumors through the phase of malignant progression and is often found in fully developed carcinomas. In HeLa cells (which are cells derived from a carcinoma of the human uterine cervix), HPV-18 integration was found to be associated with DNA rearrangement at a particular locus, and the other allele of this locus showed an altered structure of unknown origin.[265] These rearrangements could lead to a homozygous situation that was interpreted as affecting a recessive phenotype which might be involved in some aspects of tumorigenesis.

The possibility that papillomaviruses may contain transforming genes (oncogenes) should be considered, but there is only limited evidence in favor of this possibility. In general, no obvious peculiarities have been found in the genome organization of the types of papillomaviruses that are more frequently associated with malignant conversion. It is not known whether the apparently greater oncogenic potential of some specific types of papillomaviruses is due to subtle genetic differences or to a greater propensity of their target cell for neoplastic transformation, or to a combination of both.[237]

1. BPV Transforming Genes

The discovery that particular subgenomic fragments of BPV DNA can transform mouse cells *in vitro* has facilitated the studies related to the mechanisms of BPV-induced transformation.[266,267] Multiple transforming genes may be contained in the BPV genome and at least five classes of mRNAs have been identified from the transforming region of BPV-1 in C127 mouse cells transformed by the virus.[268,269] The complete nucleotide sequence and the genome organization of BPV-4 (which causes papillomas of the upper alimentary canal that may provide a focus for malignant transformation in animals eating bracken fern) indicates that the viral genome is 7261 bp long and contains several overlapping ORFs which may code for DNA replication and cell transformation functions.[270] The viral sequences that are responsible for BPV-induced transformation are discontinuous, and the sequences responsible for maintenance of multiple episomal copies are different from those that are required for transformation.[271]

At least two segments of the genome of BPV-1 possess transforming capability.[272] One of these segments, located at the 3' end of the region of the viral genome transcribed in cultured cells, can transform both mouse C127 and NIH/3T3 cell lines, whereas a second segment, located at the 5' end of the same transcribed region, can independently induce a transformed phenotype in C127 cells but cannot transform NIH/3T3 cells. The BPV-1 genomic segment capable of inducing transformation in NIH/3T3 cells has been identified as the 3' half of the E5 open reading frame (E5 ORF).[273] Translation of the E5 ORF of BPV is required for its transforming activity.[274,275] E5 ORF is a member of the E1 to E8 ORFs that are transcribed earlier in nonproductively transformed cells as well as in papillomas. The 3' half or the E5 transforming gene of BPV encodes a small polypeptide, the E5 protein, which is only 44 amino acids long and is extremely hydrophobic.[275,276] The carboxy-terminal two thirds of a chemically synthesized 44-amino acid polypeptide corresponding to the BPV-1 E5 product is able to activate cellular DNA synthesis upon microinjection into the nucleus of growth-arrested mouse C127 and NIH/3T3 cells.[277] The chemically synthesized carboxy-terminal 13-amino acid sequence of the E5 protein represents the smallest known protein fragment that can autonomously activate cellular DNA synthesis in any system.

Two other putative viral transforming proteins, termed E2 and E6, would act synergistically in the malignant transformation of certain types of BPV-infected cells.[268] Expression vectors encoding the E2 and E6 proteins have been constructed and expressed in bacteria. Antisera specifically immunoprecipitating the produced E6 protein were used to detect its presence in both nuclear and membrane fractions of BPV-transformed cells.[278] The protein encoded by the E2 ORF of BPV-1 binds specifically to the enhancer region of the virus genome.[279] Analysis of ORF-E2 mutants with microinjection of recombinant plasmids containing BPV-1 DNA into nuclei of mouse C127 cells suggests that activities encoded by the 5' portion of E2 ORF are not directly required for stimulation of DNA synthesis.[280] Further genetic and biochemical studies are required for a more precise identification of the BPV-1 gene(s) responsible for stimulation of cellular DNA synthesis and neoplastic transformation.

2. HPV Transforming Genes

The nucleotides contained in the genome of several HPVs have been completely sequenced.[241] Particular nucleotide sequence contained in specific types of HPVs would be responsible for the transforming potential of these viruses. Transfection of human keratinocytes and fibroblasts isolated from foreskin with recombinant HPV-16 DNA results in an extended or indefinite lifespan, which depends on the presence of expression of HPV-16-specific sequences.[281] Transfection of NIH/3T3 cells with a recombinant vector carrying HPV-16 DNA results in neoplastic transformation.[282] This transformation proceeds through at least two distinct phases and abundant HPV-16 gene messages representing sequences of all HPV-16 ORFs are detected in the premalignant phase. However, the quantity of HPV-16-specific mRNAs is several times lower in the tumorigenic cells, suggesting that high levels of HPV-16 gene expression are not required for the complete transformation of HPV-16-transfected cells.

Molecularly cloned DNAs of two types of human papillomaviruses, HPV-5 and HPV-1, are capable of inducing morphological transformation of mouse cells in culture, and the transformed cells contain multiple persistent episomal copies of the transfected DNA species.[283] Transfection of HPV-1a constructs containing an intact early gene region into the 3Y1 REF cell line results in induction of anchorage-independent growth and a high cloning efficiency in soft agar, and the transfected cells acquire the property of producing tumors in nude mice.[284] The cells that exhibit altered growth and tumorigenicity synthesize abundant levels of viral RNA, which suggests a correlation between expression of HPV-1a genetic information and neoplastic transformation.

The E6 and E7 regions of HPV-16 and HPV-18 are present and transcribed in human cervical cancer cell lines as well as in cervical cancer tissues.[285] Products from these regions could be responsible for the maintenance of the transformed phenotype of the cells. A 18-kDa protein from region E6 has been identified in two human cervical carcinoma cell lines (CaSki and SiHa) that harbor HPV-16 DNA as well as in mouse 3T3 fibroblasts that have been morphologically transformed with HPV-16 DNA.[286] The integration pattern observed in human cervical carcinoma cell lines usually interrupts or deletes specific regions of HPV DNA, but consistently leaves intact the E6 and E7 ORFs of the viral genome. The activity of the transcriptional promoter of the candidate E6-E7 transforming gene region of HPV-16, termed P97, can be influenced in transient transfection experiments by diffusible regulatory factors of both cellular and viral origin.[287] Positive cellular factor(s) present in uninfected human genital keratinocytes and cervical carcinoma cells and positive and negative viral factors encoded by the viral E2 ORF contribute to the regulation of P97 promoter activity. No specific functions have been assigned to the HPV E6 and E7 ORFs, but their possible role in the maintenance of a transformed phenotype is suggested by the fact that the homologous E6 of BPV is capable of inducing tumorigenic transformation of mouse cells.[268,272]

Constructed plasmids containing the E6 and E7 ORFs of HPV-18 expressed from an autologous transcriptional control region are sufficient to induce transformation of NIH/3T3 and Rat-1 cells.[288] Expression of the HPV-16 E7 ORF is sufficient to induce focal transformation of rat 3Y1 cells.[289] These results indicate that E6 and/or E7 ORFs of HPV-16 and HPV-18 may be considered, at least in some aspects, as oncogenes. However, the oncogenic potential of HPV oncogenes may not be as strong as that of the oncogenes contained in acute retroviruses.

3. Reversion of Papillomavirus-Induced Transformation

BPV-transformed hamster embryo fibroblasts revert immediately to the nontransformed phenotype and display normal growth kinetics upon exposure to the xantate compound, D609 (tricyclodecan-9-yl-xantogenate).[290] After six population doublings in the presence of D609, clones which display an untransformed morphology in the absence of D609 arise with high frequency (90%) and such clones reacquire limited *in vitro* lifetime and lose the ability to induce tumors in athymic nude mice. The revertant clones lose all extrachromosomal monomeric BPV DNA molecules and only high MW oligomeric BPV DNA that is probably integrated into the cellular genome is still detectable in a methylated, transcriptionally inactive state. No BPV mRNA transcripts can be detected in the revertant cells but such transcripts are stimulated by addition of phorbol ester tumor promoter (TPA) to the culture.[290] The results of this study demonstrate that the complete genetic program for a limited *in vitro* lifetime is maintained over several hundred generations in transformed cells and provide direct evidence for the complete reversibility of the property of immortality.

4. Role of Protooncogenes in Papillomavirus-Induced Neoplastic Transformation

There is limited evidence for protooncogene activation in cells transformed by HPVs. In two human carcinoma cell lines, HeLa and C4-I, HPV-18 DNA was found to be integrated in chromosome 8, on the 5′ side of the c-*myc* protooncogene.[291] In HeLa cells the HPV DNA integration is within 40 kb 5′ of the c-*myc* gene. Steady-state levels of c-*myc* mRNA are elevated in Hela and C4-I cells relative to other cervical carcinoma cell lines. In the SW756 cervical carcinoma cell line, the HPV-18 integration site was localized to chromosome 12 but in a region not closely linked to the c-K-*ras*-2 protooncogene. In primary cervical carcinoma harboring multiple HPV-16 integrations, human DNA sequences flanking the integrated proviruses were localized to chromosomes 3 and 20, at regions containing the protooncogenes c-*raf*-1 and c-*src*, respectively.[291]

In 11 of 12 patients with advanced stages of invasive squamous cell carcinomas of the uterine cervix, HPV-16 and HPV-18 were detected by molecular hybridization procedures in the tumor cells, and amplification of the c-*myc* and/or c-H-*ras* protooncogenes was detected in 9 of 12 of these tumors.[292] These results suggest that cooperation between HPV genomes and particular protooncogenes may be involved in the progression of carcinoma of the human uterine cervix.

5. Expression of Papillomaviruses in Transgenic Mice

Experiments with transgenic mice indicate that transmission of the BPV-1 genome through the germ line may result in the heritable formation of fibropapillomas of the skin.[293] However, the presence of BPV-1 genes is apparently insufficient by itself to induce tumors since the tumors observed in transgenic mice arise after a long latency period (8 to 9 months of age) and occur most frequently in areas prone to wounding.

D. CONCLUSION

Papillomaviruses are etiologically related to benign tumors, including papillomas and warts, occurring in humans and other animal species. Some of these lesions may eventually undergo malignant conversion. The possible role of HPVs in human cancer is still under discussion. Certain types of HPV, in particular HPV-16 and HPV-18, seem to act as cofactors in the etiology of human laryngeal and genital cancers, including vulvar and cervical carcinomas. The sole presence of HPVs would be insufficient for the malignant transformation of human cells *in vivo* since HPVs may be present in clinically and histologically normal tissue of patients with genital cancer.[294] A variable proportion of human cervical carcinomas, according to the geographical area, is apparently not associated with HPV infection. Thus, factors other than HPVs would be responsible for the development of human cervical carcinomas, at least in those patients in which HPV genomes are not detected in the tumors. Even in tumors associated with papillomavirus infection, various genetic and environmental factors are almost certainly important for determining the neoplastic conversion of the cell and the development of the tumor. The potential oncogenicity of papillomaviruses would depend on specific proteins encoded by the viral genome, but the functions of these proteins are unknown.

IX. SIMIAN VIRUS 40

Simian virus 40 (SV40) is one of the most thoroughly studied oncogenic DNA viruses.[295] It is a small papovavirus that produces natural infection in rhesus monkeys and other Asiatic macaques. Intravenous inoculation of SV40 into 3-week-old Syrian golden hamsters results in the development of neoplasms (leukemia, lymphoma, lymphosarcoma, reticulum cell sarcoma, osteogenic sarcoma, or anaplastic carcinoma) in 85 to 90% of the animals 3 to 6 months after inoculation.[296] The age of the host has a profound effect on the ability of SV40 to induce tumors; hamsters older than 22 d are usually resistant to tumor induction by SV40. Inoculation of SV40 into pregnant hamsters during the 8th or 12th day of gestation was found to produce subcutaneous tumors (undifferentiated sarcomas) in offspring 4 to 14 months after birth.[297] The inoculated mothers did not show any effect of the virus even after one year after inoculation. The tumors that appeared in the offspring contained SV40 antigen as well as SV40 DNA sequences integrated into tumor cell DNA and may thus represent an example of virus-induced transplacental carcinogenesis.

SV40 was first isolated as a contaminant of poliovirus vaccine produced in monkey kidney cell cultures.[298] This vaccine was administered to several thousands of children from 1955 to

1962. In general, human cells are rather resistant to malignant transformation induced by DNA viruses with oncogenic potential. There are, however, reports on successful transformation of human epithelial cells by SV40, with subsequent isolation of cloned transformed cell lines.[299] Human cells may be semipermissive for infection with SV40, as neoplastic transformation and virus production may occur simultaneously.[300] Cultured human fibroblasts or epithelial cells can be morphologically transformed by SV40 DNA cloned in molecular vectors such as chimeric viruses and plasmids,[301-304] but these cells are not tumorigenic when tested in the nude mouse assay despite the presence of SV40 T-antigen.[305] Previous evidence indicated resistance of human individuals to SV40-induced tumorigenicity since not a single cancer was reported 20 years after the inadvertent inoculation of several thousands of children with SV40 present as a contaminant in early poliomyelitis vaccine preparations.[306]

SV40 DNA, in form of unintegrated episomal structures was detected in 12 out of 37 human meningiomas and in 8 out of 35 different types of human intracranial tumors.[307,308] Moreover, SV40 genomes have been cloned from human brain tumors.[309] However, an etiological role of the virus in these tumors and other human tumors is rather unlikely.

In general, SV40 is not as potent in its transforming capabilities as some other oncogenic viruses. The appearance of SV40-induced tumors *in vivo* tends to be moderately slow and the morphological alterations induced in cells *in vitro* are relatively subtle.[310] However, genetically manipulated SV40 is capable of inducing tumors in tissues in which they never occur under natural conditions, e.g., in the ocular lens of vertebrates. Transgenic mice carrying a hybrid gene comprising the murine α A-crystallin promoter fused to a coding sequence of the SV40 T antigen develop lens tumors, which obliterate the eye cavity and even invade neighboring tissue.[311] Tumors of the β cells from the pancreatic islets of Langerhans occur in transgenic mice expressing recombinant genes composed of the upstream region of the rat preproinsulin gene II linked to sequences coding for SV40 large T antigen.[312] Significant levels of p53 antigen are produced in all β cells expressing SV40 large T antigen, while p53 is undetectable in normal β cells.[313] However, only a small fraction of the islets develop into tumors, which indicates that factors in addition to the expression of large T and p53 antigens are required for tumorigenesis. Transgenic mice that carry fusions between the transcriptional regulatory sequences of atrial natriuretic factor (a hormone that is synthesized and stored in the cardiac atria and that is involved in the regulation of blood pressure) and those encoding SV40 T antigen develop a several-hundredfold increase in mass of the right atrium associated with abnormalities in the atrial conduction system, which ultimately results in death.[314] However, tumors occurring in transgenic mice expressing the SV40 large T gene may occur in a variety of cell types.[315]

A. STRUCTURE AND EXPRESSION OF SV40

SV40 and polyoma virus are among the smallest DNA viruses. The particles of these viruses are about 45 nm in diameter and each particle contains a closed circular molecule of double-stranded DNA consisting of 5243 bp, with a mol wt of approximately 3.4×10^6 Da.[316] The coding capacity of the SV40 genome is limited to only a few proteins. In infected cells the extrachromosomal DNA of SV40 is present in form of a nucleoprotein complex which is structurally similar to mammalian cell chromatin and is referred to as the viral minichromosome.

Expression of the SV40 genome is regulated in a very precise fashion during the course of lytic infection in permissive cells. Prior to SV40 DNA replication, transcription occurs primarily in genes encoding SV40 tumor antigens, and after SV40 DNA replication mainly in genes encoding viral capsid proteins. Cellular transcription factors that specifically bind to promoter elements contained in the SV40 genome are able to stimulate transcription at separate early and late SV40 promoters. A cellular transcription factor, LSF, stimulates transcription at two initiation sites of the late SV40 promoter which are utilized after SV40 DNA replication during the SV40 lytic cycle.[317]

SV40-induced malignant transformation of cells depends on two proteins encoded by the early region of the viral genome, a 94,000-Da large tumor (T) antigen and a 17,000-Da small tumor (t) antigen. Although both of these tumor antigens seem to be involved in transformation, small t alone does not have the ability to initiate the transformation events and its role consists only in enhancing the ability of large T antigen to transform cells to anchorage independence.[318] Almost the entire early region of the SV40 genome is devoted to encoding large T antigen. Large T antigen plays an essential role in both SV40 replication and SV40-induced cell transformation.[310,319-321] The antigen can affect several host functions, including the synthesis or activation of enzymes involved in DNA metabolism, stimulation of RNA synthesis, and induction of DNA synthesis.

The SV40 large T antigen is a 708-amino acid protein of 94 kDa which is responsible for both the immortalizing and transforming properties of SV40 in particular experimental systems. This multifunctional protein is required for lytic growth of the virus and binds strongly to double-stranded DNA.[322] The vast majority (over 95%) of total cellular SV40 large T antigen is located in the nucleus, especially in the nucleoplasm, but minor amounts of the antigen are associated with the chromatin and the nuclear matrix.[310] A primary sequence near the amino terminus of the antigen directs the proteins to the nucleus. Synthetic peptides containing the amino acid sequence around lysine-128 of large T antigen have been used to demonstrate the existence of a specific transport signal sequence which interacts with the cellular factors necessary for nuclear localization of the antigen, but not other major nuclear proteins.[323]

SV40 large T antigen extracted from nuclei of infected or transformed cells may appear as monomers, dimers, tetramers, or higher aggregates. The antigen is subjected to posttranslational modification including acylation, glycosylation, and phosphorylation at multiple sites.[321] Large T antigen is a DNA-binding protein with a marked preference for single-stranded over double-stranded DNA. The antigen binds with relatively high affinity to double-stranded DNA regions that include as a particular motif the pentamer GAGGC. The DNA-binding region of SV40 large T antigen lies approximately between lysine-131 and lysine-371 of the protein, corresponding to DNA sequences located between 0.51 and 0.37 map units.[324] RNA is covalently linked to a specific large T antigen peptide through a phosphodiester bond between a serine residue and the 5′ hydroxyl of an invariant CMP residue.[325]

The large T antigens of both papovaviruses, SV40 and polyoma virus, are composed of a set of consensus structural elements and include an ATP binding site.[326] T antigen has an enzymatic activity, being capable of hydrolyzing ATP, dATP, and, to a lesser extent, other nucleoside triphosphates.[321] The ATPase activity of large T antigen is probably required for the DNA unwinding (helicase) activity displayed by the antigen. SV40 large T antigen is able to unwind DNA duplices several thousand base-pairs long, preferentially moving in the 3′ to 5′ direction of the strand to which it is bound. The helicase activity of antigen may be present at DNA replication forks and appears to be essential for the initiation of DNA replication.

Active SV40 large T antigen is required for the transcriptional activation of the late viral genes. Transcription of the SV40 genome depends on 72-bp tandem-repeated sequences but these sequences are apparently not virus-specific because they can be artificially replaced by nonhomologous repeated sequences derived from the LTR of cloned M-MuSV.[327] Sequences homologous to the regulatory region around the origin of replication of SV40 are present in monkey genomic DNA.[328]

B. MECHANISMS OF SV40-INDUCED TRANSFORMATION

In spite of numerous studies, the mechanisms responsible for SV40-induced neoplastic transformation of susceptible cells remain little understood at present. Three activities have been identified in large T antigen by mutations on different portions of the gene: (1) activity indispensable for transformation of primary and established cells, (2) activity essential for transformation of primary cells but not for transformation of established cells, and (3) activity sufficient to induce immortalization of primary cells in culture.[329] These findings suggest that transformation of primary cells by SV40 requires at least two distinct activities of large T antigen and that one of them can be replaced by some cellular function in immortalized cells. Studies with SV40 deletion mutants indicate that the terminal 81 amino acids of large T antigen are not needed for efficient transformation or tumorigenicity and that independent functions may be required for these two alterations.[330] Unfortunately, the biochemical nature of the biologically defined different activities of the large T antigen is unknown.

Susceptibility of different cell types to SV40-induced neoplastic transformation exhibit great variability. Some types of cells, e.g., hamster liver parenchymal cells, are completely resistant to SV40-induced transformation, even when they are stimulated to proliferate.[296] The parameters responsible for the susceptibility or resistance of different cell types to neoplastic transformation induced by SV40 have not been defined. Maintenance of the expression of differentiated functions may be observed in some SV40-transformed cells, e.g., in cells derived form a defined location of the rabbit kidney.[331] It is thus clear that induction of immortalization and neoplastic transformation by expression of SV40 large T antigen is not incompatible with the expression of cell differentiated functions.

1. Alteration of Integrated SV40 DNA Sequences

There is no site specificity at a gross level for the integration of SV40 in human or rodent cells.[332] The integrated SV40 DNA sequences are labile and may undergo amplification and rearrangement processes, which results in heterogeneity with respect to the arrangement of viral sequences among cell populations derived from single clones.[333] It is possible that the viral DNA instability that results in the generation of diverse SV40 integration patterns could represent one of the underlying mechanisms by which transformed populations evolve in a multistep fashion toward a fully tumorigenic phenotype.[334] A similar consideration could also be valid for the integration of sequences of other types of viruses with oncogenic potentialities.

Higher MW forms of SV40 large T antigens, collectively known as super T-Ag, are frequently produced in SV40-transformed murine cells but their biological significance remains obscure. Super T-Ag is not important for tumorigenicity of SV40. These forms of large T antigen may constitute a marker of genomic rearrangements by the viral genes in transformed cells.[335]

2. Role of SV40 Enhancer DNA Sequences

DNA sequences with transcriptional enhancer activity are contained in the genome of many virus with oncogenic potential. Such sequences may be involved in the activation of genes, including genes from the host cell. It has been proposed that there is a differential requirement for the SV40 early genes in immortalization and transformation of primary rodent and human embryonic cells in culture.[336] SV40 large T antigen expression is apparently sufficient to induce choroid plexus tumors in transgenic mice which have developed from fertilized eggs injected with DNA constructs.[336] However, the SV40 enhancer DNA sequence is important for the development of such tumors because transgenic mice developed from fertilized eggs injected with DNA constructs where the enhancer has been deleted but large T antigen sequences have been preserved develop demyelinating peripheral neuropathies, hepatocellular carcinomas, and islet cell adenomas but the incidence of choroid plexus tumors is markedly reduced.[338] The potent tumor promoter phorbol ester, TPA, can specifically induce the activity of the SV40 transcriptional enhancer element in HepG2 human hepatoma cells through an effect that is independent of *de novo* protein synthesis but that requires ongoing RNA synthesis.[339]

3. Karyotypic Instability in SV40-Infected Cells

Chromosome aberrations are almost universally present in tumor cells and it is believed that these aberrations are mechanistically related to the process of malignant transformation itself. To date, transformation with either wild-type or origin-defective clones of SV40 have been always found to be associated with karyotypic instability leading to extensive heteroploidy.[300,340]

4. DNA Methylation Patterns and Gene Reactivation in SV40-Infected Cells

SV40 can induce a wide variety of tumors after inoculation into newborn or adult hamsters.[341] Mice are usually resistant to the oncogenic action of SV40 but a high percentage of transgenic mice developing from eggs microinjected with plasmids containing SV40 early region genes develop tumors of the choroid plexus.[342] These mice carry SV40 T-antigen in all of their cells and they have amplification of SV40 sequences. Different types of structural rearrangements in and around the SV40 gene integration site, as well as changes in DNA methylation, were observed in the tumor tissue of these transgenic mice but a simple, systematic alteration of the genome was not uncovered. Decreased DNA methylation rates were also detected in SV40-transformed human fibroblasts.[343]

Reactivation of inactive cellular genes may be associated with SV40-induced transformation. Localized reactivation at the hypoxanthine phosphoribosyl transferase (*HPRT*) and glucose 6-phosphate dehydrogenase (*G6PD*) loci on the inactive X chromosome of female human cells can occur following infection with SV40.[340] It is not known if this reactivation is due to changes in the pattern of DNA methylation on the X chromosome or to other mechanisms.

5. Mutagenic Activity and Translational Errors Induced by SV40

SV40 may display mutagenic activity in mammalian cells, which appears to depend on the expression of the early region of the viral genome and on a function involved in specific binding of large T antigen to DNA.[344] However, the functions of SV40-induced transformation and mutation do not seem to correlate. SV40 infection may not alter the metabolic pathways involved in DNA repair. SV40-induced transformation of normal human diploid WI-38 fibroblasts is not associated with alteration in the proliferation-dependent regulation of two base excision repair enzymes, uracil DNA glycosylase and hypoxanthine DNA glycosylase.[345] Rather, the extent of enhancement of both DNA glycosylase activities as a function of cell proliferation is increased in the SV40-transformed cells, in comparison to the parental nontransformed cells.

SV40-induced transformation is associated with an increased level of translational errors in different types of cells.[346] Mistranslation, however, is not always found in other types of neoplastic transformation and its biological significance is unclear. In any case, mistranslation does not represent a general mechanism for oncogenic processes.

6. Association of SV40 Large T Antigen with Cellular Components

Large T antigen is found in the nucleoplasm of SV40 infected cells, in association with chromatin and tightly bound to the nuclear matrix,[347] but small amounts of T antigen may become stably anchored on the cell surface by a tight linkage to membrane lipid.[348] There is no structural basis for the recognition and differential associations of large T antigen with the nucleus and the cell surface,[349] and the possible functional consequences of the latter association are unknown. Cytotoxic T lymphocytes may recognize SV40 T antigen on the surface of transformed mouse cells, which may lead to the abrogation of the virus lytic cycle, indicating that cellular immune mechanisms may have an important role in limiting SV40 infection in the natural host.[350] Within the nucleus, the localization of SV40 large T antigen may be different in lytic infection and cell transformation. The subnuclear localization of large T antigens in SV40-transformed cells is largely in nonchromatinic compartments, i.e., on peri- and interchromatin ribonucleoprotein fibrils, whereas in lytic infection large T antigen is mainly associated with the cellular chromatin.[351] The biological significance of this difference is not understood, however. The association of large T with the chromatin and the nuclear matrix is apparently mediated by protein-protein interactions rather than by sequence-specific DNA binding.[352]

DNA helicase activity may be present in SV40 large T antigen.[353] In a manner similar to that of eukaryotic DNA helicase, purified large T antigen preparations unwind DNA duplexes in a reaction which is dependent on Mg^{2+} and ATP hydrolysis. This activity is strongly inhibited by several large T antigen-specific monoclonal antibodies. Furthermore, mutant T antigens from SV40-transformed cells known to be defective in ATPase function also have reduced DNA helicase activities.[353]

A cellular factor required for DNA replication has been identified as the proliferating cell nuclear antigen (PCNA), also called cyclin.[354] PCNA/cyclin is identical with a DNA polymerase-δ accessory protein that enables this enzyme to efficiently utilize template/primers containing long stretches of single-stranded template.[355,356]

The relationship between the association of SV40 large T antigen and malignant transformation is still not clear because the artificial introduction of particular deletions or point mutations at specific sites of the viral genome may result in nonkaryophylic, cytoplasmic large T antigens that are still capable of transforming established cell lines.[357,358] Large T antigen from a mutant of SV40, termed NKLT, is nonkaryophilic due to a deletion of amino acids from positions 110 to 152. Complexes formed between NKLT and p53 antigen are localized mainly in the cytoplasm.[359] NKLT is unable to induce full transformation in primary cells but can transform established cells such as NIH/3T3 mouse fibroblasts. The NKLT is totally unable by itself to transform primary REF cells, but coexpression of NKLT with either polyoma virus middle T antigen or an activated c-H-*ras* gene results in the transformation of REF cells.[360]

7. Phosphorylation of SV40 Large T Antigen

A stepwise phosphorylation of the amino-terminal region of SV40 large T antigen occurs in SV40-infected cells,[361] but its possible connection with the tumorigenic properties of this antigen is not understood. In addition to its role in the initiation and maintenance of SV40-induced transformation, the T antigen displays an ensemble of regulatory actions, including regulation of gene expression, induction of several enzymes and of host RNA and DNA synthesis. Phosphorylation inactivates at least two distinct DNA-binding activities of the T antigen polypeptide chain which may correspond to separate regions of the antigen molecule.[362] It is conceivable that the stepwise post-translational modification of large T antigen through phosphorylation processes is related to the multifunctional properties of this protein.

8. Induction of Phosphoproteins in SV40-Infected Cells

Phosphorylation of cellular proteins may be closely related to SV40-induced neoplastic transformation. Cells transformed by SV40 are characterized by the reproducible presence of two phosphoproteins of cellular origin, with molecular weights of 48,000 and 50,000 Da, respectively.[363] These proteins are encoded by different cellular genes and the 48,000-Da protein is present mainly in the nucleus of SV40-infected cells but the functions of these proteins have not been established. Studies with a *ts* mutant of SV40 indicate that SV40-induced transformation correlates with hyperphosphorylation of some cellular proteins, including large T antigen and p53 protein, and that this phosphorylation is dependent on protein synthesis and occurs early during the expression of the transformed phenotype.[364] A possible relationship between some of these proteins and protooncogene products should be considered. The kinase activity of SV40 large T antigen is mediated by a cellular kinase which can be separated from the T antigen.[365]

9. Association of SV40 Large T Antigen with the p53 Cellular Antigen

SV40 large T antigen rapidly forms a stable complex with the cellular antigen p53 within the nucleus.[351,366,367] Antigen p53 is a phosphoprotein which is predominantly located in the nucleus in both transformed and nontransformed cells.[368] Overproduction or alteration of p53 protein could contribute to SV40-induced transformation. The transformation of rat embryo fibroblasts by wild-type SV40 is enhanced two- to threefold by cotransfection of a plasmid overexpressing mouse p53.[369] Stabilization of p53 during SV40-induced transformation is mediated by a cellular process and may represent an additional step in transformation induced by the virus.[370]

The p53 domain involved in formation of the SV40 large T antigen-p53 protein complex has been identified.[371] Large T antigen occurs in various structural forms such as monomers and different homologous oligomers, and p53 binds to all the structural subclasses of the antigen.[372] The p53 antigen is a phosphoprotein which lacks protein kinase activity, and its phosphorylation at specific serine residues increases in SV40-transformed NIH/3T3 cells, as compared with that of normal parental cells.[373] Both the SV40 large T antigen and antigen p53 are associated with RNA.[325] A gene homologous to the mouse p53 gene is present in human cells, from where it has been cloned and expressed.[374]

Since the cellular gene encoding for p53 has been considered as a protooncogene and the p53 protein may have some role in growth regulation of normal cells and participates in transformation of normal embryonic cells,[375,376] it seems likely that cell proliferation may become deregulated after formation of the p53-SV40 T antigen complex. However, p53 is expressed at a constant level during the cell cycle of actively growing normal cells, like FR 3T3 rat cells.[377] The SV40 T large antigen/p53 complex is associated with the cell surface,[378] and it has been suggested that a cooperation between p53 and *ras* oncogene products may contribute to cellular transformation.[379] Transfection into adult rat chondrocytes of a cDNA clone encoding p53 is capable of inducing cellular immortality and susceptibility to transformation by a mutant T24 c-H-*ras* oncogene.[380] However, in baby mouse kidney (BMK) cells activation of p53 synthesis occurs too late to be involved in the first virus-induced round of cellular replication.[381] Apparently, SV40 large T antigen is able to trigger at least the first round of cellular DNA replication through a p53-independent pathway in SV40-infected BMK cells. Moreover, the relatively late activation of p53 expression in these cells appear to be controlled at a level other than transcription.

It has been suggested that, although SV40 large T antigen alone can induce cell immortalization, its association with the cellular p53 antigen would be determinant for SV40 to cause neoplastic transformation.[382] However, BALB 3T12 spontaneously transformed mouse cells when infected with SV40 become positive for the presence of large T antigen but contain mostly free, uncomplexed p53 protein.[383] These results suggest that "the tumorigenic phenotype or the anchorage-independent growth of cells is not influenced by large T antigen/p53 complex formation or by the absence of complex formation of the p53 protein to the (large) T antigen" and that "the changes upon SV40 infection and (large) T antigen expression are all explainable by known effects of expression of (large) T antigen in these cell systems."[383] Thus, the biological significance of large T antigen complexing to p53 protein is not understood. Mutant mouse p53 protein complex not to large T antigen but exclusively to heat shock proteins HSP72/73 in SV40-infected COS cells.[384]

10. Association of SV40 Large T Antigen with DNA Polymerase α

Large T antigen forms a complex *in vitro* with DNA polymerase α, an enzyme implicated in cellular DNA replication.[385,386] The biological significance of this association is not understood but the DNA sequences involved (residues 335 to 626) with the p53 binding site on the viral genome.[387]

11. Interaction between SV40 and Acute Transforming Retroviruses

Human epithelial cells (keratinocytes) in tissue culture develop aneuploidy and acquire indefinite lifespan but do not undergo malignant transformation (tumorigenic properties) after infection with a hybrid of Ad12 and SV40 (which expresses only substantial amounts of SV40 mRNA). Superinfection of early passage Ad12-SV40-altered cells with K-MuSV results in morphological changes and acquisition of tumorigenic properties upon inoculation into nude mice, with formation of squamous cell carcinomas.[388] This result represents the first reported induction of human epithelial cancer cells in culture.

12. Production of Growth Factors in SV40-Infected Cells

Endogenous production of growth factors may be associated with SV40-induced transformation. NIH/3T3 cells transformed with SV40 produce a factor which shares many biological properties with PDGF but which may be different from PDGF itself.[389] In particular, the factor produced by SV40-transformed cells is apparently different from the c-*sis* protein product and is also different from other known transforming growth factors.

13. Specific Tolerance to SV40 Large T Antigen in Transgenic Mice

The ability to mount a cellular immune response to epitopes of SV40 antigen has been implicated in the control of SV40-induced tumor cell growth in normal immunocompetent mice. Recently, mouse lines have been derived by the zygotic injection of SV40 early-region gene constructs, and mice from many, but not all, of these lines develop tumors at specific sites. For example, mice from two SV40 transgenic lines bearing identical SV40-carrying plasmid constructs may markedly differ in the development of choroid plexus tumors.[390] Specific immune tolerance to SV40 large T antigen is an invariant feature of mice from the SV40 transgenic line that consistently develops tumor expressing this viral gene product. In contrast, the majority of mice from the SV40 transgenic line that remains essentially tumor-free generate a normal cellular response to SV40 after immunization with the virus.[390] In general, these results indicate that the development of an adequate immune response to viral gene products with oncogenic potential may be of paramount importance for the animals to evade tumor development.

14. Protooncogene Expression in SV40-Infected Cells

Infection or transformation of cells by papovaviruses may not result in significant alterations in protooncogene expression. In none of a wide variety of SV40- and polyoma virus-induced rat fibroblast transformants was the expression of any of ten different protooncogenes tested higher than the constitutive level detected in the parental cells, with the possible exception of a slight increase in c-*sis* expression.[391] No v-*myc* transcripts were detected in the kidney tissue of transgenic mouse containing SV40 and v-*myc* sequences but cell lines derived from different tissues of this mouse became transformed and expressed significantly more c-*myc* mRNA than the control untransformed cell line.[392] There is evidence that high levels of expression of the c-*myc* gene product creates within SV40-infected human lymphoid cells a permissive environment for replication of the SV40 genome.[393]

In contrast to transformation induced by BPV, transformation induced by SV40 is apparently independent of the action of c-*ras* proteins. Microinjection into BPV-transformed NIH/3T3 cells of a monoclonal antibody neutralizing c-*ras* proteins results in reversion of the transformed phenotype, but such a reversion is not observed in SV40-transformed cells.[394] Mouse embryo fibroblasts infected by SV40 show a marked quantitative and qualitative change in the EGF receptor on the plasma membrane,[395] and this receptor is structurally related to the protein product of the c-*erb*-B oncogene.[396]

C. CONCLUSION

The ability of SV40 to transform cells depends on the synthesis of a specific protein, the large T antigen, which is encoded by the early region of the virus genome. Many structures and functions may become altered in cells infected with the virus, or transfected with specific SV40 genomic sequences, but the mechanisms responsible for SV40-induced malignant transformation are not known. Some types of cells are completely resistant to SV40-induced neoplastic transformation even when they are stimulated to proliferate. Little evidence exists for the participation of protooncogenes in SV40-induced neoplastic transformation.

X. POLYOMA VIRUS

Polyoma virus is a papovavirus that can induce several types of tumors when injected into newborn mice.[397] Tumors frequently induced by injection of polyoma virus in mice include those of the salivary glands, thymus, mammary glands, prostate, bone, and vasculature. Depending on the type of cell infected *in vitro,* polyoma virus may lead to either a lytic cycle with virus production or transformation of a part of the infected cells.[398] A strain of polyoma virus, Py(L), is unusual in causing acute morbidity and early death after inoculation into newborn mice.[399] The animals die of kidney failure associated with extensive, virus-mediated destruction of renal tissue. The Py(L) strain infects baby mouse kidney cell cultures more efficiently than do other polyoma virus strains.

A. STRUCTURE AND EXPRESSION OF POLYOMA VIRUS

A physical map of the polyoma virus genome was first constructed with the aid of restriction enzymes and allowed to determine the location of the origin of DNA replication in the viral genome.[400] The complete DNA sequence of the polyoma virus genome, which is composed of 5292 bp, was also determined.[401] In transformed cells the viral DNA is integrated into the cellular genome and replicates as a cellular gene. From the functional point of view, the polyoma virus genome comprises two halves: the early region, which is expressed early in the productive infection cycle prior to the onset of DNA replication, and the late region, which is transcribed after this.[402] The early region encodes three protein products called tumor (T) antigens: large T, middle T, and small T. These proteins result from translation of mRNAs generated by the alternate splicing of the primary early region transcript.[403] The late region encodes three capsid proteins, termed VP1, VP2, and VP3.

The polyoma virus genome can integrate into the host genome in tandem and nontandem arrangements, but tandem integration is the most efficient mechanism of viral DNA insertion leading to polyoma virus-induced transformation.[404]

1. Polyoma Virus Enhancer DNA Sequences

An enhancer sequence is located within a 246 bp segment at the 3' side of the polyoma virus genome.[405] Mutations within the polyoma virus enhancer sequence can affect the host range properties of the virus. Wild-type polyoma virus does not productively infect murine tera-tocarcinoma stem cells (embryonal carcinoma cells), but several host range mutants capable of infecting these cells have been characterized, and these mutants, designated PyEC mutants, have DNA sequence alterations within the polyoma virus enhancer.[406] Nuclear extracts of F9 embryonal carcinoma cells contain an activity that binds to an specific small region within the polyoma virus enhancer sequence. However, it is not known how specific sequence alterations within the polyoma virus enhancer can lead to different host range properties of the virus. One of the cellular factors required for polyoma virus enhancer function is almost undetectable in embryonal carcinoma cells but is induced after differentiation of these cells into parietal endoderm.[407] The induced protein may be important not only for the regulation of viral gene expression during cellular differentiation but may also have a more general role in the control of gene expression during early embryonic development. Two nuclear proteins present in mouse 3T3 cells recognize a 22-bp sequence contained in the polyoma virus enhancer, and one of these proteins can also interact with enhancers related to controlling the expression of SV40 and the c-*fos* protooncogene.[408]

2. The Polyoma Virus Large T and Middle T Antigens

The transforming potential of polyoma virus resides in the early region of the genome, which encodes the large T antigen (100 kDa), the middle T antigen (56 kDa), and the small T antigen (22 kDa). Each of these proteins may contribute to cell transformation independently of the other two. Large T antigen may be involved in the induction of immortalization and middle T antigen is mainly responsible for the maintenance of transformed state. The construction of site-directed mutants of the polyoma virus genome indicates that at least one of the activities of large T necessary for DNA replication is not required for transformation or immortalization.[409] The small T antigen is localized in the nucleus and has a growth factor-like activity capable of stimulating the growth of NIH/3T3 cells beyond their saturation density in monolayer culture.[410,411] Small T antigen can cooperate with middle T antigen in the transformation of established cell lines. However, the oncogenic potential of polyoma virus is largely due to the middle T antigen.[319,398,402] The large T antigens of both papovaviruses, SV40 and polyoma virus, are composed of consensus structural elements and contain an ATP binding site.[326]

Analysis of polyoma virus mutants indicates that their middle T antigen is crucially involved in neoplastic transformation induced by the virus and that this protein comprises three functional domains.[402] One is the amino-terminal half of the protein, which appears to contain the pp60^{c-src}-binding domain of the antigen. The second domain is the putative membrane-binding region of middle T (amino acids 394 to 421), which is important for the correct localization of the protein as well as for interaction with pp60^{c-src}. The third domain is the intervening stretch of amino acids (192 to 393) that may represent a spacer region between the other two domains, since much of it can be deleted and mutated without total loss of transforming ability.

The polyoma virus gene encoding for middle T gene has been considered as an oncogene, designated *pmt*. The phenotype of polyoma virus-transformed cells reflects the endogenous level of middle T antigen and correlates with the abundance of *pmt* RNA transcripts.[412] The *pmt* gene can act as a dominant transforming gene, i.e., as an oncogene capable of inducing transformation of NIH/3T3 mouse fibroblasts, when the gene is inserted into an MuLV vector.[413] The constructed recombinant, replication-defective virus is analogous to other acutely transforming retroviruses. Rat cells transformed by a plasmid carrying the *pmt* gene are capable of switching to the normal state with rates ranging from 10^{-3} to 10^{-2} per cell per generation, and the reversion occurs by a mechanism involving a transcriptional block of the *pmt* gene.[414] Injection of a constructed retrovirus vector carrying the *pmt* gene into newborn and adult mice results in the rapid appearance of cavernous hemangiomas.[415] Chimeric mouse embryos obtained by blastocyst injection of individual embryonal stem cells expressing the *pmt* gene are specifically arrested at midgestation, when multiple hemangiomas interrupt blood vessel formation. The results of these experiments suggest that *pmt* acts in endothelial cells as a single-step oncogene.

The polyoma virus gene coding for large T antigen, termed *plt*, is capable of conferring on rat embryo fibroblasts the property of immortality, i.e., the ability to grow in long-term culture without entering crisis.[416] Other transforming genes, including *pmt* and activated *ras* genes,[417] as well as tumor promoters such as TPA,[418] can then readily transform the *plt*-immortalized fibroblast cells. The *plt* gene may be involved in activating *pmt* expression, but continuous expression of *plt* is not required for the maintenance of *pmt* expression and hence the maintenance of a transformed state.[419] It thus seem that *plt* is capable of activating *pmt* expression by a kind of "hit-and-run" mechanism, which could be associated with recombination in the vicinity of the *pmt* locus.

3. Homology of Polyoma Virus Middle T Antigen with Gastrin

A region of the middle T antigen of polyoma virus shows significantly high homology with gastrin,[420] a hormone which stimulates acid secretion by the stomach and acts as a growth factor for the gastric mucosa. Homology is especially apparent around the sole tyrosine residue of gastrin. The biological meaning of this homology is unknown but acquisition of the gastrin DNA sequence could have conferred a selective advantage on the virus. The possible significance of the gastrin homology and surrounding sequences in polyoma virus middle T antigen in relation to cell transformation has been discussed recently.[421] Although these sequences can influence the physical properties of middle T antigen, its presence does not ensure the biological activity of the protein. Hence, more subtle structural elements outside of these immediate sequences must be of considerable importance for the transforming ability of the virus.

B. MECHANISMS OF POLYOMA VIRUS-INDUCED TRANSFORMATION

Both the large T and the middle T proteins act in the control of cellular growth but only the middle T antigen is required for maintaining transformation of established cell lines.[416,422-425] A quantitative correlation exists between the level of middle T expression and different transformation parameters.[426,427] Morphological aspects of transformation are the most sensitive to middle T expression while anchorage-independent growth and tumorigenicity require much higher levels of this expression. A constructed recombinant RSV DNA in which the v-*src* gene was replaced by the coding sequences for polyoma virus middle T antigen is able to efficiently induce transformation of primary CEF cells without requiring prior immortalization of the transfected cells.[428] Middle T antigen can be produced in large scale by using genetically engineered tumor tissues.[429]

The construction of a family of recombinant retroviruses transducing genes for individual polyoma virus antigens allowed to demonstrate that, whereas polyoma virus at best stably transforms 1% of infected cells, every cell infected by a retroviral vector carrying the gene coding for polyoma virus middle T antigen is transformed.[430] The constructed recombinant retroviral vectors are technically superior to other polyoma virus vectors, such as transfectable plasmid constructs, facilitating the efficient and stable introduction of each of the T antigens into cells. These retroviral vectors can thus permit genetic analysis of the relationship between tumorigenesis by polyoma virus T antigens and the alteration of cellular growth and differentiation. However, in unestablished rat fibroblasts, efficient polyoma virus gene expression does not necessarily ensure expression of the fully transformed phenotype, which indicates that polyoma virus-mediated transformation may require additional alterations beyond the acquisition of transforming viral genes.[427]

Elevation of the intracellular concentration of cAMP may totally block the proliferation of polyoma virus-transformed rat 3T3 cells.[431] This elevation does not have a significant effect on the proliferation of parental normal rat 3T3 cells or transformants induced by SV40, and its activity requires an intact polyoma virus middle T protein. The biological significance of this difference as well as the mechanism involved in the inhibition of polyoma virus-transformed cells by cAMP are unknown.

1. Protein Phosphorylation

Polyoma virus middle T antigen has been shown to be phosphorylated *in vivo* on serine, threonine, and tyrosine residues.[432-435] Phosphorylation of middle T on serine is stimulated by TPA, probably through activation of protein kinase C.[436,437] Phosphorylation of several cellular proteins on tyrosine residues, including an 85-kDa protein,[438] is increased in cells transformed by polyoma virus. The biological significance of these phosphorylations is little understood.

Polyoma virus middle T antigen-associated protein kinase activity may depend on the formation of a complex between the antigen and endogenous protooncogene products that possess tyrosine-specific protein kinase activity, including pp60$^{c\text{-}src}$.[425,439-441] The formation of this complex would enhance the tyrosyl kinase activity associated with c-*src* gene protein, pp60$^{c\text{-}src}$, which could be an essential step in polyoma virus-induced neoplastic transformation.[442,443] It is not the overall level of middle T antigen present in the cells which correlates with transformation parameters and tumorigenicity but rather the variable and usually small fraction of the antigen which can be isolated in a complex with pp60$^{c\text{-}src}$.[426] The carboxy-terminal domain of pp60$^{c\text{-}src}$ is apparently required for middle T antigen association.[444] It is possible that middle

T antigen activates the pp60^{c-src} kinase by binding directly to the region of the molecule that contains the tyrosine-527 residue, thus preventing the phosphorylation of this residue which is known to be involved in regulation of pp60^{c-src} activity *in vivo*.

Maintenance of a transformed phenotype by polyoma virus middle T antigen in established cell lines depends, at least in part, on a minimal threshold level of pp60^{c-src} protein.[445] The pp60^{c-src} protein would acquire enhanced kinase activity upon its binding to polyoma virus middle T antigen and this change may be responsible for the reduction in cell-to-cell communication (reduced junctional permeability) which is observed in rat cells transfected with an inducible middle T recombinant DNA or infected with a conditional mutant virus.[446] Deficiency in junctional permeability is common to various types of tumor cells, including RSV-transformed cells.

Phorbol ester (TPA) enhances the association of polyoma virus middle T antigen with pp60^{c-src} and increases the phosphorylation of the antigen on tyrosine residues.[437] The TPA-induced enhanced association between middle T antigen and the pp60^{c-src} kinase is apparently due to activation of protein kinase C and results in an increased ability of middle T antigen to transform cells.[447]

Interestingly, an increase in the intracellular levels of pp60^{c-src} 15-fold over normal endogenous levels by means of a c-*src*-carrying retroviral vector is not accompanied by a proportionate increase in the amount of middle T antigen-pp60^{c-src} complex, since the majority of the components of the complex remains unassociated.[448] Double infection of CEF cells with a molecular vector carrying DNA sequences coding for polyoma virus middle T antigen and a viral vector expressing pp60^{c-src} at high level do not result in enhancement of morphological cell transformation, and the phosphorylation of middle T antigen in the doubly infected cells is not increased in proportion to the overexpression of the c-*src* protein product.[428]

Protein pp60^{c-src} associated with polyoma virus middle T antigen contains altered sites of tyrosine phosphorylation, including a site within the amino-terminal portion which is clearly distinct from that on the carboxy-terminal half of the molecule that is phosphorylated when pp60^{c-src} is not bound to the polyoma virus middle T antigen.[449,450] The possible biological significance of this qualitative difference is not understood.

The artificial introduction of deletions into the amino-terminal coding region of the polyoma virus middle T antigen shows that truncated middle T antigen may be associated with the cell membrane but do not have protein kinase activity and fail to transform rat or mouse cells.[451] Middle T antigen of a polyoma virus transformation-defective mutant (NG59) is associated with pp60^{c-src},[452] and mutations around the NG59 lesion indicate that an active association of polyoma virus middle T antigen with pp60^{c-src} is required for polyoma virus-induced cell transformation.[453] There appears to be a conformational constraint on the amino-terminal half of the polyoma virus middle T antigen with regard to both its interaction with pp60^{c-src} and its ability to induce neoplastic transformation.[454] Studies with antisense RNA (anti-mRNA) complementary to mRNA for pp60^{c-src} also indicate that a significant proportion of the alterations which correspond to the phenotype of middle T antigen-transformed rodent cells is dependent upon the activity of the endogenous c-*src* gene protein product.[455]

However, the role of pp60^{c-src} in polyoma virus-induced transformation of cells is not totally clear, and there is evidence that tyrosine phosphorylation in the middle T antigen of polyoma virus may not be required for transformation.[456] Elevation of pp60^{c-src} kinase activity is not required for the transformation of hamster embryo cells by other DNA oncogenic viruses (SV40, Ad2, and BPV-1).[457] An interaction between pp60^{c-src} and DNA virus-encoded proteins is probably not a general mechanism responsible for DNA virus-induced neoplastic transformation. The level of phosphotyrosine in polyoma virus-transformed cells is the same as in nontransformed cells,[458] which indicates that an overall increase in tyrosine phosphorylation is not responsible for polyoma virus-induced transformation.

Polyoma virus middle T antigen may be associated with cellular protein-tyrosine kinases other than pp60^{c-src}. Using antibody raised against a fusion protein between β-galactosidase and amino-terminal sequences of p90$^{gag-yes}$ protein from Y73 ASV (anti-*yes* antibody), it was found that polyoma virus middle T antigen can associate with and be phosphorylated by the c-*yes* protooncogene protein product.[459] This product is a protein of 62 kDa, p62-$^{c-yes}$, which possesses tyrosine-specific kinase activity. It has been calculated that approximately 5 to 10% of the total immunoprecipitable pp60^{c-src} molecules in polyoma virus-transformed cells are stably associated with middle T antigen, and that 10 to 15% of the detectable middle T antigen molecules are stably associated with pp60^{c-src} in the same cells.[460] Between 50 and 75% of the total middle T antigen-associated cellular tyrosine kinase activity would represent the enzymatic activity of pp60^{c-src}, while the remaining 25 to 50% would represent the activity of other cellular kinases, including the p62^{c-yes} kinase.

The possible contribution of protooncogene-encoded tyrosine kinases to polyoma virus-induced neoplastic transformation remains to be determined. Treatment of polyoma virus-transformed cells with sodium orthovanadate (an inhibitor of phosphotyrosine phosphatases), allow the detection of phosphotyrosine-containing proteins by preventing the turnover of phosphate on substrates phosphorylated by activated cellular protein-tyrosine kinases associated with polyoma virus middle T antigen, including the pp60^{c-src} and p62^{c-yes} kinases.[461] The results of these studies support the hypothesis that tyrosine phosphorylation of cellular proteins may be involved in the events that are responsible for polyoma virus-induced neoplastic transformation.

2. Phosphoinositide Metabolism

Increased phosphatidylinositol kinase activity is observed in cells transformed by polyoma virus.[438,462] It has been suggested that phosphatidylinositol kinase activity, in addition to tyrosine protein kinase activity, is associated with middle T antigen-pp60^{c-src} complexes.[463] However, these types of kinase activities reside in different molecular species and tyrosine-specific protein kinases do not possess phosphatidylinositol kinase activity.[464,465] No significant phosphatidylinositol kinase activity is present in purified preparations of polyoma virus middle T antigen-pp60^{c-src} complexes.[466] The phosphatidylinositol kinase activity observed in immunoprecipitates of middle T antigen/pp60^{c-src} complexes is likely to be derived from a cellular enzyme whose activity could be altered by such complexes.[462,467] A protein of 81 kDa (p81) may be responsible for the phosphatidylinositol kinase activity which is associated with the middle T antigen/pp60^{c-src} complex.[468]

3. Association of Middle T Antigen with Cellular Proteins

In addition to its association with the products of the c-*src* and c-*yes* protooncogenes, polyoma virus middle T antigen is associated with three cellular proteins with apparent MWs of 88,000 (88K protein), 61,000 (61K protein), and 37,000 (37K protein).[469] Although the role, if any, of the association of middle T antigen with these cellular proteins in polyoma virus-induced neoplastic transformation is unknown, a much larger fraction of middle T antigen is bound to 88K, 61K, and 37K proteins than to pp60^{c-src}.

4. Cooperation of Middle T Antigen with Hormones and Growth Factors

Cooperation between hormones, peptide growth factors and protooncogene protein products may be important in the induction of neoplastic transformation by DNA viruses with oncogenic potential. There is evidence that mitogenic growth factors may cooperate with polyoma virus middle T antigen in the transformation of secondary cultured rat cells.[470] Polyoma virus-induced transformation of the rat fibroblast cell line NRK-49F results in abrogation of the requirement for the exogenous supply of insulin and retinoic acid, but not EGF and fibronectin.[471] In contrast, transformation of the NRK-49F cells by by Ad5 does not result in abrogation of these factors. The biological basis of this difference is not understood.

5. Polyoma Virus Mutants

The study of spontaneous or induced mutants of polyoma virus, especially of sequences encoding the middle T antigen, may contribute to define the structural and functional requirements for polyoma virus-induced neoplastic transformation.[402] In general, the results of these studies indicate that middle T antigen is crucially involved in transformation induced by polyoma virus and that the association of middle T antigen with the cellular protein pp60[c-src] is of major importance in this transformation.

A constructed polyoma virus mutant, Py808A, expressing large T and small T but no detectable middle T, is unable to induce complete transformation of cultured rat embryo fibroblasts but has a mitogenic effect on resting cells.[403] This mutant induces changes of the cell surface associated with transformation but no detectable alterations of the microfilament or extracellular fibronectin. Thus, changes on the cell surface associated with transformation are not necessarily coupled to changes in cytoskeletal organization. Another mutant of polyoma virus, an *mlt* mutant, contains a 12-bp deletion between nucleotides 1347 and 1360 (a region which encodes parts of the large T and middle T antigens) is capable of transforming rat cells in culture, but has a much lower tumorigenic potential when injected into newborn rats.[472] These results are interesting because they show that the transformation markers, as determined in cultured cells, can be segregated from the tumorigenic markers, which are responsible for tumor growth in the animal.

Mutations introduced into the gene of the DNA binding domain of polyoma virus large T antigen (between amino acids 290 and 310 of the antigen) result in proteins that no longer bind to the high-affinity binding sites of the polyoma virus genome and that are not able to initiate DNA replication from the viral origin.[473] However, introduction of these mutant genes into REF cells facilitates the establishment of these cells in long-term culture at an efficiency indistinguishable from that of the wild-type protein. It is thus apparent that the product of *plt*, and perhaps the products of other genes, including oncogenes, can activate the expression of cellular genes related with acquisition of immortality and/or transformation without specific interaction with DNA sequences. However, localization of these products to the nucleus would be necessary for exerting such regulatory changes in the cell genome.

6. Viral and Host Genetic Determinants

Induction of tumors in mice by polyoma virus involves viral genetic determinants that are, at least in part, different from those involved in cell transformation *in vitro*.[474] Molecularly cloned polyoma virus strains may show profoundly different abilities to induce tumors in mice, despite being equally efficient in the transformation of cells in culture. The PTA strain of polyoma virus is a high-tumor strain which induces multiple tumors in 90 to 100% of recipient animals. The tumors are of epithelial as well as mesenchymal origin and lead to a moribund condition of the host within a period of about 12 weeks. The RA low-tumor strain of the virus induces usually single tumors in a small fraction of the animals. These tumors are exclusively of mesenchymal origin and lead to a moribund condition after an average survival time of over 40 weeks. Constructed recombinant viruses between PTA and RA strains revealed two classes of genetic determinants present in PTA, deriving from noncoding and coding regions, that contribute to a high frequency and broad spectrum of tumors.[474] In addition, these studies indicated the interaction of a cellular factor(s) with noncoding viral sequences.

The study of transgenic mice carrying replication-defective polyoma virus early region regulatory sequences linked to cDNAs encoding either polyoma virus large T or middle T has yield interesting results.[475] While transgenic mice expressing large T sequences have no phenotypic alterations, the mice expressing middle T sequences develop multifocal tumors of the vascular endothelium, but these mice do not develop tumors of other tissues. The restricted specificity of tumors in the transgenic mice indicates that the polyoma virus middle T antigen alone is not sufficient to recapitulate the broad tumor spectrum of the virus. Expression analysis of the transgenic animals showed that detectable levels of transgene RNA and protein were found only in the vascular tumors and the testes, but the testes did not exhibit any detectable abnormality. Thus, local tissue factors, in addition to viral factors, are importantly involved in determining the final consequence of the expression of polyoma virus genes with oncogenic potential and in some tissues this expression may be inconsequential. Moreover, not every endothelial cell expressing the polyoma virus middle T antigen undergoes proliferative expansion associated with transformation.

7. Cooperation between Polyoma Virus Antigens and Oncogene Products

Although the large T antigen of polyoma virus may induce immortalization of primary REF cells, the viral middle T protein is required for expression of tumorigenicity in these cells. However, efficient transformation of REF cells can be achieved by transfer of molecular vectors containing the *plt* gene and two forms of the *myc* oncogene, i.e., *gag-myc* fused gene from MC29 AMCV or rearranged c-*myc* sequences from a mouse plasmacytoma cell line.[476] A comparable efficiency of transformation was obtained when the *plt* gene was cotransferred with the human c-H-*ras* oncogene. Focus formation can be obtained in REF cells after transfer of the *plt* gene (or a v-*myc* oncogene) when the cells are subsequently treated with the phorbol ester TPA.[418]

Neither the T24 c-H-*ras* gene nor the polyoma virus middle T gene, *pmt*, are able to induce observable alterations in the growth or morphology of BRK cells, but either of both genes induce phenotypes associated with oncogenic transformation when cotransfected with plasmids containing the adenovirus E1A region.[184] Thus, expression of E1A-encoded functions, which are probably associated with an extended growth potential of cultured primary cells, enables BRK cells to respond to the oncogenic potential of the polyoma virus *pmt* gene.

8. Induction of Alterations in the Host Genome Cell Genome

The possible role of host cell genome alterations in polyoma virus-induced neoplastic transformation is not clear. Expression of the *plt* gene of polyoma virus by transfection of a *plt*-containing bacterial plasmid into fertilized mouse eggs resulted in transgenic mice which exhibited genetic instability favoring the occurrence of DNA transpositions and specific recombination events.[477] Integration of polyoma virus into chromosomal DNA in the transformed rat cell line LPT caused a 3.0-kb deletion of cellular DNA next to the virus inserts.[478] The LPT cells with polyoma virus inserts were heterozygous with respect to both the virus inserts and the cellular DNA deletion. Integration of polyoma virus into the genome of mouse embryo cells (Cyp cell line) is associated with a major rearrangement of host cell DNA near the sites of viral DNA insertion.[479] This rearrangement could exert an important influence on the expression of integrated polyoma virus DNA in Cyp cells.

9. Protooncogene Alterations

The possible role of protooncogene alterations in polyoma virus-induced neoplastic transformation is little known. Infection of BALB/c 3T3 mouse cells with polyoma virus is associated with accumulation of c-*myc* and c-*fos* mRNAs in a biphasic pattern.[480] The initial phase of polyoma virus-induced mRNA accumulation is rapid, does not require protein synthesis, and is effected by virions or capsids in a dose-responsive manner, which suggests that it may result from virus (or capsid) attachment to a cell membrane receptor. The second phase of c-*myc* and c-*fos* mRNA accumulation is associated with the expression of early viral proteins, i.e., the polyoma virus T antigens. It is possible that these viral antigens act in the regulation of protooncogene expression.

Amplification of c-*myc* associated with the presence of chromosome abnormalities (DMs and HSRs) was detected in mouse SEWA tumor cells, which are derived from an osteosarcoma induced in A.SW mouse by polyoma virus infection.[481] SEWA cells contain three to five copies of polyoma virus but it is unclear which function, if any, of these polyoma virus sequences contributes to the malignant phenotype in the presence of amplified c-*myc* gene.

Transformation of neonatal rat hepatocytes in primary cultures by transfection with a constructed plasmid containing polyoma virus early gene sequences was associated with elevated levels of expression of the c-*neu/erb*-B-2 protooncogene.[482] However, the expression of c-*neu/erb*-B-2 was not related to the maintenance of the transformed state and exhibited variation among different clones of the transformed cells.

10. Expression of Mitochondrial Genes

Increased levels of the mitochondrial RNA encoding subunit II of cytochrome oxidase have been found in rat fibroblasts immortalized by transfer of the *plt* gene.[211] A similar alteration has been observed after transfer of adenovirus E1A genes or a rearranged c-*myc* protooncogene into the same cells. The molecular mechanisms involved in this alteration are unknown.

11. Immunologic Factors

It has been suggested that one of the functions of the early T antigens of DNA viruses with oncogenic potential is the regulation of the level of susceptibility or resistance of cells transformed by these agents to host cellular immune rejection.[483] Of course, this hypothesis leaves open the question of the generation of the transformed cells.

12. BK Virus

BK virus (BKV) is a human papovavirus isolated from the urine of an immunosuppressed renal transplant recipient.[484] Since then, BKV has been frequently isolated from immunosuppressed or immunodeficient patients but only rarely from human tumors. More recently, BKV DNA was detected in 19 of 74 human brain tumors of different histological types as well as in 4 of 9 tumors of human pancreatic islets.[485] No BKV DNA was detected in several tumors of other sites or in normal human tissues. Curiously, BKV RNA transcripts were detected in three tumors that were apparently free of BKV DNA. The potential oncogenicity of BK virus is indicated by the induction of malignant undifferentiated sarcomas in newborn Syrian hamsters by subcutaneous inoculation of a recombinant vector containing BK virus early region gene and the activated (T24) human c-H-*ras* protooncogene.[486]

XI. SUMMARY

Several DNA viruses which are ubiquitous in certain human populations may possess oncogenic potential under experimental conditions. The possible etiological role of these viruses in cancer occurring spontaneously in humans and other animal species remains controversial. In spite of the efforts of numerous investigators, the evidence for an etiological role of DNA viruses in human cancer is based mainly on epidemiological data and these data, although useful for guiding other types of studies, are generally incapable *per se* of establishing secure causal associations. Since neoplastic transformation of cells associated with infection by DNA viruses is at most a fortuitous event, the name oncogenic DNA viruses should be used only in a restricted sense.

The mechanisms responsible for the neoplastic transformation of cells induced by DNA viruses under either natural or experimental conditions remain poorly characterized. The results obtained with different types of experimental procedures, including the use of natural or induced virus mutants, indicate that distinct sequences of the genomes of DNA viruses may be responsible for the oncogenic potential exhibited by these viruses under specific experimental conditions. Unfortunately, the cellular mechanisms of action of the proteins coded by these sequences are unknown. Protooncogene alterations in cells infected with DNA viruses with oncogenic potential have been little characterized and their possible role in the expression of a transformed phenotype is unknown. In any case, cellular alterations in addition to those directly introduced by the viral functions may be critically required for the acquisition of tumorigenic properties by cells infected with DNA viruses with oncogenic potentialities. Other environmental factors, including chemical and/or physical carcinogenic agents, as well as host factors, including hormonal and/or immunologic factors, may have a critical role in the origin and fate of tumors associated with infection by potentially oncogenic DNA viruses.

REFERENCES

1. Pimentel, E., Human oncovirology, *Biochim. Biophys. Acta,* 560, 169, 1979.
2. Rapp, F., Viral carcinogenesis, *Int. Rev. Cytol.,* Suppl. 15, 203, 1983.
3. Rapp, F., The challenge of herpesviruses, *Cancer Res.,* 44, 1309, 1984.
4. Tocci, M.J. and St. Jeor, S.C., Susceptibility of lymphoblastoid cells to infection with human cytomegalovirus, *Infect. Immun.,* 23, 418, 1979.
5. Pottathil, R., Pottathil, I.R., Cheung, K.-S., and Lang, D.J., Enhanced replication of murine cytomegalovirus in murine leukemic lymphocytes, *Cancer Res.,* 46, 124, 1986.
6. Purtilo, D.T. and Linder, J., Oncological consequences of impaired immune surveillance against ubiquituous viruses, *J. Clin. Immunol.,* 3, 197, 1983.
7. Purtilo, D.T., Defective immune surveillance in viral carcinogenesis, *Lab. Invest.,* 51, 373, 1984.
8. Calnek, B.W., Marek's disease — a model for herpesvirus oncology, *Crit. Rev. Microbiol.,* 12, 293, 1986.
9. Rowe, W.P., Genetic interactions between tumor viruses and host cells, *Cancer,* 49, 1958, 1982.
10. Jones, K.W., Kinross, J., Maitland, N., and Norval, M., Normal human tissues contain RNA and antigens related to infectious adenovirus type 2, *Nature,* 277, 274, 1979.
11. Puga, A., Cantin, E.M., and Notkins, A.L., Homology between murine and human cellular DNA sequences and the terminal repetition of the S component of herpes simplex virus type 1 DNA, *Cell,* 31, 81, 1982.
12. Arrand, J.R., Walsh-Arrand, J.E., and Rymo, L., Cytoplasmic RNA from normal and malignant human cells shows homology to the DNAs of Epstein-Barr virus and human adenovirus, *EMBO J.,* 2, 1673, 1983.
13. Blomquist, M.C., Hunt, L.T., and Barker, W.C., Vaccinia virus 19-kilodalton protein: relationship to several mammalian proteins, including two growth factors, *Proc. Natl. Acad. Sci. U.S.A.,* 81, 7363, 1984.
14. Brown, J.P., Twardzik, D.R., Marquardt, M., and Todaro, G.J., Vaccinia virus encodes a polypeptide homologous to epidermal growth factor and transforming growth factor, *Nature,* 313, 491, 1985.
15. Twardzik, D.R., Brown, J.P., Ranchalis, J.E., Todaro, G.J., and Moss, B., Vaccinia virus-infected cells release a novel polypeptide functionally related to transforming and epidermal growth factors, *Proc. Natl. Acad. Sci. U.S.A.,* 82, 5300, 1985.
16. Stroobant, P., Rice, A.P., Gullick, W.J., Cheng, D.J., Kerr, I.M., and Waterfield, M.D., Purification and characterization of vaccinia virus growth factor, *Cell,* 42, 383, 1985.
17. Chang, W., Upton, C., Hu, S.-L., Purchio, A.F., and McFacden, G., The genome of Shope fibroma virus, a tumorigenic poxvirus, contains a growth factor gene with sequence similarity to those encoding epidermal growth factor and transforming growth factor alpha, *Mol. Cell. Biol.,* 7, 535, 1987.
18. Sugden, B., Epstein-Barr virus: a human pathogen inducing lymphoproliferation *in vivo* and *in vitro, Rev. Infect. Dis.,* 4, 1048, 1982.
19. Klein, G. and Klein, E., The changing faces of EBV research, *Progr. Med. Virol.,* 30, 87, 1984.
20. Frizzera, G., The clinico-pathological expressions of Epstein-Barr virus infection in lymphoid tissues, *Virchows Arch. B,* 53, 1, 1987.
21. Hanto, D.W., Frizzera, G., Gajl-Peczalska, K.J., and Simmons, Epstein-Barr virus, immunodeficiency, and B cell lymphoproliferation, *Transplantation,* 39, 461, 1985.
22. de Thé, G., Epstein-Barr virus and Burkitt's lymphoma worldwide: the causal relationship revisited, in *Burkitt's Lymphoma: A Human Cancer Model,* Lenoir, G., O'Conor, G., and Olweny, C.L.M., Eds., International Agency for Research on Cancer, Lyon, France, 1985, 165.
23. Purtilo, D.T., Manolov, G., Manolova, Y., Harada, S., Lipscomb, H., and Tatsumi, E., Role of Epstein-Barr virus in the etiology of Burkitt's lymphoma, in *Burkitt's Lymphoma: A Human Cancer Model,* Lenoir, G., O'Conor, G., and Olweny, C.L.M., Eds., International Agency for Research on Cancer, Lyon, France, 1985, 231.
24. Tugwood, J.D., Lau, W.-H., O, S.-K., Tsao, S.-Y., Martin, W.M., Shiu, W., Desgranges, C., Jones, P.H., and Arrand, J.R., Epstein-Barr virus-specific transcription in normal and malignant nasopharyngeal biopsies and in lymphocytes from healthy donors and infectious mononucleosis patients, *J. Gen. Virol.,* 68, 1081, 1987.
25. Sculley, T.B., Moss, D.J., Hazelton, R.A., and Pope, J.H., Detection of Epstein-Barr virus strain variants in lymphoblastoid cell lines "spontaneously" derived from patients with rheumatoid arthritis, infectious mononucleosis and controls, *J. Gen. Virol.,* 68, 2069, 1987.

26. Jones, J.F., Shurin, S., Abramowsky, C., Tubbs, R.R., Sciotto, C.G., Wahl, R., Sands, J., Gottman, D., Katz, B.Z., and Sklar, J., T-cell lymphomas containing Epstein-Barr viral DNA in patients with chronic Epstein-Barr virus infections, *N. Engl. J. Med.,* 318, 733, 1988.

27. Baer, R., Bankier, A.T., Biggin, M.D., Deininger, P.L., Farrell, P.J., Gibson, T.J., Hatfull, G., Hudson, G.S., Satchwell, S.C., Séguin, C., Tuffnell, P.S., and Barrell, B.G., DNA sequence and expression of the B95-8 Epstein-Barr virus genome, *Nature,* 310, 207, 1984.

28. Diala, E.S. and Hoffman, R.M., Epstein-Barr HR-1 virion DNA is very highly methylated, *J. Virol.,* 45, 482, 1983.

29. Nemerow, G.R. and Cooper, N.R., Infection of B lymphocytes by a human herpesvirus, Epstein-Barr virus, is blocked by calmodulin antagonists, *Proc. Natl. Acad. Sci. U.S.A.,* 81, 4955, 1984.

30. Janssen, O. and Kabelitz, D., Tumor necrosis factor selectively inhibits activation of human B cells by Epstein-Barr virus, *J. Immunol.,* 140, 125, 1988.

31. Luka, J., Kreofsky, T., Pearson, G.R., Hennessy, K., and Kieff, E., Identification and characterization of a cellular protein that cross-reacts with the Epstein-Barr virus nuclear antigen, *J. Virol.,* 52, 833, 1984.

32. Gross, T.G., Sakai, K., and Volsky, D.J., Transfer of the Epstein-Barr virus (EBV) DNA fragment coding for EBNA-1, the putative transforming antigen of EBV, into normal human lymphocytes: gene expression without cell transformation, *Biochem. Biophys. Res. Commun.,* 134, 1260, 1986.

33. Liebowitz, D., Kopan, R., Fuchs, E., Sample, J., and Kieff, E., An Epstein-Barr virus transforming protein associates with vimentin in lymphocytes, *Mol. Cell. Biol.,* 7, 2299, 1987.

34. zur Hausen, H., Bornkamm, G.W., Schmidt, R., and Hecker, E., Tumor initiators and promoters in the induction of Epstein-Barr virus, *Proc. Natl. Acad. Sci. U.S.A.,* 76, 782, 1979.

35. Sample, J., Tanaka, A., Lancz, G., and Nonoyama, M., Identification of Epstein-Barr virus genes expressed during the early phase of virus replication and during lymphocyte immortalization, *Virology,* 139, 1, 1984.

36. Stoerker, J., Holliday, J.E., and Glaser, R., Identification of a region of the Epstein-Barr virus (B95-8) genome required for transformation, *Virology,* 129, 199, 1983.

37. Gordon, J., Ley, S.C., Melamed, M.D., English, L.S., and Hughes-Jones, N.C., Immortalized B lymphocytes produce B-cell growth factor, *Nature,* 310, 145, 1984.

38. Heller, M., Flemington, E., Kieff, E., and Deininger, P., Repeat arrays in cellular DNA related to the Epstein-Barr virus IR3 repeat, *Mol. Cell. Biol.,* 5, 457, 1985.

39. Tosato, G. and Blaese, R.M., Epstein-Barr virus infection and immunoregulation in man, *Adv. Immunol.,* 37, 99, 1985.

40. Stevenson, M., Volsky, B., Hedenskog, M., and Volsky, D.J., Immortalization of human T lymphocytes after transfection of Epstein-Barr virus DNA, *Science,* 233, 980, 1986.

41. Adldinger, H.K., Delius, H., Freese, U.K., Clarke, J., and Bornkamm, G.W., A putative transforming gene of Jijoye virus differs from that of Epstein-Barr virus prototypes, *Virology,* 141, 221, 1985.

42. Mark, W. and Sugden, B., Transformation of lymphocytes by Epstein-Barr virus requires only one-fourth of the viral genome, *Virology,* 122, 431, 1982.

43. Alfieri, C. and Joncas, J.H., Biomolecular analysis of a defective nontransforming Epstein-Barr virus (EBV) from a patient with chronic active EBV infection, *J. Virol.,* 61, 3306, 1987.

44. Nilsson, K., Giovanella, B.C., Stehlin, J.S., and Klein, G., Tumorigenicity of human hematopoietic cell lines in athymic nude mice, *Int. J. Cancer,* 19, 337, 1977.

45. Nilsson, K. and Klein, G., Phenotypic and cytogenetic characteristics of human B-lymphoid cell lines and their relevance for the etiology of Burkitt's lymphoma, *Adv. Cancer Res.,* 37, 319, 1982.

46. Matsuo, T., Heller, M., Petti, L., O'Shiro, E., and Kieff, E., Persistence of the entire Epstein-Barr virus genome integrated into human lymphocyte DNA, *Science,* 226, 1322, 1984.

47. Bornkamm, G.W., Knoebel-Doeberitz, M.V., and Lenoir, G.M., No evidence for differences in the Epstein-Barr virus genome carried in Burkitt lymphoma cells and nonmalignant lymphoblastoid cells from the same patient, *Proc. Natl. Acad. Sci. U.S.A.,* 81, 4930, 1984.

48. Zimber, U., Adldinger, H.K., Lenoir, G.M., Vuillaume, M., Knebel-Doeberitz, M.V., Laux, G., Desgranges, C., Wittmann, P., Freese, U.-K., Schneider, U., and Bornkamm, G.W., Geographical prevalence of two types of Epstein-Barr virus, *Virology,* 154, 56, 1986.

49. Epstein-Barr virus strain-specific differences in transformed cell lines demonstrated in growth characteristics, induction of viral antigens and ADCC susceptibility, *Int. J. Cancer,* 30, 393, 1982.

50. Griffin, B.E. and Karran, L., Immortalization of monkey epithelial cells by specific fragments of Epstein-Barr virus DNA, *Nature,* 309, 78, 1984.

51. Swendeman, S. and Thorley-Lawson, D.A., The activation antigen BLAST-2, when shed, is an autocrine BCGF for normal and transformed B cells, *EMBO J.,* 6, 1637, 1987.

52. Blomhoff, H.K., Smeland, E., Mustafa, A.S., Godal, T., and Ohlsson, R., Epstein-Barr virus mediates a switch in responsiveness to transforming growth factor, type beta, in cells of the B cell lineage, *Eur. J. Immunol.,* 17, 299, 1987.

53. Hutt-Fletcher, L.M., Synergistic activation of cells by Epstein-Barr virus and B-cell growth factor, *J. Virol.,* 61, 774, 1987.

54. Tosato, G., Seamon, K.B., Goldman, N.D., Sehgal, P.B., May, L.T., Washington, G.C., Jones, K.D., and Pike, S.E., Monocyte-derived human B-cell growth factor identified as interferon-β_2 (BSF-2, IL-6), *Science,* 239, 502, 1988.

55. Birx, D.L., Redfield, R.R., and Tosato, G., Defective regulation of Epstein-Barr virus infection in patients with acquired immunodeficiency syndrome (AIDS) or AIDS-related disorders, *N. Engl. J. Med.,* 314, 874, 1986.

56. Ablashi, D.V., Flagader, A., Markham, P.D., and Salahuddin, S.Z., Isolation of transforming Epstein-Barr virus from plasma of HTLV-III/LAV-infected patients, *Intervirology,* 17, 25, 1987.

57. Kenney, S., Kamine, J., Markovitz, D., Fenrick, R., and Pagano, J., An Epstein-Barr virus immediate-early gene product trans-activates gene expression from the human immunodeficiency virus long terminal repeat, *Proc. Natl. Acad. Sci. U.S.A.,* 85, 1652, 1988.

58. Tomei, L.D., Noyes, I., Blocker, D., Holliday, J., and Glaser, R., Phorbol ester and Epstein-Barr virus dependent transformation of normal primary human skin epithelial cells, *Nature,* 329, 73, 1987.

59. Hirayama, T. and Ito, Y., A new view of the etiology of nasopharyngeal carcinoma, *Prev. Med.,* 10, 614, 1981.

60. Glazer, P.M. and Summers, W.C., Oncogene expression in isogenic, EBV-positive and -negative Burkitt lymphoma cell lines, *Intervirology,* 23, 82, 1985.

61. Lacy, J., Summers, W.P., Watson, M., Glazer, P.M., and Summers, W.C., Amplification and deregulation of *MYC* following Epstein-Barr virus infection of a human B-cell line, *Proc. Natl. Acad. Sci. U.S.A.,* 84, 5838, 1987.

62. Wennborg, A., Aman, P., Saranath, D., Pear, W., Sümegi, J., and Klein, G., Conversion of the lymphoma line "BJAB" by Epstein-Barr virus into phenotypically altered sublines is accompanied by increased c-*MYC* mRNA levels, *Int. J. Cancer,* 40, 202, 1987.

63. Cleary, M.L., Epstein, M.A., Finerty, S., Dorfman, R.F., Bornkamm, G.W., Kirkwood, J.K., Morgan, A.J., and Sklar, J., Individual tumors of multifocal EB virus-induced malignant lymphomas in tamarins arise from different B-cell clones, *Science,* 228, 722, 1985.

64. Cheah, M.S.C., Ley, T.J., Tronick, S.R., and Robbins, K.C., *fgr* proto-oncogene mRNA induced in B lymphocytes by Epstein-Barr virus infection, *Nature,* 319, 238, 1986.

65. Nishizawa, M., Semba, K., Yoshida, M.C., Yamamoto, T., Sasaki, M., and Toyoshima, K., Structure, expression, and chromosomal location of the human c-*fgr* gene, *Mol. Cell. Biol.,* 6, 511, 1986.

66. Weller, T.H., The cytomegaloviruses: ubiquitous agents with protean clinical manifestations, *N. Engl. J. Med.,* 285, 203, 1971.

67. Lamberson, H.V., Cytomegalovirus (CMV): the agent, its pathogenesis, and its epidemiology, *Progr. Clin. Biol. Res.,* 182, 149, 1985.

68. Rapp, F., Cytomegalovirus and carcinogenesis, *J. Natl. Cancer Inst.,* 72, 783, 1984.

69. Detels, R., Vischer, B.R., Fahey, J.L., Schwartz, K., Greene, R.S., Madden, D.L., Sever, J.L., and Gottlieb, M.S., The relation of cytomegalovirus and Epstein-Barr virus antibodies to T-cell subsets in homosexually active men, *JAMA,* 251, 1719, 1984.

70. Giraldo, G., Beth, E., and Buonaguro, F.M., Kaposi's sarcoma: a natural model of interrelationships between viruses, immunologic responses, genetics, and oncogenesis, *Antibiot. Chemother.,* 32, 1, 1984.

71. Huang, E.-S., Cytomegalovirus: its oncogenes and Kaposi's sarcoma, *Antibiot. Chemother.,* 32, 27, 1984.

72. Nelson, J.A., Fleckenstein, B., Jahn, G., Galloway, D.A., and McDougall, J.K., Structure of the transforming region of human cytomegalovirus AD169, *J. Virol.,* 49, 109, 1984.

73. Pande, H., Baak, S.W., Riggs, A.D., Clark, B.R., Shively, J.E., and Zaia, J.A., Cloning and physical mapping of a gene fragment coding a 64-kilodalton major late antigen of human cytomegalovirus, *Proc. Natl. Acad. Sci. U.S.A.,* 81, 4965, 1984.

74. Beck, S. and Barrell, B.G., Human cytomegalovirus encodes a glycoprotein homologous to MHC class-I antigens, *Nature,* 331, 269, 1988.

75. Rasmussen, R.D., Staprans, S.I., Shaw, S.B., and Spector, D.H., Sequences in human cytomegalovirus which hybridize with the avian retrovirus oncogene v-*myc* are G+C rich and do not hybridize with the human c-*myc* gene, *Mol. Cell. Biol.,* 5, 1525, 1985.

76. Clanton, D.J., Jariwalla, R.J., Kress, C., and Rosenthal, L.J., Neoplastic transformation by a cloned human cytomegalovirus DNA fragment uniquely homologous to one of the transforming regions of herpes simplex virus type 2, *Proc. Natl. Acad. Sci. U.S.A.,* 80, 3826, 1983.

77. Sergiescu, D., Activation of an endogenous mouse type C virus by UV-irradiated murine cytomegalovirus, *Int. J. Cancer,* 29, 459, 1982.

78. Fletcher, K., Cordiner, J.W., and MacNab, J.C.M., Detection of sequences that hybridize to human cytomegalovirus DNA in cervical neoplastic tissue, *Disease Markers,* 4, 219, 1986.

79. Desgranges, C., Seigneurin, J.-M., Baccard, M., and Nejmi, S., Cytomegalovirus isolations from cell cultures derived from Epstein-Barr virus-associated nasopharyngeal carcinoma, *J. Natl. Cancer Inst.,* 71, 39, 1983.

80. Huang, E.-S., Cytomegalovirus: its oncogenes and Kaposi's sarcoma, *Antibiot. Chemother.,* 32, 27, 1984.

81. Roizman, B., Carmichael, L.E., Deinhardt, F., de-Thé. G., Nahmias, A.J., Plowright, W., Rapp, F., Sheldrick, P., Takahashi, M., and Wolf, K., Herpesviridae: definition, provisional nomenclature, and taxonomy, *Intervirology,* 16, 201, 1981.

82. Granoff, A., Herpesvirus and the frog renal adenocarcinoma, *Fed. Proc. Fed. Am. Soc. Exp. Biol.,* 31, 1626, 1972.

83. Naegele, R.F., Granoff, A., and Darlington, R.W., The presence of the Lucké herpesvirus genome in induced tadpole tumors and its oncogenicity: Koch-Henle postulates fulfilled, *Proc. Natl. Acad. Sci. U.S.A.,* 71, 830, 1974.

84. Naegele, R.F. and Granoff, A., Viruses and renal carcinoma of *Rana pipiens.* XV. The presence of virus-associated membrane antigen(s) on Lucké tumor cells, *Int. J. Cancer,* 19, 414, 1977.

85. Wildy, P., Herpesvirus, Intervirology, 25, 117, 1986.

86. Vonka, V., Kanka, J., Hirsch, I., Zavadova, H., Krcmar, M., Suchankova, A., Rezacova, D., Broucek, J., Press, M., Domorazkova, E., Svoboda, B., Havrankova, A., and Jelinek, J., Prospective study of the relationship between cervical neoplasia and herpes simplex virus type-2 virus. II. Herpes simplex type-2 antibody presence in sera taken at enrolment, *Int. J. Cancer,* 33, 61, 1984.

87. Prakash, S.S., Reeves, W.C., Sisson, G.R., Brenes, M., Godoy, J., Bacchetti, S., de Britton, R.C., and Rawls, W.E., Herpes simplex virus type 2 and human papillomavirus type 16 in cervicitis, dysplasia and invasive cervical carcinoma, *Int. J. Cancer,* 35, 51, 1985.

88. Berman, P.W., Gregory, T., Crase, D., and Lasky, L.A., Protection from genital herpes simplex virus type 2 infection by vaccination with cloned type 1 glycoprotein D, *Science,* 227, 1490, 1985.

89. Umene, K., Sakaki, Y., Morl, R., and Takagi, Y., Isolation of human DNAs homologous to the *Bam*HI-Z fragment of *Herpesvirus simplex* type 1 DNA, *Gene,* 31, 9, 1984.

90. Galloway, D.A., Nelson, J.A., and McDougall, J.K., Small fragments of herpesvirus DNA with transforming activity contain insertion sequence-like structures, *Proc. Natl. Acad. Sci. U.S.A.,* 81, 4736, 1984.

91. Puga, A., Gomez-Marquez, J., Brayton, P.R., Cantin, E.M., Long, L.K., Barbacid, M., and Notkins, A.L., The immediate-early enhancer element of herpes simplex virus type 1 can replace a regulatory region of the c-Ha-*ras* 1 oncogene required for transformation, *J. Virol.,* 54, 879, 1985.

92. Huszar, D. and Bacchetti, S., Is ribonucleotide reductase the transforming function of herpes simplex virus 2?, *Nature,* 301, 76, 1983.

93. Hayashi, Y., Iwasawa, T., Smith, C.C., Aurelian, L., Lewis, G.K., and Ts'o, P.O.P., Multistep transformation by defined fragments of herpes simplex virus type 2 DNA: oncogenic region and its gene product, *Proc. Natl. Acad. Sci. U.S.A.,* 82, 8493, 1985.

94. Jariwalla, R.J., Tanczos, B., Jones, C., Ortiz, J., and Salimi-Lopez, S., DNA amplification and neoplastic transformation mediated by a herpes simplex DNA fragment containing cell-related sequences, *Proc. Natl. Acad. Sci. U.S.A.,* 83, 1738, 1986.

95. Bejcek, B. and Conley, A.J., A transforming plasmid from HSV-2 transformed cells contains rat DNA homologous to the HSV-1 and HSV-2 genomes, *Virology,* 154, 41, 1986.

96. Manservigi, R., Cassai, E., Deiss, L.P., Di Luca, D., Segala, V., and Frenkel, N., Sequences homologous to two separate transforming regions of herpes simplex virus DNA are linked in two human genital tumors, *Virology,* 155, 192, 1986.

97. Macnab, J.C.M. and La Thangue, N.B., Cellular proteins expressed in herpes simplex virus transformed cells also accumulate on herpes simplex virus infection, *EMBO J.,* 3223, 1985.

98. Kemp, L.M., Preston, C.M., Preston, V.G., and Latchman, D.S., Cellular gene induction during herpes simplex virus infection can occur without viral protein synthesis, *Nucleic Acids Res.,* 14, 9261, 1986.

99. Goswami, B.B., Transcriptional induction of proto-oncogene *fos* by HSV-2, *Biochem. Biophys. Res. Commun.,* 143, 1055, 1987.

100. Johnson, F.B., Chemical interactions with herpes simplex type 2 virus: enhancement of transformation by selected chemical carcinogens and procarcinogens, *Carcinogenesis,* 3, 1235, 1982.

101. Kamine, J., Bakker, A., and Desrosiers, R.C., Mapping of RNA transcribed from a region of the *Herpesvirus saimiri* genome required for oncogenicity, *J. Virol.,* 52, 532, 1984.

102. Desrosiers, R.C., Bakker, A., Kamine, J., Falk, L.A., Hunt, R.D., and King, N.W., a region of the *Herpesvirus samiri* genome required for oncogenicity, *Science,* 228, 184, 1985.

103. Schat, K.A., Marek's disease: a model for protection against herpesvirus-induced tumours, *Cancer Surv.,* 6, 1, 1987.

104. Salahuddin, S.Z., Ablashi, D.V., Markham, P.D., Josephs, S.F., Sturzenegger, S., Kaplan, M., Halligan, G., Biberfeld, P., Wong-Staal, F., Kramarsky, B., and Gallo, R.C., Isolation of a new virus, HBLV, in patients with lymphoproliferative disorders, *Science,* 234, 596, 1986.

105. Josephs, S.F., Buchbinder, A., Streicher, H.Z., Ablashi, D.V., Salahuddin, S.Z., Guo, H.-G., Wong-Staal, F., Cossman, J., Raffeld, M., Sundeen, J., Levine, P., Biggar, R., Krueger, G.R.F., Fox, R.I., and Gallo, R.C., Detection of human B-lymphotropic virus (human herpesvirus 6) sequences in B cell lymphoma tissues of three patients, *Leukemia,* 2, 132, 1988.

106. Josephs, S.F., Salahuddin, S.Z., Ablashi, D.V., Schachter, F., Wong-Staal, F., and Gallo, R.C., Genomic analysis of the human B-lymphotropic virus (HBLV), *Science,* 234, 601, 1986.

107. Szmuness, W., Hepatocellular carcinoma and the hepatitis B virus: evidence for a causal association, *Progr. Med. Virol.,* 24, 40, 1978.

108. Shafritz, D.A., Hepatitis B virus DNA molecules in the liver of HBsAg carriers: mechanistic considerations in the pathogenesis of hepatocellular carcinoma, *Hepatology,* 2, 35S, 1982.

109. Blumberg, B.S. and London, W.T., Hepatitis B virus: pathogenesis and prevention of primary cancer of the liver, *Cancer,* 50, 2657, 1982.

110. Eisenburg, J., Die Virus-induzierten Lebererkrankungen des Menschen. III. Chronische Hepatitis, *Naturwissenschaften,* 70, 79, 1983.

111. Blumberg, B.S. and London, W.T., Hepatitis B virus and the prevention of primary cancer of the liver, *J. Natl. Cancer Inst.,* 74, 267, 1985.

112. Grob, P.J., Leberzellkarzinom, Hepatitis-B-Virus, und Immunsystem, *Schweiz. Med. Wochenschr.,* 116, 1133, 1986.

113. Bréchot, C., Hepatitis B virus and hepatocellular carcinoma, *Bull. Inst. Pasteur (Paris),* 85, 125, 1987.

114. Beasley, R.P., Hepatitis B virus — the major etiology of hepatocellular carcinoma, *Cancer,* 61, 1942, 1988.

115. Hsu, H.-C., Wu, M.-Z., Chang, M.-H., Su, I.-J., and Chen, D.-S., Childhood hepatocellular carcinoma develops exclusively in hepatitis B surface antigen carriers in three decades in Taiwan: report of 51 cases strongly associated with rapid development of liver cirrhosis, *J. Hepatol.,* 5, 260, 1987.

116. Melbye, M., Skinhoj, P., Nielsen, N.H., Vestergaard, B.F., Ebbesen, P., Hansen, J.P.H., and Biggar, R.J., Virus-associated cancers in Greenland: frequent hepatitis B virus infection but low primary hepatocellular carcinoma incidence, *J. Natl. Cancer Inst.,* 73, 1267, 1984.

117. Zhou, Y.-Z., Butel, J.S., Li, P.-J., Finegold, M.J., and Melnick, J.L., Integrated state of subgenomic fragments of hepatitis B virus DNA in hepatocellular carcinoma from mainland China, *J. Natl. Cancer Inst.,* 79, 223, 1987.

118. Wogan, G.N., Dietary factors and special epidemilogical situation of liver cancer in Thailand and Africa, *Cancer Res.,* 35, 3499, 1975.

119. Ono, Y., Onda, H., Sasada, R., Igarashi, K., Sugino, Y., and Nishioka, K., The complete nucleotide sequences of the cloned hepatitis B virus DNA, subtype adr and adw, *Nucleic Acids Res.,* 11, 1747, 1983.

120. Summers, J. and Mason, W.S., Replication of the genome of a hepatitis B-like virus by reverse transcription of an RNA intermediate, *Cell,* 29, 403, 1982.

121. Miller, R.H. and Robinson, W.S., Common evolutionary origin of hepatitis B virus and retroviruses, *Proc. Natl. Acad. Sci. U.S.A.,* 83, 2531, 1986.

122. Miller, R.H., Close evolutionary relatedness of the hepatitis B virus and murine leukemia virus polymerase gene sequences, *Virology,* 164, 147, 1988.

123. Will, H., Salfeld, J., Pfaff, E., Manso, C., Theilmann, L., and Schaler, H., Putative reverse transcriptase intermediates of human hepatitis B virus in primary liver carcinomas, *Science,* 231, 594, 1986.

124. Yaginuma, K., Kobayashi, H., Kobayashi, M., Morishima, T., Matsuyama, K., and Koike, K., Multiple integration site of hepatitis B virus DNA in hepatocellular carcinoma and chronic active hepatitis tissues from children, *J. Virol.,* 61, 1808, 1987.

125. Esumi, M., Arikata, T., Arii, M., Suzuki, K., Tanikawa, K., Mizuo, H., Mima, T., and Shikata, T., Clonal origin of human hepatoma determined by integration of hepatitis B virus DNA, *Cancer Res.,* 46, 5757, 1986.

126. Bowyer, S.M., Dusheiko, G.M., Schoub, B.D., and Kew, M.C., Expression of the hepatitis B virus genome in chronic hepatitis B carriers and patients with hepatocellular carcinoma, *Proc. Natl. Acad. Sci. U.S.A.,* 84, 847, 1987.

127. Siddiqui, A., Hepatitis B virus DNA in Kaposi sarcoma, *Proc. Natl. Acad. Sci. U.S.A.,* 80, 4861, 1983.

128. Yaginuma, K., Kobayashi, M., Yoshida, E., and Koike, K., Hepatitis B virus integration in hepatocellular carcinoma DNA: duplication of cellular flanking sequences at the integration site, *Proc. Natl. Acad. Sci. U.S.A.,* 82, 4458, 1985.

129. Ziemer, M., Garcia, P., Shaul, Y., and Rutter, W.J., Sequence of hepatitis B virus DNA incorporated into the genome of a human hepatoma cell line, *J. Virol.,* 53, 885, 1985.

130. Tur-Kaspa, R., Burk, R.D., Shaul, Y., and Shafritz, D.A., Hepatitis B virus DNA contains a glucocorticoid-responsive element, *Proc. Natl. Acad. Sci. U.S.A.,* 83, 1627, 1986.

131. Ou, J. and Rutter, W.J., Hybrid hepatitis B virus-host transcripts in a human hepatoma cell, *Proc. Natl. Acad. Sci. U.S.A.,* 82, 83, 1985.

132. Rogler, C.E., Sherman, M., Su, C.Y., Shafritz, D.A., Summers, J., Shows, T.B., Henderson, A., and Kew, M., Deletion in chromosome 11p associated with a hepatitis B integration site in hepatocellular carcinoma, *Science,* 230, 319, 1985.

133. Yunis, J.J. and Ramsay, N.K.C., Familial occurrence of the aniridia-Wilms' tumor syndrome with deletion 11p13-14.1, *J. Pediat.,* 96, 1027, 1980.

134. Kaneko, Y., Egues, M.C., and Rowley, J.D., Interstitial deletion of short arm of chromosome 11 limited to Wilms' tumor cells in a patient without aniridia, *Cancer Res.,* 41, 4577, 1981.

135. Hino, O., Shows, T.B., and Rogler, C.E., Hepatitis b virus integration site in hepatocellular carcinoma at chromosome 17;18 translocation, *Proc. Natl. Acad. Sci. U.S.A.,* 83, 8338, 1986.

136. Mizusawa, H., Taira, M., Taginuma, K., Kobayashi, M., Yoshida, E., and Koire, K., Inversely repeating integrated hepatitis B virus DNA and cellular flanking sequences in the human hepatoma-derived cell line huSP, *Proc. Natl. Acad. Sci. U.S.A.,* 82, 208, 1985.

137. Dejean, A., Bougueleret, L., Grzeschik, K.-H., and Tiollais, P., Hepatitis B virus DNA integration in a sequence homologous to v-*erb-A* and steroid receptor genes in a hepatocellular carcinoma, *Nature,* 322, 70, 1986.

138. Morizane, T., Nakamura, T., Saito, H., Watanabe, T., Inagaki, Y., Satoh, I., Tsuchimoto, K., and Tsuchiya, M., Transformation of NIH/3T3 cells by DNA from a human hepatoma cell line with integrated hepatitis B virus DNA, *Eur. J. Cancer Clin. Oncol.,* 23, 163, 1987.

139. Ogston, C.W., Jonak, G.J., Rogler, C.E., Astrin, S.M., and Summers, J., Cloning and structural analysis of integrated woodchuck hepatitis virus sequences from hepatocellular carcinomas of woodchucks, *Cell,* 29, 385, 1982.

140. Möröy, T., Marchio, A., Etiemble, J., Trépo, C., Tiollais, P., and Buendia, M.-A., Rearrangement and enhanced expression of c-*myc* in hepatocellular carcinoma of hepatitis virus infected woodchucks, *Nature,* 324, 276, 1986.

141. McBride, W.D. and Wiener, A., *In vitro* transformation of hamster kidney cells by human adenovirus type 12, *Proc. Soc. Exp. Biol. Med.,* 115, 870, 1964.

142. Flint, S.J., Organization and expression of viral genes in adenovirus-transformed cells, *Int. Rev. Cytol.,* 76, 47, 1982.

143. Graham, F.L., Rowe, D.T., McKinnon, R., Bacchetti, S., Ruben, M., and Branton, P.E., Transformation by human adenoviruses, *J. Cell. Physiol.,* Suppl. 3, 151, 1984.

144. Bernards, R. and van der Eb, A.J., Adenovirus: transformation and oncogenicity, *Biochim. Biophys. Acta,* 783, 187, 1984.

145. Branton, P.E., Bayley, S.T., and Graham, F.L., Transformation by human adenoviruses, *Biochim. Biophys. Acta,* 780, 67, 1985.

146. Ivankovic, S., Entstehung von subcutanen Sarkomen bei Nachkommen von syrischen Goldhamstern nach Behandlung mit Adeno 12 Virus während der Schwangerschaft, *Z. Krebsforsch.,* 88, 323, 1977.

147. Huebner, R.J., Adenovirus-directed tumor and T-antigens, *Persp. Virol.,* 5, 147, 1967.

148. Bos, J.L. and van der Eb, A.J., Adenovirus region EIA: transcription modulator and transforming agent, *Trends Biochem. Sci.,* 10, 310, 1985.

149. Jonsson, N. and Ankerst, J., Studies on adenovirus type 9 induced mammary fibroadenomas in rats and their malignant transformation, *Cancer,* 39, 2513, 1977.

150. Brusca, J.S., Jannun, R., and Chinnadurai, G., Efficient transformation of rat 3Y1 cells by human adenovirus type 9, *Virology,* 136, 328, 1984.

151. Woodworth, C.D. and Isom, H.C., Transformation of differentiated rat hepatocytes with adenovirus and adenovirus DNA, *J. Virol.,* 61, 3570, 1987.

152. Mukai, N., Kalter, S.S., Cummins, L.B., Matthews, V.A., Nishida, T., and Nakajima, T., Retinal tumor induced in the baboon by human adenovirus 12, *Science,* 210, 1023, 1980.

153. Mak, S., Mak, I., Gallie, B.L., Godbout, R., and Phillips, R.A., Adenovirus-12 genes undetectable in human retinoblastoma, *Int. J. Cancer,* 30, 697, 1982.

154. Berk, A.J., Functions of adenovirus E1A, *Cancer Surv.,* 5, 367, 1986.

155. Stillman, B., Functions of the adenovirus E1B tumour antigens, *Cancer Surv.,* 5, 389, 1986.

156. Grand, R.J.A., The structure and functions of the adenovirus early region I proteins, *Biochem. J.,* 241, 25, 1987.

157. Nevins, J.R., Regulation of early adenovirus gene expression, *Microbiol. Rev.,* 51, 419, 1987.

158. Dery, C.V., Herrmann, C.H., and Mathews, M.B., Response of individual adenovirus promoters to the products of the E1A gene, *Oncogene,* 2, 15, 1987.

159. Stabel, S., Argos, P., and Philipson, L., The release of growth arrest by microinjection of adenovirus E1A DNA, *EMBO J.,* 4, 2329, 1985.

160. Boeuf, H., Zajchowski, D.A., Tamura, T., Hauss, C., and Kédinger, C., Specific cellular proteins bind to critical promoter sequences of the adenovirus early EIIa promoter, *Nucleic Acids Res.,* 15, 509, 1987.

161. Herrmann, C.H., Dery, C.V., and Mathews, M.B., Transactivation of host and viral genes by the adenovirus E1B 19K tumor antigen, *Oncogene,* 2, 25, 1987.

162. Rosenfeld, P.J., O'Neill, E.A., Wides, R.J., and Kelly, T.J., Sequence-specific interactions between cellular DNA-binding proteins and the adenovirus origin of DNA replication, *Mol. Cell. Biol.,* 7, 875, 1987.

163. Schellner, J., Stüber, K., and Doerfler, W., Computer analyses on the structure of junction sites between adenovirus DNA and cellular DNA, *Biochim. Biophys. Acta,* 867, 114, 1986.

164. Schulz, M., Freisem-Rabien, U., Jessberger, R., and Doerfler, W., Transcriptional activities of mammalian genomes at sites of recombination with foreign DNA, *J. Virol.,* 61, 344, 1987.

165. Lichtenberg, U., Zock, C., and Doerfler, W., Insertion of adenovirus type 12 DNA in the vicinity of an intracisternal A particle genome in Syrian hamster tumor cells, *J. Virol.,* 61, 2719, 1987.

166. Casto, B.C., Pieczynski, W.J., and DiPaolo, J.A., Enhancement of adenovirus transformation by treatment of hamster embryo cells with diverse chemical carcinogens, *Cancer Res.,* 34, 72, 1974.

167. Mak, I., Galet, H., and Mak, S., Adenovirus 12 nononcogenic mutants: oncogenicity of transformed cells and viral proteins synthesized *in vivo* and *in vitro, J. Virol.,* 52, 687, 1984.

168. Montell, C., Courtois, G., Eng, C., and Berk, A., Complete transformation by adenovirus 2 requires both E1A proteins, *Cell,* 36, 951, 1984.

169. Cone, R.D., Grodzicker, T., and Jaramillo, M., A retrovirus expressing the 12S adenoviral E1A gene product can immortalize epithelial cells from a broad range of rat tissues, *Mol. Cell. Biol.*, 8, 1036, 1988.

170. Senear, A.W. and Lewis, J.B., Morphological transformation of established rodent cell lines by high-level expression of the adenovirus type 2 E1a gene, *Mol. Cell. Biol.*, 6, 1253, 1986.

171. Kelekar, A. and Cole, M.D., Tumorigenicity of fibroblast lines expressing the adenovirus E1a, cellular p53, or normal c-*myc* genes, *Mol. Cell. Biol.*, 6, 7, 1986.

172. Byrd, P., Brown, K.W., and Gallimore, P.H., Malignant transformation of human embryo retinoblasts by cloned adenovirus 12 DNA, *Nature*, 298, 69, 1982.

173. Jochemsen, A.G., Peltenburg, L.T.C., te Pas, M.F.W., de Wit, C.M., Bos, J.L., and van der Eb, A.J., Activation of adenovirus 5 E1A transcription by region E1B in transformed primary rat cells, *EMBO J.*, 6, 3399, 1987.

174. Feldman, L.T., Imperiale, M.J., and Nevins, J.R., Activation of early adenovirus transcription by herpesvirus immediate early gene: evidence for a common cellular control factor, *Proc. Natl. Acad. Sci. U.S.A.*, 79, 4952, 1982.

175. Perricaudet, M., Akusjarvi, G., Virtanen, A., and Peterson, U., Structure of two spliced mRNAs from the transforming region of human subgroup C adenoviruses, *Nature*, 281, 694, 1979.

176. Kaczmarek, L., Ferguson, B., Rosenberg, M., and Baserga, R., Induction of cellular DNA synthesis by purified adenovirus E1A proteins, *Virology*, 152, 1, 1986.

177. Zerler, B., Roberts, R.J., Mathews, M.B., and Moran, E., Different functional domains of the adenovirus E1A gene are involved in regulation of host cell cycle products, *Mol. Cell. Biol.*, 7, 821, 1987.

178. Hurwitz, S., and Chinnadurai, G., Evidence that a second tumor antigen coded by adenovirus early gene region E1A is required for efficient cell transformation, *Proc. Natl. Acad. Sci. U.S.A.*, 82, 163, 1985.

179. Babiss, L.E., Liaw, W.-S., Zimmer, S.G., Godman, G.C., Ginsberg, H.S., and Fisher, P.B., Mutations in the *E1a* gene of adenovirus type 5 alter the tumorigenic properties of transformed cloned rat embryo fibroblast cells, *Proc. Natl. Acad. Sci. U.S.A.*, 83, 2167, 1986.

180. Murphy, M., Opalka, B., Sajaczkowski, R., and Schulte-Holthausen, H., Definition of a region required for transformation in E1a of adenovirus 12, *Virology*, 159, 49, 1987.

181. Jochemsen, H., Daniels, G.S.G., Hertoghs, J.J.L., Schrier, P.I., van den Elsen, P.J., and van der Eb, A.J., Identification of adenovirus-type 12 gene products involved in transformation and oncogenesis, *Virology*, 122, 15, 1982.

182. Moran, E., Grodzicker, T., Roberts, R.J., Mathews, M.B., and Zerler, B., Lytic and transforming functions of individual products of the adenovirus E1A gene, *J. Virol.*, 57, 765, 1986.

183. Ruley, H.E., Adenovirus early region 1A enables viral and cellular transforming genes to transform primary cells in culture, *Nature*, 304, 602, 1983.

184. Zerler, B., Moran, B., Maruyama, K., Moomaw, J., Grodzicker, T., and Ruley, H.E., Adenovirus E1A coding sequences that enable *ras* and *pmt* oncogenes to transform cultured primary cells, *Mol. Cell. Biol.*, 6, 887, 1986.

185. Moran, B. and Zerler, B., Interactions between cell growth-regulating domains in the products of the adenovirus E1A oncogene, *Mol. Cell. Biol.*, 8, 1756, 1988.

186. Jochemsen, A.G., Bernards, R., van Kranen, H.J., Houweling, A., Bos, J.L., and van der Eb, A.J., Different activities of the adenovirus types 5 and 12 E1A regions in transformation with the EJ Ha-*ras* oncogene, *J. Virol.*, 59, 684, 1986.

187. Braithwaite, A.W., Lejeune, S., and Naora, H., Adenoviruses have homology with a reiterated sequence in genomic DNA, *DNA*, 3, 223, 1984.

188. Ralston, R. and Bishop, J.M., The protein products of the *myc* and *myb* oncogenes and adenovirus E1a are structurally related, *Nature*, 306, 803, 1983.

189. McLachlan, A.D. and Boswell, D.R., Confidence limits for homology in protein or gene sequences: the c-*myc* oncogene and adenovirus E1a protein, *J. Mol. Biol.*, 185, 39, 1985.

190. Ghrist, B.F.D. and Ricciardi, R.P., How reliable is amino acid sequence homology in predicting similarity of structure and function of c-myc and Ad12 E1A oncogenic proteins?, *J. Mol. Evol.*, 23, 177, 1986.

191. Krippl, B., Ferguson, B., Jones, N., Rosenberg, M., and Westphal, H., Mapping of functional domains in adenovirus E1A proteins, *Proc. Natl. Acad. Sci. U.S.A.*, 82, 7480, 1985.

192. Lyons, R.H., Ferguson, B.Q., and Rosenberg, M., Pentapeptide nuclear localization signal in adenovirus E1a, *Mol. Cell. Biol.*, 7, 2451, 1987.

193. Schmitt, R.C., Fahnenstock, M.L., and Lewis, J.B., Differential nuclear localization of the major adenovirus type 2 E1a proteins, *J. Virol.*, 61, 247, 1987.

194. Blair Zajdel, M.E., Barker, M.D., Dixon, S.C., and Blair, G.E., The use of monoclonal antibodies to study the proteins specificied by the transforming region of human adenoviruses, *Biochem. J.*, 225, 649, 1985.

195. La Thangue, N.B. and Rigby, P.W.J., An adenovirus E1A-like transcription factor is regulated during the differentiation of murine embryonal carcinoma stem cells, *Cell*, 49, 507, 1987.

196. Subramanian, T., Kuppuswamy, M., Nasr, R.J., and Chinnadurai, G., An N-terminal region of adenovirus E1a essential for cell transformation and induction of an epithelial cell growth factor, *Oncogene*, 2, 105, 1988.

197. Kuppuswamy, M.N. and Chinnadurai, G., Relationship between the transforming and transcriptional regulatory functions of adenovirus 2 E1a oncogene, *Virology*, 159, 31, 1987.

198. Chatterjee, P.K. and Flint, S.J., Partition of E1A proteins between soluble and structural fractions of adenovirus-infected and -transformed cells, *J. Virol.*, 60, 1018, 1986.

199. Kao, H.-T. and Nevins, J.R., Alteration of cellular gene expression in adenovirus transformed cells by post-transcriptional mechanisms, *Nucleic Acids Res.*, 14, 7253, 1986.

200. Zantema, A., Schrier, P.I., Davis-Olivier, A., van Laar, T., Vaessen, R.T.M.J., and van der Eb, A.J., Adenovirus serotype determines association and localization of the large E1B tumor antigen with cellular tumor antigen p53 in transformed cells, *Mol. Cell. Biol.*, 5, 3084, 1985.

201. Subramanian, T., Kuppuswamy, M., Mak, S., and Chinnadurai, G., Adenovirus *cyt*⁺ locus, which controls cell transformation and tumorigenicity, is an allele of lp⁺ locus, which codes for a 19-kilodalton tumor antigen, *J. Virol.*, 52, 336, 1984.

202. Takemori, N., Cladara, C., Bhat, B., Conley, A.J., and Wold, W.S.M., *cyt* gene of adenoviruses 2 and 5 is an oncogene for transforming function in early region E1B and encodes the E1B 19,000-molecular-weight polypeptide, *J. Virol.*, 52, 793, 1984.

203. Liu, H.T., Baserga, R., and Mercer, W.E., Adenovirus type 2 activates cell cycle-dependent genes that are a subset of those activated by serum, *Mol. Cell. Biol.*, 5, 2936, 1985.

204. Braithwaite, A.W., Fry, K.E., LeJeune, S., and Naora, H., Altered regulation of c-*myc* expression in adenovirus-transformed cells, *Can. J. Genet. Cytol.*, 28, 712, 1986.

205. Wu, B.J. and Morimoto, R.I., Transcription of the human *hsp70* gene is induced by serum stimulation, *Proc. Natl. Acad. Sci. U.S.A.*, 82, 6070, 1985.

206. Grand, R.J.A. and Gallimore, P.H., Modulation of the level of expression of cellular genes in adenovirus 12-infected and transformed human cells, *EMBO J.*, 5, 1253, 1986.

207. Wu, B.J., Hurst, H.C., Jones, N.C., and Morimoto, R.I., The E1A 13S product of adenovirus 5 activates transcription of the cellular human HSP70 gene, *Mol. Cell. Biol.*, 6, 2994, 1986.

208. Webster, K.A., Muscat, G.E.O., and Kedes, L., Adenovirus E1A products suppress myogenic differentiation and inhibit transcription from muscle-specific promoters, *Nature*, 332, 553, 1988.

209. Schneider, J.F., Fisher, F., Goding, C.R., and Jones, N.C., Mutational analysis of the adenovirus E1a gene: the role of transcriptional regulation in transformation, *EMBO J.*, 6, 2053, 1987.

210. Eager, K.B., Sawicki, J.A., and Ricciardi, R.P., Cellular protein differences between nontumorigenic Ad5 and tumorigenic Ad12 transformed mouse cells, *Virology*, 152, 487, 1986.

211. Glaichenhaus, N., Léopold, P., and Cuzin, F., Increased levels of mitochondrial gene expression in rat fibroblast cells immortalized or transformed by viral and cellular oncogenes, *EMBO J.*, 5, 1261, 1986.

212. Babiss, L.E., Zimmer, S.G., and Fisher, P.B., Reversibility of progression of the transformed phenotype in Ad5-transformed rat embryo cells, *Science*, 228, 2099, 1985.

213. Vogel, S., Rosahl, T., and Doerfler, W., Chromosomal localization of integrated adenovirus DNA in productively infected and transformed mammalian cells, *Virology*, 152, 159, 1986.

214. Blair, G.E. and Russell, W.C., Identification of a protein kinase activity associated with human adenovirus, *Virology*, 86, 157, 1978.

215. Tsuzuki, J. and Luftig, R.B., An unexpected effect of divalent cations on the adenovirus endogenous protein kinase: alteration in the specificity of phosphorylation, *Virus Res.*, 2, 95, 1985.

216. Milo, G.E., Jr., Schaller, J.P., and Yohn, D.S., Hormonal modification of adenovirus transformation of hamster cells *in vitro*, *Cancer Res.*, 32, 2338, 1972.

217. Kelekar, A. and Cole, M.D., Immortalization by c-*myc*, H-*ras*, and E1a oncogenes induces differential cellular gene expression and growth factor responses, *Mol. Cell. Biol.*, 7, 3899, 1987.

218. Sircar, S. and Weber, J.M., Normalization of epidermal growth factor receptor and transforming growth factor production in drug resistant variants derived from adenovirus transformed cells, *J. Cell. Physiol.*, 134, 467, 1988.

219. Babiss, L.E., Ginsberg, H.S., and Fisher, P.B., Cold-sensitive expression of transformation by a host-range mutant of type 5 adenovirus, *Proc. Natl. Acad. Sci. U.S.A.*, 80, 1352, 1983.

220. Guernsey, D.L., Duigou, G.J., Babiss, L.E., and Fisher, P.B., Regulation of thyroidal inducibility of Na,K-ATPase and binding of epidermal growth factor in wild-type and cold-sensitive E1a mutant type 5 adenovirus-transformed CREF cells, *J. Cell. Physiol.*, 133, 507, 1987.

221. Cook, J.L., Walker, T.A., Lewis, A.M., Jr., Ruley, H.E., Graham, F.L., and Pilder, S.H., Expression of the adenovirus *E1A* oncogene during cell transformation is sufficient to induce susceptibility to lysis by host inflammatory cells, *Proc. Natl. Acad. Sci. U.S.A.*, 83, 6965, 1986.

222. Bernards, R., Schrier, P.I., Houweling, A., Bos, J.L., van der Eb, A.J., Zijlstra, M., and Melief, C.J.M., Tumorigenicity of cells transformed by adenovirus type 12 by evasion of T-cell immunity, *Nature*, 305, 776, 1983.

223. Vasavada, R., Eager, K.B., Barbanti-Brodano, G., Caputo, A., and Ricciardi. R.P., Adenovirus type 12 early region 1a proteins repress class I HLA expression in transformed human cells, *Proc. Natl. Acad. Sci. U.S.A.*, 83, 5257, 1986.

224. Tanaka, K., Isselbacher, K.J., Khoury, G., and Jay, G., Reversal of oncogenesis by the expression of a major histocompatibility complex class I gene, *Science*, 228, 26, 1985.

225. Tanaka, K., Hayashi, H., Hamada, C., Khoury, G., and Jay, G., Expression of major histocompatibility complex class I antigens as a strategy for the potentiation of immune recognition of tumor cells, *Proc. Natl. Acad. Sci. U.S.A.*, 83, 8723, 1986.

226. Haddada, H., Lewis, A.M., Jr., Sogn, J.A., Coligan, J.E., Cook, J.L., and Walker, T.A., Tumorigenicty of hamster and mouse cells transformed by adenovirus types 2 and 5 is not influenced by the level of class I major histocompatibility antigens expressed on the cells, *Proc. Natl. Acad. Sci. U.S.A.*, 83, 9684, 1986.

227. Hen, R., Borrelli, E., and Chambon, P., Repression of the immunoglobulin heavy chain enhancer by the adenovirus-2 E1A products, *Science*, 230, 1391, 1985.

228. Montano, X. and Lane, D.P., The adenovirus E1a gene induces differentiation of F9 teratocarcinoma cells, *Mol. Cell. Biol.*, 1782, 1987.

229. Müller, R. and Wagner, E.F., Differentiation of F9 teratocarcinoma stem cells after transfer of c-*fos* proto-oncogenes, *Nature*, 311, 438, 1984.

230. Gissmann, L., Papillomaviruses and their association with cancer in animals and in man, *Cancer Surv.*, 3, 161, 1984.

231. Smith, K.T. and Campo, M.S., The biology of papillomaviruses and their role in oncogenesis, *Anticancer Res.*, 5, 31, 1985.

232. McCance, D.J., Human papillomaviruses and cancer, *Biochim. Biophys. Acta*, 823, 195, 1986.

233. Brescia, R.J., Jenson, A.B., Lancaster, W.D., and Kurman, R.J., The role of human papillomaviruses in the pathogenesis and histologic classification of precancerous lesions of the cervix, *Hum. Pathol.*, 17, 552, 1986.

234. Giri, I. and Danos, O., Papillomavirus genomes: from sequence data to biological properties, *Trends Genet.*, 2, 227, 1986.

235. Syrjänen, K.J., Biology of human papillomavirus (HPV) infections and their role in squamous cell carcinogenesis, *Med. Biol.*, 65, 21, 1987.

236. zur Hausen, H., Papillomaviruses in human cancer, *Cancer*, 59, 1692, 1987.

237. Campo, M.S., Papillomas and cancer in cattle, *Cancer Surv.*, 6, 39, 1987.

238. Pfister, H., Human papillomavirus and genital cancer, *Adv. Cancer Res.*, 48, 113, 1987.

239. Muñoz, N., Bosch, X., and Kaldor, J.M., Does human papillomavirus cause cervical cancer? The state of the epidemiological evidence, *Br. J. Cancer*, 57, 1, 1988.

240. Jarrett, W.F.H., Campo, M.S., O'Neil, B.W., Lairo, H.M., and Coggins, L.W., A novel bovine papillomavirus (BPV-6) causing true epithelial papillomas of the mammary gland skin: a member of a proposed new BPV subgroup, *Virology*, 136, 255, 1984.

241. Ostrow, R.S. and Faras, A.J., The molecular biology of human papillomaviruses and the pathogenesis of genital papillomas and neoplasms, *Cancer Metast. Rev.*, 6, 383, 1987.

242. Beaudenon, S., Kremsdorf, D., Obalek, S., Jablonska, S., Pehau-Arnaudet, G., Croissant, O., and Orth, G., Plurality of genital human papillomaviruses: characterization of two new types with distinct biological properties, *Virology*, 161, 374, 1987.

243. Kleiner, E., Dietrich, W., and Pfister, H., Differential regulation of papilloma virus early gene expression in transformed fibroblasts and carcinoma cell lines, *EMBO J.*, 5, 1945, 1986.

244. Gloss, B., Bernard, H.U., Seedorf, K., and Glock, G., The upstream regulatory region of the human papilloma virus-16 contains an E2 protein-independent enhancer which is specific for cervical carcinoma cells and regulated by glucocorticoid hormones, *EMBO J.*, 6, 3735, 1987.

245. zur Hausen, H., Gissmann, L., and Schlehofer, J.R., Viruses in the etiology of human genital cancer, *Progr. Med. Virol.*, 30, 170, 1984.

246. Coleman, D.V. and Richman, P.I., Human papillomavirus infection and cancer of the uterine cervix, *J. Pathol.*, 145, 207, 1985.

247. Beaudenon, S., Kremsdorf, D., Croissant, O., Jablonska, S., Wain-Hobson, S., and Orth, G., A novel type of human papillomavirus associated with genital neoplasias, *Nature*, 321, 246, 1986.

248. Lorincz, A.T., Temple, G.F., Kurman, R.J., Jenson, A.B., and Lancaster, W.D., Oncogenic association of specific papillomavirus types with cervical neoplasia, *J. Natl. Cancer Inst.*, 79, 671, 1987.

249. Gupta, J., Pilotti, S., Rilke, F., and Shah, K., Association of human papillomavirus type 16 with neoplastic lesions of the vulva and other genital sites by *in situ* hybridization, *Am. J. Pathol.*, 127, 206, 1987.

250. Schwarz, E., Freese, U.K., Gissmann, L., Mayer, W., Roggenbuck, B., Stremlau, A., and zur Hausen, H., Structure and transcription of human papillomavirus sequences in cervical carcinoma cells, *Nature*, 314, 111, 1985.

251. Crum, C.P., Ikenberg, H., Richart, R.M., and Gissman, L., Human papillomavirus type 16 and early cervical neoplasia, *N. Engl. J. Med.*, 310, 880, 1984.

252. Di Luca, D., Pilotti, S., Stefanon, B., Rotola, A., Monini, P., Tognon, M., De Palo, G., Rilke, F., and Cassai, E., Human papillomavirus type 16 DNA in genital tumours: a pathological and molecular analysis, *J. Gen. Virol.*, 67, 583, 1986.

253. Tomita, Y., Kubota, K., Kasai, T., Sekiya, S., Takamizawa, H., and Simizu, Detection of human papillomavirus DNA in genital warts, cervical dysplasias and neoplasias, *Intervirology*, 25, 151, 1986.

254. Pater, M.M., Dunne, J., Hogan, G., Ghatage, P., and Pater, A., Human papillomavirus types 16 and 18 sequences in early cervical neoplasia, *Virology,* 155, 13, 1986.

255. Toon, P.G., Arrand, J.R., Wilson, L.P., and Sharp, D.S., Human papillomavirus infection of the uterine cervix of women without cytological signs of neoplasia, *Br. Med. J.,* 293, 1261, 1986.

256. Fuchs, P.G., Girardi, F., and Pfister, H., Human papillomavirus DNA in normal, metaplastic, preneoplastic and neoplastic epithelia of the cervix uteri, *Int. J. Cancer,* 41, 41, 1988.

257. Reeves, W.C., Caussy, D., Brinton, L.A., Brenes, M.M., Montalvan, P., Gomez, B., de Britton, R.C., Morice, E., Gaitan, E., Loo de Lao, S., and Rawls, W.E., Case-control study of human papillomaviruses and cervical cancer in Latin America, *Int. J. Cancer,* 40, 450, 1987.

258. Ostrow, R.S., Manias, D.A., Clark, B.A., Okagaki, T., Twiggs, L.B., and Faras, A.J., Detection of human papillomavirus DNA in invasive carcinomas of the cervix by *in situ* hybridization, *Cancer Res.,* 47, 649, 1987.

259. Kjaer, S.K., de Villiers, E.-M., Haugaard, B.J., Christensen, R.B., Teisen, C., Moller, K.A., Poll, P., Jensen, H., Vestergaard, B.F., Lynge, E., and Jensen, O.M., Human papillomavirus, herpes simplex virus and cervical cancer incidence in Greenland and Denmark. A population-based cross-sectional study, *Int. J. Cancer,* 41, 518, 1988.

260. Dürst, M., Dzarlieva-Petrusevska, R.T., Boukamp, P., Fusenig, N.E., and Gissmann, L., Molecular and cytogenetic analysis of immortalized human primary keratinocytes obtained after transfection with human papillomavirus type 16 DNA, *Oncogene,* 1, 251, 1987.

261. Noda, T., Yajima, H., and Ito, Y., Progression of the phenotype of transformed cells after growth stimulation of cells by a human papillomavirus type 16 gene function, *J. Virol.,* 62, 313, 1988.

262. Groff, D.E. and Lancaster, W.D., Evidence that integration of virus DNA may not be necessary for maintenance of cell transformation, *Progr. Med. Virol.,* 29, 218, 1984.

263. Campo, M.S., Moar, M.H., Sartirana, M.L., Kennedy, I.M., and Jarrett, W.F.H., The presence of bovine papillomavirus type 4 DNA ius not required for the progression to, or the maintenance of, the malignant state in cancers of the alimentary canal in cattle, *EMBO J.,* 4, 1819, 1985.

264. Smith, K.T. and Campo, M.S., "Hit and run" transformation of mouse C127 cells by bovine papillomavirus type 4: the viral DNA is required for the initiation but not for maintenance of the transformed phenotype, *Virology,* 164, 39, 1988.

265. Lazo, P.A., Rearrangement of both alleles of human chromosome 8 in HeLa cells, one of them as a result of papillomavirus DNA integration, *J. Biol. Chem.,* 263, 360, 1988.

266. Lowy, D.R., Dvoretzky, I., Shober, R., Law, M.F., Engel, L., and Howley, P.M., In vitro tumorigenic transformation by a defined subgenomic fragment of bovine papillomavirus DNA, *Nature,* 287, 72, 1980.

267. Howley, P.M., The molecular biology of papillomavirus transformation, *Am. J. Pathol.,* 113, 414, 1983.

268. Yang, Y.-C., Okayama, H., and Howley, P.M., Bovine papillomavirus contains multiple transforming genes, *Proc. Natl. Acad. Sci. U.S.A.,* 82, 1030, 1985.

269. Stenlund, A., Zabielski, J., Ahola, H., Moreno-Lopez, J., and Pettersson, U., Messenger RNA from the transforming region of bovine papilloma virus type I, *J. Mol. Biol.,* 182, 541, 1985.

270. Patel, K.R., Smith, K.T., and Campo, M.S., The nucleotide sequence and genome organization of bovine papillomavirus type 4, *J. Gen. Virol.,* 2117, 1987.

271. Nakabayashi, Y., Chattopadhyay, S.K., and Lowy, D.R., The transforming function of bovine papillomavirus DNA, *Proc. Natl. Acad. Sci. U.S.A.,* 80, 5832, 1983.

272. Schiller, J.T., Vass, W.C., and Lowy, D.R., Identification of a second transforming region in bovine papillomavirus DNA, *Proc. Natl. Acad. Sci. U.S.A.,* 81, 7880, 1984.

273. Schiller, J.T., Vass, W.C., Vousden, K.H., and Lowy, D.R., E5 open reading frame of bovine papillomavirus type 1 encodes a transforming gene, *J. Virol.,* 57, 1, 1986.

274. DiMaio, D., Guralski, D., and Schiller, J.T., Translation of open reading frame E5 of bovine papillomavirus is required for its transforming activity, *Proc. Natl. Acad. Sci. U.S.A.,* 83, 1797, 1986.

275. Burckhardt, A., DiMaio, D., and Schlegel, R., Genetic and biochemical definition of the bovine papillomavirus E5 transforming protein, *EMBO J.,* 6, 2381, 1987.

276. Schlegel, R., Wade-Glass, M., Rabson, M.S., and Yang, Y.-C., The E5 transforming gene of bovine papillomavirus encodes a small hydrophobic polypeptide, *Science,* 233, 464, 1986.

277. Green, M. and Loewenstein, P.M., Demonstration that a chemically synthesized BPV1 oncoprotein and its C-terminal domain function to induce cellular DNA synthesis, *Cell,* 51, 795, 1987.

278. Androphy, E.J., Schiller, J.T., and Lowy, D.R., Identification of the protein encoded by the E6 transforming gene of bovine papillomavirus, *Science,* 230, 442, 1985.

279. Moskaluk, C. and Bastia, D., The *E2* "gene" of bovine papillomavirus encodes an enhancer-binding protein, *Proc. Natl. Acad. Sci. U.S.A.,* 84, 1215, 1987.

280. Jaskulski, D., Kaczmarek, L., and DiMaio, D., Stimulation of cellular DNA synthesis by wild type and mutant bovine papillomavirus DNA, *Biochem. Biophys. Res. Commun.,* 148, 86, 1987.

281. Pirisi, L., Yasumoto, S., Feller, M., Doniger, J., and DiPaolo, J.A., Transformation of human fibroblasts and keratinocytes with human papillomavirus type 16 DNA, *J. Virol.,* 61, 1061, 1987.

282. Yasumoto, S., Doniger, J., and DiPaolo, J.A., Differential early viral gene expression in two stages of human papillomavirus type 16 DNA-induced malignant transformation, *Mol. Cell. Biol.,* 7, 2165, 1987.

283. Watts, S.L., Phelps, W.C., Ostrow, R.S., Zachow, K.R., and Faras, A.J., Cellular transformation by human papillomavirus DNA *in vitro, Science,* 225, 634, 1984.

284. Green, M., Brackman, K.H., and Loewenstein, P.M., Rat embryo fibroblast cells expressing human papillomavirus 1a genes exhibit altered growth properties and tumorigenicity, *J. Virol.,* 60, 868, 1986.

285. Takebe, N., Tsunokawa, Y., Nozawa, S., Terada, M., and Sugimura, T., Conservation of E6 and E7 regions of human papillomavirus types 16 and 18 present in cervical cancers, *Biochem. Biophys. Res. Commun.,* 143, 837, 1987.

286. Androphy, E.J., Hubbert, N.L., Schiller, J.T., and Lowy, D.R., Identification of the HPV-16 E6 protein from transformed mouse cells and human cervical carcinoma cell lines, *EMBO J.,* 6, 989, 1987.

287. Cripe, T.P., Haugen, T.H., Turk, J.P., Tabatai, F., Schmid, P.G., III, Dürst, M., Gissmann, L., Roman, A., and Turek, P., Transcriptional regulation of the human papillomavirus-16 E6-E7 promoter by a keratinocyte-dependent enhancer, and by viral E2 *trans*-activator and repressor gene products: implications for cervical carcinogenesis, *EMBO J.,* 6, 3745, 1987.

288. Bedell, M.A., Jones, K.H., and Laimins, L.A., The E6-E7 region of human papillomavirus type 18 is sufficient for transformation of NIH 3T3 and Rat-1 cells, *J. Virol.,* 61, 3635, 1987.

289. Kanda, T., Furuno, A., and Yoshike, K., Human papillomavirus type 16 open reading frame E7 encodes a transforming gene for rat 3Y1 cells, *J. Virol.,* 62, 610, 1988.

290. Amtmann, E., Müller, K., Knapp, A., and Sauer, G., Reversion of bovine papillomavirus-induced transformation and immortalization by a xanthate compound, *Exp. Cell Res.,* 161, 541, 1985.

291. Dürst, M., Croce, C.M., Gissmann, L., Schwarz, E., and Huebner, K., Papillomavirus sequences integrate near cellular oncogenes in some cervical carcinomas, *Proc. Natl. Acad. Sci. U.S.A.,* 84, 1070, 1987.

292. Riou, G., Barrois, M., Tordjman, I., Dutroquay, V., and Gerard, O., Presence de genomes de papillomavirus et amplification des oncogenes c-*myc* et c-Ha-*ras* dans des cancers envahissants du col de l'uterus, *C.R. Acad. Sci. Paris,* 299, 575, 1984.

293. Lacey, M., Alpert, S., and Hanahan, D., Bovine papillomavirus genome elicits skin tumours in transgenic mice, *Nature,* 322, 609, 1986.

294. Macnab, J.C.M., Walkinshaw, S.A., Cordiner, J.W., and Clements, J.B., Human papillomavirus in clinically and histologically normal tissue of patients with genital cancer, *N. Engl. J. Med.,* 315, 1052, 1986.

295. Butel, J.S. and Melnick, J.L., The state of the viral genome in cells transformed by simian virus 40: a review, *Exp. Mol. Pathol.,* Aug 1972.

296. Diamandopoulos, G.T., Neoplastic transformation in vivo and in vitro of regenerating hamster hepatic cells by oncogenic DNA simian virus 40, *J. Natl. Cancer Inst.,* 52, 139, 1974.

297. Rachlin, J., Wollmann, R., and Dohrmann, G., Inoculation of simian virus 40 into pregnant hamsters can induce tumors in offspring, *Lab. Invest.,* 58, 26, 1988.

298. Sweet, B.H. and Hilleman, M.R., The vacuolating virus, SV40, *Proc. Soc. Exp. Biol. Med.,* 105, 420, 1960.

299. Chang, S.E., Keen, J., Lane, B.E., and Taylor-Papadimitriou, J., Establishment and characterization of SV40-transformed human breast epithelial cell lines, *Cancer Res.,* 42, 2040, 1982.

300. Sack, G.H., Jr., Human cell transformation by simian virus 40 — a review, *In Vitro,* 17, 1, 1981.

301. Van Doren, K. and Gluzman, Y., Efficient transformation of human fibroblasts by adenovirus-simian virus 40 recombinants, *Mol. Cell. Biol.,* 4, 1653, 1984.

302. Woodworth, C., Secott, T., and Isom, H.C., Transformation of rat hepatocytes by transfection with simian virus 40 DNA to yield proliferating differentiated cells, *Cancer Res.,* 46, 4018, 1986.

303. Chang, P.L., Gunby, J.L., Tomkins, D.J., Mak, I., Rosa, N.E., and Mak, S., Transformation of human cultured fibroblasts with plasmids carrying dominant selection markers and immortalizing potential, *Exp. Cell Res.,* 167, 407, 1986.

304. Reddel, R.R., Ke, Y., Gerwin, B.I., McMenamin, M.G., Lechner, J.F., Su, R.T., Brash, D.E., Park, J.-B., Rhim, J.S., and Harris, C.C., Transformation of human bronchial epithelial cells by infection with SV40 or adenovirus-12 SV40 hybrid virus, or transfection via strontium phosphate coprecipitation with a plasmid containing SV40 early region genes, *Cancer Res.,* 48, 1904, 1988.

305. Sager, R., Tanaka, K., Lau, C.C., Ebina, Y., and Anisowicz, A., Resistance of human cells to tumorigenesis induced by cloned transforming genes, *Proc. Natl. Acad. Sci. U.S.A.,* 80, 7601, 1983.

306. Mortimer, E., Lepow, M.L., Gold, E., Robbins, F.C., Burton, G.J., and Fraumeni, J.F., Jr., Long-term follow-up of persons inadvertently inoculated with SV40 as neonates, *N. Engl. J. Med.,* 305, 1517, 1981.

307. Scherneck, S., Lubbe, L., Geissler, E., Nisch, G., Rudolph, M., Wahlte, H., Weickmann, F., and Zimmermann, W., Detection of simian virus 40 related T-antigen in human meningiomas, *Zentralbl. Neurochir.,* 40, 121, 1979.

308. Krieg, P., Amtmann, E., Jonas, D., Fischer, H., Zang, K., and Sauer, G., Episomal simian virus 40 genomes in human brain tumors, *Proc. Natl. Acad. Sci. U.S.A.,* 78, 6446, 1981.

309. Krieg, P. and Scherer, G., Cloning of SV40 genomes from human brain tumors, *Virology,* 138, 336, 1984.

310. Butel, J.S., SV40 large T-antigen: dual oncogene, *Cancer Surv.,* 5, 343, 1986.

311. Mahon, K.A., Chepelinsky, A.B., Khillan, J.S., Overbeek, P.A., Piatigorsky, J., and Westphal, H., Oncogenesis of the lens in transgenic mice, *Science,* 235, 1622, 1987.

312. Hanahan, D., Heritable formation of pancreatic beta-cell tumours in transgenic mice expressing recombinant insulin/simian virus 40 oncogenes, *Nature,* 315, 115, 1985.

313. Efrat, S., Baekkeskov, S., Lane, D., and Hanahan, D., Coordinate expression of the endogenous p53 gene in beta cells of transgenic mice expressing hybrid insulin-SV40 T antigen genes, *EMBO J.,* 6, 2699, 1987.

314. Field, L.J., Atrial natriuretic factor-SV40 T antigen transgenes produce tumors and cardiac arrhythmias in mice, *Science,* 239, 1029, 1988.

315. Suda, Y., Aizawa, S., Hirai, S., Inoue, T., Furuta, Y., Suzuki, M., Hirohashi, S., and Ikawa, Y., Driven by the same Ig enhancer and SV40 T promoter *ras* induced lung adenomatous tumors, *myc* induced pre-B cell lymphomas and SV40 large T gene a variety of tumors in transgenic mice, *EMBO J.,* 6, 4055, 1987.

316. Crawford, L.V., Proteins of polyoma virus and SV40, *Br. Med. Bull.,* 29, 253, 1973.

317. Kim, C.H., Heath, K.C., Bertuch, A., and Hansen, U., Specific stimulation of simian virus 40 late transcription *in vitro* by a cellular factor binding the simian virus 40 21-base-pair repeat promoter element, *Proc. Natl. Acad. Sci. U.S.A.,* 84, 6025, 1987.

318. Chang, L.-S., Pater, M.M., Hutchinson, N.I., and Di Mayorca, G., Transformation by purified early genes of simian virus 40, *Virology,* 133, 341, 1984.

319. Weinberg, R.A., How does T antigen transform cells?, *Cell,* 11, 243, 1977.

320. Butel, J.S. and Jarvis, D.L., The plasma-membrane-associated form of SV40 large tumor antigen: biochemical and biological properties, *Biochim. Biophys. Acta,* 865, 171, 1986.

321. Stahl, H. and Knippers, R., The simian virus 40 large tumor antigen, *Biochim. Biophys. Acta,* 910, 1, 1987.

322. Carroll, R.B., Hager, L., and Dulbecco, R., Simian virus 40 T antigen binds to DNA, *Proc. Natl. Acad. Sci. U.S.A.,* 71, 3754, 1974.

323. Yoneda, Y., Arioka, T., Imamoto-Sonobe, N., Sugawa, H., Shimonishi, Y., and Uchida, T., Synthetic peptides containing a region of SV40 large T-antigen involved in nucelar localization direct the transport of proteins to tne nucleus, *Exp. Cell Res.,* 170, 439, 1987.

324. Simmons, D.T., DNA-binding region of the simian virus 40 tumor antigen, *J. Virol.,* 57, 776, 1986.

325. Carroll, R.B., Samad, R.B., Mann, A., Harper, J., and Anderson, C.W., RNA is covalently linked to SV40 large T antigen, *Oncogene,* 2, 437, 1988.

326. Bradley, M.K., Smith, T.F., Lathrop, R.H., Livingston, D.M., and Webster, T.A., Consensus topography in the ATP binding site of the simian virus 40 and polyomavirus large tumor antigens, *Proc. Natl. Acad. Sci. U.S.A.,* 84, 4026, 1987.

327. Levinson, B., Khoury, G., Vande Woude, G., and Gruss, P., Activation of SV40 genome by 72-base pair tandem repeats of Moloney sarcoma virus, *Nature,* 255, 568, 1982.

328. Lord, S.T. and Singer, M.F., Transcriptionally active monkey genomic segment homologous to the regulatory region of simian virus 40 is associated with DNase I-hypersensitive sites, *Mol. Cell. Biol.,* 4, 1635, 1984.

329. Sugano, S. and Yamaguchi, N., Two classes of transformation-deficient, immortalization-positive simian virus 40 mutants constructed by making three-base insertions in the T antigen gene, *J. Virol.,* 52, 884, 1984.

330. Tevethia, M.J., Pipas, J.M., Kierstead, T., and Cole, C., Requirements for immortalization of primary mouse embryo fibroblasts probed with mutants bearing deletions in the 3′ end of SV40 gene A, *Virology,* 162, 76, 1988.

331. Scott, D.M., MacDonald, C., Brzeski, H., and Kinne, R., Maintenance of expression of differentiated function of kidney cells following transformation by SV40 early region DNA, *Exp. Cell Res.,* 166, 391, 1986.

332. Hwang, S.-P. and Kucherlapati, R., Localization and organization of integrated simian virus 40 sequences in a human cell line, *Virology,* 105, 196, 1980.

333. Hiscott, J., Murphy, D., and Defendi, V., Amplification and rearrangement of integrated SV40 DNA sequences accompany the selection of anchorage-independent transformed mouse cells, *Cell,* 22, 535, 1980.

334. Hiscott, J.B., Murphy, D., and Defendi, V., Instability of integrated viral DNA in mouse cells transformed by simian virus 40, *Proc. Natl. Acad. Sci. U.S.A.,* 78, 1736, 1981.

335. Butel, J.S., Wong, C., and Evans, B.K., Fluctuation of simian virus 40 (SV40) super T-antigen expression in tumors induced by SV40-transformed mouse mammary epithelial cells, *J. Virol.,* 60, 817, 1986.

336. Chang, L.-S., Pan, S., Pater, M.M., and Di Mayorca, G., Differential requirement for SV40 early genes in immortalization and transformation of primary rat and human embryonic cells, *Virology,* 146, 246, 1985.

337. Palmiter, R.D., Chen, H.Y., Messing, A., and Brinster, R.L., SV40 enhancer and large-T antigen are instrumental in development of choroid plexus tumours in transgenic mice, *Nature,* 316, 457, 1985.

338. Messing, A., Chen, H.Y., Palmiter, R.D., and Brinster, R.L., Peripheral neuropathies, hepatocellular carcinomas, and islet cell adenomas in transgenic mice, *Nature,* 316, 461, 1985.

339. Imbra, R.J. and Karin, M., Phorbol ester induces the transcriptional stimulatory activity of the SV40 enhancer, *Nature,* 323, 555, 1986.

340. Beggs, A.H., Axelman, J., and Migeon, B.R., Reactivation of X-linked genes in human fibroblasts transformed by origin-defective SV40, *Somat. Cell Mol. Genet.,* 12, 585, 1986.

341. Diamandopoulos, G.T., Incidence, latency and morphological types of neoplasms induced by simian virus 40 inoculated intravenously into hamsters of three inbred strains and one outbred stock, *J. Natl. Cancer Inst.,* 60, 445, 1978.

342. Brinster, R.L., Chen, H.Y., Messing, A., van Dyke, T., Levine, A.J., and Palmiter, R.D., Transgenic mice harboring SV40 T-antigen genes develop characteristic brain tumors, *Cell,* 37, 367, 1984.

343. Levitt, L.J., Boss, G.R., and Erbe, R.W., Decreased methylation rates of DNA in SV40-transformed human fibroblasts, *Cancer,* 57, 764, 1986.

344. Theile, M., Krause, H., and Geissler, E., Simian virus 40-induced mutagenesis: action of the early viral region, *J. Gen. Virol.,* 68, 233, 1987.

345. Dehayza, P., Bell, J., and Sirover, M.A., Proliferation-dependent regulation of base excision repair in normal and SV-40 transformed human cells, *Carcinogenesis,* 7, 621, 1986.

346. Pollard, J.W., Harley, C.B., Chamberlain, J.W., Goldstein, S., and Stanners, C.P., Is transformation associated with an increased error frequency in mammalian cells?, *J. Biol. Chem.,* 257, 5977, 1982.

347. Staufenbiel, M. and Deppert, W., Different structural systems of the nucleus are targets for SV40 large T antigen, *Cell,* 33, 173, 1983.

348. Lange-Mutschler, J. and Henning, R., Cell surface binding simian virus 40 large T antigen become anchored and stably linked to lipid of the target cells, *Virology,* 136, 404, 1984.

349. Jarvis, D.L., Cole, C.N., and Butel, J.S., Absence of a structural basis for intracellular recognition and differential localization of nuclear and plasma membrane-associated forms of simian virus 40 large tumor antigen, *Mol. Cell. Biol.,* 6, 758, 1986.

350. Bates, M.P., Jennings, S.R., Tanaka, Y., Tevethia, M.J., and Tevethia, S.S., Recognition of simian virus 40 T antigen synthesized during viral lytic cycle in monkey kidney cells expressing mouse H-2K^b- and H-2D^b-transfected genes by SV40-specific cytotoxic T lymphocytes leads to the abrogation of virus lytic cycle, *Virology,* 162, 197, 1988.

351. Caron de Fromentel, C., Viron, A., Puvion, E., and May, P., SV40 large T-antigen and transformation related protein p53 are associated in situ with nuclear RNP structures containing hnRNA of transformed cells, *Exp. Cell Res.,* 164, 35, 1986.

352. Hinzpeter, M. and Deppert, W., Analysis of biological and biochemical parameters for chromatin and nuclear matrix association of SV40 large T antigen in transformed cells, *Oncogene,* 1, 119, 1987.

353. Stahl, H., Dröge, P., and Knippers, R., DNA helicase activity of SV40 large tumor antigen, *EMBO J.,* 5, 1939, 1986.

354. Prelich, G., Kostura, M., Marshak, D.R., Mathews, M.B., and Stillman, B., The cell-cycle regulated proliferating cell nuclear antigen is required for SV40 DNA replication *in vitro, Nature,* 326, 471, 1987.

355. Bravo, R., Frank, R., Blundell, P.A., and Macdonald-Bravo, H., Cyclin/PCNA is the auxiliary protein of DNA polymerase-delta, *Nature,* 326, 515, 1987.

356. Prelich, G., Tan, C.-T., Kostura, M., Mathews, M.B., So, A.G., Downey, K.M., and Stillman, B., Functional identity of proliferating cell nuclear antigen and a DNA polymerase-delta auxiliary protein, *Nature,* 326, 517, 1987.

357. Kalderon, D., Richardson, W.D., Markham, A.F., and Smith, A.E., Sequence requirements for nuclear location of simian virus 40 large-T antigen, *Nature,* 311, 33, 1984.

358. Fischer-Fantuzzi, L. and Vesco, C., Deletion of 43 amino acids in the NH$_2$-terminal half of the large tumor antigen of simian virus 40 results in a non-karyophilic protein capable of transforming established cells, *Proc. Natl. Acad. Sci. U.S.A.,* 82, 1891, 1985.

359. Montenarh, M., Vesco, C., and Scheidtmann, K.H., Dimers and complexes with p53 are the prevalent oligomeric forms of a transforming nonkaryophilic T antigen of simian virus 40, *J. Virol.,* 61, 940, 1987.

360. Fischer-Fantuzzi, L. and Vesco, C., A nonkaryophilic T antigen of SV40 can either immortalize or transform rodent cells, and cooperates better with cytoplasmic than with nuclear oncoproteins, *Oncogene Res.,* 1, 229, 1987.

361. Simmons, D.T., Stepwise phosphorylation of the NH$_2$-terminal region of the simian virus 40 large T antigen, *J. Biol. Chem.,* 259, 8633, 1984.

362. Simmons, D.T., Chou, W., and Rodgers, K., Phosphorylation downregulates the DNA-binding activity of simian virus 40 T antigen, *J. Virol.,* 60, 888, 1986.

363. Melero, J.A., Tur, S., and Carroll, R.B., Host nuclear proteins expressed in simian virus 40-transformed and -infected cells, *Proc Natl. Acad. Sci. U.S.A.,* 77, 97, 1980.

364. Stürzbecher, H.-W., Montenarh, M., and Henning, R., Enhanced protein phosphorylation in SV40-transformed and -infected cells, *Virology,* 160, 445, 1987.

365. Walser, A. and Deppert, W., The kinase activity of SV40 large T antigen is mediated by a cellular kinase, *EMBO J.,* 5, 883, 1986.

366. Schmieg, F.L. and Simmons, D.T., Intracellular location and kinetics of complex formation between simian virus 40 T antigen and cellular protein p53, *J. Virol.,* 52, 350, 1984.

367. O'Reilly, D.R., p53 and transformation by SV40, *Biol. Cell,* 57, 187, 1986.

368. Yewdell, J.W., Gannon, J.V., and Lane, D.P., Monoclonal antibody analysis of p53 expression in normal and transformed cells, *J. Virol.,* 59, 444, 1986.

369. Michalovitz, D., Eliyahu, D., and Oren, M., Overproduction of protein p53 contributes to simian virus 40-mediated transformation, *Mol. Cell. Biol.,* 6, 3531, 1986.

370. Deppert, W., Haug, M., and Steinmayer, T., Modulation of p53 protein expression during cellular transformation with simian virus 40, *Mol. Cell. Biol.,* 7, 4453, 1987.

371. Tan, T.-T., Wallis, J., and Levine, A.J., Identification of the p53 protein domain involved in formation of the simian virus 40 large T-antigen-p53 protein complex, *J. Virol.,* 59, 574, 1986.

372. Montenarh, M., Kohler, M., and Henning, R., Complex formation of simian virus 40 large T antigen with cellular protein p53, *J. Virol.,* 60, 761, 1986.

373. Meek, D.W. and Eckhart, W., Phosphorylation of p53 in normal and simian virus 40-transformed NIH 3T3 cells, *Mol. Cell Biol.,* 8, 461, 1988.

374. Matlashewsky, G., Lamb, P., Pim, D., Peacock, J., Crawford, L., and Benchimol, S., Isolation and characterization of a human p53 cDNA clone: expression of the human p53 gene, *EMBO J.,* 3, 3257, 1984.

375. Mercer, W.E., Avignolo, C., and Baserga, A., Role of the p53 protein in cell proliferation as studied by microinjection of monoclonal antibodies, *Mol. Cell. Biol.,* 4, 276, 1984.

376. Eliyahu, D., Raz, A., Gruss, P., Givol, D., and Oren, M., Participation of p53 cellular tumor antigen in transformation of normal embryonic cells, *Nature,* 312, 646, 1984.

377. Coulier, F., Imbert, J., Albert, J., Jeunet, E., Lawrence, J.-J., Crawford, L., and Birg, F., Permanent expression of p53 in FR 3T3 rat cells but cell cycle-dependent association with large-T antigen in simian virus 40 transformants, *EMBO J.,* 4, 3413, 1985.

378. Santos, M. and Butel, J.S., Surface T-antigen expression in simian virus 40-transformed mouse cells: correlation with cell growth rate, *Mol. Cell. Biol.,* 5, 1051, 1985.

379. Parada, L.F., Land, H., Weinberg, R.A., Wolf, D., and Rotter, V., Cooperation between gene encoding p53 tumour antigen and *ras* in cellular transformation, *Nature,* 312, 649, 1984.

380. Jenkins, J.R., Rudge, K., and Currie, G.A., Cellular immortalization by a cDNA clone encoding the transformation-associated phosphoprotein p53, *Nature,* 312, 651, 1984.

381. Duthu, A., Ehrhart, J.-C., Benchimol, S., Chandrasekaran, K., and May, P., p53-Transformation-related protein: kinetics of synthesis and accumulation in SV40-infected primary mouse kidney cell cultures, *Virology,* 147, 275, 1985.

382. Montenarh, M., Kohler, M., Aggeler, G., and Henning, R., Structural prerequisites of simian virus 40 large T antigen for the maintenance of cell transformation, *EMBO J.,* 4, 2941, 1985.

383. Thathamangalam, U., Chandrasekaran, K., Hoffman, J.C., McFarland, V.W., Parott, C., Dale Smith, C.A., Simmons, D.T., and Mora, P.T., The transformation-related protein p53 is not bound to the SV40 T antigen in BALB 3T12 cells expressing T antigen, *Virology,* 155, 132, 1986.

384. Stürzbecher, H.-W., Chumakov, P., Welch, W.J., and Jenkins, J.R., Mutant p53 proteins bind hsp 72/73 cellular heat shock-related proteins in SV40-transformed monkey cells, *Oncogene,* 1, 201, 1987.

385. Smale, S.T. and Tjian, R., T antigen-DNA polymerase alpha complex implicated in simian virus 40 DNA replication, *Mol. Cell. Biol.,* 6, 4077, 1986.

386. Gannon, J.V. and Lane, D.P., p53 and DNA polymerase alpha compete for binding to SV40 T antigen, *Nature,* 329, 456, 1987.

387. Schmieg, F.I. and Simmons, D.T., Characterization of the *in vitro* interaction between SV40 T antigen and p53: mapping the p53 binding site, *Virology,* 164, 132, 1988.

388. Rhim, J.S., Jay, G., Arnstein, P., Price, F.M., Sanford, K.K., and Aaronson, S.A., Neoplastic transformation of human epidermal keratinocytes by AD12-SV40 and Kirsten sarcoma viruses, *Science,* 227, 1250, 1985.

389. Bleiberg, I., Harvey, A.K., Smale, G., and Grotendorst, G.R., Identification of a PDGF-like mitoattractant produced by NIH/3T3 cells after transformation with SV40, *J. Cell. Physiol.,* 123, 161, 1985.

390. Faas, S.J., Pan, S., Pinkert, C.A., Brinster, R.L., and Knowles, B.B., Simian virus 40 (SV40)-transgenic mice that develop tumors are specifically tolerant to SV40 T antigen, *J. Exp. Med.,* 165, 417, 1987.

391. Winberry, L., Priehs, C., Friderici, K., Thompson, M., and Fluck, M., Expression of proto-oncogenes in normal and papovavirus-transformed or -infected rat fibroblasts, *Virology,* 147, 154, 1985.

392. Small, J.A., Blair, D.G., Showalter, S.D., and Scangos, G.A., Analysis of a transgenic mouse containing simian virus 40 and v-*myc* sequences, *Mol. Cell. Biol.,* 5, 642, 1985.

393. Classon, M., Henriksson, M., Sümegi, J., Klein, G., and Hammaskjöld, M.-L., Elevated c-*myc* expression facilitates the replication of SV40 DNA in human lymphoma cells, *Nature,* 330, 272, 1987.

394. Smith, M.R., DeGudicibus, S.J., and Stacey, D.W., Requirement for c-*ras* proteins during viral oncogene transformation, *Nature,* 320, 540, 1986.

395. Berhanu, P. and Hollenberg, M.D., Epidermal growth factor-urogastrone receptor: selective alteration in simian virus 40 transformed mouse fibroblasts, *Arch. Biochem. Biophys.,* 203, 134, 1980.

396. Downward, J., Yarden, Y., Mayes, E., Scrace, G., Totty, N., Stockwell, P., Ullrich, A., Schlessinger, J., and Waterfield, M.D., Close similarity of epidermal growth factor receptor and v-*erb*-B oncogene protein sequences, *Nature,* 307, 521, 1984.

397. Cuzin, F., The polyoma virus oncogenes: coordinated functions of three distinct proteins in the transformation of rodent cells in culture, *Biochim. Biophys. Acta,* 781, 193, 1984.

398. Lemieux, L., All three polyoma early genes are involved in transformation of rat embryo fibroblast cells, *Anticancer Res.,* 6, 413, 1986.

399. Bolen, J.B., Fisher, S.E., Chowdhury, K., Shan, T.-C., Williams, J.E., Dawe, C.J., and Israel, M.A., A determinant of polyomavirus virulence enhances virus growth in cells of renal origin, *J. Virol.,* 53, 335, 1985.

400. Griffin, B.E., Fried, M., and Cowie, A., Polyoma DNA: a physical map, *Proc. Natl. Acad. Sci. U.S.A.,* 71, 2077, 1974.

401. Soeda, E., Arrand, R., Smolar, N., Walsh, J.E., and Griffin, B.E., Coding potential and regulatory signals of the polyoma virus genome, *Nature,* 283, 445, 1980.

402. Markland, W. and Smith, A.E., Mutants of polyomavirus middle-T antigen, *Biochim. Biophys. Acta,* 907, 299, 1987.

403. Liang, T.J., Carmichael, G.G., and Benjamin, T.L., A polyoma mutant that encodes small T antigen but not middle T antigen demonstrates uncoupling of cell surface and cytoskeletal changes associated with cell transformation, *Mol. Cell. Biol.,* 4, 2774, 1984.

404. Della Valle, G., Fenton, R.G., and Basilico, C., Polyoma large T antigen regulates the integration of viral DNA sequences into the genome of transformed cells, Cell, 23, 347, 1981.

405. de Villiers, J. and Schaffner, W., A small segment of polyoma virus DNA enhances the expression of a cloned beta-globin gene over a distance of 1,400 base pairs, *Nucleic Acids Res.,* 9, 6251, 1981.

406. Fujimura, F.K., Nuclear activity from F9 embryonal carcinoma cells binding specifically to the enhancers of wild-type polyoma virus and PyEC mutant DNAs, *Nucleic Acids Res.,* 14, 2845, 1986.

407. Kryszke, M.-H., Piette, J., and Yaniv, M., Induction of a factor that binds to the polyoma virus A enhancer on differentiation of embryonal carcinoma cells, *Nature,* 328, 254, 1987.

408. Piette, J. and Yaniv, M., Two different factors bind to the alpha-domain of the polyoma virus enhancer, one of which also interacts with the SV40 and c-*fos* enhancers, *EMBO J.,* 6, 1331, 1987.

409. Roberge, C. and Bastin, M., Site-directed mutagenesis of the polyomavirus genome: replication-defective large T mutants with increased immortalization potential, *Virology,* 162, 144, 1988.

410. Noda, T., Satake, M., Robins, T., and Ito, Y., Isolation and characterization of NIH 3T3 cells expressing polyomavirus small T antigen, *J. Virol.,* 60, 105, 1986.

411. Noda, T., Satake, M., Yamaguchi, Y., and Ito, Y., Cooperation of middle and small T antigens of polyomavirus in transformation of established fibroblast and epitheliallike cell lines, *J. Virol.,* 61, 2253, 1987.

412. Gélinas, C. and Bastin, M., Malignant transformation of rat cells by the polyomavirus middle T gene, *Virology,* 146, 233, 1985.

413. Donoghue, D.J., Anderson, C., Hunter, T., and Kaplan, P.L., Transmission of the polyoma virus middle T gene as the oncogene of a murine retrovirus, *Nature,* 308, 748, 1984.

414. Bouchard, L., Mathieu, F., and Bastin, M., High-frequency changes in transcriptional activity in polyomavirus-transformed cell lines, *J. Virol.,* 61, 2448, 1987.

415. Williams, R.L., Courtneidge, S.A., and Wagner, E.F., Embryonic lethalities and endothelial tumors in chimeric mice expressing polyoma virus middle T oncogene, *Cell,* 52, 121, 1988.

416. Rassoulzadegan, M., Naghashfar, Z., Cowie, A., Carr, A., Grisoni, M., Kamen, R., and Cuzin, F., Expression of the large T protein of polyoma virus promotes the establishment in culture of "normal" rodent fibroblast cell lines, *Proc. Natl. Acad. Sci. U.S.A.,* 80, 4354, 1983.

417. Land, H., Parada, L.F., and Weinberg, R.A., Tumorigenic conversion of primary embryo fibroblasts require at least two cooperating oncogenes, *Nature,* 304, 596, 1983.

418. Connan, G., Rassoulzadegan, M., and Cuzin, F., Focus formation in rat fibroblasts exposed to a tumour promoter after transfer of polyoma *plt* and *myc* oncogenes, *Nature,* 314, 277, 1985.

419. Bouchard, L., Mathieu, F., and Bastin, M., Polyoma large T can activate middle T expression by a hit-and-run mechanism, *Oncogene,* 2, 379, 1987.

420. Baldwin, G.S., Gastrin and the transforming protein of polyoma virus have evolved from a common ancestor, *FEBS Lett.,* 137, 1, 1982.

421. Clark, K.L. and Folk, W.R., Significance of the gastrin homology and surrounding sequences in polyomavirus middle T antigen for cell transformation, *J. Virol.,* 57, 237, 1986.

422. Novak, U., Dilworth, S.M., and Griffin, B.E., Coding capacity of a 35% fragment of the polyoma virus genome is sufficient to initiate and maintain cellular transformation, *Proc. Natl. Acad. Sci. U.S.A.,* 77, 3278, 1980.

423. Treisman, R., Novak, U., Favaloro, J., and Kamen, R., Transformation of rat cells by an altered polyoma virus genome expressing only the middle-T protein, *Nature,* 292, 595, 1981.

424. Rassoulzadegan, M., Cowie, A., Carr, A., Glaichenhaus, N., Kamen, R., and Cuzin, F., The roles of individual polyoma virus early proteins in oncogenic transformation, *Nature,* 300, 713, 1982.

425. Courtneidge, S.A., Activation of the pp60^{c-src} kinase by middle T antigen binding or by dephosphorylation, *EMBO J.,* 4, 1471, 1985.

426. Raptis, L., Lamfrom, H., and Benjamin, T.L., Regulation of cellular phenotype and expression of polyomavirus middle T antigen in rat fibroblasts, *Mol. Cell. Biol.,* 5, 2476, 1985.

427. Bouchard, L., Vass-Marengo, J., and Bastin, M., Expression of the malignant phenotype in rat fibroblasts transfected with the polyomavirus transforming genes, *Virology,* 155, 1, 1986.

428. Kornbluth, S., Cross, F.R., Harbison, M., and Hanafusa, H., Transformation of chicken embryo fibroblasts and tumor induction by the middle T antigen of polyomavirus carried in an avian retroviral vector, *Mol. Cell. Biol.,* 6, 1545, 1986.

429. Kaplan, D.R., Bockus, B., Roberts, T.M., Bolen, J., Israel, M., and Schaffhausen, B.S., Large-scale production of polyoma middle T antigen by using genetically engineered tumors, *Mol. Cell. Biol.,* 5, 1795, 1985.

430. Cherington, V., Morgan, B., Spiegelman, B.M., and Roberts, T.M., Recombinant retroviruses that transduce individual polyoma tumor antigens: effects on growth and differentiation, *Proc. Natl. Acad. Sci. U.S.A.,* 83, 4307, 1986.

431. Kamech, N., Seif, R., and Pantaloni, D., Cyclic AMP specifically blocks proliferation of rat 3T3 cells transformed by polyomavirus, *J. Virol.,* 61, 1546, 1987.

432. Schaffhausen, B.S. and Benjamin, T.L., Phosphorylation of polyoma T antigens, *Cell,* 18, 935, 1979.

433. Schaffhausen, B.S. and Benjamin, T.L., Comparison of phosphorylation of two polyoma virus middle T antigens *in vivo* and *in vitro, J. Virol.,* 40, 184, 1981.

434. Segawa, K. and Ito, Y., Differential subcellular localization of *in vivo*-phosphorylated and non-phosphorylated middle-sized tumor antigen of polyoma virus and its relationship to middle-sized tumor antigen phosphorylating activity *in vitro, Proc. Natl. Acad. Sci. U.S.A.,* 79, 6812, 1982.

435. Balmer-Hofer, K. and Benjamin, T.L., Phosphorylation of polyoma middle T antigen and cellular proteins in purified plasma membranes of polyoma virus-infected cells, *EMBO J.,* 4, 2321, 1985.

436. Matthews, J.T. and Benjamin, T.L., 12-*O*-tetradecanoylphorbol-13-acetate stimulates phosphorylation of the 58,000-M_r form of polyomavirus middle T antigen in vivo: implications for a possible role of protein kinase C in middle T function, *J. Virol.,* 58, 239, 1986.

437. Raptis, L., Boynton, A.L., and Whitfield, J.F., Protein kinase C promotes the phosphorylation of immunoprecipitated middle T antigen from polyoma-transformed cells, *Biochem. Biophys. Res. Commun.,* 136, 995, 1986.

438. Kaplan, D.R., Whitman, M., Schaffhausen, B., Pallas, D.C., White, M., Cantley, L., and Roberts, T.M., Common elements in growth factor stimulation and oncogenic transformation: 85 kd phosphoprotein and phosphatidylinositol kinase activity, *Cell,* 50, 1021, 1987.

439. Courtneidge, S.A. and Smith, A.E., Polyoma virus transforming protein associates with the product of the c-*src* cellular gene, *Nature,* 303, 435, 1983.

440. Courtneidge, S.A. and Smith, A.E., The complex of polyoma virus middle-T antigen and pp60^{c-src}, *EMBO J.,* 3, 585, 1984.

441. Bolen, J.B. and Israel, M.A., *In vitro* association and phosphorylation of polyoma virus middle T antigen by cellular tyrosil kinase activity, *J. Biol. Chem.,* 259, 11686, 1984.

442. Bolen, J.B., Thiele, C.J., Israel, M.A., Yonemoto, W., Lipsich, L.A., and Brugge, J.S., Enhancement of cellular *src* gene product associated tyrosyl kinase activity following polyoma virus infection and transformation, *Cell,* 38, 767, 1984.

443. Bolen, J.B., Lewis, A.M., Jr., and Israel, M.A., Stimulation of pp60^{c-src} tyrosyl kinase activity in polyoma virus-infected mouse cells is closely associated with polyoma middle tumor antigen synthesis, *J. Cell. Biochem.,* 27, 157, 1985.

444. Cheng, S.H., Piwnica-Worms, H., Harvey, R.W., Roberts, T.M., and Smith, A.E., The carboxy terminus of pp60^{c-src} is a regulatory domain and is involved in complex formation with the middle-T antigen of polyomavirus, *Mol. Cell. Biol.,* 8, 1736, 1988.

445. Bolen, J.B., Amini, S., DeSeau, V., Reddy, S., and Shalloway, D., Analysis of polyomavirus middle-T-antigen-transformed rat cell variants expressing different levels of pp60^{c-src}, *J. Virol.,* 61, 1079, 1987.

446. Azarnia, R. and Loewenstein, W.R., Polyomavirus middle T antigen downregulates junctional cell-to-cell communication, *Mol. Cell. Biol.,* 7, 946, 1987.

447. Raptis, L. and Whitfield, J.F., Protein kinase C stimulation increases the transforming ability of the polyoma virus middle T antigen, *Biochem. Biophys. Res. Commun.,* 140, 1106, 1986.

448. Piwnica-Worms, H., Kaplan, D.R., Whitman, M., and Roberts, T.M., Retrovirus shuttle vector for study of kinase activities of pp60^{c-src} synthesized *in vitro* and overproduced *in vivo, Mol. Cell. Biol.,* 6, 2033, 1986.

449. Yonemoto, W., Jarvis-Morar, M., Brugge, J.S., Bolen, J.B., and Israel, M.A., Tyrosine phosphorylation within the amino-terminal domain of pp60^{c-src} molecules associated with polyoma virus middle-sized tumor antigen, *Proc. Natl. Acad. Sci. U.S.A.,* 82, 4568, 1985.

450. Cartwright, C.A., Kaplan, P.L., Cooper, J.A., Hunter, T., and Eckhart, W., Altered sites of tyrosine phosphorylation in pp60^{c-src} associated with polyoma virus middle tumor antigen, *Mol. Cell. Biol.,* 6, 1562, 1986.

451. Templeton, D. and Eckhart, W., N-terminal amino acid sequences of the polyoma middle-size T antigen are important for protein kinase activity and cell transformation, *Mol. Cell. Biochem.,* 4, 817, 1984.

452. Bolen, J.B. and Israel, M.A., Middle tumor antigen of polyoma virus transformation-defective mutant NG59 is associated with pp60^{c-src}, *J. Virol.,* 53, 114, 1985.

453. Cheng, S.H., Markland, W., Markham, A.F., and Smith, A.E., Mutations around the NG59 lesion indicate an active association of polyoma virus middle-T antigen with pp60^{c-src} is required for cell transformation, *EMBO J.,* 5, 325, 1986.

454. Markland, W. and Smith, A.E., Mapping of the amino-terminal half of polyomavirus middle-T antigen indicates that this region is the binding domain for pp60^{c-src}, *J. Virol.,* 61, 285, 1987.

455. Amini, S., DeSeau, V., Reddy, S., Shalloway, D., and Bolen, J.B., Regulation of pp60^{c-src} synthesis by inducible RNA complementary to c-*src* mRNA in polyomavirus-transformed rat cells, *Mol. Cell. Biol.,* 6, 2305, 1986.

456. Mes-Mason, A.-M., Schaffhausen, B., and Hassell, J.A., The major site of tyrosine phosphorylation in polyomavirus middle T antigen is not required for transformation, *J. Virol.,* 52, 457, 1984.

457. Amini, S., Lewis, A.M., Jr., Israel, M.A., Butel, J.S., and Bolen, J.B., Analysis of pp60^{c-src} protein kinase activity in hamster embryo cells transformed by simian virus 40, human adenoviruses, and bovine papillomavirus 1, *J. Virol.,* 57, 357, 1986.

458. Sefton, B.M., Hunter, T., Beemon, K., and Eckhart, W., Evidence that the phosphorylation of tyrosine is essential for cellular transformation by Rous sarcoma virus, *Cell,* 20, 807, 1980.

459. Kornbluth, S., Sudol, M., and Hanafusa, H., Association of the polyomavirus middle-T antigen with c-*yes* protein, *Nature,* 325, 171, 1987.

460. Bolen, J.B., DeSeau, V., O'Shaughnessy, J., and Amini, S., Analysis of middle tumor antigen and pp60^{c-src} interactions in polyomavirus-transformed rat cells, *J. Virol.,* 61, 3299, 1987.

461. Yonemoto, W., Filson, A.J., Queral-Lustig, A.E., Wang, J.Y.J., and Brugge, J.S., Detection of phosphotyrosine-containing proteins in polyomavirus middle tumor antigen-transformed cells after treatment with a phosphotyrosine phosphatase inhibitor, *Mol. Cell. Biol.,* 7, 905, 1987.

462. Kaplan, D.R., Whitman, M., Schaffhausen, B., Raptis, L., Garcea, R.L., Pallas, D., Roberts, T.M., and Cantley, L., Phosphatidylinositol metabolism and polyoma-mediated transformation, *Proc. Natl. Acad. Sci. U.S.A.,* 83, 3624, 1986.

463. Whitman, M., Kaplan, D.R., Schaffhausen, B., Cantley, L., and Roberts, T.M., Association of phosphatidylinositol kinase activity with polyoma middle-T competent for transformation, *Nature,* 315, 239, 1985.

464. MacDonald, M.L., Kuenzel, E.A., Glomset, J.A., and Krebs, E.G., Evidence from two transformed cell lines that the phosphorylations of peptide tyrosine and phosphatidylinositol are catalyzed by different proteins, *Proc. Natl. Acad. Sci. U.S.A.,* 82, 3993, 1985.

465. Sugano, S. and Hanafusa, H., Phosphatidylinositol kinase activity in virus-transformed and nontransformed cells, *Mol. Cell. Biol.,* 5, 2399, 1985.

466. Koch, W., Carbone, A., and Walter, G., Purified polyoma virus medium T antigen has tyrosine-specific protein kinase activity but no significant phosphatidylinositol kinase activity, *Mol. Cell. Biol.,* 6, 18966, 1986.

467. Whitman, M., Kaplan, D., Cantley, L., Roberts, T.M., and Schaffhausen, B., Phosphoinositide kinase activity and transformation, *Fed. Proc. Fed. Am. Soc. Exp. Biol.,* 45, 2647, 1986.

468. Courtneidge, S.A. and Heber, A., An 81 kd protein complexed with middle T antigen and pp60^{c-src}: a possible phosphatidylinositol kinase, *Cell,* 50, 1031, 1987.

469. Grussenmeyer, T., Carbone-Wiley, A., Scheidtmann, K.H., and Walter, G., Interactions between polyomavirus medium T antigen and three cellular proteins of 88, 61, and 37 kilodaltons, *J. Virol.,* 61, 3902, 1987.

470. Segawa, K., Cooperation of mitogenic growth factors with polyoma virus middle T antigen in transformation of secondary cultured rat cells, *Biochem. Biophys. Res. Commun.,* 136, 921, 1986.

471. El-Enanany, T.M. and Dubes, G.R., The set of growth factors stimulatory for a transformed rat cell of line NRK-49F depends on the identity of the transforming virus, *Tumour Biol.,* 7, 49, 1986.

472. Gelinas, C., Chartrand, P., and Bastin, M., Polyoma virus mutant with normal transforming ability but impaired tumorigenic potential, *J. Virol.,* 43, 1072, 1982.

473. Cowie, A., de Villiers, J., and Kamen, R., Immortalization of rat embryo fibroblasts by mutant polyomavirus large T antigens deficient in DNA binding, *Mol. Cell. Biol.,* 6, 4344, 1986.

474. Freund, R., Mandel, G., Carmichael, G.G., Barncastle, J.P., Dawe, C.J., and Benjamin, T.L., Polyomavirus tumor induction in mice: influences of viral coding and noncoding sequences on tumor profiles, *J. Virol.,* 61, 2232, 1987.

475. Bautch, V.L., Toda, S., Hassell, J.A., and Hanahan, D., Endothelial cell tumors develop in transgenic mice carrying polyoma virus middle T oncogene, *Cell,* 51, 529, 1987.

476. Mougneau, E., Lemieux, L., Rassoulzadegan, M., and Cuzin, F., Biological activities of v-*myc* and rearranged c-*myc* oncogenes in rat fibroblast cells in culture, *Proc. Natl. Acad. Sci. U.S.A.,* 81, 5758, 1984.

477. Léopold, P., Mougneau, E., Vailly, J., Cerni, C., Rassoulzadegan, M., and Cuzin, Genetic instabilities at the chromosomal and molecular levels induced by the *plt* oncogene of polyoma virus, *Ann. Clin. Res.,* 18, 304, 1986.

478. Neer, A., Baran, N., and Manor, H., Integration of polyoma virus DNA into chromosomal DNA in transformed rat cells causes deletion of flanking cell sequences, *J. Gen. Virol.,* 64, 69, 1983.

479. Allard, D., Delbecchi, L., Bourgaux-Ramoisy, D., and Bourgaux, P., Major rearrangement of cellular DNA in the vicinity of integrated polyomavirus DNA, *Virology,* 162, 128, 1988.

480. Zullo, J., Stiles, C.D., and Garcea, R.L., Regulation of c-*myc* and c-*fos* mRNA levels by polyomavirus: distinct roles for the capsid protein VP₁ and the viral early proteins, *Proc. Natl. Acad. Sci. U.S.A.*, 84, 1210, 1987.

481. Schwab, M., Ramsay, G., Alitalo, K., Varmus, H.E., Bishop, J.M., Martinsson, T., Levan, G., and Levan, A., Amplification and enhanced expression of the c-*myc* oncogene in mouse SEWA tumour cells, *Nature*, 315, 345, 1985.

482. Höhne, M., Piasecki, A., Ummelmann, E., and Paul, D., Transformation of differentiated neonatal rat hepatocytes in primary culture by polyoma virus early region sequences, *Oncogene*, 1, 337, 1987.

483. Lewis, A.M., Jr. and Cook, J.L., A new role for DNA virus early proteins in viral carcinogenesis, *Science*, 227, 15, 1985.

484. Gardner, S.D., Field, A.M., Coleman, D.V., and Hulme, B., New human papovavirus (B.K.) isolated from urine after renal transplantation, *Lancet*, 1, 1253, 1971.

485. Corallini, A., Pagnani, M., Viadana, P., Silini, E., Mottes, M., Milanesi, G., Gerna, G., Vettor, R., Trapella, G., Silvani, V., Gaist, G., and Barbanti-Brodano, G., Association of BK virus with human brain tumors and tumors of pancreatic islets, *Int. J. Cancer*, 39, 60, 1987.

486. Corallini, A., Pagnani, M., Viadana, P, Camellin, P., Caputo, A., Reschiglian, P., Rossi, S., Altavilla, G., Selvatici, R., and Barbanti-Brodano, G., Induction of malignant subcutaneous sarcomas in hamsters by a recombinant DNA containing BK virus early region and the activated human c-Harvey-*ras* oncogene, *Cancer Res.*, 47, 6671, 1987.

Chapter 6

VIRAL AND CELLULAR ONCOGENES

I. INTRODUCTION

Oncogenes (transforming genes) can be defined as genes with potential capability for the induction of neoplastic (malignant) cell transformation in either natural or experimental conditions. Most oncogenes have been isolated from acute transforming retroviruses, which act as oncogene transducers,[1,2] although these viruses do not usually transmit cancer under natural conditions in any animal species. The viral oncogenes derive from cellular DNA sequences, the cellular oncogenes, or protooncogenes.

A. HISTORICAL DEVELOPMENT OF THE ONCOGENE CONCEPT

The existence of potentially transforming sequences in the genome of vertebrates was postulated as a possible general mechanism for the process of oncogenesis in the viral oncogene hypothesis.[3,4] According to this hypothesis, all vertebrates would contain in their DNA endogenous genetic information related to nucleotide sequences present in RNA tumor viruses. These sequences were named virogenes, and the activation of a portion of a virogene, the oncogene, would be responsible for transforming a normal cell into a tumor cell. Various exogenous agents (radiations, chemical carcinogens, viruses) would be capable of activating the endogenous oncogenic information. The viral oncogene hypothesis postulated, however, a genetic linkage between the oncogene sequence and endogenous viral sequences, which was not confirmed in later studies.

1. The *Tr* Genes

The existence of a number of structural cellular genes, termed *Tr* genes, whose unscheduled activation would lead to neoplasia was discussed later as a general theory of carcinogenesis.[5] The *Tr* genes would be involved in the normal control of growth but would code for products with transforming potential, and would be contained in all cells of the multicellular organisms. These genes would normally be active during embryogenesis, being specifically repressed thereafter in particular tissues by the action of regulatory genes. Spontaneous tumors, or tumors induced by chemicals or radiation, would arise as the result of mutation of regulatory genes releasing the suppression of the corresponding *Tr* genes and leading to transformation. According to the same hypothesis, oncogenic viruses evolved by the extraction of host *Tr* genes with their conversion to viral transforming genes. Moreover, the reintroduction of *Tr* genes into susceptible cells would produce their malignant transformation. The *Tr* genes remained, however, uncharacterized.

2. The *Tu* Gene

The existence of a cellular tumor gene, named the *Tu* gene, was postulated in experiments of selective crosses of *Xiphophorus* fishes.[6-10] Furthermore, in some experiments the *Tu* gene was successfully transferred into fish embryos, where its heritable expression was observed.[11] Regrettably, the structure of both the *Tu* gene and its putative product, as well as their respective normal functions, was not elucidated.

3. Viral and Cellular Oncogenes

The unexpected presence of avian tumor virus RNA- and protein-related sequences was detected in uninfected chicken embryo cells.[12-14] Furthermore, cellular DNA and RNA sequences homologous to acute transforming retroviruses (K-MuLV and H-MuLV) were found in rat tumors as well as in rat normal tissues.[15,16] Mouse DNA and RNA were found to contain sequences specific for M-MuSV.[17] It was demonstrated that the cells of uninfected chickens contain in their genome nucleotide sequences that are homologous to the transforming gene of ASVs but that are not linked to endogenous viral sequences.[18-25] Since that time, cellular oncogenes (protooncogenes) have been found in all vertebrate species studied so far,[26-28] as well as in invertebrates such as the fruit fly, *Drosophila melanogaster*.[29-34] Protooncogenes are apparently present and expressed in all multicellular animals, including sponges.[35-38] At least some protooncogenes are present and expressed in yeasts such as *Saccharomyces cerevisiae* and *S. pombe* as well as in a slime mold, the simple eukaryotic microbe *Dictyostelium discoideum*.[39-42] DNA sequences and proteins related to v-*myb* and v-*myc* have been detected in Archaebacteriae,[43,44] which are primitive organisms representing a kind of bridge between prokaryotes and eukaryotes.[45]

4. Oncogenes in Plants

A phenomenon that evokes the autonomous, growth factor-independent proliferation of animal tumor cells is observed in tumors occurring in plants. Dicotyledoneous plants may be affected by a neoplastic disease, crown gall, which is induced by the soil bacterium *Agrobacterium tumefaciens*.[46] Virulent strains of *A. tumefaciens* contain a large plasmid of approximately 200 kbp, the Ti plasmid. Central to the development of crown gall disease are the transfer of a part of this plasmid, the T-DNA, and the integration of this segment into the nuclear genome.[47,48] The T-DNA of Ti plasmid carries genes (T-*aux*-1, T-*aux*-2, and T-*cyt*) that specify enzymes required for the biosynthesis of the phytohormones auxin and cytokinin.[49] These hormones have an important role in the regulation of transcriptional functions in plant tissues.[50] Integration of the T-DNA into the host cell genome of the plant may result in autonomous growth in the absence of phytohormones.[51,52] the genes T-*aux*-1, T-*aux*-2, and T-*cyt* may thus be considered as oncogenes. The T-DNA of *A. tumefaciens* contains, in addition to T-*aux*-1, T-*aux*-2, and T-*cyt*, genes that specify the biosynthesis of unusual amino acid derivatives called opines (octopine, nopaline, and agropine). These derivatives cannot be catabolized by the plant cells and may be accumulated inside the cells, whereas the bacteria can use them as sole sources of carbon and nitrogen.

The T-DNA transfer process of *A. tumefaciens* is activated by induction of the expression of the Ti plasmid virulence (*vir*) loci by plant signal molecules such as acetosyringone.[53] The *vir* gene products act in *trans* to mobilize the T-DNA element from the bacterial plasmid. The T-DNA is bounded by 25-kb direct repeat sequences which are essential for transfer and are specifically nicked by acetosyringone after *vir* gene activation. Integration of the T-DNA in the plant cell genome may be associated with rearrangement of plant DNA sequences.[54] As it occurs in animal cells, such DNA rearrangements of the cellular genome may have an important role in the pathogenesis of oncogenic processes.

B. ISOLATION AND NOMENCLATURE OF ONCOGENES

Oncogenes have been isolated from acute transforming retroviruses of avian, rodent, feline, and primate origin, but they are genes of eukaryotic cellular origin, not of viral origin, i.e., these viruses act only as oncogene transducers. The presence of oncogenes in such viruses is generally attributed to recombinational events that occurred between retroviruses and eukaryotic cells. Some oncogenes, or oncogene-related sequences, have not been found as yet in retroviruses and have been isolated only from the genome of different types of cells. Cellular oncogenes are also named protooncogenes or c-*onc* genes, whereas their viral counterparts are named v-*onc* genes. Each oncogene is usually represented by a three-letter symbol related to the name of the retrovirus or the cell from which it was originally defined.[55] An international system for human gene nomenclature proposed recently should be applied to the designation of protooncogenes.[56]

C. DEFINITION OF ONCOGENES AND PROTOONCOGENES

The definition of the oncogenes is still under discussion. Oncogenes of either viral or cellular origin have been defined as "genes capable of contributing directly to the conversion of a normal cell to a tumorigenic one", and protooncogenes, the cellular genomic sequences from where the viral oncogenes derive, have been defined as "cellular genes convertible to oncogenes by mutations or rearrangements."[58] However, only viral oncogenes are capable of inducing the rapid conversion of normal cells into malignant cells, and the potential to directly convert a normal cell into a tumorigenic one may possibly not exist in any cellular gene under natural conditions. Consequently, the term oncogene should be more conveniently applied to viral oncogenes (v-*onc* genes) and the term "protooncogene" should be used to designate the so-called cellular oncogenes (c-*onc* genes). However, it has become a common practice to use the term oncogene for designating both the viral oncogenes and the protooncogenes. Although it is difficult to change this practice by now, it should always be remembered that protooncogenes are normal cellular genes and that a general causal association between protooncogene activation and cancer has yet to be firmly established.

It is mòst difficult to achieve a proper definition of protooncogenes. At least five different criteria have been used to define these genes. Protooncogenes were initially defined through their homology with genomic sequences present in certain retroviruses with acute transforming capability (acute retroviruses) which were isolated from tumors occurring in animals that had been inoculated with infectious retroviruses lacking this capability (chronic retroviruses) or treated with chemical carcinogens. The potent and rapid transforming ability of the oncogene sequences contained in acute retroviruses was ascertained in experiments performed both *in vitro* and *in vivo*. A second class of protooncogenes was detected by the transforming ability of discrete cellular genomic sequences in experiments performed in test systems *in vitro*, especially by transfection of cellular DNA into NIH/3T3 mouse fibroblast cells, which are especially sensitive to oncogenic transformation. A third class of protooncogenes has been detected by their activation when chronic retroviruses infecting cells are inserted in their vicinity, which may result in the neoplastic transformation of susceptible cells. A fourth class of protooncogenes has been recognized by the results of their expression through recombinational events or artificial manipulations that subjugate them to new powerful regulatory signals. Finally, a fifth class of putative protooncogenes has been defined on the basis of their DNA sequence homology with known protooncogenes. A strict definition of protooncogenes would include only the first three of these classes. If only strict criteria are accepted for their definition, protooncogenes are limited in number. Less than 40 different protooncogenes have been detected so far in vertebrates, including humans, and there are probably not many more. A list of viral oncogenes with their respective isolation origin appears in Chapter 2, Table 2. Many reviews on different aspects of this subject have been published recently.[1,2,22-25,59-97]

II. CHROMOSOME LOCALIZATION OF PROTOONCOGENES

A precise knowledge of the chromosomal localization and sublocalization of protooncogenes is important for understanding the possible role of protooncogenes in neoplastic processes occurring in human and nonhuman animal species. Since it is known that specific chromosomal rearrangements are associated with several kinds of human malignant diseases,[98-107] it is important to compare the chromosomal breakpoints occurring in such neoplasias with the localization of protooncogenes within chromosomes of the neoplastic cell populations. It has been proposed that chromosomal rearrangements are associated with certain forms of neoplasia through translocation-mediated activation of specific protooncogenes.[99,102,108-114]

A. HUMAN PROTOONCOGENES

High-resolution techniques for the induction of chromosome binding in conjunction with *in*

TABLE 1
Chromosomal Location of Human Protooncogenes

Chromosome	Location	Protooncogene	Ref.
1	1p11-p13	N-*ras*	119,120
1	1p31-p32	*jun*	121
1	1p32	L-*myc*	122
1	1p32	B-*lym*-1	123
1	1p32-p35	*lck/lsk/tck*	124
1	1p36.1-p36.2	*fgr*	125
1	1q22-q24	*ski*	126
1	1q24-q25	*arg*	127
2	2p12-p13	*rel*	128
2	2p23-p24	N-*myc*	129
3	3p21-pter	*erb*-A-2	130
3	3p25	*raf*-1/*mil*	131
4	4q11-q12	*kit*	132
5	5q34	*fms*	133
6	6p21	*pim*	134
6	6q21	*fyn/syn/slk*	135
6	6q22	*ros*-1	136
6	6q22-q23	*myb*	137
7	7p11.4-q21	*raf*-2	138
7	7p12-p14	*erb*-B	139
7	7p15-p22	*ral*	140
7	7q21-q31	*met*	141
8	8q11-q22	*mos*	142,143
8	8q24	*myc*	142
9	9q34.1	*abl*	144
11	11p14.1	H-*ras*-1	145
11	11q13	*int*-2	146
11	11q13	*hst*	147
11	11q13	*bcl*-1	148
11	11q23-q24	*ets*	149
12	12p11.1-p12.1	K-*ras*-2	120
12	12q13	*int*-1	150
13	13q12	*ros*-2/*flt/frt*	136
14	14q24.3-q31	*fos*	151
15	15q26.1	*fes/fps*	144
17	17p13	p53	152
17	17q11.2	*erb*-A-1	153
17	17q21	*neu/erb*-B-2	154
18	18q21	*bcl*-2	155
18	18q21.3	*yes*-1	156
19	19p13.2-q13.2	*mel*	157
20	20q11-q12	*hck*	158
20	20q12-q13	*src*	159
21	21q22.1-q22.3	*ets*-2	160
22	22q13.1	*sis*	144
X	Xp21-q11	A-*raf*-1	138
X	Xq27	*mcf*-2	161

situ molecular hybridization with specific nucleic acid probes have been applied for establishing the localization of protooncogenes in the human karyotype.[115,116] All of the known human protooncogenes have been assigned already to specific chromosomes and the sublocalization to particular regions of human chromosomes is known for most of them (Table 1 and Figure 1).[117,118]

B. NONHUMAN PROTOONCOGENES

Data related to chromosome localization of protooncogenes in nonhuman animal species are

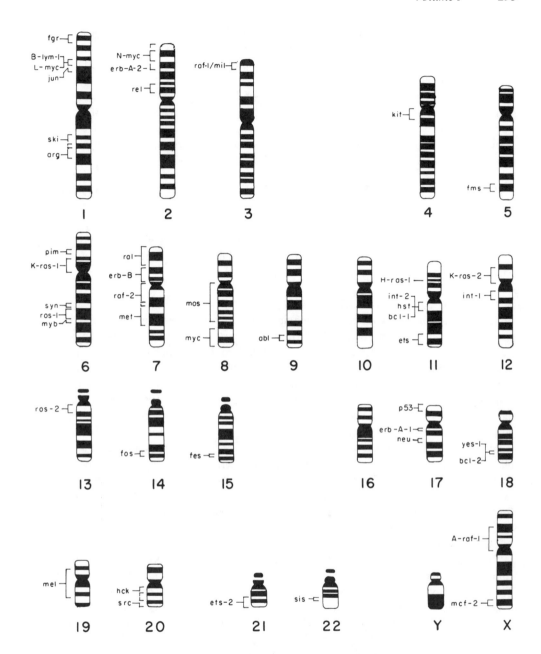

FIGURE 1. Chromosomal location of human protooncogenes.

still fragmentary. In the mouse c-*src* is localized on chromosome 2,[162,163] c-*raf* and c-K-*ras* are on chromosome 6,[162-166] c-*fes* and c-H-*ras* on chromosome 7,[162,163,167] c-*myb* on chromosome 10,[162] c-*sis* and c-*myc* on chromosome 15,[168-170] c-*ets*-1 and c-*ets*-2 are on chromosomes 9 and 16, respectively,[160,171] c-*rel* is on chromosome 11,[172] c-*abl* on chromosome 2,[173] and *pim*-1 on chromosome 17.[174,175] The protooncogenes c-*erb*-A and c-*erb*-B are asyntenic in man but syntenic in the mouse, both being located on chromosome 11.[176,177] The c-*fes* and albumin genes are syntenic in the owl monkey (*Aotus trivirgatus*).[178]

The protooncogenes c-H-*ras* and c-K-*ras* are located on hamster chromosomes 3 and 8, respectively.[179] The genes c-*myc*, N-*myc*, and L-*myc* have been mapped to rat chromosomes 7, 6, and 5, respectively.[180] Three c-*ras* protooncogenes have been assigned to rat chromosomes 1, 4, and X, respectively.[181] The c-H-*ras*-1 gene has been assigned to rat chromosome region

1q43.[182] The X chromosome linked c-*ras* gene of the rat is an intronless pseudogene and it was suggested that no functional protooncogenes exist in the mammalian X chromosome.[183] However, an actively transcribed gene of the c-*raf* protooncogene group is located on the X chromosome in mouse and human.[138]

Three c-*ras* genes are present in the genome of *Drosophila* and have been assigned to positions 85D, 64B, and 62B on chromosome 3.[33] *Drosophila* DNA sequences homologous to v-*abl* and v-*src* are located on chromosome positions 73B and 64B, respectively.[30] The *Drosophila* homolog of the murine and human *int*-1 gene is represented by a single locus at position 28A1-2 on chromosome 2.[184]

III. DETECTION AND CHARACTERIZATION OF ONCOGENES

Oncogenes of either viral or cellular origin can be detected and characterized by means of DNA transfection experiments or by biochemical and/or immunological procedures operating at the DNA, RNA, or protein levels. Virological methods are required for the isolation of oncogenes present in acute transforming retroviruses.

A. DNA TRANSFECTION EXPERIMENTS

The detection of genes with transforming capability in the genome of eukaryotic cells is based on experiments demonstrating that DNA from RSV-transformed rat fibroblasts can be artificially transferred (transfected) into chicken embryo fibroblasts, which resulted in transformation of the transfected cells.[185-187] Thereafter, the possible presence of transforming sequences in the genome of vertebrate tumor cells was suggested by the results of transfection of DNA extracted from experimental or spontaneous tumors into normal cells cultured *in vitro,* inducing the appearance of a transformed phenotype. Preliminary positive results were obtained with normal human fibroblasts continuously exposed *in vitro* to DNA extracted from human leukemic cells.[188] The normal cells exposed to DNA from tumor cells expressed a transformed phenotype, and the acquired alteration appeared to be heritable. No alteration was observed in comparative studies using DNA extracted from human nonleukemic cells. However, this test system was apparently not efficient and more clear results were obtained with a test system using for transfection DNA coprecipitated with calcium phosphate crystals.[189-191]

1. The NIH/3T3 Assay System

The cells used as recipients in most transfection experiments are NIH/3T3 cells, which are fibroblasts of murine (mouse) origin maintained as a contact-inhibited, nontumorigenic cell line. These cells have been considered as normal cells because they grow in sheets with the characteristic flattened appearance of fibroblasts, forming a confluent monolayer in Petri dishes, after which there is no more growth. NIH/3T3 cells acquire typical neoplastic characteristics a few weeks after being transfected with high molecular weight (>30 kb) DNA from tumor cells containing "active" protooncogenes. The transfected cells may appear as foci of morphologically transformed cells on top of the confluent monolayer, becoming more round and piling up on one another, as can be observed with a light microscope.[192-197] It has been suggested that NIH/3T3 cells maintained in a hormonally defined culture medium may be conveniently used, since it would select the growth of oncogene-transformed cells.[198]

The efficiency of transformation with the NIH/3T3 DNA transfection assay is comparable to that of transformation induced by DNA of virus-transformed cells (0.1 to 1 transformant per microgram DNA). In contrast, high molecular weight DNA of normal cells do not display transforming ability, although low molecular weight fragments of normal cell DNAs (0.5 to 5 kb) induces a low efficiency of transformation (0.003 transformants per microgram DNA).[193,199] Putative transforming genes can also be transfected into NIH/3T3 cells by using a cosmid rescue strategy for cloning.[200]

Cells transformed by activated *ras* protooncogenes show unrestrained growth and acquire tumorigenic properties, including the expression of a metastatic phenotype upon implantation in nude mice.[201-203] Moreover, NIH/3T3 cells containing different transfected *ras* genes, which may be either activated or inactivated, rapidly acquire phenotypes that enable them to form lung tumors after tail vein injection into nude mice.[204] Whereas the focus-forming activity of different *ras* genes may differ by two orders of magnitude, the metastatic activity varies much less. The mechanism by which both activated and inactivated *ras* oncogenes can confer intrinsic metastatic ability in *in vivo* experimental metastasis assays is unknown. It is also unknown whether such artificial manipulations of *ras* genes are relevant for the natural carcinogenic processes occurring in humans and other animals.

The foci of transformed cells can be picked up and single cells from them can be cloned in semisolid media. Clonal cells can be grown to mass culture and their DNAs can be analyzed for detection of repetitive sequences, e.g., human *Alu* sequences.[205,206] The putative oncogenes present in donor DNA can be studied by transformation assays of DNA fragments obtained by digestion with restriction enzymes.[197] Since the transforming ability of extracted DNA is somewhat variable, it is convenient to monitor the donor DNA with some well-characterized marker in parallel assays. The most used of these markers is the thymidine kinase (tk) gene, which is assayed in murine LMtk⁻ cells, the tk⁺ colonies being selected in HAT medium.[207] Variability in the results obtained with DNA transfection assay may be circumvented, at least in part, by improving some of the experimental conditions.[208]

2. Mechanisms of Transformation in the NIH/3T3 Assay System

Cellular DNA can acquire transforming ability in transfection experiments through different changes leading to oncogenic activation.[62,209] Some of these changes may occur during manipulations related to the transfection experiment itself.[209,210] They could consist in DNA fragmentation, removal of the 5′ flanking sequences of oncogenes, association of transferred protooncogenes with efficient promoters in the recipient cells, breakages in protooncogene exons and/or introns, and other structural or functional changes.[62] Spontaneous activation of human c-*ras* protooncogenes has been observed during transfection experiments.[211,212] Protooncogenes other than those of the c-*ras* family, e.g., c-*ros* and c-*raf*-1, can also be activated by rearrangement-associated mechanisms that may occur during the manipulations related to gene transfer procedures.[213-215] Obviously, such artificially activated genes are not related to the neoplastic transformation that occurred in the original tumor cells but represent epiphenomena suggesting a particular susceptibility of those cells for structural alteration of protooncogene DNA sequences.

A very high frequency of spontaneous mutation has been observed in experimental systems involving DNA transfection into mammalian cells, including mouse, monkey, and human cells.[216,217] It is conceivable that these changes occur more frequently in malignant donor cells than in donor cells from the respective normal tissues. A general instability of the genome is frequently associated with malignant transformation of cells,[218] which could predispose to the occurrence of different kinds of genomic changes, especially under unusual environmental conditions such as those related to DNA transfection. Destabilization of the recipient cell genome induced by the DNA transfection procedure itself may lead to neoplastic transformation in a rather unspecific manner.[219] Nonspecific effects of DNA transfection may affect the metastatic potential of the recipient cells. The high efficiency of the NIH/3T3 system for transfection/transformation assays (as compared to the low efficiency observed in other assay systems) could be related to some peculiarity intrinsinc to the genome of NIH/3T3 cells, which would make these cells more susceptible to transformation in the presence of foreign DNA, especially if the DNA comes from certain malignant cells.

Integration of donor DNA during transfection into NIH/3T3 cells appears to proceed by a pathway which is nonspecific for both donor and recipient DNA sequences.[220] Both homologous and nonhomologous recombination events occur at high efficiency in DNA molecules transfected into mammalian cells but the rate of nonhomologous recombination may be two- to threefold higher than the rate of homologous recombination.[221] The sites of insertion of donor DNA into the genome of NIH/3T3 cells appear to be completely random, but all the foreign DNA taken up by one cell is probably fixed at a unique site.[222] Thus, the location of foreign DNA is unique in each clone, but varies from clone to clone. However, the possibility of slight preferences for certain genomic sites during the process of integration cannot be totally discarded. Some cellular DNA sequences could be rearranged and/or amplified during or after the process of protooncogene integration,[223] and these events may constitute critical steps in the multistage phenomenon of neoplastic transformation. Spontaneous amplification of genes encoding two different human myeloid cell surface antigens (gp150 and p67) has been observed after DNA-mediated gene transfer of cellular DNA from the human myeloid leukemia cell line HL-60 into NIH/3T3 mouse fibroblasts.[224] Cotransfection of "normal" DNA from NIH/3T3 cells and retroviral LTR sequences (M-MuLV 3′-LTR sequences) has been suggested as a possible strategy for the detection of potential cellular oncogenes.[225]

The genomic sites where protooncogenes are initially integrated into the genome of NIH/3T3 cells have not been characterized. Moreover, protooncogenes are integrated with some carried segments from the donor cells, and the possible role of these nononcogene DNA segments in the process of malignant transformation is not understood.

3. Molecular Changes Involved in the DNA Transfection Assay

Many molecular phenomena at both genetic and epigenetic levels could occur between the transfection of DNA and the appearance of foci of transformed cells, and the details of these events are little understood. At least one step of the multiple stages of DNA transfection-induced oncogenic transformation of NIH/3T3 cells is susceptible to inhibition by protease inhibitors such as antipain, leupeptin, α_1-antitripsin, and ε-aminocaproic acid, but the molecular mechanisms of this inhibitory effect are not understood.[226] Examination of the integration sites resulting from the transfer of purified gene fragments introduced into mouse cells gave the following results: there are no direct or indirect repeats or specific DNA sequences at the sites of integration; there is no detectable sequence homology between cellular and exogenous DNAs near the junctions; integration is always accompanied by rearrangements or deletions of host DNA; and integration occurs preferentially at repetitive DNA elements of the host.[227] Marked enhancement in the frequency of foci formation is observed when 3-methoxybenzamide (an inhibitor of the enzyme ADP-ribosyl transferase) was added to NIH/3T3 cells during or after DNA transfection but there was no effect when cells were only pretreated with the inhibitor.[228] ADP-ribosyl transferase catalyzes the formation and attachment of poly(ADP-ribose) moieties to nuclear proteins but its possible role in DNA transfection experiments is not understood. Addition of tumor promoters such as phorbol esters may induce modifications in the specific growth response on *ras*-transformed embryo fibroblasts.[229]

DNA transfected to mammalian cells suffers mutation with an extremely high frequency. These mutations include base substitutions and deletions as well as insertions from the recipient genome.[217] The mutations are introduced early, rather than continually, during replication and they may be the explanation, at least in some cases, for the detection of mutated oncogenes after DNA transfection. DNA fragments from normal human lymphocytes may acquire transforming activity as a consequence of spontaneous activation of c-*ras* genes.[212] The increased susceptibility of c-*ras* genes derived from tumor cells for mutagenic processes occurring during DNA transfection experiments could be related to some conformational changes present in genes which are actively transcribed in the population of tumor cells. It seems thus clear that some protooncogenes, and possibly also other cellular genes, can undergo different types of structural changes during transfection experiments and that these changes may result in an artificial activation of the oncogenic potential of the particular genes. Introduction of homologous DNA sequences into mammalian cells may frequently result in the occurrence of mutations in the cognate gene.[230] This event may depend not only on homology but also on mismatched base pairs between the newly introduced DNA sequence and the corresponding sequence residing in the recipient cell genome.

Reversible DNA amplification may play a central role in the expression of transfected genes.[231] A position effect would provide an explanation for amplification of integrated gene if the integration occurs into a region close to an origin of replication. Moreover, this phenomenon raises the possibility that other genes in the amplifying unit may play a role in either maintaining or regulating the growth state of the cells for transfection assays.[231] New, small circular DNA molecules appear a short time (42 h) after DNA transfection into cells.[232] These molecules are apparently generated by rearrangement of the transfected DNA and induction of small circles of cellular DNA. The circular DNA could have autonomous transcriptional functions or could act as intermediates in DNA amplification or rearrangements occurring in the genome of transfected cells.

Nonspecific effects of the DNA transfection procedure may result in marked alterations in the malignant behavior of the recipient cells, including their metastatic capability.[219] An enhancement of the metastatic behavior of cells can be achieved after transfection with DNA from highly metastasizing tumor cells but also with DNA from rat muscle or *Drosophila* cells. The treatment of cells with calcium phosphate alone may also strongly enhance their metastatic capability.

4. DNA Transfection and Multistage Oncogenic Transformation

Immortalization of human senescing embryonic cells can be obtained with viral (SV40) and nonviral (salmon sperm) DNA,[233] which suggests that acquisition of an infinite growth potential and a transformed phenotype are complex multistage phenomena, and that they are not equivalent. Mouse cells (fibroblasts) are more prone to transformation than human cells. Embryonal mouse fibroblasts, such as the NIH/3T3 cells, as well as foreskin cells, may represent a state in which differentiation is not yet complete and which is phenotypically similar to transformation *in vitro*.[234] Apparently, these cells are genotypically highly sensitive to a variety of carcinogenic insults. Acquisition of an infinite lifespan is a very rare event in normal human cells. It has been observed only in human embryonic or newborn fibroblasts and, in one instance, with cultured cells from human adult neuroretina after infection with SV40.[235]

Modification of the DNA of donor cells within the tumor cells, and/or the recipient cells or their descendants, may be required for positive results in the NIH/3T3 assay. While DNAs prepared from 4-dimethylaminoazobenzene (DAB)- or AAF-induced rat hepatomas do not induce the formation of transformed foci in the NIH/3T3 transfection assay, DNAs from transplanted hepatomas display transforming activity in the assay.[236] Acquisition of transforming potential following repeated transplantation may be related to tumor cell progression or selection which may implicate the activation of cellular genes with transforming capability.

The transformation events occurring in NIH/3T3 cells after DNA transfection are probably not a simple consequence of activation of a transfected protooncogene. Fibroblast immortality is a prerequisite for transformation by oncogene products *in vitro*.[237] Immortality of cell lines, itself, is probably a phenotypic trait that may result from different events, or sets of events, occurring in the genetic program that limits the division of normal cell populations.[238] Experimental induction of cell fusion between immortal cell lines of different origin may result in hybrids with finite division capacity. Thus, the events leading to cellular immortality are recessive and heterogeneous at the genetic level.

Sublines of NIH/3T3 cells cultured in different laboratories may exhibit great variation in susceptibility to oncogenic transformation in transfection experiments.[239] Moreover, certain sublines of mouse 3T3 cells may be tumorigenic, as can be shown when these cells are attached to glass beds and injected into mice, which results in the appearance of malignant hemangioendotheliomas.[240] EK-3, a subline derived from NIH/3T3 cells, differs from the parental cell line with respect to loss of tumorigenicity in nude mice and to inefficient transformation *in vitro* by an activated c-*ras* gene alone.[241] EK-3 cells require both *myc* and *ras* genes for *in vitro* transformation, which suggests that they have lost a function which is analogous to that of *myc* and that this function is present in the parental cell lines. When carefully tested, untransfected NIH/3T3 cultures contain subpopulations of cells that are already tumorigenic as judged by their ability to produce tumors in mice at two anatomical locations, to form pulmonary metastases from a primary tumor growing in the footpad, and to generate lung colonies following i.v. injection.[242] Thus, it is clear that NIH/3T3 cells should be considered at least as premalignant cells.

5. DNA Transfection and Induction of Endogenous Proviruses

Transformation of NIH/3T3 cells by DNA transfected from a human mammary carcinoma cell line induces expression of an endogenous MuLV provirus.[243] Four MuLV proteins (gp86, gp72, p70, and p19) can be detected in NIH/3T3 cells after transfection of DNA from human and mouse mammary carcinomas. The possible role of these proteins in the oncogenic transformation of NIH/3T3 cells after DNA transfection is not understood. In general, the possible role of endogenous proviruses in cell transformation is not understood. In any case, the expression of oncogenes may not be tightly associated with transformation as is observed when cells are treated with butyrate, which permits oncogene expression but prevents formation of foci of transformed cells.[244]

6. Inhibition of Oncogenic Transformation in the DNA Assay

Interferon (IFN) is capable of inhibiting the transformation of mouse cells by exogenous cellular or viral genes.[245] Mouse interferon inhibits the development of transformed foci in NIH/3T3 cells transfected with v-H-*ras*, v-*mos*, or EJ/T24 c-*ras* DNA.[246] Moreover, prolonged treatment with mouse IFN-α/β induces phenotypic reversion in NIH/3T3 cells transformed with an LTR-activated human c-H-*ras*-1 gene (clonal line RS485), but no reversion is observed with IFN-treated RS504 cells, an NIH/3T3 cell line transformed with the mutant EJ c-H-*ras* gene.

The mechanisms responsible for these inhibitory actions of interferon have not been characterized. Treatment with interferon may reduce the amount of c-H-*ras*-specific mRNA and p21 protein expressed in NIH/3T3 cells transformed by an LTR-activated human c-H-*ras* gene or may inhibit the stabilization or integration of protooncogene sequences transfected into the same cells.[246-248] In contrast to the reversibility of cellular changes seen with exposure to IFN for several days, the phenotypic reversion of RS485 cells established after 1 to 2 months of IFN treatment may persist long after treatment is discontinued.[249] The persistent revertants express high levels of p21[c-*ras*] yet are not tumorigenic. Moreover, while the persistent revertants resist retransformation by a variety of viral or cellular oncogenes, they are readily retransformed after exposure to DNA demethylating drugs such as 5-azacytidine. These results suggest that DNA methylation processes may be involved in the expression of a transformed phenotype in transfected cells. However, this expression is not necessarily associated with changes in protooncogene expression.[250] Most probably, other cellular genes participate in these changes.

7. Biological Significance and Limitations of the NIH/3T3 Assay System

A better characterization of the molecular events involved in DNA transfection/transformation experiments with the NIH/3T3 system is needed. As stated above, NIH/3T3 cells cannot be strictly considered as normal cells but are probably preneoplastic cells because they have genetic alterations caused by their maintenance in continuous cell culture in the laboratory for many years. NIH/3T3 cells are aneuploid and, under appropriate conditions, can form malignant neoplasms upon transplantation into normal or nude (athymic) mice.[242,251] The process of $Ca_3(PO_4)_2$-mediated DNA transfection is itself associated with disturbances in the expression of recipient cell genes which may result in profound alterations in tumorigenic or metabolic behavior.[219,252] Furthermore, at least some of these changes are heritable. Thus, there appears that, upon transfection of DNA from foreign tumor cells, the transfected cells are occasionally forced further in their state of neoplastic progression rather than initiated as new neoplastic cells. A possible explanation for this phenomenon would be that the genome of NIH/3T3 cells, like that of other preneoplastic cells, is unstable and that it is, consequently, very susceptible to transfection by appropriate "active" protooncogenes from different sources. However, an activated (T24) c-H-*ras* gene is also able to confer tumorigenic and metastatic phenotype upon its transfection into early passage, diploid rodent fibroblasts.[253] An alternative murine recipient cell line, C127, was tumorigenic but not metastatic when transformed with an activated *ras* protooncogene, which indicates that an undefined factor present in NIH/3T3 cells is absent in C127 cells.[253] *In vitro* establishment (immortality) may not be a sufficient prerequisite for transformation by activated *ras* genes since these genes morphologically transform other established cell lines (REF52 cells) only at low frequencies and the adenovirus E1A region collaborates with the activated *ras* genes to convert REF52 cells to a tumorigenic phenotype.[254]

Transfection of NIH/3T3 cells with plasmids carrying nononcogene sequences such as the protein kinase C-I gene may result in altered growth behavior and acquisition of tumorigenic potential upon inoculation into nude mice.[255] Cells expressing the protein kinase C-I gene exhibit reduced dependence on serum for sustained growth but their morphological alterations are less striking that those of NIH/3T3 cells transfected with activated *ras* oncogenes and are unable to form foci in the assay system *in vitro*. The changes observed in these cells are somewhat similar to those produced by transfection of c-*myc*, E1A, or p53 gene. In any case, it is clear that nononcogene genes can induce altered growth when transfected into NIH/3T3 cells.

Cultivation of tumor cell populations *in vitro* may be accompanied by selection of the particular subsets of malignant cells which may constitute an extremely small subpopulation in the patient's tumor.[256] It is also possible that other subsets of the tumor cell population disappear during cocultivation. Thus, the colonies obtained *in vitro* may not be a representative sample of the tumor cell population *in vivo*.

Experiments involving DNA transfection into NIH/3T3 cells are unable to demonstrate that activation of a single and specific protooncogene is an event crucially involved in transformation of a normal cell into a neoplastic cell. On the contrary, the latter is highly unlikely. Even the expression of a v-H-*ras* oncogene may not be sufficient for induction of a transformed phenotype. When NIH/3T3 cells adapted to grow in a medium containing 5 m*M* butyrate are infected with H-MuSV, addition of butyrate to the medium does not prevent the expression of the p21[v-ras] oncogene product on the inner aspect of the plasma membrane, but the appearance of foci of transformed cells is reversibly inhibited by butyrate.[244] In general, the expression of genes introduced into cells by retroviral infection is much more efficient than that of genes introduced by calcium phosphate-mediated DNA transfection procedures, which may be attributed to DNA methylation occurring in the integrated gene when it is introduced by transfection but not when introduced by viral infection.[257]

Transfection of DNA sequences with transforming capability would occur not only *in vitro* but also *in vivo*.[258] The study of cultures initiated from a human small-cell lung carcinoma growing as a xenograft in nude mice indicated the presence of mouse cell lines expressing a transformed as well as a differentiated phenotype.[259] The transformed mouse cells contained human DNA sequences and expressed both mouse- and human-specific histocompatibility antigens. These observations implicate that human genetic information was transferred to primary mouse host fibroblasts*in vivo*. The results further suggest the possible use of the nude mice to study the oncogenic process as it relates to spontaneous or natural DNA transfection.

8. Detection of Activated Protooncogenes in the NIH/3T3 DNA Transfection Assay

An intriguing fact is that only one family of protooncogenes, the *ras* family, gives regular positive results in DNA transfection experiments using the NIH/3T3 assay.[260] Moreover, mutations that selectively affect codons 12 and 61 of c-*ras* genes are almost exclusively found in positive results obtained with this assay. An interesting possibility is that mutations occurring at sites other than codons 12 or 61 of c-*ras* genes would have remained undetected in the commonly used NIH/3T3 DNA transfection assay. Mutations of the N-*ras* protooncogene at codon 13 were detected in the tumor cells of four out of five patients with AML.[261] The mutations substituted asparagine or valine for glycine at this codon but such mutations are relatively weak for inducing foci of transformed cells in the NIH/3T3 assay.

Protooncogenes other than c-*ras* are usually little able, or totally unable, to induce transformation of NIH/3T3 cells, although there are some exceptions to this general rule.[262] The putative human B-*lym*-1 protooncogene may be responsible for positive transformation results in the NIH/3T3 assay system obtained with DNA from Burkitt's lymphoma, but the mechanisms involved in this activation remain unknown.[263] No mutational changes or increased expression of B-*lym*-1 genes have been detected in Burkitt's lymphoma cells. More recently, it has been clearly demonstrated that B-*lym*-1 genes are structurally related to the human long interspersed (LINE) repetitive sequence, which is highly conserved in mammalian evolution.[264,265]

A protooncogene that can be detected in the NIH/3T3 transfection assay is c-*neu*, but the oncogenic activation of this gene is apparently not associated with gross structural alteration in its DNA sequences, as judged by extensive restriction endonuclease mapping.[266] A putative protooncogene, *mel*, was detected in the human malignant melanoma cell line NK14.[267] An unidentified putative transforming gene, apparently not related to c-*ras* genes or other previously described oncogenes, was detected in the human pancreatic adenocarcinoma cell line HPAF.[268]

An oncogenically activated gene, *hst*, was detected in 3 of 58 samples of DNA obtained from of a total of 26 patients with stomach cancer.[269,270] The *hst* gene exhibited oncogenic activity not only in the tumor samples from two patients but also in a sample obtained from a noncancerous portion of the stomach from one of these two patients. None of the 58 samples of DNAs in this study of stomach cancer contained activated c-*ras* genes, and the mechanism of activation of *hst* was not characterized. An activated *hst* gene, detected in a human hepatoma by means of a tumorigenicity assay in nude mice using transfected NIH/3T3 cells, was associated with a DNA rearrangement event that occurred during or after the transfection procedure.[271] A putative protooncogene identified by the NIH/3T3 DNA transfection assay in Kaposi's sarcoma may be similar or identical to *hst*.[272,273] The *hst* gene encodes a protein related to the FGF family of growth factors. The possible role of the *hst* protein in tumorigenic processes is unknown.

Combination of the NIH/3T3 DNA transfection assay with subsequent injection of the cells into nude mice was used to detect a putative protooncogene, *mas*, in a human epidermoid carcinoma.[274]

9. Oncogenic Activation of Genomic Sequences during the DNA Transfection Procedure

Oncogenic activation of cellular genomic sequences, as assessed in the NIH/3T3 DNA transfection/transformation assay, can occur during the transfection procedure. Spontaneous activation of an N-*ras* gene associated with mutation (G-T transversion) at codon 12 occurred during the transfection of DNA from chemically induced rat intestinal adenocarcinomas into NIH/3T3 cells.[275] The original tumor DNA did not contain the mutated allele but hybridized only with an oligonucleotide probe representing the normal cells. Activation of a putative transforming gene, *ret*, occurred during transfection of NIH/3T3 cells with human lymphoma DNA.[276] The transforming sequence was apparently not originated by mutation but by rearrangement of normal human DNA during transfection. A putative transforming gene, *mcf*-3, isolated from nude mouse tumors obtained upon transfection of NIH/3T3 cells with DNA from the human mammary carcinoma cell line MCF-7, arose by recombination of a normal human c-*ros* protooncogene during the DNA transfection procedure.[213] Another gene, *mcf*-2, was identified using cotransfection of DNA from the human mammary carcinoma cell line MCF-7 and a G418 antibiotic resistance gene into NIH/3T3 cells, followed by tumor formation in athymic mice.[161] The transforming sequence was mapped to human chromosome X, at region Xq27.

Activation of the protooncogene c-*raf* occurred during transfection of DNA from a rat hepatocellular carcinoma induced by the carcinogen, 2-amino-3-methylimidazo(4,5-*f*)quinoline.[277] The activation of c-*raf* during transfection occurred not by point mutation but by DNA recombination in the 5′ terminal region of the gene with rat genomic sequences, which resulted in transcription of an abnormally fused mRNA in which the 5′ half of the sequence was replaced by an unknown rat sequence.[277,278] The fused c-*raf*-related mRNA coded for a hybrid c-*raf*-related protein. Connection of the rearranged, but not the normal, c-*raf* sequence to RSV LTR resulted in a vector capable of transforming NIH/3T3 cells.[214] An activated c-*raf*-1-related gene present in NIH/3T3 cell transformants derived from the GL-5-JCK human glioblastoma DNA transfection consisted of three portions of human DNA sequences, with the 3′ half of the c-*raf*-1 gene at its middle portion.[279] The c-*raf*-1-derived sequence was 20 kb long and contained exons 8 to 17 and the poly(A) addition site. This rearranged c-*raf*-1 gene was present in the transforming DNA of NIH/3T3 cells but was not present in the original GL-5-JCK tumor DNA, and was probably generated by rearrangement of c-*raf*-1 sequences that occurred during the process of tumor DNA transfection. Two transformants of NIH/3T3 cells, obtained by transfection of human colon cancer and normal colon DNAs, contained activated c-*raf*-1 gene.[215] In both the activated c-*raf*-1 genes, the 5′ half of the c-*raf*-1 DNA sequence was replaced by sequences other than c-*raf*-1 as a result of recombination which occurred at the intron between exons 7 and 8. These recombinations were apparently responsible for the oncogenic activation of c-*raf*-1 but they occurred during the transfection procedure and were not present in the original cells. Although these results should bring caution in the interpretation of DNA transfection assays, they are interesting in themselves in the sense that they demonstrate that particular recombinations of cellular DNA sequences may result in the creation of novel sequences with oncogenic capability.

A putative protooncogene, *dbl*, was isolated following transfection of NIH/3T3 cells with DNAs from a human diffuse B-cell lymphoma and a human nodular poorly differentiated lymphoma.[280,281] The *dbl* gene was apparently activated by a structural rearrangement that occurred during the process of gene transfer *in vitro* and affected the 5′ end sequences of the gene. The normal product of the human *dbl* gene corresponds to a protein of 66 kDa, p66*dbl*, which is located in the cytoplasm and is phosphorylated on serine residues.[282,283] The normal function of p66*dbl* is unknown.

Transfection analysis of seven established human AML cell lines indicated the presence of activated N-*ras* genes in three lines and five putative novel transforming genes in the other four lines.[284] However, the data suggested that the transforming sequences reported became activated during the transfection procedure and were not present in the original cell lines. The putative protooncogene *mas* was activated during transfection of human AML DNA.[285] Transcripts of the *mas* gene could not be detected in normal cells. In any case, the detection of cellular DNA sequences that are accidentally activated during the transfection assay may serve to identify potential protooncogenes whose structural alteration and/or inappropriate expression may contribute to neoplastic transformation *in vivo*.

An active transforming gene, *trk*, detected in a human colon carcinoma, was generated not by mutation but by somatic recombination of a truncated tyrosine kinase receptor gene with the tropomyosin gene.[262] The truncated kinase sequences of the *trk* gene can also be activated by recombination with other genomic sequences.[286] Transfection of NIH/3T3 cells with cDNA containing the entire coding sequences of the tyrosine protein kinase domain of the human *trk* gene results in the frequent generation of transforming genes, which involves acquisition of cellular DNA sequences.[287] The high frequency with which *trk* DNA sequences acquire transforming properties by recombination with other sequences appears to be a distinctive feature of this locus.

10. Transforming Gene(s) in Atherosclerotic Plaques

Proliferation of smooth muscle cells is an early event in the development of atherosclerotic plaques. According to the monoclonal hypothesis, human atherosclerotic plaques are monoclonal in origin and could arise via mutational or viral events.[288] These plaques would represent benign muscle cell tumors of the artery wall. It is thus most interesting that human atherosclerotic plaque DNA is capable of completing the oncogenic transformation of NIH/3T3 cells via DNA transfection, giving origin to foci of transformed cells.[289,290] Moreover, the cells from such foci contain human DNA and are capable of eliciting the appearance of tumors after injection into nude mice. The human gene(s) responsible for such oncogenic events derived from atherosclerotic plaques have not been identified but are not members of the c-*ras* family of protooncogenes. The possible role of this gene(s) in the origin and/or development of human atherosclerotic plaques is unknown.

11. Assay Systems other than the NIH/3T3 Assay

The sensitivity of NIH/3T3 cells for obtaining positive results in DNA transfection/ transformation experiments is intriguing. Negative results have been obtained frequently with many other indicator cells when DNA from tumor cells, or even cloned protooncogenes, are tested. However, positive results in DNA transfection/transformation experiments may be obtained with a number of cell lines derived from several animal species.

C3H/10T1/2 cells represent an immortal cell line which was originally derived from C3H mouse embryos and which has been widely used for the *in vitro* assessment of the possible carcinogenic effects of environmental agents. Transfection of C3H/10T1/2 cells with a plasmid containing a cloned mutant c-H-*ras* gene results in neoplastic transformation as judged by colony morphology and tumorigenic growth in nude mice.[291] The phorbol ester TPA, which is a potent tumor promoter, causes an approximately fivefold increase in the number of transformed foci obtained in C3H10T1/2 cells transfected with the mutant T24 c-H-*ras* oncogene.[292]

Cultured secondary REF cells do not yield detectable foci of transformed cells after transfection of the cloned v-H-*ras* oncogene but foci of transformed cells appear when v-H-*ras* and v-*myc* cloned oncogenes are applied together to REF cultures.[65] Thus, at least in the REF test system, a synergistic cooperation of two oncogenes, the viral *ras* and *myc* genes, is necessary for the expression of a transformed phenotype. Augmented expression of normal c-*myc* is sufficient for cotransformation of REF cells with a mutant EJ c-*ras* gene.[293] The N-*myc* gene, which shows sequence homology to c-*myc*, is also able to cooperate with a mutant c-H-*ras* gene for the induction of transformation in REF cells.[294] Foci of transformed cells are also observed in REF cells when transfer of a v-*myc* oncogene is followed by treatment with the phorbol ester, TPA.[295]

The mouse C127 cell line is an immortal but morphologically nontransformed line derived from a mammary tumor of an RIII mouse. This line may be a robust and reliable alternative to NIH/3T3 cells in selection for the malignant phenotype elicited by either DNA- or chromosome-mediated gene transfer.[296] Transfection of C127 cells with mitotic chromosomes from EJ human bladder carcinoma (which contain a mutant c-H-*ras* gene) gave rise, at high frequency, to foci of transformed cells. The transformants may thereafter be selected for tumorigenicity in an assay *in vivo*.

Cotransfection of a mutant T24 c-H-*ras* gene and an adenovirus (Ad2) E1A gene, using a constructed plasmid, results in about ten times greater efficiency of transformation of REF cells in comparison to transfection of the *ras* gene alone.[297] However, the cotransfected cells do not generate metastases after subcutaneous injection and have a diminished ability to induce lung metastases after i.v. injection into 4-week-old nude mice.

The rat cell line EL2 is highly susceptible to transformation by several oncogenes.[298] EL2 cells were isolated from primary REF cultures after transfection with recombinant plasmids encoding polyoma virus middle-T and large-T antigens but, after repeated passages, they do not contain any detectable polyoma virus or plasmid sequences. When these cells are transfected with human DNA containing an activated protooncogene (c-*ras* from T24 bladder carcinoma cell line) they yield more foci of transformed cells (15 foci per 20 μg of DNA) than NIH/3T3 cells (5 foci per 20 μg of DNA). T24-transformed EL2 cells are tumorigenic when injected into young Fisher rats but, as it occurs with NIH/3T3 cells, the molecular mechanisms involved in their oncogenic transformation are not understood. The transcriptional activity of two endogenous protooncogenes (c-*myc* and c-*sis*) is similar in normal and transformed EL2 cells.

Transformation of a rat cell line (Rat 1 cells) has also been achieved by chromosome-mediated gene transfer.[299] In these experiments it was demonstrated that it is possible to transfer the malignant phenotype of anchorage independence from human AML cells to anchorage-dependent rat cells, using isolated chromosomes as the source of genetic information. Chromosomes isolated from human leukemic cells lines are capable of transferring the transformed phenotype, whereas chromosomes derived from the lymphocytes of normal individuals are not active in this assay. Using Southern blot analysis of the DNA from transfectants, it was shown that the same segment of DNA is active in this transfection assay and that an active N-*ras* protooncogene is probably responsible for the positive results obtained with this procedure.

A procedure proposed for the isolation of protooncogenes is based on the cocultivation of cells that release endogenous viruses with other cells, which would result in production of recombinant retroviruses.[300] Cocultivation of the rat embryonic cell line SD1-T, which releases endogenous rat leukemia viruses, with normal rat kidney cells transformed by cloned v-*mos* DNA, the rat mammary tumor cell line 63SP, or NRK cells transformed by 63SP DNA results within 1 month in the release of oncogenic retroviruses that can be recovered from the coculture supernatants.

DNA sequences with transforming capability that are not detected by DNA transfer into NIH/3T3 cells might be detected with JB6 mouse epidermal cells.[301] Transfection of DNA from a human leukemia cell line (Reh) into mouse primary lymphocytes can produce cell lines with the capacity of proliferate continuously in culture.[302] However, it is not known whether this DNA contains a protooncogene previously defined in other systems, a new protooncogene, or another type of gene involved in the control of cell proliferation.

In an alternate method proposed for transfection assay, the tumorigenic properties of a line of mouse mammary epithelial cells (NMuMg) is tested in nude mice after DNA transfection.[303] In initial experiments it was shown that NMuMg cells are capable of taking up and expressing a mutant c-H-*ras* oncogene cloned from the EJ human bladder carcinoma cell line. Upon injection into nude mice, the cells transfected with the activated oncogene grew and produced invasive carcinomas.

Subcutaneous injection of NIH/3T3 cells transfected with DNA from a primary human cutaneous squamous cell carcinoma not only induced tumors at the site of injection but also metastasized spontaneously to the lungs in all of the nude mice injected.[304] Southern blot hybridization with *ras*-specific probes revealed that both the primary tumors and the metastases that occurred in the injected mice contained a highly amplified c-H-*ras* gene. However, at least part of this amplification could take place during or after the gene transfer procedure.

Mammary tumors are very rare in rabbits, and rabbit mammary cells appear to be unable to undergo spontaneous transformation. However, an assay system has been proposed using rabbit cell lines established by microinjecting SV40 DNA.[305] A fully transformed cell line was obtained in this system by coinjecting SV40 DNA and a plasmid containing the activated EJ c-H-*ras* protooncogene. The proliferation rate of these cells was high and their growth was anchorage independent. The cells were tumorigenic in nude mice but had no metastatic potential.

An assay system using human cells would be most appropriate for testing the possible oncogenic activity of human protooncogenes. However, human cells incorporate much less exogenous DNA than rodent cells in transfection experiments.[306] Human diploid fibroblasts are completely resistant to transformation by a cloned mutant oncogene, the EJ c-*ras* gene, which is highly active in the NIH/3T3 assay. The resistance occurs in spite of high levels of the altered p21[c-*ras*] oncogene product.[307] The same cells are also resistant to oncogenic transformation by SV40 DNA despite the presence of T antigen, which indicates that the normal gene products of human cells can override the oncogenic action of protein products that are highly oncogenic in cellular systems from nonhuman species. However, transformation of human embryo kidney (HEK) cells to anchorage independence (growth in soft agar) can be achieved by transfection with a combination of the EJ c-H-*ras*-1 gene and human papovavirus BK.[308] More recently, morphological transformation of normal diploid human foreskin fibroblasts in culture was achieved by using a plasmid vector (pH06T1) containing the T24 c-H-*ras* gene with 5′ and 3′ enhancer sequences.[309] However, the transfected human cells were nontumorigenic in athymic mice and they reverted to a normal phenotype as the cells were passaged in culture. It may be concluded that normal human cells are relatively resistant to transformation induced by mutant c-*ras* genes.

A test system with human neonatal foreskin fibroblasts has been proposed for detection of transforming genes.[310] It is possible that the human cell transformation system allows the detection of transforming genes not effective in the NIH/3T3 system. A permanent human lymphoblast cell line (MOLT-4) and a human multiple myeloma cell line (GM 1312), whose DNAs were inefficient in transforming NIH/3T3 cells, were effective in inducing anchorage independence, but not foci, in the human foreskin fibroblast system.[310,311] Since human cells take up DNA poorly, the cells are treated with polyethylene glycol to facilitate the uptake of coprecipitated DNA-calcium phosphate. DNAs from human tumor cells can transform these human recipient cells to anchorage-independent growth, whereas DNAs from normal human tissues are apparently unable to induce this alteration. However, the recipient transformed human cells are not immortal nor tumorigenic, and the possible role of human protooncogenes in the results obtained with this assay remains uncharacterized. More recently, a DNA transfection assay has been proposed using the nontumorigenic, revertant human osteosarcoma cell line HOS, which may be transformed to tumorigenicity in athymic nude mice by active human protooncogenes with latency periods as short as 3 weeks.[312]

B. BIOCHEMICAL AND IMMUNOLOGICAL PROCEDURES

The NIH/3T3 DNA transfection/transformation assay and other similar biological assays have only limited sensitivity for the detection of oncogenically activated protooncogenes in tumor cells.[313] Protooncogenes, or their RNA and protein products, can also be detected by different procedures acting at the DNA, RNA, or protein levels.

1. Studies at the DNA Level

Analytical approaches involving recombinant DNA techniques and nucleic acid hybridization procedures have been applied with excellent results to the study of human genetic diseases and can also be applied to the direct analysis of oncogenes and protooncogenes.[314-317] Many protooncogenes of human and nonhuman origin have been isolated from recombinant DNA libraries derived from either normal cells or tumor cells. cDNA segments containing protooncogene sequences can be cloned in molecular vectors, their nucleotide sequences can be determined, and the products expressed in bacteria or other cells transformed by such vectors may be purified and characterized.

The semiquantitative "spot" or "dot-blot" technique can be used for the detection of oncogenes and protooncogenes.[318] In this technique, hybridization of target DNA immobilized as spots on a filter is used for demonstration of the presence (or absence) of a nucleic acid (DNA or RNA) sequence of interest. When information on the size of specific DNA fragments is desired, the Southern blotting technique can be conveniently used.[319-322] This technique involves extraction of double-stranded cellular DNA, digestion with selected restriction enzymes, electrophoresis on agarose gels, transference onto nitrocellulose filters, blot hybridization with labeled probes, and autoradiography.

These procedures have been applied to the detection and characterization of human protooncogenes. In one of the earliest applications of these procedures to the study of DNA from several vertebrate species, it was found that human DNA contains the sequences c-*sis* (homologous to the SSV oncogene), c-*fes* (homologous to the FeSV oncogene), and c-H-*ras* (homologous to the H-MuSV oncogene).[323] Thereafter, more than 20 protooncogenes have been detected and characterized in the genome of men and other animal species. Some protooncogenes with apparently no homologous sequences present in acute transforming retroviruses have been isolated and characterized directly from the animal genome, including the chicken and human B-*lym* and T-*lym* protooncogenes and the human N-*ras* protooncogene.[324-327] The DNA probes obtained from molecular vectors and representing protooncogene sequences have been used for the detection and characterization of mRNAs transcribed from protooncogenes such as the human c-*myc* gene.[328]

DNA probes with specificity for particular human chromosomes, or for protooncogene sequences contained within particular chromosomes, are increasingly used with excellent results for the diagnosis and molecular analysis of structural chromosome alterations, especially translocations, which due to their size or other characteristics cannot be easily recognized with the current cytogenetic techniques. Such molecular probes are being used for the study of human leukemias and lymphomas.[329,330] Polymorphic DNA probes assigned to specific human chromosome regions may be extremely useful for the detection and chromosomal localization of genomic sequences that undergo loss of constitutional heterozygosity at specific loci in different types of human tumors.[331-340] Such sequences may correspond to tumor suppressor genes (antioncogenes).

Mutational changes occurring in protooncogene sequences can be detected by restriction endonucleases when they result in production of RFLPs.[341] This method has been applied, for example, for the detection of single point mutations of somatic origin in the c-K-*ras* gene in human lung cancer cells.[342] The main limitation of this method consists in that only a fraction of the possible mutations occurring in a given gene produce nucleotide changes that can be recognized by the available restriction enzymes.

Protooncogene mutations can be conveniently detected with the aid of synthetic oligonucleotide probes.[343] The assay is based on the fact that a fully matched DNA:DNA hybrid has a higher thermal stability than a hybrid with a mismatched base pair. By using a selective washing procedure, nonperfectly matching hybrids can melt off, whereas a fully matched hybrid molecule remains stable. This method has been applied as a screening test to detect mutations in codon 61 of the N-*ras* gene and codon 12 of the c-K-*ras* gene of various human tumor cell lines.[343,344] The advantages of the method consist in that it is applied directly on the genomic DNA, avoiding the possibility of mutations such as that occurring in the transfection procedure, and that it detects both the mutated and the normal alleles. In addition, its sensitivity does not depend on the transforming capacity of the affected gene. Some of the mutations detected with synthetic oligonucleotide probes have only weak transforming capacity and may remain undetected in the usual NIH/3T3 DNA transfection assay. The disadvantages are that the level of detection is limited, especially when the major part of the tissue sample is constituted by nonneoplastic cells, as frequently occurs in biopsy samples, and that it recognizes only specific point mutations.

A main limitation of molecular hybridization methods represented by their inadequate sensitivity for biological applications has been circumvented recently with the aid of oligonucleotide primers and DNA polymerase which produce an increase in the number of detectable target molecules in the sample *in vitro*.[345] In this procedure, called the polymerase chain reaction (PCR), target DNA is denatured, primers are hybridized to both strands of the target, and new strands of are synthesized by primer extension with DNA polymerase. The cycle, lasting only about 5 min, is repeated 20 times, resulting in 2×10^5-fold amplification of the target DNA.[314]

Amplification of DNA by the PCR method, combined with direct sequence analysis, is very useful for the detection of mutant protooncogenes.[346] PCR-induced amplification of *ras*-specific sequences results in a more than 10^4-fold increase in the sequence that might contain a point mutation, thus producing a considerable improvement in the sensitivity of the method used for the detection of c-*ras* point mutations.[347] Furthermore, it is no longer necessary to use high molecular weight DNA, and paraffin-embedded material may be a suitable source for DNA, which permits the analysis of archival samples in retrospect. Mutations in multiple alleles of the rat c-K-*ras* gene were detected by using a technique for direct sequence analysis of a 90-bp region of the gene produced by PCR DNA amplification.[348] The combined PCR amplification-direct sequencing methodology provides a rapid and sensitive means for the detection and characterization of mutations occurring in c-*ras* and other genes.[349] The use of a combination of techniques, including the application of PCR to small fresh or archival sections of formalin-fixed, paraffin-embedded tissue, and mutation detection by cleavage at single base mismatches by RNAse A in DNA:RNA and RNA:RNA heteroduplexes, allowed the detection of mutations at codon 12 of the c-K-*ras* gene in 21 of 22 primary carcinomas of the human exocrine pancreas.[350]

Virological methods are required for the isolation of viral oncogenes. According to a suggestion, viral oncogenes, as well as other viral genes, can be detected not only by hybridization nucleic acid probes labeled with radioisotopes but also by probe DNA fragments cloned in phages with direct enzyme labels which can be detected by highly sensitive and rapid colorimetric methods.[351]

2. Studies at the RNA Level

The transcriptional activity of oncogenes and protooncogenes can be examined by molecular hybridization procedures. In the semiquantitative spot or dot-blot technique, a mixture of RNA molecules containing the putative oncogene transcripts is immobilized in a solid matrix (usually a filter of nitrocellulose), and a radioactively labeled DNA probe containing known v-*onc* or c-*onc* sequences is then applied. If the DNA mixture contains protooncogenes, or protoonco-gene-like sequences, the radioactive DNA sticks to the immobilized dot of RNA, and this can be detected by overlaying the nitrocellulose filter with a piece of roentgenographic film, which would result in the appearance of a dot-blot in the film. The sizes of these dot blots, under specific experimental conditions, are roughly proportional to the concentrations of the particular protooncogene transcripts.

For determining the size (approximate molecular weight) of oncogene or protooncogene transcripts, a procedure of Northern blotting could be applied. This technique involves separation of the different RNA species from the mixture by electrophoresis in semisolid agarose gels, transference of the separated RNAs to nitrocellulose filters, hybridization to radioactive single-stranded DNA probes containing the oncogene sequences, and detection of the radioactive bands by autoradiography.[352] However, the detection of some protooncogene mRNAs may be difficult because they may be present at very low levels and may be unstable.

A sensitive method for the detection and quantitation of RNA from oncogenes or other genes may be represented by a solution hybridization technique.[353,354] Steps of this procedure include dissolving cells in concentrated guanidine thiocyanate, hybridizing with RNA probe at room temperature in the same solution, and measuring hybrid formed. Purification of cellular RNA or DNA is not required in this method. The PCR method can also be applied at the RNA level.

An analysis of protooncogene expression in individual cells from malignant tumors requires the application of *in situ* molecular hybridization procedures in order to determine whether this expression is associated with the malignant phenotype or whether it originates from cells infiltrating the tumor.[314,355] *In situ* hybridization is done directly on intact cells or tissues fixed on a support and enables the localization of target sequences within the cell. *In situ* DNA-mRNA hybridization techniques have been successfully applied to the detection of oncogene transcripts in cells transformed with viral oncogenes.[357] Following *in situ* hybridization with ^{32}P-labeled v-*src* and v-H-*ras* probes, *src*- and H-*ras*-related mRNAs were identified in cell lines transfected with v-*src* and v-H-*ras* oncogenes, respectively. A comparison of the level of oncogene-related mRNA by *in situ* hybridization using radioautography and by filter hybridization indicated that the *in situ* hybridization technique is not as sensitive as filter hybridization in revealing quantitative differences in the expression of oncogene transcripts. However, *in situ* hybridization may be more sensitive than immunofluorescence for the detection of virus-infected cells. *In situ* hybridization can be used for studying the expression of viral or cellular oncogenes in experimental and spontaneous tumors. Moreover, adaptation of the method to tissue specimens may allow the detection of oncogene and protooncogene expression in single cells using relatively small amounts of tissue.[357] *In situ* chromosomal hybridization techniques can be used for the study of translocations and deletions involving protooncogene sequences.[358-361]

A powerful method for the detection of mutant products of protooncogenes (or other cellular genes) is based on the ability of pancreatic ribonuclease (RNAse A) to cleave RNA heteroduplexes containing simple base mismatches.[362] Using this method it has been shown that certain human tumor cells contain mutant c-K-*ras* genes and the nature and position of these mutations have been defined.[363] The method can be applied only for genes that are expressed at least in some tissues. Another method based on the ribonuclease cleavage at mismatches in RNA:DNA duplexes can be used for the detection of single base substitutions in genes that are either expressed or unexpressed.[364] Both methods are simple and rapid but they allow the detection of only a part of all the possible point mutational events.

3. Characterization of Protooncogene Protein Products

The protein products of different protooncogenes have been totally or partially characterized. Their physicochemical properties, including molecular weight and amino acid sequence, may be deduced from the nucleotide sequences of the respective cDNA or mRNA when such data are available. Protooncogene-encoded proteins can be identified by *in vitro* translation of mRNAs from the cloned genes.[365,366] Electrophoretic analysis, assays for enzymatic activity, and immunological methods have been widely applied for the study of protooncogene protein products.

4. Electrophoretic Analysis

The electrophoretic mobility of protooncogene protein products can be used for the detection of possible qualitative changes (amino acid substitutions). For example, a tumor isolated from a woman with serous cystadenocarcinoma of the ovary contained an activated c-K-*ras* gene detected by DNA transfection assay and the 21,000-Da (p21) protein product of this protooncogene displayed an electrophoretic mobility in sodium dodecyl sulfate (SDS)-polyacrylamide gels that differed from the mobilities of c-K-*ras* proteins present in other tumors, thus indicating the possible occurrence of protooncogene mutation in the tumor cells.[367]

High-resolution two-dimensional polyacrylamide gel electrophoresis is a powerful method for the separation of proteins from normal and malignant cells.[368-371] Several hundreds of different polypeptides may be detected by this method in cultured cells such as HeLa cells.[372] An approximate 20% *de novo* synthesis of polypeptides has been detected by the same method in SV40- and K-MuSV-transformed cells but the polypeptide synthesis was similar irrespective of whether the cells were transformed with any of these two viruses.[373] Many of the differences detected between normal and transformed cells by two-dimensional electrophoresis may be related to alterations in the carbohydrate content of membrane glycoproteins.[374] The method is potentially useful for the study of protein products whose synthesis depends on the activity of protooncogenes or other genes which may have an enhanced transcriptional activity in transformed cells. In an extensive study with giant two-dimensional electrophoresis, about 2700 proteins from chick fibroblasts transformed by two acute transforming retroviruses (RSV UR2 ASV) were examined.[375] Although these two viruses possess different oncogenes and code for different transforming proteins, it was found that they modulate nearly identical sets of cellular proteins in transformed fibroblasts. Changes in protein phosphorylation were relatively small and affected only proteins already phosphorylated in nontransformed cells. In contrast, large changes in nonphosphorylated proteins were detected, and some of them appeared to be specifically related to the maintenance of the transformed state.[375] Further studies would be required for the characterization of these proteins and for establishing their possible relation to or association with protooncogene protein products.

5. Assays for Kinase Activity

Phosphorylation of cellular proteins is a major mechanism for biological regulation.[376,377] Unfortunately, quantitative analysis of the phosphorylation of specific cellular proteins *in vivo* is difficult to perform. Methods used for this analysis include those measuring protein-bound phosphate directly by chemical or physical means, and indirectly by isotopic labeling or evaluation of protein functional changes.[378] The phosphorylation can affect tyrosine or nontyrosine (serine and/or threonine) residues in a diversity of cellular proteins,[379-382] but the physiologically significant substrates of these phosphorylations remain little characterized.[383] There is a partial overlapping of the cellular substrates of oncogene and protooncogene products with protein kinase activity and those related to the mechanisms of action of hormones and growth factors at the receptor and postreceptor levels.[384-386]

6. Immunological Methods

A number of oncogene and protooncogene protein products do not have protein kinase activity and different types of analytical procedures must be applied for their detection and characterization. Immunological methods have been extensively applied for the detection and separation of these products. Monoclonal or polyclonal antisera against the native protein or against synthetic oligopeptides corresponding to specific portions of the protein can be used for immunoprecipitation. Indirect immunoprecipitation using antisera against specific oncogene protein products can be used for the analysis of normal or tumor cells.[387]

Antisera against synthetic oligopeptides corresponding to sequences from different parts of the carboxyl terminus of the c-*myc* and v-*myc* polypeptides have been used for the detection of these proteins.[196,388-392] Similar methods have been applied to the detection and identification of c-*myb* and v-*myb* protein products.[393] A radioimmunoassay for the human c-*myc* protein was developed by using a synthetic amino-terminal sequence of the c-*myc* protein (amino acids 11 to 24).[394] Antisera prepared in mice, rats, and rabbits by immunization with synthetic peptides corresponding to regions of high variability located near the carboxyl termini of *ras* protein react uniquely with H-*ras* and K-*ras* gene protein products in immunoblots and immunoprecipitation reactions.[395] For an unknown reason, an antisera generated in rabbits against a synthetic oligopeptide corresponding to the carboxy-terminal region of the N-*ras* p21 protein failed to react with this protein in spite of its positive reactivity with the N-*ras* peptide.[396] Antisera generated against a set of chemically synthesized peptides spanning position 12 of p21^{ras} protein (residues 5 to 17) are able to distinguish between different forms of p21 according to the amino acid replacing glycine at the 12th codon position.[397]

Antisera to synthetic peptides predicted from nucleic acid sequences of oncogenes have been used to screen the urine of cancer patients, pregnant women, and normal controls for the presence of immunologically related proteins.[398,399] Increased levels of oncogene-related proteins were found in cancer patients as well as in pregnant women. In another study using immunoblotting technique and sheep antisera against a conserved region of the *ras* protein, a 55-kDa protein (p55), immunologically related to the *ras* product, was detected in the urine from 16 of 26 patients with transitional cell carcinoma of the bladder.[400] The expression of p55 tended to correlate with tumor grade and stage and was elevated in patients with a history of multiple tumor recurrences.

Although the production of antibodies to synthetic peptides is a simple and versatile tool for the study of oncogene and protooncogene protein products, there are still some questions about the design of peptides for the production of useful antibodies.[401] Factors such as the length of the peptides, their hydrophilicity, their location in the native molecule, and the secondary and tertiary configuration of peptides may all be important in generating useful antibodies. In a study of 35 different peptides from several viral and cellular oncogene protein products, more than one half of the antipeptide antisera reacted with their respective oncoproteins derived from virus-transformed cell lines.[401] However, among four anti-*myc*-peptide antisera with high titers (1:10⁴) to peptides, only one reacted with the protein p110$^{gag\text{-}myc}$ while four out of five anti-*fes*-peptide antisera reacted with the p85$^{gag\text{-}fes}$ protein. These reactivity differences may depend on whether or not the selected peptide corresponds to an antigenic domain of the native protein molecule. Similar peptides differing in a single or a few amino acids could elicit antisera of markedly different reactivities. A rabbit antiserum prepared against a cyclic 19-amino acid peptide predicted from the sequence of the v-*mos* oncogene recognized not only the v-*mos* product but also a normal cellular protein of 55,000-mol wt (p55) which was identical to the intermediate filament protein, vimentin.[402] In any case, both positive and negative results obtained with immunological methods based on the use of synthetic oligopeptides should be evaluated with proper criticism.

Combination of immunologic and histologic or cytologic methods can give important results in relation to the expression of oncogene and protooncogene products in individual cells of primary tumors or their metastases as well as in normal animal tissues. Immunocytochemical techniques can be used to demonstrate the subcellular localization of oncogene and protoonco-gene products, e.g., the presence of *ras* products in the area of the cell membrane.[403] Immunohistochemical methods using immunoperoxidase staining have been applied to the study of paraffin-embedded, formalin-fixed tissue sections in relation to the expression of c-*ras* gene proteins in human mammary, gastric, pulmonary, thyroidal, and colonic carcinomas.[404-415] Similar methods have been applied to the study of the expression of c-*myc* protein in human gastric, mammary, and testicular tumors as well as in lymphomas,[416-420] c-*erb*-B/EGF receptor protein in gastric carcinomas and lung tumors,[421,422] and c-*neu/erb*-B-2 in breast tumors and various types of adenocarcinoma.[423-425] Immunohistochemical methods are useful for evaluating the expression of specific protooncogene proteins in tumor cell populations *in vivo,* which is frequently characterized by its heterogeneity from one cell to another within the same tumor. Immunocytochemical methods can also be applied to the study of smears obtained from suspected malignant lesion, for example, to brush smears obtained by fiberoptic endoscopy from human gastric and colonic lesions.[426] Expression of c-*ras* gene in the smears can be detected by using the monoclonal antibody RAP-5, which specifically recognizes both mutated and unaltered forms of p21$^{c\text{-}ras}$ proteins.

In order to refine the qualitative or semiquantitative results obtained with indirect immunofluorescence assays, quantitative methods can be applied to the study of protooncogene protein products. A sensitive and quantitative enzyme-linked immunosorbance assay (ELISA) has been proposed for the evaluation of c-*myc* and N-*myc* protein expression.[427] This assay was applied to the study of c-*myc* protein expression in human colon carcinoma cell lines.[428]

Flow cytometric assay can be used to study the expression of protooncogene protein products in isolated nuclei from normal or tumor tissues by using fluorescein-labeled polyclonal or monoclonal antibodies. This method was applied to the study of c-*myc* expression in archival biopsies of uterine cervix and colon cancers as well as in testicular tumors and in normal and neoplastic hematopoietic cells.[429-432] The method may be used to define quantitative differences in the expression of protooncogene proteins in different stages of cell differentiation.

After precipitation of the oncogene or protooncogene protein product, different protein analytical procedures can be applied, including tryptic peptide mapping, SDS-polyacrylamide gel electrophoresis, gel filtration, and gradient sedimentation analysis. The cellular localization and sublocalization of oncogene protein products can be determined by radioisotope labeling, immunofluorescence, or cell fractionation analysis. Intracellular oncogene or protooncogene antigens, e.g., p21^{ras} proteins, can be detected by cell permeabilization using lysolecithin, followed by immunofluorescence staining and flow cytometry.[433] The use of flow microfluorometry may allow an analysis on a cell-by-cell basis, as opposed to a total cell population. Therefore, not only can the percentage of cells expressing the oncogene or protooncogene protein product be determined, but the relative expression of the product within each cell can be assessed.[433] This technique can thus circumvent the need for physical separation of cells in samples of body fluids or in suspensions derived from solid tissues.

Monoclonal antibodies have been applied for studying the expression of polypeptide products of tumor viruses and are also useful tools for the detection and study of proteins coded by viral or cellular oncogenes.[434-440] Not only the native protein but also synthetic peptides corresponding to specific portions of the protein molecule can be used as effective and specific immunogens for the production of monoclonal antibodies capable of recognizing the protein with high specificity and sensitivity. Monoclonal antibodies have been produced against a synthetic peptide corresponding to the six carboxyl terminus amino acids of pp60^{v-src}, and this antibody reacts with native pp60^{v-src} and binds the protein in a competition test.[441] More than 20 different monoclonal antibodies against pp60^{src} were obtained recently by means of mouse hybridoma clones.[442] All these antibodies reacted with pp60^{v-src} produced by different RSV strains, ten of them cross-reacted strongly with pp60^{c-src} from chicken embryo cells, and two monoclonal antibodies detected enzymatically active pp60^{c-src} from a variety of rodent and human cells. Monoclonal antibodies against the normal and mutant (T24) human c-H-*ras* gene products have been prepared using synthetic oligopeptides corresponding to amino acid positions 10 to 17 of the respective human c-*ras* products as immunogens.[443] These antibodies, as well as other similar monoclonal antibodies,[444] react with the p21^{ras} protein and have been applied to study the expression of p21^{ras} in human colon and mammary carcinomas using immunocytochemical methods.[412] Monoclonal antibodies with specificity for activated, mutant c-*ras* proteins have also been developed.[445] Mouse hybridoma clones producing monoclonal antibodies reactive with p21^{ras} proteins have also been established by using bacterially expressed *ras* protein and an ELISA assay.[446] Flow cytometry using a monoclonal antibody to p21^{ras} (antibody Y13-259) has been applied as a method with sufficient sensitivity to differentiate between cellular and viral p21^{ras} levels, to detect small subpopulations of virus-transformed cells, and to monitor changes in p21 expression in response to physiologic variables.[447] The monoclonal antibody NCC-RAS-004, produced by using recombinant c-H-*ras* p21 as an immunogen, was found to be extremely sensitive when used in immunoblotting analysis, facilitating semiquantitative detection of c-H-*ras*, c-K-*ras*, and N-*ras* p21 in cell and tissue lysates.[448] In cells carrying a point mutationally activated c-*ras* gene, p21 with abnormal mobility could be easily detected with NCC-RAS-004 upon SDS-polyacrylamide gel electrophoresis.

Monoclonal antibodies made against a synthetic peptide from the v-*sis* oncogene protein sequence have been used to identify bacterial colonies in which the protein is being produced after transformation with a v-*sis* expression vector.[449] Monoclonal antibodies have also been produced against the human c-*myc* protooncogene protein.[450] Methods using monoclonal or polyclonal antibodies can be applied for establishing radioimmunoassays for the determination of specific protooncogene protein products in tumor tissues or body fluids.[394,451] Studies using human cell lines should always be compared with those obtained directly from fresh tumor specimens.

IV. STRUCTURE OF ONCOGENES

The general structure and the complete or partial nucleotide sequences of many viral and cellular oncogenes and their flanking regions have been reported, including the human protooncogenes c-*sis*,[452-460] c-*src*,[461-464] c-*fes/fps*,[465-467] c-*fgr*,[468,469] c-*mos*,[470] c-H-*ras*, c-K-*ras*, N-*ras*, and R-*ras*,[452,471-483] c-*myc* and N-*myc*,[484-493] c-*abl*,[494-496] c-*myb*,[497,498] B-*lym*-1,[325,326] c-*fms*,[499] c-*raf* and A-*raf*-1,[500-502] c-*ros*,[213,503] c-*yes*,[504] c-*neu/erb*-B-2,[505,506] and c-*jun*.[507]

Similar studies have been performed in other animal species. The general organization, structure, and nucleotide sequences of several chicken protooncogenes have been determined, including the protooncogenes c-*src*,[508] c-*myc*,[509-511] c-*fps*,[512-514] c-*mil*,[515,516] c-*myb*,[517-519] c-*erb*-A,[520] c-*ros*,[521] c-*fos*,[522,523] and c-*ets*.[524] Other protooncogenes whose structure has been characterized include c-*rel* (turkey),[525,526] c-*abl* (mouse and cat),[527,528] c-*mos*, c-H-*ras*, and c-*myc* (rat),[529-535] c-*myb*, c-K-*ras*, c-*sis*, and c-*fms*, and c-*myc*, N-*myc*, and L-*myc* (mouse),[483,536-543] N-*ras* (guinea pig),[544,545] c-*fms*, c-*myc*, c-*sis*, and c-*fes/fps* (cat),[458,459,546-549] and c-*src* (*Drosophila*).[550,551] Three c-*ras* genes have been detected in *Drosophila* and two of them have been sequenced.[33] One of the two c-*raf*-related genes present in the *Drosophila* genome was also sequenced.[552]

A. STRUCTURAL CONSERVATION OF PROTOONCOGENES

The structure of cellular oncogenes is similar to that of their viral counterparts. An important difference is the presence of introns or intervening sequences in the cellular oncogenes, such sequences being absent in viruses. At least seven introns are present, for example, in the human c-*abl* gene, and more than 90% of this gene of approximately 32 kb represents noncoding sequences.[494] Unlike other protooncogenes, c-*mos* has no intervening sequences.[470]

In addition to intervening sequences, viral and cellular homologous oncogenes may have differences in nucleotide sequences, although such differences are usually small. For example, the human c-H-*ras* gene differs from the viral v-H-*ras* gene (derived from rat) at only 3 out of 189 amino acid positions, and the human c-K-*ras* gene differs from the viral v-K-*ras* gene (also derived from rat) at only 7 out of 189 positions.[476] Moreover, certain "constant" regions of the *ras* genes (and other oncogenes) are more preserved in structure than other, "variable" regions. The coding sequences (exons) of protooncogene are highly conserved even in distantly related species, which suggests the evolutionary importance of their respective polypeptide products. For example, the protein product of the c-*src* protooncogene, pp60[c-*src*], of either human or murine origin is closely related in its primary structure to the homologous protein present in chicken.[26] The protein products of the three c-*ras* protooncogenes (c-H-*ras*, c-K-*ras*, and N-*ras*) contained in the vertebrate genome are highly homologous in their molecular weights and amino acid sequences, the most variable sequences being clustered in two regions, between amino acid positions 121-132 and 164-184, but these variable regions are conserved, for example, between human and rat.[476] Moreover, the c-*ras* genes of *Drosophila* are highly homologous to their vertebrate counterparts and display variability in the same regions as the vertebrate c-*ras* genes.[33] On the other hand, the size of protooncogenes, even of members of the same family, may show great variation. For example, the c-H-*ras*-1 gene is contained in a 4.5-kbp DNA sequence, whereas the c-K-*ras*-2 gene, also of human origin, is much larger, spanning 35 to 45 kbp and containing 4 exons interrupted by intervening sequences.[476,477] In spite of these differences, the p21[*ras*] protein products of both protooncogenes are similar in size.

The coding exons of the c-*myc* genes of chicken, mouse and human are highly conserved. In the chicken, c-*myc* is composed of three exons and two introns, analogous to the structure of the human and mouse c-*myc* genes, but the transcript of the first exon is apparently not translated.[510] This exon, composed of approximately 500 bp, is located at 1.6 kbp upstream of the coding exons and is separated from them by an intron 700 to 800 bp. The nucleotide sequence of this exon reveals the absence of an ATG codon and the presence of multiple termination codons in all of three reading frames.[510] The function of this unusually untranslated exon is unknown but it could play a role in the transcriptional and/or posttranscriptional regulation of c-*myc* expression. In murine plasmacytoma and human Burkitt's lymphoma, loss of this 5' exon is frequently, but not invariably, associated with translocations involving c-*myc*.[553]

B. POLYMORPHISM OF PROTOONCOGENES

Protooncogene DNA sequences have been well conserved during evolution and polymorphisms could not be frequent among them. However, RFLPs have been detected in several protooncogene sequences, particularly in the respective noncoding regions. The study of RFLPs of protooncogene and nonprotooncogene sequences has been proposed as a method for the evaluation of human cancer risk.[554] However, there is no definite proof for the general validity of this method.[555]

1. Polymorphism of the c-*fms* Protooncogene

Polymorphism of the *fms* protooncogene has been detected with three restriction endonucleases (*Eco*RI, *Hin*dIII, and *Bam*HI) in a human population of 48 adults and 38 children.[556] The detected polymorphisms are more easily explained on the basis of the existence of two *fms* alleles, *a* and *b*, in the human population. The data are compatible with a distribution of 75% homozygotes *bb*, 23% heterozygotes *ab*, and 2% homozygotes *aa*. It was found that 74% of children from the couples (*ab* x *bb*) were heterozygotes which, when compared with the 50% expected frequency of heterozygotes, suggests the existence of some selective advantage for heterozygotes.[556] Unfortunately, the c-*fms* gene is located on human chromosome 5, region 5q34, about which little information useful for linkage studies is available and no rearrangements affecting human chromosome region 5q34 have been described.

The biological significance of the c-*fms* polymorphism, including its possible relation to malignant diseases, is unknown. Among 12 cancer patients, an abnormal RFLP pattern affecting the c-*fms* locus was detected in an individual with ALL and congenital hypothyroidism.[557,558] The abnormal allele of the c-*fms* gene present in the patient contained a deletion 426 bp in size located in close proximity to a putative c-*fms* exon. The patient was homozygous for the abnormal allele which was inherited from each parent. The possible relationship between the genetic finding and the clinical condition of the patient remains undetermined.

2. Polymorphism of the c-*erb* Protooncogenes

An RFLP has been detected in the 3' end of the human c-*erb*-A protooncogene.[559] The frequency of the rarer allele was around 3.0% in a normal population of 107 unrelated individuals and did not significantly differ in DNA samples from patients with breast tumors or acute leukemias. Polymorphism has also been found in the chicken c-*erb*-B gene, where at least seven different *Eco*RI-digestion patterns were identified and both homozygous and heterozygous animals for two alleles of c-*erb*-B (α and β alleles) were detected.[560,561] The restriction endonuclease *Pvu*II identified two alleles of the human c-*erb*-A-1 gene with population frequencies of 0.11 (A1) and 0.89 (A2), respectively.[562]

3. Polymorphism of the c-*mos* Protooncogene

Polymorphism has been reported for human c-*mos*.[563] An RFLP at the 3' side of c-*mos* was detected in 6 of 75 human breast tumor DNA samples as well as in lymphocyte DNA from 3 of these cancer patients. The same polymorphism was detected in 1 of 73 human leukemic cell DNAs but was not found in a series of 69 lymphocyte DNAs from the unaffected population.[563] The polymorphism was also detected in the normal and tumor tissue of two patients from 12 with esophageal cancer.[564] In a breast cancer patient, RFLP in the 3' end of the c-*mos* locus was due to a single nucleotide substitution. (T instead of C), resulting in the disappearance of an *Eco*RI restriction enzyme site.[565] The biological significance of this molecular change, if any, is obscure. The study of patients with gynecological tumors and lymphomas and a control group indicated that the *Eco*RI polymorphism of c-*mos* is not significantly associated with malignant diseases.[566]

4. Polymorphism of the c-*ras* Protooncogenes

Restriction endonuclease analysis has demonstrated the existence of individual alleles of the c-H-*ras*-1 gene that can be distinguished in the human population.[567] Different restriction endonucleases (*Bam*HI, *Msp*I/*Hpa*II, *Ava*II, and *Taq*I) have been used to detect DNA polymorphisms associated with the human c-H-*ras*-1 gene. Variation in the number of 28-kb variable tandem repeat consensus sequences occurring approximately 1 kb 3' to the poly(A) signal of the c-H-*ras*-1 gene are responsible for the RFLP that distinguish individual c-H-*ras* alleles. In addition, a polymorphism in the 5'-flanking region of the gene has been detected.[569]

It was suggested that specific RFLP alleles of the c-H-*ras* gene are more frequent in patients with various cancers, especially with melanoma, than in DNA from unaffected individuals.[567-569] These results were not confirmed in other studies.[570-573] However, a significant association between some rare c-H-*ras*-1 alleles and human bladder cancer was detected in a recent study.[574] Further studies using large populations of cancer patients and appropriate control cases, as well as experimental studies in nonhuman animal species, are required for the elucidation of this issue. An *Eco*RI RFLP occurring in a region of the murine genome containing the first exon of the c-K-*ras*-2 protooncogene showed correlation with the inherited susceptibility to urethan-induced pulmonary adenomas.[575] The genetic factor influencing pulmonary adenoma incidence in mice could be either the c-K-*ras*-2 locus itself or a closely linked genetic element.

5. Polymorphism of the c-*sis* Protooncogene

A *Hin*dIII-RFLP was detected in human DNA samples from ten unrelated individuals, including five leukemic patients.[576] Six of these individuals had an additional *Hin*dIII sensitive site in one allele and the other four were homozygous for the absence of this site. No individual was found to possess the *Hin*dIII site in both alleles. The site was localized in the middle of the DNA region homologous to v-*sis*.

6. Polymorphism of the c-*abl* Protooncogene

An RFLP caused by a deletion within the human c-*abl* gene has been detected in 67 unrelated human individuals.[577] The polymorphism is generated by the existence of two alleles, *a* and *b*, due to a deletion of about 500 bp in an intron located downstream of the codon for the phosphate acceptor tyrosine residue of the c-*abl* gene product. The two alleles *a* and *b* are in Hardy-Weinberg equilibrium, with allelic frequencies of 94.8 and 5.2%, respectively. In the population studied, 10% were heterozygotes *ab* and 90% homozygotes *aa*; no homozygotes *bb* were detected.[577] The results were consistent with Mendelian inheritance of the alleles. Similar results were obtained in an independent study.[578] The possible relationship, if any, between this polymorphism and the development of CML (which is associated with c-*abl* gene translocation) is unknown.

7. Polymorphism of the c-*myb* Protooncogene

An RFLP of the human c-*myb* locus was detected in the tumor cell line 7060, which was derived from a human rectal carcinoma.[579] The 7060-transformed epithelial cells were homozygous for the detected polymorphic change, whereas normal fibroblasts from the same patient were heterozygous. In addition to this change, the tumor cells contained a mutated N-*ras* protooncogene affecting codon 61 of the p21 protein. The murine c-*myb* gene also exhibits an RFLP.[580]

8. Polymorphism of the N-*myc* and L-*myc* Genes

Two RFLPs were detected in the Japanese population using Southern blot hybridization with

N-*myc* probes.[581] Two alleles, S1 and S2, were accounted for by the presence or absence, respectively, of an *Sph*I restriction site in the second intron of the N-*myc* gene. Other two alleles, P1 and P2, were related to the presence or absence, respectively, of a *Pvu*II site in the 3' region of the gene. Whereas P1, P2, and S1 alleles exhibited no significant differences in their distribution among the normal population and neuroblastoma patients, N-*myc* amplification was strictly associated with S2 allele in neuroblastomas associated with amplification of this protooncogene. Recently, a close correlation was detected between RFLPs of the human L-*myc* gene and the clinical characteristics of lung cancer, especially the production of metastases to the lymph nodes and other organs.[582]

9. Polymorphism of the c-*raf*-1 Protooncogene

Polymorphic variation of the c-*raf*-1 protooncogene was found in a study of 21 individuals, including 17 with non-Hodgkin's lymphomas and 3 healthy controls.[583] Three alleles of c-*raf*-1 (*a*, *b*, and *c*) were recognized in this study, but the short number of controls did not allow any conclusion about the possible association of some particular c-*raf*-1 allele(s) with lymphoma.

10. Polymorphism of the c-*ets*-1 Protooncogene

An RFLP involving the c-*ets*-1 protooncogene was identified during the study of 24 samples of DNA from 23 normal individuals and leukemic patients.[584] Four samples from unrelated individuals lacked an *Xba*I site, giving rise to a longer restriction fragment detectable by Southern hybridization analysis. No association could be found between the c-*ets*-1 RFLP and disease among the individuals included in this study. Pedigree analysis of a cohort demonstrated Mendelian inheritance consistent with a somatic polymorphism. Two other different RFLPs involving the c-*ets*-1 locus had been identified previously.[585,586]

11. Conclusion

Polymorphic changes have been detected in a number of protooncogenes by analysis with restriction endonucleases. The biological significance of RFLPs affecting protooncogenes is obscure at present. Whereas most of these polymorphisms do not appear to convey an increased risk for cancer, conflictive results obtained in certain clinical studies where specific types of RFLPs appeared to correlate with particular types of human tumors may warrant the prosecution of well controlled studies on this subject.

V. EVOLUTION OF PROTOONCOGENES

Protooncogenes, or protooncogene-related DNAs, RNAs, and proteins, have been found in all multicellular animals studied so far, including fish such as *Xiphophorus* and insects such as *Drosophila*.[10,34,37,587] At least some protooncogenes are present in sponges,[36] yeast,[39,588] fungi,[589] and even in Archaebacteriae,[43,44] which are primitive organisms representing a kind of bridge between prokaryotes and eukaryotes.[45] The widespread distribution of protooncogenes in nature indicates that their protein products have essential biological roles. In general, protooncogenes and the associated linkage groups have been conserved during mammalian evolution.[590]

Cellular oncogenes, as all genes, are subjected to continuous evolutionary changes and data obtained from studies at either the DNA or the protein levels may contribute to delineate the phylogeny of protooncogenes and to define the functional properties of the respective protein products. The protooncogene protein domains which are more highly conserved in evolution are probably those which have a more crucial role for preservation of the essential functional properties of the protooncogene protein in different species. Such domains may be recognized by comparative studies of either the nucleotide or amino acid sequences from the gene or the protein, respectively.[37]

Whereas the rates of evolution of cellular oncogenes is slow and comparable to that of many functional genes in the genome, suggesting some important biological functions played by these genes, the rates of evolution of viral oncogenes (or other RNA viral genes) are several orders of magnitude higher. For example, the rates of nucleotide substitution of the protooncogene c-*mos* is 1.71×10^{-9} per site per year, in comparison with the rates for the M-MuSV *gag* and v-*mos*, which are 6.3×10^{-4} and 1.31×10^{-3} per site per year, respectively.[591] In general, the rates of nucleotide substitution for viral oncogenes are about 1 million times greater than those for their cellular counterparts.[592]

A. EVOLUTION OF PROTOONCOGENES IN THE ANIMAL KINGDOM

The distribution and relatedness of protooncogenes in the animal kingdom were studied by structural analysis at the genomic level and the following conclusions were obtained:[38] (1) the gene *ras* is probably one of the earliest protooncogenes in the evolutionary history of the animal kingdom; it can be traced from humans down to the organization of heterotrophic eukaryotes such as yeast. (2) The gene *src* has apparently evolved with the organization of the metazoa; this protooncogene occurs first in sponges. (3) The protooncogenes *abl*, *myb*, *fes*, *myc*, *raf*, *erb*-B, and *bcl*-2 appear with the Protostomia-Coelomata-Bilateria organization; they occur in *Anguillula*, *Tubifex*, cuttle-fish, *Limulus*, and *Drosophila*, i.e., they are all present at the beginning of the evolution of the Deuterostomia. (4) The protooncogene *sis* occurred probably in the early Chordata like *Amphioxus* that developed the closed system of blood pressure circulation. (5) The protooncogene *yes* occurred probably first in sharks, *erb*-A and *fos* in Teleosts such as *Xiphophorus*, *ros* in Tetrapoda such as frogs, snakes, and chicken, and *mos* in mammals. (6) The protooncogene *neu/erb*-B-2 appeared first in Teleosts, although sequences related to this gene can be traced down to Protostomia.

B. THE *SRC* GENE FAMILY

The functional aspects of protooncogene evolution are only partially understood because the normal functions of several protooncogene protein products are unknown and the functions of other products have been only partially characterized. The best delineated oncogene family is the *src* family, which is composed of several oncogenes whose product have tyrosine kinase activity (*src*, *yes*, *abl*, *fgr*, *fes/fps*, *fms*, *erb*-B, *ros*, and *kit*). Other members of the same family are probably the oldest of this particular phylogenetic tree and have not acquired tyrosine kinase activity (*raf/mil/mht* and *mos*). Three loci related to the *src* oncogene are contained in the *Drosophila* genome.[593] *Drosophila* sequences homologous to the c-*abl* gene are located near the 5′ end of a gene, *Dash*, which is transcribed to give long RNAs (5 to 6 kb) and short RNAs (3.0 kb) by alternative splicing patterns.[594] The *Drosophila* c-*abl/Dash* gene product is a protein of 1520 amino acids that exhibits high homology to the human c-*abl* protein and possesses tyrosine-specific protein kinase activity.[595] Mutants of the c-*abl/Dash* gene may have pleiotropic effect on *Drosophila* late development and may result in lethality at the pupal stage.[596] Two *raf*-related genes, *Draf*-1 and *Draf*-2, are present in the *Drosophila* genome.[552]

The reason of the diversification and maintenance of several different members of the *src* oncogene family is unknown but it is possible that at least those members with tyrosine kinase activity are engaged with subtle differences in their respective general function; for example, they may have different substrate specificities, modes of regulation, tissue distribution, or cellular localization.[37] In any case, the active site for the specific kinase activity of these oncogene products resides in their carboxyl terminal half, and the highest degree of amino acid homology is also localized on the same region of the respective proteins. Moreover, the oncogenes of the *src* family are structurally and functionally related to the catalytic subunit of cAMP-dependent protein kinase, an enzyme that has a specificity for serine.[597] The *src* oncogene family is also structurally related to the insulin receptor, which possesses tyrosine-specific protein kinase activity.[598] All of these genes, irrespective of amino acid substrate specificity of the protein kinase products, may comprise a single divergent gene family.

C. THE *RAS* GENE FAMILY

The *ras* gene family is composed of three closely related members, namely: H-*ras*, K-*ras*, and N-*ras*.[599,600] These oncogenes are highly homologous at the DNA level. The nucleotide sequences of the goldfish *ras*-related gene show extensive homology to the mammalian c-*ras* gene family.[601] The percentage of homology between the goldfish sequence and the sequences of three mammalian genes is similar to or even greater than the homologies among the three mammalian c-*ras* genes themselves. DNA sequences homologous to mammalian c-*ras* genes are present in the genome of the marine mollusk *Aplysia californica*. The nucleotide sequences of three c-*ras* genes contained in the *Drosophila* genome are highly homologous to the c-*ras* genes of vertebrates.[33] The predicted amino acid sequences of the insect and vertebrate p21$^{c\text{-}ras}$ protein products are highly homologous and display variability in the same regions. In general, these sequences are more conserved at the amino terminus, which is probably involved in guanine nucleotide binding than at the carboxy terminus, which may be involved in the determination of affinity for different cellular macromolecules and the regulatory or catalytic specificities. *ras*-related proteins are present in yeast and in the the simple eukaryote microbe *Dictyostelium discoideum*, where they are subjected to developmental regulation.[39,40,588] Yeast and mammalian c-*ras* proteins have conserved similar biochemical and physiological properties.[602,603] The extensive conservation of c-*ras*-related nucleotide and amino acid sequences in all the animal species studied so far suggests that c-*ras* proteins may play an important physiological role in cellular homeostatic processes. The evolutionary aspects of c-*ras* genes are discussed further in Chapter 7 in Volume II.

VI. EXPRESSION OF PROTOONCOGENES

Protooncogenes are genes that participate, in conjunction with many other cellular genes, in normal developmental processes. The expression of protooncogenes is variable, depending on the tissue, the cell type, the stage of differentiation, and the general or local physiological conditions.[604] Particular protooncogenes are expressed in the placenta and extraembryonic tissues or during specific stages of the embryonic and fetal development.[605,606] However, the specific functions of protooncogenes in the complex developmental processes occurring in metazoan species are little understood. There is also scarce information about the physiological significance of protooncogene expression in relation to the expression of differentiated functions by different types of cells.

The level of expression of certain protooncogenes, or protooncogene-like sequences, as well as the expression of other cellular genes, may show important variation in association with the cell cycle and may undergo significant changes in relation to cellular proliferation, for example, in regenerative processes.[607-611] Alteration in protooncogene expression may also be observed in tumor cells or in normal cells stimulated by mitogenic agents of either endogenous or exogenous origin, including hormones and growth factors.[386] Sequential expression of protooncogenes is seen during lectin-stimulated mitogenesis of normal human lymphocytes.[612] It has been postulated that certain protooncogenes may be considered, as other cellular genes, as cell cycle-dependent genes.[613-615] However, the levels of expression of certain protooncogenes, including c-*myc*, are constant throughout the cell cycle.[618,619] Moreover, persistence of the competent state for DNA replication in cells like cultured mice fibroblasts may be independent of the expression of particular protooncogenes, including c-*fos* and c-*myc*.[618] The levels of c-*fos* expression are extremely low, or even undetectable, throughout the cycle of cultured mouse fibroblasts, which suggests that c-*fos* does not contribute to the regulation of the normal cell cycle and is not required for the continuous cycling of cells.[619]

A. EXPRESSION OF INSECT PROTOONCOGENES

Cellular *ras* genes may be involved in the regulation of cell differentiation and/or cell proliferation. Expression of the three c-*ras* protooncogenes contained in the *Drosophila* genome is subjected to developmental regulation.[603] Although the three *Drosophila* c-*ras* genes are expressed in all stages during the life cycle of the insect, the different transcripts produced by these genes are expressed differentially.[620] A larger transcript of each gene is present at a constant abundance in all stages, whereas one or two smaller transcripts are found mainly in embryos. Differential expression of the c-*abl*, c-*src*, and c-*erb*-B protooncogenes is also observed in *Drosophila*.[621,551] There is a substantial maternal contribution of c-*abl* transcripts to the early embryo of *Drosophila*, which may be required for the normal development of the insect.[594-596] The putative protooncogene *int*-1 is expressed in early larval and pupal stages of *Drosophila*, but is barely detectable in adult tissues of the insect.[184,622] In general, the role of protooncogenes in the development of *Drosophila* is little understood at present.

B. EXPRESSION OF FISH PROTOONCOGENES

Fish of the genus *Xiphophorus* have represented for many years an excellent model for the analysis of genetic and environmental factors involved in normal developmental processes as well as for the study of tumorigenesis in vertebrates. Both genetic and environmental factors are involved in the causation of tumors in *Xiphophorus*.[7-9,623-628] Neoplastic development in *Xiphophorus* is mediated by the putative protooncogene *Tu*, whose expression may be associated with that of the c-*src* protooncogene.[629] Differential expression of protooncogenes is observed in different tissues of the fish during normal development.[630,631] Whereas transcripts of c-*abl*, c-*raf*/*mil*, and c-*erb*-A are not observed in normal organs of the adult fish or during embryogenesis, different types of c-*src*, c-*sis*, c-*ras*, and c-*erb*-A transcripts are synthesized during different stages of the fish development. The *src* gene is preferentially expressed in the neural tissues of the fish.

C. EXPRESSION OF CHICKEN PROTOONCOGENES

In the chicken, protooncogenes including c-*erb*, c-*myb*, and c-*myc* are differentially expressed during hematopoiesis.[632] Whereas c-*myc* and c-*myb* RNA levels are generally elevated in immature hematopoietic cells, c-*erb* is expressed in only a minority of normal hematopoietic cells.[633] A differential expression of c-*src* and c-*yes* also occurs in embryonal and adult chicken tissues.[634]

D. EXPRESSION OF RODENT PROTOONCOGENES

A stage- and tissue-specific expression of protooncogenes has been observed in the mouse.[635-640] The protooncogenes c-*myc*, c-*erb*-A, and/or c-*erb*-B, c-H-*ras*, c-*src*, and c-*sis* are expressed at appreciable levels in whole mouse embryos or fetuses and most of these genes are modulated in a consistent manner during the course of prenatal mouse development.[640] While the expression of c-*myc*, c-*erb*, and c-*src* varies in a consistent fashion when whole mouse embryos or fetuses are analyzed, c-H-*ras* and c-*sis* are expressed throughout mouse prenatal development. In contrast to the protooncogene c-*mos*, which has been found to be apparently inactive in most normal mouse cells and tissues, even during prenatal development, the protooncogenes c-H-*ras*, c-*abl*, and c-*fos* are widely expressed in pre- and postnatal mouse tissues.[635]

The levels of expression of c-*ras* genes (c-H-*ras*, c-K-*ras*, and N-*ras*) in different mouse tissues are regulated in a complex manner, but the three genes are expressed in all tissues.[641] Differences in expression of c-*ras* genes occur through mouse pre- and postnatal development, and certain adult tissues preferentially express one member of the family over the others. Although $p21^{c-ras}$ products have been found to be associated with cellular proliferation in particular systems, very high levels of c-*ras* expression may occur in nonproliferating cells. For example, c-H-*ras* is expressed at its highest levels in mouse brain and muscle, where cell division is minimal or nonexistent,[641] which suggests that p21$^{c\text{-}ras}$ proteins are associated more with the expression of differentiated functions than with the control of cell proliferation.

The *myc* family of protooncogenes is differentially expressed during murine development.[642] While the expression of c-*myc* in generalized to many tissues of the mouse at different stages of development, the expression of two other members of this family, N-*myc* and L-*myc*, is very restricted with respect to tissue and stage of development.

The protooncogene c-*abl* is expressed at high levels in the mouse embryo, especially at days 10 and 11, and it is also expressed in apparently all postnatal mouse tissues, although severalfold differences in c-*abl* expression are observed between different mouse organs and tissues. Compared to the RNAs of other protooncogenes (c-*myb*, c-*myc*, and c-*src*), the levels of c-*abl* transcripts are, in general, much higher.[604] Regulated expression of c-*abl* occurs in the mouse testis during spermatogenesis, which suggests an important function for this gene in the development of male germ cells.[643]

The gene c-*fos* is expressed at high levels in prenatal mice, especially in the placenta and during the later stages of development (after day 16 of gestation), and is also expressed, although at lower levels, in all postnatal tissues investigated so far.[635] Differential expression of c-*fos* is observed in hematopoietic cells and it correlates with differentiation of monomyelocytic cells *in vitro*.[355] Transcripts of c-*fos* accumulate to high levels during development of mouse placenta, yolk sac, and amnion.[644] The c-*fos* gene is expressed at high levels during differentiation-dependent growth processes of fetal bone and mesodermal web tissue.[645] The level of expression of the c-*fos*-related gene, r-*fos*, declines precipitously in the rat myocardium between 3 and 7 d after birth.[646] A similar decline is observed in the level of c-*myc* expression. As it is known, cardiac myocytes irreversibly lose their proliferation capacity soon after birth.

Transcripts of c-*myb* are confined in the mouse to only hematopoietic tissues, with two distinct lineages, the erythroid and T-cell lineages, expressing c-*myb* at relatively high levels.[647] Moreover, the expression of c-*myb* decreases with the successive degrees of maturation of the T-cell lineage.

The putative protooncogenes *int*-1 and *int*-2, which show homology to FGFs and are involved in MMTV-induced mammary tumorigenesis in the mouse, are differentially expressed in mouse embryonic and extraembryonic tissues, but not in the adult tissues of the animal.[648-650] While *int*-1 may have a role in the early stages of mouse central nervous system development, *int*-2 appears to be important in developmental processes including migration of early mesoderm cells and induction of the otocyst. In the adult mouse, expression of *int*-1 is restricted to postmeiotic male germ cells that undergo differentiation from round spermatids to mature spermatozoa.[651]

1. Expression of Protooncogenes in Rodent Cells during Proliferation and Differentiation

Very complex changes in the levels of expression of different protooncogenes, or protoon-cogene sets, have been observed during proliferation and differentiation processes occurring in normal rodent tissues. Comparison of the expression of 13 protooncogenes in proliferating and terminally differentiated cardiac and muscle cells of the rat indicated the existence of unique tissue- and cell-specific patterns of protooncogene expression and suggested that at least some of these genes may be involved in the regulation of cellular proliferation and terminal differentiation in striated muscle.[652]

Normal bone marrow-derived mouse cells committed to the monocytic lineage, as well as leukemic cells with a differentiated myelomonocytic phenotype, express high levels of c-*fgr* transcripts.[653] In contrast, the highly related c-*src* gene is expressed in both undifferentiated and differentiated myelomonocytic cells and the c-*yes* gene is not expressed in any of these cells. These results indicate that each one of the protooncogenes encoding tyrosine protein kinases is independently regulated in specific hematopoietic cell lineages.

2. Expression of Protooncogenes during Tissue Regeneration in Rodents

The activity of c-H-*ras* increases markedly during liver regeneration induced in rodents by partial hepatectomy or administration of carbon tetrachloride.[636,637] The transcriptional activities of c-K-*ras*, c-*myc*, c-*fos*, and other protooncogenes are modulated in a sequential manner during regeneration and compensatory growth of rat liver.[654,655] The expression of c-*myc* in rat liver is increased up to 10- to 15-fold of the normal level within 1 to 3 h after partial hepatectomy.[656] This expression begins to decrease rapidly after 4 h and returned to less than double the normal level at 8 h, but a very large increase (approximately 600-fold) occurs in the liver when protein synthesis is inhibited by an injection of cycloheximide. The latter finding suggests that expression of c-*myc* is repressed by a short-lived protein that becomes abundant soon after the onset of the proliferative process and which impedes an exaggerated expression of c-*myc*.[656] The results further suggest an involvement of c-*myc* in the control mechanisms of regenerative processes occurring in the liver and, possibly, also in other tissues.

After partial hepatectomy in the adult rat, the steady-state levels of mRNAs for c-*fos*, c-*myc*, and p53 increase sequentially in the liver during the prereplicative phase which precedes DNA synthesis.[655] Levels of c-*fos* mRNA are elevated at least fourfold within 15 min after the operation and decrease rapidly by 2 h; c-*myc* mRNA reaches maximal levels (fivefold over normal) between 30 min and 2 h after the operation. A second, transient phase of expression for both c-*fos* and c-*myc* occurs around 8 h after partial hepatectomy, and p53 mRNA levels increase fivefold between 8 and 12 h after the operation.[655] The biphasic pattern observed in c-*fos* and c-*myc* expression is similar to the pattern of changes in ornithine decarboxylase and cAMP concentrations during liver regeneration, but it is not known whether these events are interdependent. The levels of c-*ras* p21 protein increase much later, at time of active DNA replication and cell division. Actinomycin D injected at the time of partial hepatectomy blocks the increase in c-*myc* mRNA at 2 h but has no effect on c-*fos* mRNA levels, whereas injection at 6 h only partially blocks the increase in c-*myc* and p53 mRNAs at 8 h but does not affect c-*fos* mRNA.[655] The results show that expression of particular protooncogenes induced by endogenous humoral factors involved in the induction of tissue regeneration after partial hepatectomy in the adult rat is controlled by transcriptional as well as posttranscriptional mechanisms.

E. EXPRESSION OF HUMAN PROTOONCOGENES

The expression of different human protooncogenes depends on the tissue and the stage of development and differentiation. For example, the levels of expression of c-H-*ras*, c-*fms*, c-erb-B, c-*myc*, and c-*fos*, as well as the expression of the AFP gene are increased in certain stages of human fetal liver development, especially between 4 to 6 months of gestation, as compared to normal human adult liver.[657] The same genes are reexpressed at high levels in human hepatomas. In contrast, the levels of expression of other protooncogenes, including c-*rel*, c-*mos*, c-*sis*, c-*src*, c-*bas*, and c-K-*ras*, do not show any clear changes during fetal liver development and in hepatoma. Differential expression of protooncogenes is observed in normal and abnormal human hematopoietic cells.[611,658] In a study with fresh cells isolated from the human bone marrow, low levels of expression of c-*myc*, c-*myb*, c-*fes*, and c-*raf* were detected, whereas c-*fos* was expressed at higher levels and c-*sis* was not expressed at all.[659] Altered levels of expression of some of these protooncogenes were found in human leukemic cells. The biological significance of the complex changes of protooncogene expression occurring in normal and neoplastic cells is not clear at present.

1. Expression of the Human c-*src* Gene

The protooncogene c-*src* is active in most normal human tissues.[660] The product of this gene is the protein pp60[c-*src*], which is present in normal human tissues, with highest levels being observed in the brain, followed by kidney, lung, muscle and connective tissue. The levels of pp60[c-*src*] in human fetal muscle are two- or threefold higher than in adult muscle, and they were also found to be increased in about one third of 30 human tumors examined.[660]

2. Expression of the Human c-*fos* and c-*fms* Genes

The expression of c-*fos* and c-*fms* was studied in human tissues at different stages of differentiation.[355,661] The c-*fos* gene is expressed in at least two different cell types, where it appears to be correlated with cellular differentiation, namely, in the bone marrow and in cells of the fetal membranes. Apparently, the expression of c-*fos* is a common property of mature hematopoietic cells and in the mononuclear phagocyte lineage it is restricted to differentiated cells.[355] A rapid induction of c-*fos* expression occurs during human monocyte differentiation induced by phorbol esters in hematopoietic cell lines.[662] In such cell lines c-*fos* transcripts increase within 10 min after treatment with the inducer and attain maximum levels by 30 min. Expression of c-*fos* occurs only when the cell lines are induced to enter the macrophage differentiation pathway, not when the cells differentiate to granulocytes. Expression of c-*fms* is also regulated during human monocytic differentiation.[663] In the human amnion c-*fos* transcripts increase as gestation proceeds and they are 100-fold greater in human amniotic and chorionic cells than in other normal human tissues and cells (kidney, liver, lymph nodes, lung). The levels of expression of c-*fos* and c-*fms* are greater in human term placenta than in other normal human tissues.[661]

3. Expression of the Human c-*myc* and c-*ras* Genes

The spatial and temporal pattern of c-*myc* expression in developing human placenta suggest that the protein product of this gene is involved in processes related to embryonic cell proliferation. Transcripts of c-*myc* are especially abundant in first trimester human placentas and are localized in the cytotrophoblast layer, which is very active in proliferation.[664,665] Interestingly, the distribution of c-*myc* expression is uneven within the first trimester cytotrophoblast layer, and only every third to fifth cytotrophoblast cell contains abundant c-*myc* transcripts. Coexpression of the c-*myc* and c-*sis* protooncogenes occurs in human placenta and the c-*sis* transcripts are translated into a PDGF-like protein, which suggests an autocrine type of control of trophoblastic growth.[666] Both c-*myc* and c-*ras* protooncogenes were found to be expressed in hydatiform moles and in a malignant trophoblast cell line (BeWo), as well as in early villous normal trophoblast at 4 weeks after conception.[667] No expression of c-*myc* and c-*ras* was detected in decidual tissue or term placenta.

Expression of c-*myc* correlates to the rate of proliferation of some types of cells. Levels of c-*myc* mRNA are usually low in quiescent cells such as growth-arrested mouse BALB/c 3T3 fibroblasts or lymphoid cells as well as in terminally differentiated endoderm cells but show an early and marked increase in mitogen-stimulated cells.[668-672] Cardiac myocyte hypertrophy is associated with altered c-*myc* gene expression.[673] Although expression of both c-*myc* and c-K-*ras* is dependent upon the cellular growth state, c-*myc*, but not c-K-*ras*, may be expressed constitutively in chemically transformed mouse cells.[674] A relaxed regulation of protooncogene expression could contribute to loss of growth control in neoplastic transformation.

In somatic mammalian cells the level of c-*myc* transcription is not restricted to particular cell types but may correlate closely with the rate of cell division. Transcription of c-*myc* involves the use of two promoters and results in the production of two mRNA species that are differentially represented in different tissues. In contrast to somatic cells, mitotically and meiotically dividing germ cells have very few c-*myc* transcripts and appear to proliferate in the absence of c-*myc* transcription.[675]

4. Expression of the Human c-*fes* Gene

The protooncogene c-*fes* is expressed at detectable levels in human hematopoietic cells but only in myeloid, not in lymphoid, cell populations.[676] Among normal human tissues the highest levels of c-*fes* expression are consistently found in macrophages, followed by bone marrow.[677] The c-*fes* protooncogene is also expressed in mature peripheral blood monocytes and granulocytes but at lower levels than in the bone marrow cell precursors, which suggests that the levels decrease during cell maturation.

5. Expression of Protooncogenes in Human Hematopoietic Tissues

According to their transcriptional activity in human hematopoietic cells, protooncogenes can be classified in three groups: (1) protooncogenes that are almost universally active in different cells and different stages of differentiation (c-*abl*, c-*myc*, c-*ras*); (2) protooncogenes that are active only in certain cells and in certain stages of differentiation (c-*myb*), and (3) protooncogenes that are apparently inactive in most cells (c-*fes*, c-*sis*).[59] However, expression of the human c-*fes* gene occurs normally in human myeloid cell populations.[678]

Differential activation of protooncogenes may be involved in the regulation of hematopoietic processes, as demonstrated by *in situ* hybridization studies of human bone marrow with radiolabeled probes.[658] The protooncogenes c-*myc*, c-*myb*, and c-*fes* are expressed at relatively high levels in early precursors of the myeloid, erythroid, and megakaryocytic lineages (myeloblasts, promyelocytes, basophilic erythroblasts, and megakaryoblasts). Expression of c-*myc* and c-*myb*, but not c-*fes*, decreases in more advanced stages of maturation of the myeloid lineage. No expression of c-*myc*, c-*myb*, and c-*fes* is detectable in erythroblasts beyond the basophilic stage, whereas mature megakaryocytes show high levels of mRNAs from all three protooncogenes.[658] The results suggest that c-*myc* and c-*myb* expression is related in some way to the cellular proliferation of myeloid and erythroid precursors, whereas c-*fes* expression is more restricted to myeloid differentiation. In the 12-week-old human fetus, the highest levels of c-*fgr* expression were found in the liver, which may reflect a specific role of the product of this gene in the development of hematopoietic cells.[469] A protooncogene that may be involved in regulating the growth and differentiation of lymphoid cells is c-*ets*.[679]

F. REGULATION OF PROTOONCOGENE EXPRESSION

The mechanisms involved in the regulation of protooncogene expression under different physiological conditions are very complex. Both transcriptional and posttranscriptional control mechanisms may participate in regulating the levels of protooncogene expression in specific types of cells under different physiological conditions, e.g., the expression of c-*fos* and c-*myc* in normal lymphocytes under basal conditions and at various times after mitogenic stimulation.[680] Chromatin structural modifications, flanking DNA sequence elements, DNA methylation patterns, and posttranscriptional phenomena may be important for the regulation of protooncogene expression. The relative importance of each mechanism may depend, at least in part, on the influence of specific environmental factors.

1. Chromatin Structural Modifications

Chromatin structural modifications in the protooncogene sequences and their vicinity may be importantly involved in the regulation of protooncogene transcriptional activity.[681] These modifications would depend on structural changes of the chromatin-associated proteins as well as on changes in the local physical state of the DNA. Phosphorylation of protein chromatin components induced by different cellular kinases may have profound consequences on the expression of different genes, including protooncogenes, according to the cell type and the predominant physiologic conditions.

2. Flanking DNA Sequences

Flanking DNA sequences may also have an important role for determining the activity or inactivity of specific protooncogenes. Structural homology has been detected between the flanking regions of c-*myc* and c-*fos* and the region located immediately 5′ to the gene coding for IL-2, a protein involved in the control of T-cell proliferation.[682] Moreover, the region of homology, represented by the consensus sequence TGGANNGNANCCAA, is also shared with sequences of viruses with oncogenic properties, including the LTRs of HTLV-I and HTLV-II and region E1A of Ad5.[682] The presence of the consensus sequence in these cellular and viral genomes suggests the existence of common mechanisms related to the control of cell proliferation. A negative transcriptional control element is located upstream of the murine c-*myc* gene.[683]

Differential regulation of the c-*myc*, N-*myc*, and c-*src* genes is observed in embryonal carcinoma cells undergoing neuronal differentiation.[684] The molecular mechanisms involved in the differential regulation of protooncogene expression are not understood but would be similar to that of other cellular genes.

Activation of c-*mos* in the mouse is prevented by normal DNA sequences located upstream to the protooncogene.[685] This region, termed upstream mouse sequence (UMS), is approximately 1 kb length and is located 0.8 to 1.8 kb upstream from the first initiation codon (ATG) in the open reading frame of c-*mos*. However, c-*mos* can be activated by the insertion of an endogenous retrovirus-like DNA element (IAP) within or upstream to the coding region of c-*mos*, in particular, when IAP LTR insertion occurs between the UMS region of the c-*mos* locus.[686] UMS can also prevent enhancement of the transforming activity of v-*mos*. A 95% reduction in the transforming efficiency of a cloned v-*mos* gene was obtained by inserting UMS 20 bp upstream from the first ATG in v-*mos* but no reduction was observed when UMS was inserted 441 bp from v-*mos*.[685]

3. DNA Methylation Patterns

Specific patterns of DNA methylation may contribute to the regulation of protooncogene expression.[687-691] In general, DNA hypermethylation of oncogene sequences is associated with their transcriptional silence,[692,693] whereas undermethylation of these sequences is associated with their transcriptional activation.[694] The c-K-*ras* protooncogene is hypermethylated in both hepatocytes and nonparenchymal cells isolated from rat liver, which suggests that it is, at most, minimally expressed in normal rat liver.[695] The c-H-*ras*-1 gene is extensively methylated in human leukocytes and sperm, with the former exhibiting a highly specific methylation pattern.[569] In fetal fibroblasts and immortal cell lines, individual alleles of the c-H-*ras*-1 are differentially methylated at a variable tandem repeat region located 1 kb downstream of the polyadenylation signal sequence.

Regional patterns of methylation within oncogenes may be important for regulation of the oncogene transcriptional activity. The sequence 5′-CCGG-3′ in the third exon of the c-*myc* gene is fully methylated in normal cell strains but was found to be hypomethylated in three of five human tumor cell lines exhibiting a reduction in total DNA methylation, whereas other CCGG sequences of the same oncogene (first exon, first intron, and second exon) were hypomethylated in all cell types tested, regardless of whether normal or oncogenically transformed.[696]

4. Posttranscriptional Regulatory Phenomena

Protooncogene expression may also be regulated at the level of posttranscriptional events. In all human cells tested, including normal human embryonic fibroblasts and different types of transformed cell lines of various origins (HeLa cervix carcinoma cells, MCF7 mammary carcinoma cells, Daudi Burkitt's lymphoma cells, and HL60 promyelocytic leukemia cells), c-*myc* transcripts are extremely unstable, with a half-life of approximately 10 to 15 min.[697] Differential efficiencies are observed in the *in vitro* translation of c-*myc* transcripts differing in the 5′ untranslated region.[698] These results suggest that c-*myc* expression may also be regulated by posttranscriptional events affecting the efficiency of c-*myc* mRNA translation and/or degradation of the c-*myc* mRNA.

G. PROTOONCOGENE EXPRESSION IN STIMULATED CELLS

Stimulation of susceptible cells by mitogenic agents may result in sequential changes in the expression of specific protooncogenes and other genes. The c-*myc* gene is expressed when human T lymphocytes of the T4 phenotype, but not the T8 phenotype, are stimulated with the mitogenic agent PHA.[699] Normal human T lymphocytes stimulated with PHA exhibit particular changes in the pattern of expression of several protooncogenes.[612,672,700] Whereas some protooncogenes (N-*ras*, c-*abl*, c-*ets*, and c-*yes*) are expressed in unstimulated lymphocytes, protooncogenes encoding nuclear proteins (c-*myc*, c-*myb*, c-*fos*, and p53) are expressed following PHA stimulation. In addition, the genes coding for IL-2 and the IL-2 receptor are expressed in the stimulated cells. The expression of some of these genes (the c-*myc* and c-*fos* protooncogenes and the genes for IL-2 and the IL-2 receptor) shows an early response to PHA stimulation, whereas other genes (the c-*myb* and N-*ras* protooncogenes and the gene for transferrin receptor) behave as late response genes. Expression of the c-*myb* protein, p80[c-myb], in PHA-stimulated human T lymphocytes occurs only after initiation of the S phase of the cell cycle.[701] Expression of the putative protooncogene *bcl*-2 is also stimulated by mitogens in B and T lymphocytes.[702] The functions of protooncogene products in the stimulated lymphocytes are unknown but they could be related to some differentiated functions of the cells.

Responses of different protooncogenes may exhibit variation among different types of mitogen-stimulated cells, as demonstrated with the use of specific inhibitors. Specific inhibitors of the nuclear enzyme ADP-ribosyltransferase block differentiation of several eukaryotic cells, including an early event in lymphocyte activation. In PHA-stimulated human lymphocytes, ADP-ribosyltransferase inhibitors completely block the proliferative response and the increase in c-*myc* gene expression without affecting c-*fos* significantly.[703] Conversely, in fibroblasts the serum-induced growth is not affected by the ADP-ribosyltransferase inhibitor, and both protooncogenes are superinduced. Hence, there are differences between the early responses of lymphocytes and fibroblasts to mitogenic stimulation, and also between the regulation of c-*fos* and c-*myc* expression. These results support the concept that different protooncogenes serve different functions in different types of cells.

A set of responsive genes, called TPA-induced sequences, has been identified in cells stimulated by phorbol esters and other external stimuli.[704,705] The protooncogene c-*fos* is included among TPA-induced sequences. TPA and the calcium ionophore A23187 induce a transient expression of both c-*fos* and c-*myc* mRNA in human peripheral blood lymphocytes.[706] The physiologic role of c-*fos* and c-*myc* gene expression in the stimulated human lymphocytes is not known but their induction is not sufficient by itself to commit the cells to DNA synthesis.[707] Phorbol ester and calcium ionophore, as well as synthetic diacylglycerol, induce c-*fos* mRNA in normal peritoneal macrophages with a peak at 30 min, but this induction is not associated with cell proliferation or the expression of differentiated macrophage functions.[708] Moreover, treatment of macrophages with either IFN-β or IFN-γ, which are potent macrophage activators eliciting tumoricidal activity, does not alter the levels of c-*fos* mRNA. Thus, c-*fos* mRNA augmentation would represent a stimulus-specific rather than a function-specific response and is apparently connected to activation of protein kinase C. Growth factor-induced activation of phosphoinositide breakdown, with the ensuing activation of protein kinase C and release of Ca^{2+}, is associated with the induction of c-*fos* gene expression in both fibroblasts and macrophages.[709] Induction of c-*fos* and c-*myc* mRNA by EGF or calcium inophore is dependent on an increase in the intracellular concentration of cAMP.[710] cAMP-dependent protein kinases may have a direct role in the induction of gene expression in mammalian cells.[711]

The plant lectin concanavalin A, the phorbol ester TPA, and the calcium ionophore A23187 each causes a rapid increase in both c-*fos* and c-*myc* mRNAs when added to cultured quiescent murine thymocytes.[712] The activation of both protooncogenes is completely dependent on the extracellular Ca^{2+} concentration for A23187 and is independent of this concentration for TPA. Calcitriol inhibits the accumulation of mRNA for c-*myc*, as well as mRNAs for IL-2 and IFN-γ, in human T lymphocytes activated by mitogens or differentiation-inducing agents such as phorbol esters or A23187.[713]

Expression of protooncogenes in blood cells other than lymphocytes may also be altered as a consequence of specific stimulation. For example, treatment of murine peritoneal macrophages with bacterial lipopolysaccharide (LPS) alters expression of the c-*fos* and c-*myc* genes.[714] Adenosine diphosphate (ADP), which is the most potent mitogen described for monkey kidney epithelial cells maintained in culture (BSC-1 cell line), activates the expression of c-H-*ras* and c-*myc* protooncogenes in these cells before the initiation of DNA synthesis.[715]

Activity of the adenylate cyclase system has an important role in the regulation of cell proliferation and differentiation. Either stimulation of inhibition of these processes may be associated with cAMP accumulation, depending on the cell type and the physiological conditions.[716] Changes of cAMP concentration may be accompanied by altered expression of protooncogene products. For example, treatment of the human B precursor cell line Reh (derived from acute lymphocytic leukemia cells) with the adenylate cyclase activator forskolin resulted in greatly augmented concentrations of intracellular cAMP, and this change was associated with reduced proliferation and accumulation of the Reh cells in the G_1 phase of the cycle, but without the appearance of differentiation markers.[717] The production of both c-*myc* and c-H-*ras* protein was inhibited during the first 3 h of forskolin treatment but it was reestablished during the next 20 h.

1. Influence of Hormones and Growth Factors in the Regulation of Protooncogene Expression

Hormones and growth factors have an important role in the regulation of protooncogene expression in their respective target cells and tissues. Addition of specific hormones or growth factors to the culture medium of particular cell types or treatment of intact animals with these agents may result in marked changes in protooncogene expression. The altered protooncogene expression may or may not be followed by increased DNA synthesis and cell division. Complex interactions between hormones, growth factors, and protooncogene products operate in regulating the metabolism as well as the differentiation and proliferation of normal cells and may also be of great importance in tumorigenic processes. The complex relationships between hormones, growth factors, and protooncogene products are extensively discussed in a recent book.[386]

2. Influence of Aging on Protooncogene Expression

The levels of expression of some protooncogenes may decline in aging cells. Expression of both c-*myc* and c-*ras* is significantly lower in late passage human IMR-90 fibroblasts than in early passage cells.[718,719] However, c-*myc* transcripts have been found to be markedly elevated in the liver of aging Fischer rats.[720] On the other hand, c-*sis* and c-*src* transcripts do not exhibit alterations in the aging animals. Changes in tissue-specific patterns of DNA methylation may be associated with gene expression and such changes have been found to occur during the aging process of mice.[721] Expression of several protooncogenes was examined in fibroblasts cultured from seven different primate species, looking for a possible correlation between the level of expression and the maximal achievable lifespan.[722] The only protooncogene whose level of expression was found to be higher in fibroblasts derived from three relatively long-lived species (the human, gorilla, and chimpanzee) was c-*erb*-B. No significant difference was found in the level of expression of the c-K-*ras*, c-*myc*, or c-*src* protooncogenes. These findings suggest that certain protooncogenes may participate in a coordinate manner in the molecular phenomena leading to the senescent phenotype.

H. PROTOONCOGENE EXPRESSION IN INDUCED DIFFERENTIATION OF NEOPLASTIC CELL LINES

The expression of certain protooncogenes may be altered during differentiation-related phenomena induced in neoplastic cell lines by experimental manipulations *in vitro*.[723-725] The expression of c-*myc* and c-*myb* genes decreases when differentiation is induced in neoplastic human hematopoietic cell lines by treatment with a diversity of compounds including the vitamin D derivative 1,25-dihydroxycholecalciferol (calcitriol), dimethyl sulfoxide (DMSO), retinoic acid, phorbol esters such as TPA and PMA, inhibitors of poly(ADP-ribose)-polymerase, and neplanocin A.[726-734] In cultured cells from human medullary thyroid carcinoma, phorbol esters produce 80% decreased c-*myc* mRNA levels and increased calcitonin gene transcription.[735] In a human neuroblastoma cell line, decreased expression of the N-*myc* gene precedes retinoic acid-induced morphological differentiation.[736,737] In the human neuroblastoma cell line SH-SY5Y, TPA-induced differentiation is associated with decreased expression of both c-*myc* and N-*myc* genes and increased levels of c-*fos*.[738] Retinoic acid-induced differentiation of SH-SY5Y cells is also associated with down regulation of c-*myc* and N-*myc* expression but no expression of c-*fos* is detected. However, decreased expression of c-*myc* is not universally observed in cells induced to differentiate by particular types of inducers. Terminal differentiation of THP-1 human monocytic leukemia cells induced by phorbol ester or retinoic acid is associated with induction of c-*fos* and down regulation of c-*myb*, but the level of expression of c-*myc* remains unaltered.[739] Not a decrease but a small increase of c-*myc* mRNA may occur following PMA-induced differentiation in the human B-cell line JD38, which was derived from an undifferentiated lymphoma and contains an (8;14) translocation involving the c-*myc* protooncogene.[740] These results indicate that the (8;14) translocation is not necessarily associated with a permanent block of differentiation. Additional examples of differentiation-related processes elicited by specific inducers in neoplastic cell lines are discussed next.

1. Human Promyelocytic Leukemia Cells HL-60

The human promyelocytic leukemia cell line HL60, which was derived from a patient with acute promyelocytic leukemia (APL), can be induced to differentiate along either the monocytic or the myeloid pathways, depending on the chemical inducer used.[723,741-743] However, the chemically induced mature cellular forms derived from HL-60 cells do not completely resemble the normally differentiated terminal cells of the respective pathways of maturation. HL-60 cells are rich in azurophilic granules containing myeloperoxidase and induction of differentiation of these cells into more mature granulocytes by DMSO is associated with decreased activity of myeloperoxidase and decreased expression of myeloperoxidase mRNA.[744] Differentiation of HL-60 cells induced by retinoic acid, DMSO, or calcitriol is associated with superoxide formation and an early and marked increase in the expression of a 47-kDa protein (P47) whose function is unknown.[745]

Changes in the expression of protooncogenes encoding nuclear phosphoproteins (c-*myc*, c-*myb*, and c-*fos*), but not other protooncogenes like c-H-*ras* or c-*fes*, may be associated with calcitriol-induced monocytic differentiation of HL-60 cells.[746,747] Numerous studies have indicated that induction of differentiation of HL-60 cells by either TPA or calcitriol (monocytic pathway) or by DMSO (myeloid pathway) is accompanied by a decrease in the levels of c-*myc* mRNA.[732,748-751] The decrease of c-*myc* gene expression may be causally related to cessation of DNA synthesis and differentiation of the induced HL-60 cells. Introduction of a plasmid vector carrying an antisense human c-*myc* gene into HL-60 cells resulted in the production of high levels of antisense c-*myc*-specific transcripts and inhibition of endogenous c-*myc* mRNA and protein synthesis, which were associated with cessation of cellular DNA synthesis and differentiation of the cells through the monocytic pathway.[752] However, not decreased but increased c-*myc* mRNA levels may be associated with the precommitment stage during the differentiation of HL-60 cells.[753] Changes in c-*myc* expression in HL-60 cells induced to differentiation by treatment with DMSO are apparently caused by the differentiation process itself and not by the simultaneously occurring inhibition of cell proliferation since c-*myc* expression remains elevated in HL-60 growth-inhibited but undifferentiated cells.[731]

Decreased transcriptional activity of the c-*myc* protooncogene is frequently seen in HL-60 cells during the process of differentiation induced by various agents. In the continuous presence of phorbol ester, the rate of c-*myc* transcription in HL-60 cells is significantly decreased. The cell-permeable 1,2-diacylglycerol analogue, *sn*-1,2-dioctanoylglycerol, causes a rapid decrease in c-*myc* transcription in HL-60 cells, suggesting that prolonged stimulation of protein kinase C is required for persistent inhibition of c-*myc* transcription in these cells.[754] Protein kinase C is normally activated *in vivo* by 1,2-diacylglycerol that is generated in response to receptor-mediated stimulation of membrane-bound phospholipase C. The Ca^{2+}/phospholipid-dependent enzyme, protein kinase C, is a cellular receptor for phorbol esters. However, the role of protein kinase C in the down-regulation effect of phorbol ester in HL-60 cell differentiation is not clear. The macrocytic lactone bryostatin, isolated from the marine bryozoan *Bugula neritina*, can activate protein kinase C without inducing differentiation of HL-60 cells, and the effect of bryostatin is not associated with down regulation of c-*myc* gene expression.[755]

Exposure of HL-60 cells to calcitriol, which induces their differentiation into monocyte-like cells, is associated with a significant decrease in the level of c-*myc* mRNA expression due to inhibition of c-*myc* gene transcriptional activity.[756,757] A similar inhibition of c-*myc* gene expression is observed when HL-60 cells are induced to differentiate along the monocytic pathway by treatment with the cyclic nucleotide analogue, dibutyryl cAMP.[758] Decreased c-*myc* expression, accompanied by increased membrane-bound tyrosine-specific protein kinase activity, was observed in HL-60 cells induced to differentiate by the synergistic action of retinoic acid and the calcium ionophore A23187.[759] Growth factors can induce differentiation of HL-60 cells. Recombinant TNF-α selectively inhibits the expression of c-*myc* in HL-60 cells and concomitantly induces a process of differentiation that may account for the decreased growth rate observed in TNF-α-treated HL-60 cells.[760] The action of TNF-α on c-*myc* gene expression occurs primarily at the level or transcription and is independent of *de novo* protein synthesis. Down regulation of c-*myc* gene expression induced by TNF-α and phorbol esters in HL-60 cells is due, at least in part, to interruption of transcription.[761] Differentiation of HL-60 cells by two new benzoic acid derivatives is associated with more than 90% inhibition of c-*myc* expression.[762]

The role of inhibited c-*myc* gene expression in relation to the process of differentiation induced in HL-60 cells is unknown. The action of some differentiation inducers is apparently independent of changes in c-*myc* expression. IFN-γ-induced differentiation of HL-60 cells is not associated with reduced expression of c-*myc*.[761] Moreover, although IFN-γ and TNF-α have synergistic effects in inducing HL-60 cell differentiation, this synergy is not reflected in dose regulation of *myc* gene expression. Exposure of HL-60 cells to phorbol dibutyrate under appropriate culture conditions results in differentiation to macrophage-like cells in 95% of the population. Studies with a subclone of HL-60 cells (HL-60 1E3), which is partially resistant to differentiation along the monocyte and granulocyte pathway, indicate that early (4 to 6 h) down regulation of c-*myc* transcriptional expression is not sufficient to terminally commit HL-60 cells to phorbol butyrate-induced differentiation.[763] However, additional regulation of the c-*myc* gene at later stages could be part of the mechanisms which allow terminal differentiation events to occur.

Expression of the c-*fos* protooncogene may also be altered, although not always, during differentiation-like events induced in HL-60 cells. A rapid increase in c-*fos* expression is observed when HL-60 cells are induced to differentiate by treatment with the TPA but not when the induction is performed by treatment with calcitriol or retinoic acid.[764] Treatment of HL-60 cells with TPA results in induction of macrophage-like differentiation, which is associated with c-*fos* gene expression and rising levels of class I MHC antigens, whereas treatment with DMSO results in differentiation into granulocyte-like cells and this is not accompanied by c-*fos* expression and is followed by declining MHC antigen levels.[765] These results indicate that altered c-*fos* gene expression is not an obligatory step in the differentiation of leukemic cells. Moreover, HL-60 cell variants resistant to TPA can be induced to differentiate in the absence of detectable c-*fos* expression.[748] In any case, c-*myc* and c-*fos* would have different roles in relation to the processes of differentiation induced in HL-60 cells. Phorbol ester-induced inactivation of c-*myc* gene expression in HL-60 cells is associated with reassembly of nucleosomal particles at the c-*myc* locus, whereas activation of c-*fos* expression in the same cells is associated with relaxation of nucleosomal particles at the c-*fos* locus.[766]

Expression of other protooncogenes may also be modulated at either the transcriptional or posttranscriptional levels in differentiating HL-60 cells. Induction of c-*sis* gene expression and synthesis of PDGF is observed in HL-60 cells during differentiation along the monocytic pathway.[767] Phorbol ester-induced differentiation of HL-60 cells along the monocytic pathway is associated with the expression of c-*fms*/CSF-1 receptor and CSF-1 transcripts, which are not detectable in uninduced HL-60 cells.[768,769] Proteins regulated by the c-*ets* protooncogene, or related to the products of this gene, are generated during differentiation of HL-60 cells.[770] The protooncogene c-H-*ras* is expressed at an increased rate in HL-60 cells induced to differentiate along the granulocytic pathway by treatment with DMSO.[771] The transcription rate and steady-state levels of c-H-*ras* mRNA are increased in the DMSO-treated cells, and correlate with the acquisition of the phenotypic markers of differentiation. The activity of $pp60^{c\text{-}src}$ protooncogene protein kinase is increased in HL-60 cells induced to differentiate, but the change in enzyme activity is apparently not associated with increased transcriptional activity of the c-*src* gene.[772,773] The expression of the N-*ras* gene is not altered during the differentiation of HL-60 cells induced by different agents.[733]

The role of altered protooncogene expression in relation to differentiation-like events induced in HL-60 cells is not clear at all. IFN-γ is capable of inducing the differentiation of HL-60 cells into monocyte-like cell but the IFN-γ-induced changes in protooncogene expression occur after the appearance of multiple markers of the monocytic phenotype.[774] In the IFN-γ-treated cells, c-*myc* expression decreases as a later event after 72 h and c-*fos* transcripts remain undetectable until 5 d of treatment. Furthermore, c-*fms* mRNA is induced only after 7 d and expression of the c-*sis* protooncogene at the RNA and protein levels remains undetectable after induction with IFN-γ. These findings strongly suggest that declines in c-*myc* expression, as well as induction of c-*fos*, c-*fms*, and c-*sis* expression, are not requisite events in the commitment of HL-60 cells to differentiation induced by IFN-γ, and may possibly also not be required for the differentiation induced in these cells by other agents.

Induction of differentiation of HL-60 cells by calcitriol is associated with an early inhibition of DNA synthesis which precedes down regulation of c-*myc* gene expression.[775] Moreover, calcitriol directly inhibits DNA synthesis in isolated nuclei of HL-60 cells. The results of these studies suggest that an altered expression of the c-*myc* gene is apparently not a requisite for the inhibition of DNA synthesis which precedes the monocytic differentiation of HL-60 cells induced by calcitriol. The delayed inhibition of DNA synthesis induced by calcitriol in HL-60 cells is accompanied by an elevated expression of the c-*fos* and c-*fms* protooncogenes, as well as by reduced calmodulin concentration, which could be related to the monocytic differentiation of these cells.[776]

The mechanisms responsible for altered protooncogene expression in HL-60 cells induced to differentiate are little understood. HL-60 cells have a markedly amplified c-*myc* protooncogene which is overexpressed in comparison with that of normal cells.[777,778] Decreased c-*myc* gene transcription observed in HL-60 cells during differentiation is not associated with detectable changes in the primary structure or methylation of the gene but following the differentiation one of four S1 nuclease-sensitive sites contained in c-*myc* is not detectable and the remaining three sites appear to be qualitatively decreased.[779] DMSO-induced differentiation of HL-60 cells is is accompanied by the loss of a single DNase I hypersensitive site 0.9 kb upstream of the gene.[780] Such changes are suggestive of alterations in the physical state of the c-*myc* gene, which may be closely related to its transcriptional activity. A block to transcript elongation may be largely responsible for decreased transcription of c-*myc* gene in HL-60 cell differentiation induced by either retinoic acid or DMSO.[781,782]

In conclusion, altered expression of distinct protooncogenes is observed frequently, but not always, during the process of differentiation induced by treatment of HL-60 cells with various agents. Many of the changes observed in protooncogene expression in the treated cells are agent specific rather than differentiation specific and their possible role in the molecular events related to the phenotypic differentiation of HL-60 cells remains unknown.

2. Mouse Erythroleukemia Cells

Mouse erythroleukemia (MEL) cells are also called Friend cells because they have been isolated from the spleen of mice infected with the F-MuLV complex. The cells resemble proerythroblasts and can be induced by exposure to particular chemical agents to undergo a program of differentiation events which is very similar to that of the final stages of normal erythropoiesis, including the expression of adult- and embryonic-type globin gene transcripts.

Sequential expression of protooncogenes in the order c-*fos*, c-*myb*, c-*myc*, and c-K-*ras* occurs during the first 48 h in cultured MEL cells induced to differentiate by exposure to DMSO.[783] The levels of both c-*myc* and c-*myb* mRNA show a biphasic pattern of expression after DMSO-induced differentiation of MEL cells, with a marked decrease (20-fold) during the first 14 h after induction, followed by an increase between 24 to 72 h and a final gradual decrease coincident with a progressive rise in α-globin RNA, which indicates a state of terminal differentiation.[784,785] Whereas the DMSO-induced decline of c-*myc* expression does not absolutely require new protein synthesis, the reappearance of c-*myc* mRNA is dependent on continued protein synthesis, which suggests the existence of both negative and positive regulatory mechanisms of c-*myc* expression.

A cell cycle-dependent change in the level of c-*myc* expression is observed in differentiation of MEL cells induced by hypoxanthine hexamethylenebisacetamide (HMBA).[786] Prior to inducer treatment the level of c-*myc* mRNA is relatively constant throughout the cell cycle but upon treatment with the differentiation inducer c-*myc* levels abruptly decline. When the c-*myc* mRNA level is restored at different times in inducer-treated cells, according to the type of inducer used, it is more highly restricted to cells in the G_1 phase of the cycle. Thus, treatment with inducers of differentiation may lead to a change in the cell cycle regulation of c-*myc* gene transcriptional activity.

Introduction of additional copies of c-*myc* by transfecting MEL cells with recombinant plasmids carrying the c-*myc* gene indicates that altering the time of c-*myc* reexpression in these cells to earlier times correlates with a shortening of the latent differentiation period.[787] These results support the view that c-*myc* may have, at appropriate times of expression, a positive effect on the rate of differentiation in particular types of cells. Moreover, deregulated expression of c-*myc* in MEL cells may prevent their differentiation.[788,789] Introduction of a plasmid vector containing a full-length mouse c-*myc* cDNA into MEL cells can produce a complete or partial inhibition of DMSO-induced MEL cell differentiation. Interestingly, at least one response to DMSO, i.e., modulation of endogenous c-*myc* protooncogene expression, occurs in the MEL cells transfected with a viral promoter-driven c-*myc* gene even though the cells do not show the final differentiated phenotype in response to induction.[788]

Different types of differentiation inducers may have different effects on MEL cells, including different patterns of protooncogene expression. During the initial 4 h of culture, HMBA causes a marked decrease not only in c-*myc* but also in c-*myb* mRNA levels, whereas c-*fos* mRNA levels are increased.[790] During this early period the cells are not irreversibly committed to differentiation but commitment occurs with continued culture in the presence of HMBA. With continued culture, the decrease in c-*myb* and the increase in c-*fos* mRNA persists, while the c-*myc* mRNA returns to control levels before the time that MEL cells begin to show irreversible differentiation.[790] Dexamethasone, which block expression of HMBA-induced MEL cell differentiation, does not alter the early pattern of changes in protooncogene expression nor the sustained elevation of c-*fos* mRNA, but it inhibits the continued suppression of c-*myb* expression, allowing c-*myb* to return toward control levels. This result suggests that the continued suppression of c-*myb* gene expression is critical for HMBA-induced MEL cell commitment to terminal erythroid differentiation. Hemin, which induces MEL cells to accumulate globin molecules but does not initiate commitment to terminal cell division, does not alter the expression of c-*myc*, c-*myb*, or c-*fos* protooncogenes.[790]

3. Daudi Human Lymphoblastoid Cell Line

The Daudi human lymphoblastoid cell line was derived from an African Burkitt's lymphoma.

A selective reduction of c-*myc* mRNA levels is observed in Daudi cells under the influence of human IFN-β and a close link would exist between reduction of c-*myc* expression and interferon-induced arrest of cells at a specific phase (G_0/G_1) of the cell cycle.[791,792] IFN-β regulates c-*myc* expression in Daudi cells not at the transcriptional level but at the posttranscriptional level, reducing the half-life of c-*myc* mRNA.[793,794] Although the steady-state level of c-*myc* mRNA is reduced by 60% in IFN-β-treated cells within 3 h, the rate of c-*myc* gene transcription is virtually unaffected even at 24 h of IFN exposure.[793] Since c-*myc* mRNA reduction is observed in Daudi cells whose protein synthesis is inhibited by more than 95% with cycloheximide or emetine, it may be concluded that neither sustained nor IFN-induced protein synthesis is required for the c-*myc* mRNA regulation in these cells.[795]

It is not known at which posttranscriptional level the c-*myc* transcripts are regulated in Daudi cells. In other human leukemic cell lines (HL-60 and U937) IFN fails to reduce the c-*myc* mRNA level.[792] The basis of this difference between Daudi cells and other leukemic cell lines is unknown. HL-60 and U937 cells display normal induction of other IFN-regulated activities and show a decline in c-*myc* gene expression when they become arrested in the G_0/G_1 phase of the cycle as part of their terminal differentiation.[296] IFN-γ and calcitriol may reduce the expression of c-*myc* in HL-60 cells in a cooperative manner related to inhibition of cell proliferation.[796]

In some clones of Daudi cells selected for resistance to the antiproliferative action of IFN, the level of c-*myc* mRNA does not change significantly following IFN treatment, but a subclone of the IFN-resistant cells which had reverted to almost complete sensitivity to the antiproliferative action of IFN remained refractory to IFN-induced modulation of c-*myc* expression.[797] These results suggest that a reduced level of c-*myc* mRNA may not be a prerequisite for inhibition of cell proliferation in IFN-treated cells. Thus, the exact relationship between c-*myc* gene expression and the control mechanisms of cell proliferation remains undetermined.

4. Human Leukemia Cell Line K-562

The K-562 early blast human leukemia cell line was derived from CML and contains a translocated and decapitated c-*abl* protooncogene.[496] Moreover, an amplified copy number of the c-*abl* gene is present in K-562 CML cells. These cells can be induced to erythroid differentiation by treatment with particular types of chemical inducers. Hemin-mediated erythroid induction and proliferation of K-562 cells is associated with changes in the expression of the c-*abl* and c-*myc* protooncogenes.[798] The cytosine analogue 1-β-D-aribinofuranosylcytosine (ara-C) irreversibly induces the coordinate expression of differentiation markers in K-562 cells, including hemoglobin synthesis, and this differentiation is associated with a marked decrease of c-*myc* mRNA expression after the first 4 h of induction.[799] Differentiation induced in the K-562 cell line by phorbol ester is associated with transcriptional expression of the c-*sis* protooncogene.[800]

5. Murine Myeloid Leukemia Cell Line WEHI-3B

The WEHI-231 cell line was derived from a murine B-cell lymphoma. Treatment of WEHI-231 cells with either TPA or antisera directed against the surface immunoglobulin inhibits proliferation and results in an initial increase in c-*myc* mRNA level followed by a precipitous drop.[801] The early increase in c-*myc* mRNA is due to both an increase in c-*myc* gene transcription and c-*myc* mRNA stabilization, whereas the later decrease results from both a shutdown in c-*myc* transcription and a return to the normal lability of the cytoplasmic c-*myc* mRNA. In WEHI-3B cells the transcriptional expression of c-*myc* and c-*myb* decreases after the cells reach the monocyte stage in differentiation induced by treatment with granulocyte colony-stimulating factor (G-CSF) plus a low concentration of actinomycin D.[802] Transcripts of other protooncogenes are either unaltered (c-*abl*, c-K-*ras*, and c-*fes*) or are not detectable (c-*src*, c-*sis*, c-*mos*, c-*erb*-A, and c-*erb*-B) during the process of differentiation induced in the same cells. In contrast, there is a marked increase in the expression of c-*fos*, which is apparently associated with monocyte differentiation.

6. Human Chronic Lymphocytic Leukemia Cell Line I-73

In contrast to the cell lines HL-60 and U-937, I-73 human chronic lymphocytic leukemia cells, which have phenotypic features similar to those of resting normal B lymphocytes, display a marked increase in the expression of both c-*myc* and c-*fos* genes upon PMA-induced differentiation into Ig-secreting lymphoblasts and plasmablasts.[803] The induced differentiation of I-73 cells is associated with a transition of the cells from the G_0 to G_1 phase of the cycle, without entering into the S phase.

7. Mouse Plasmacytoid Lymphosarcoma Cell Lines

Treatment of A-MuLV-induced mouse plasmacytoid lymphosarcoma cell lines with PMA results in various degrees of growth arrest, presumably due to myelomonocytic differentiation, but this arrest is not accompanied by reduced c-*myc* or c-*myb* gene expression.[804] Thus, a switching-off of these two protooncogenes is not obligatory for the cells to become growth arrested.

8. Murine Embryonal Carcinoma Cells

Levels of expression of several several protooncogenes may show important changes during either spontaneous or induced differentiation of murine teratocarcinoma stem cells (embryonal carcinoma cell lines), but partially contradictory results have been obtained in different studies on this subject. The level of N-*myc* mRNA decreases by 85% when PCC7 embryonal carcinoma is induced by retinoic acid and cAMP treatment to form nerve-like cells.[684] After 6 d of induction, the PCC7 cells change into aggregates of neurofilament-positive cells with massive neurite outgrowths. The decreased N-*myc* expression in induced PCC7 cells is paralleled by 300 to 500% increase in the level of c-*src* expression. Since slowing of cell multiplication by serum starvation is not accompanied by changes in N-*myc* and c-*src* mRNA levels, such changes are thus most probably related to cell differentiation than to cell proliferation. Moreover, c-*myc* gene is not expressed in PCC7 cells even at exponential rate of proliferation. Chemical induction of F9 cells to form visceral or parietal endoderm results in markedly reduced levels of N-*myc* and c-*myc* transcripts, whereas no *src* transcripts are detectable in proliferating or differentiated F9 cells.[684] However, decreased levels of expression of c-*myc* were not found in another study on F9 cells induced to differentiate by treatment with retinoic acid.[805] In this study, a decreased expression of c-*myb* was detected, a later increase in c-*src* transcripts was associated with decreasing cell growth rate, and induction and maintenance of elevated c-*abl* mRNA levels were dependent on the presence of retinoic acid in the medium. Increased levels of c-*fos* transcripts were seen only in late stages of differentiation in monolayer cultures.

Induction of differentiation of F9 embryonal carcinoma cells into parietal endoderm-like cells in response to treatment with retinoic acid and dibutyryl cAMP was not found to be accompanied by any large transient increase in c-*fos* gene expression.[644] These results demonstrate that c-*fos* expression is not an obligatory step in the induction of differentiation of neoplastic cells. Regulation of c-*myc* expression during retinoic acid-induced differentiation of F9 cells occurs at a posttranscriptional level and is associated with growth arrest.[806] It is thus clear that complex and varied patterns in the levels of expression of different protooncogenes may be observed during chemically induced differentiation in embryonal carcinoma cells.

9. Human Teratocarcinoma Cells

The teratocarcinoma cell clone Tera-2cl.13 was clonally derived from the Tera-2 cell line, which was established from the pulmonary metastasis of a human testicular teratoma. Exposure of of Tera-2cl.13 cells in monolayer culture to retinoic acid results in terminal differentiation and the formation of a mixture of cell types expressing characteristic markers. This differentiation process is initially associated, within the first 3 d, with a drop in c-*myc* mRNA levels, followed by a persistent increase of these levels which lasts until the cells differentiate and cease division.[207]

10. Human Colon Carcinoma Cell Line HT29

The human colon carcinoma cell line HT29 is undifferentiated in standard culture conditions but can be induced to differentiate by treatment with 5 mM sodium butyrate. Cell populations that emerge from this treatment may express in standard culture medium stable characteristics of differentiation, including mucus secretion. Cloned differentiated cells derived from HT29 cells exhibit a fivefold increase in the expression of the c-H-*ras* protooncogene.[808] Expression of c-K-*ras* is also increased but to a lower extent, whereas no increase is observed in the expression of other protooncogenes (c-*myc*, N-*myc*, c-*myb*, c-*sis*, and c-*mos*) in the differentiated cells. Interestingly, c-*ras* gene has been found to be expressed at high levels in the most differentiated cells of the colon mucosa at the top of colonic crypts. It is thus apparent that c-*ras* expression does not correlate with proliferation and malignancy of colon mucosa cells *in vitro* or *in vivo*.

11. Rat Pheochromocytoma Cell Line PC12

Treatment of PC12 rat pheochromocytoma cells with the specific growth factor NGF results in ceasing of mitosis and induction of differentiated characteristics such as the appearance of branched neuronal-like processes.[809] These effects are associated with a rapid and specific stimulation of c-*fos* mRNA expression.[810-813] However, the role of c-*fos* induction in NGF-induced differentiation of PC12 cells is uncertain. Expression of c-*fos* may be unnecessary for PC12 cell differentiation.[814]

In contrast to most types of transformed cells in which induction of differentiation is associated with decreased expression of the c-*myc* gene, NGF-induced differentiation of PC12 cells is not accompanied by reduced transcription and steady-state levels of c-*myc* mRNA.[812] Introduction of a c-*myc* gene driven by an SV40 promoter, or transfection of an adenovirus E1A gene, into PC12 cells inhibits NGF-induced differentiation of these cells and, when expressed constitutively, the c-*myc* and E1A genes allowed NGF to act as a mitogenic stimulus.

Microinjection of antibody to p21^{ras} protein inhibits NGF-induced differentiation of PC12 cells.[814] Studies using a construct containing a mouse N-*ras* gene linked to a dexamethasone-inducible promoter indicate that N-*ras* expression promotes neuronal differentiation of PC12 cells, inducing the extension of neuritic processes and arresting cell proliferation.[814] However, the phenotype induced by the transfected N-*ras* is in several respects not identical to that induced by NGF.

12. Modulation of Protooncogene Expression during *In Vivo*-Induced Differentiation

Therapy of premalignant or malignant human diseases with differentiation inducers is an area of active investigation but its place among other forms of cancer treatment has not been established. Protocols using synergistic combinations of differentiation inducers may represent an interesting modality of this type of treatment, especially for acute myeloid leukemia and myelodysplastic syndromes.[816]

The level of expression of particular protooncogenes may be altered not only *in vitro* but also during *in vivo*-induced differentiation. However, little evidence exists in favor of this possibility. In a patient with CML, treatment with the RNA synthesis inhibitor mithramycin resulted in reduction of previously enhanced levels of c-*abl* and c-*myc* transcripts, followed soon after by evidence of differentiation, as reflected in a substantial increase in the number of myelocytes and metamyelocytes before a decrease in the total white cells in the peripheral blood.[817] The results suggest the possibility of using the level of protooncogene expression as a clinically useful parameter for the evaluation of agents with *in vivo* differentiation capability as well as for the prediction of a therapeutic response.

13. Conclusion

Expression of particular protooncogenes may be correlated with differentiation phenomena induced by different types of agents in neoplastic cell lines. A possible role of protooncogene products in regulation of genomic functions related to cell differentiation is suggested by the predominant nuclear localization of c-*fos*, c-*myb*, and c-*myc* products, whose expression has been found to be most frequently correlated with induced differentiation phenomena. However, there are remarkable exceptions to this rule and the exact role of protooncogene products in differentiation processes occurring under either experimental or natural conditions remains to be established.

Studies with the immortal, nontumorigenic Syrian hamster embryo cell line DES-4 under-score the complex relationships existing between oncogene expression and induced cell differentiation.[818] Transfection of these cells with cloned v-*src* or v-H-*ras* oncogenes results in their malignant transformation. Retinoic acid inhibits the expression of the transformed phenotype in DES-4 cells expressing the v-*src* oncogene but, in contrast, enhances the expression of the transformed phenotype in DES-4 cells that express the v-H-*ras* oncogene. The role of endogenous protooncogenes in retinoic acid-induced phenotypic changes is not under-stood. The level of expression of pp60[c-*src*] and p21[c-*ras*] is not affected in DES-4 cells treated with retinoic acid, and the activity of the pp60[c-*src*] kinase remains unchanged in these cells.[818] The results of this study and other studies discussed above indicate that there is no simple correlation between the expression of oncogenes or protooncogenes and the differentiation of neoplastic cells induced by chemical agents.

REFERENCES

1. Bishop, J.M., Cellular oncogenes and retroviruses, *Annu. Rev. Biochem.*, 52, 301, 1983.
2. Bishop, J.M., Viral oncogenes, *Cell*, 42, 23, 1985.
3. Huebner, R.J. and Todaro, G.J., Oncogenes of RNA tumor viruses as determinants of cancer, *Proc. Natl. Acad. Sci. U.S.A.*, 64, 1087, 1969.
4. Todaro, G.J. and Huebner, R.J., The viral oncogene hypothesis: new evidence, *Proc. Natl. Acad. Sci. U.S.A.*, 69, 1009, 1972.
5. Comings, D.E., A general theory of carcinogenesis, *Proc. Natl. Acad. Sci. U.S.A.*, 70, 3324, 1973.
6. Anders, F., Anders, A., and Vielkind, U., Regulation of tumor expression in the Gordon-Kosswig melanoma system and the origin of malignancy, in Abstr. XI Int. Cancer Congr., Vol. 3, Florence, Italy, 1974, 305.
7. Anders, A. and Anders, F., Etiology of cancer as studied in the platyfish-swordtail system, *Biochim. Biophys. Acta*, 516, 61, 1978.
8. Anders, F., Schartl, M., and Barnekow, A., *Xiphophorus* as an *in vivo* model for studies on oncogenes, *Natl. Cancer Inst. Monogr.*, 65, 97, 1984.
9. Anders, F., Schartl, M., Barnekow, A., and Anders, A., *Xiphophorus* as an *in vivo* model for studies on normal and defective control of oncogenes, *Adv. Cancer Res.*, 42, 191, 1984.
10. Anders, F., Anders, A., Schartl, M., Gronau, T., Lüke, W., Schmidt, C.-R., and Barnekow, A., Oncogenes in development, neoplasia, and evolution, in *New Experimental Modalities in the Control of Neoplasia*, Chandra, P., Ed., Plenum Press, New York, 1986, 15.
11. Vielkind, J., Haas-Andela, H., and Anders, F., DNA-mediated transformation in the platyfish-swordtail melanoma system, *Experientia*, 32, 1043, 1976.
12. Leong, J., Garapin, A., Jackson, N., Fanshier, L., Levinson, W., and Bishop, J.M., Virus-specific ribonucleic acid in cells producing Rous sarcoma virus: detection and characterization, *J. Virol.*, 9, 891, 1972.
13. Hayward, W.S. and Hanafusa, H., Detection of avian tumor virus RNA in uninfected chicken embryo cells, *J. Virol.*, 11, 157, 1973.

14. Chen, J.H., Hayward, W.S., and Hanafusa, H., Avian tumor virus proteins and RNA in uninfected chicken embryo cells, *J. Virol.,* 14, 1419, 1974.

15. Anderson, G.R. and Robbins, K.C., Rat sequences of the Kirsten and Harvey murine sarcoma virus genomes: nature, origin, and expression in rat tumor RNA, *J. Virol.,* 17, 335, 1976.

16. Scolnick, E.M., Goldberg, R.J., and Williams, D., Characterization of rat genetic sequences of Kirsten sarcoma virus: distinct class of endogenous rat type C viral sequences, *J. Virol.,* 18, 559, 1976.

17. Frankel, A.E. and Fischinger, P.J., Nucleotide sequence in mouse DNA and RNA specific for Moloney sarcoma virus, *Proc. Natl. Acad. Sci. U.S.A.,* 73, 3705, 1976.

18. Stehelin, D., Varmus, H.E., Bishop, J.M., and Vogt, P.K., DNA related to the transforming gene(s) of avian sarcoma viruses is present in normal avian DNA, *Nature,* 260, 170, 1976.

19. Spector, D.H., Varmus, H.E., and Bishop, J.M., Nucleotide sequences related to the transforming gene of avian sarcoma virus are present in the DNA of uninfected vertebrates, *Proc. Natl. Acad. Sci. U.S.A.,* 75, 4100, 1978.

20. Bishop, J.M., Retroviruses, *Annu. Rev. Biochem.,* 47, 35, 1978.

21. Bishop, J.M., Enemies within: the genesis of retrovirus oncogenes, *Cell,* 23, 5, 1981.

22. Bishop, J.M., Retroviruses and cancer genes, *Adv. Cancer Res.,* 37, 1, 1982.

23. Graf, T. and Stehelin, D., Avian leukemia viruses, oncogenes and genome structure, *Biochim. Biophys. Acta,* 651, 245, 1982.

24. Varmus, H.E., Viruses, genes, and cancer. I. The discovery of cellular oncogenes and their role in neoplasia, *Cancer,* 55, 2324, 1985.

25. Bishop, J.M., Viruses, genes, and cancer. II. Retroviruses and cancer genes, *Cancer,* 55, 2329, 1985.

26. Sefton, B.M., Hunter, T., and Beemon, K., Relationship of polypeptide products of the transforming gene of Rous sarcoma virus and the homologous gene of vertebrates, *Proc. Natl. Acad. Sci. U.S.A.,* 77, 2059, 1980.

27. Langbeheim, H., Shih, T.Y., and Scolnick, E.M., Identification of a normal vertebrate cell protein related to the p21 *src* of Harvey murine sarcoma virus, *Virology,* 106, 292, 1980.

28. Ellis, R.W., DeFeo, D., Shih, T.Y., Gonda, M.A., Young, H.A., Tsuchida, N., Lowy, D.R., and Scolnick, E.M., The p21 *src* genes of Harvey and Kirsten sarcoma viruses originate from divergent members of a family of normal vertebrate genes, *Nature,* 292, 506, 1981.

29. Shilo, B. and Weinberg, R.A., DNA sequences homologous to vertebrate oncogenes are conserved in *Drosophila melanogaster,* *Proc. Natl. Acad. Sci. U.S.A.,* 78, 6789.1981.

30. Hoffman-Falk, H., Einat, P., Shilo, B.-Z., and Hoffmann, F., *Drosophila melanogaster* DNA clones homologous to vertebrate oncogenes: evidence for a common ancestor to the *src* and *abl* cellular genes, *Cell,* 32, 589, 1983.

31. Hoffmann, F.M., Fresco, L.D., Hoffman-Falk, H., and Shilo, B.-Z., Nucleotide sequences of the Drosophila *src* and *abl* homologs: conservation and variability in the *src* family of oncogenes, *Cell,* 35, 393, 1983.

32. Lev, Z., Leibovitz, N., Segev, O., and Shilo, B-Z., Expression of the *src* and *abl* cellular oncogenes during development of *Drosophila melanogaster,* *Mol. Cell. Biol.,* 4, 982, 1984.

33. Neuman-Silberberg, F.S., Schejter, E., Hoffmann, F.M., and Shilo, B.-Z.., The Drosophila *ras* oncogenes: structure and nucleotide sequence, *Cell,* 37, 1027, 1984.

34. Shilo, B.-Z. and Hoffmann, F.M., *Drosophila melanogaster* cellular oncogenes, *Cancer Surv.,* 3, 299, 1984.

35. Schartl, M. and Barnekow, A., The expression in eukaryotes of a tyrosine kinase which is reactive with pp60$^{v\text{-}src}$ antibodies, *Differentiation,* 23, 109, 1982.

36. Barnekow, A. and Schartl, M., Cellular *src* gene product detected in the freshwater sponge *Spongilla lacustris,* *Mol. Cell. Biol.,* 4, 1179, 1984.

37. Shilo, B.-Z., Evolution of cellular oncogenes, *Adv. Viral Oncol.,* 4, 29, 1984.

38. Anders, F., Burg, O., Kaiser, P., Schleenbecker, U., Zechel, C., Schmidt, D., Gröger, H., Pfütz, M., and Schartl, M., Oncogenes in the evolution of the animal kingdom, in *Abstr. Annu. Meet. German Genetics Society,* Resch-Verlag, Munich, 1988, 3.

39. DeFeo-Jones, D., Scolnick, E.M., Koller, R., and Dhar, R., *ras*-Related gene sequences identified and isolated from *Saccharomyces cerevisiae,* *Nature,* 306, 707, 1983.

40. Temeles, G.L., DeFeo-Jones, D., Tatchell, K., Ellinger, M.S., and Scolnick, E.M., Expression and characterization of *ras* mRNAs from *Saccharomyces cerevisiae,* *Mol. Cell. Biol.,* 4, 2298, 1984.

41. Fukui, Y. and Kaziro, Y., Molecular cloning and sequence analysis of a *ras* gene from *Schizosaccharomyces pombe,* *EMBO J.,* 4, 687, 1985.

42. Prakash, K. and Seligy, V.L., Oncogene related sequences in fungi: linkage of some to actin, *Biochem. Biophys. Res. Commun.,* 133, 293, 1985.

43. Perbal, B. and Kohiyama, M., Existence de séquences homologues de l'oncogène v-*myb* dans le génome des archaebactéries, *C.R. Acad. Sci. Paris,* 300, 177, 1985.

44. Ben-Mahrez, K., Perbal, B., Kryceve-Martinerie, C., Thierry, D., and Kohiyama, M., A protein of *Halobacterium halobium* immunologically related to the v-*myc* gene product, *FEBS Lett.,* 227, 56, 1988.

45. Wais, A.C., Archaebacteria: the road to the universal ancestor, *BioEssays,* 5, 75, 1986.

46. Smith, E.F. and Townsend, C.O., A plant tumor of bacterial origin, *Science,* 25, 671, 1907.

47. Memelink, J., de Pater, B.S., Hoge, J.H.C., and Shilperoort, R.A., T-DNA hormone biosynthetic genes: phytohormones and gene expression in plants, *Dev. Genet.*, 8, 321, 1987.
48. Weiler, E.W. and Schröder, J., Hormone genes and crown gall disease, *Trends Biochem.*, 12, 271, 1987.
49. Buchmann, I., Marner, F.J., Schröder, G., Waffenschmidt, S., and Schröder, J., Tumour genes in plants: T-DNA encoded cytokinin biosynthesis, *EMBO J.*, 4, 853, 1985.
50. Hagen, G. and Guilfoyle, T.J., Rapid induction of selective transcription by auxins, *Mol. Cell. Biol.*, 5, 1197, 1985.
51. Nester, E.W. and Kosuge, T., Plasmids specifying plant hyperplasias, *Annu. Rev. Microbiol.*, 35, 531, 1981.
52. Bevan, M.W. and Chilton, M.D., T-DNA of the *Agrobacterium* Ti and Ri plasmids, *Annu. Rev. Genet.*, 16, 357, 1982.
53. Wang, K., Stachel, S.E., Timmerman, B., Van Montagu, M., and Zambryski, P.C., Site-specific nick in the T-DNA border sequence as a result of *Agrobacterium vir* gene expression, *Science*, 235, 587, 1987.
54. Gheysen, G., Van Montagu, M., and Zambryski, P., Integration of *Agrobacterium tumefaciens* transfer DNA (T-DNA) involves rearrangements of target plant DNA sequences, *Proc. Natl. Acad. Sci. U.S.A.*, 84, 6169, 1987.
55. Coffin, J.M., Varmus, H.E., Bishop, J.M., Essex, M., Hardy, W.D., Martin G.S., Rosenberg, N.E., Scolnick, E.A., Weinberg, R.A., and Vogt, P.K., A proposal for naming host cell-derived inserts of retrovirus genomes, *J. Virol.*, 40, 953, 1981.
56. Shows, T.B., McAlpine, P.J., Boucheix, C., Collins, F.S., Conneally, P.M., Frezal, J., Gershowitz, H., Goodfellow, P.N., Hall, J.G., Issitt, P., Jones, C.A., Knowles, B.B., Lewis, M., McKusick, V.A., Meisler, M., Morton, N.E., Rubinstein, P., Schanfield, M.S., Schmickel, R.D., Skolnick, M.H., Spence, M.A., Sutherland, G.R., Traver, M., Van Cong, N., and Willard, H.F., An international system for human gene nomenclature (ISGN, 1987), *Cytogenet. Cell Genet.*, 46, 11, 1987.
57. Varmus, H. and Bishop, J.M., Introduction, *Cancer Surv.*, 5, 153, 1986.
58. Duesberg, P.H., Transforming genes of retroviruses, *Cold Spring Harbor Symp. Quant. Biol.*, 44, 13, 1980.
59. Gallo, R.C. and Wong-Staal, F., Retroviruses as etiologic agents of some animal and human leukemias and lymphomas and as tools for elucidating the molecular mechanisms of leukemogenesis, *Blood*, 60, 545, 1982.
60. Robinson, H.L., Retroviruses and cancer, *Rev. Infect. Dis.*, 4, 1015, 1982.
61. Weinberg, R.A., Oncogenes of spontaneous and chemically induced tumors, *Adv. Cancer Res.*, 36, 149, 1982.
62. Cooper, G.M., Cellular transforming genes, *Science*, 217, 801, 1982.
63. Duesberg, P.H., Retroviral transforming genes in normal cells?, *Nature*, 304, 219, 1983.
64. Kurth, R., Oncogenes in retroviruses and cells, *Naturwissenschaften*, 70, 439, 1983.
65. Land, H., Parada, L.F., and Weinberg, R.A., Cellular oncogenes and multistep carcinogenesis, *Science*, 222, 771, 1983.
66. Hehlmann, R., Schetters, H., Kreeb, G., Erfle, V., Schmidt, J., and Luz, A., RNA-tumorviruses, oncogenes, and their possible role in human carcinogenesis, *Klin. Wochenschr.*, 61, 1217, 1983.
67. Levy, J.-P., Les oncogènes, *Nouv. Rev. Fr. Hematol.*, 26, 1 and 57, 1984.
68. Busch, H., Onc genes and other new targets for cancer chemotherapy, *J. Cancer Res. Clin. Oncol.*, 107, 1, 1984.
69. Bartram, C.R., Oncogenes: clues to carcinogenesis, *Eur. J. Pediat.*, 141, 134, 1984.
70. Willecke, K. and Schäfer, R., Human oncogenes, *Hum. Genet.*, 66, 132, 1984.
71. Cooper, G.M. and Lane, M.-A., Cellular transforming genes and oncogenesis, *Biochim. Biophys. Acta*, 738, 9, 1984.
72. Paul, J., Oncogenes, *J. Pathol.*, 143, 1, 1984.
73. Hall, A., Oncogenes — implications for human cancer, *J. R. Soc. Med. (London)*, 77, 410, 1984.
74. Cline, M.J., Slamon, D.J., and Lipsick, J.S., Oncogenes: implications for the diagnosis and treatment of cancer, *Ann. Int. Med.*, 101, 223, 1984.
75. Sinkovics, J.G., Retroviral and human cellular oncogenes, *Ann. Clin. Lab. Sci.*, 14, 343, 1984.
76. Hunter, T., Oncogenes and proto-oncogenes: how do they differ?, *J. Natl. Cancer Inst.*, 73, 773, 1984.
77. Varmus, H.E., The molecular genetics of cellular oncogenes, *Annu. Rev. Genet.*, 18, 553, 1984.
78. Marshall, C.J. and Rigby, P.W.J., Viral and cellular genes involved in oncogenesis, *Cancer Surv.*, 3, 183, 1984.
79. Pimentel, E., Oncogenes and human cancer, *Cancer Genet. Cytogenet.*, 14, 347, 1985.
80. Duesberg, P.H., Activated proto-onc genes: sufficient or necessary for cancer?, *Science*, 228, 669, 1985.
81. Gordon, H., Oncogenes, *Mayo Clin. Proc.*, 60, 697, 1985.
82. Ratner, L., Josephs, S.F., and Wong-Staal, F., Oncogenes: their role in neoplastic transformation, *Annu. Rev. Microbiol.*, 39, 419, 1985.
83. Garrett, C.T., Oncogenes, *Clin. Chim. Acta*, 156, 1, 1986.
84. Lacey, S.W., Oncogenes in retroviruses, malignancy, and normal tissues, *Am. J. Med. Sci.*, 291, 39, 1986.
85. Pimentel, E., Proto-oncogenes as human tumor markers, *J. Tumor Marker Oncol.*, 1, 27, 1986.
86. Barbacid, M., Oncogenes and human cancer: cause or consequence?, *Carcinogenesis*, 7, 1037, 1986.
87. Marshall, C.J., Oncogenes, *J. Cell Sci.*, Suppl. 4, 417, 1986.
88. Colb, M. and Krontiris, T.G., Oncogenes, *Adv. Int. Med.*, 31, 47, 1986.

89. Ascione, R., Sacchi, N., Watson, D.K., Fisher, R.J., Fujiwara, S., Seth, A., and Papas, T.S., Oncogenes: molecular probes for clinicla application in malignant diseases, *Gene Anal. Technol.,* 3, 25, 1986.

90. Pimentel, E., Update on proto-oncogenes and human cancer, in *Human Tumor Markers: Biology and Clinical Applications,* Cimino, F., Birkmayer, G.D., Klavins, J.V., Pimentel, E., and Salvatore, F., Eds., Walter de Gruyter, Berlin, 1987, 49.

91. Bishop, J.M., The molecular genetics of cancer, *Science,* 235, 305, 1987.

92. Duesberg, P.H., Cancer genes: rare recombinants instead of activated oncogenes, *Proc. Natl. Acad. Sci. U.S.A.,* 84, 2117, 1987.

93. Nishimura, S. and Tekiya, T., Human cancer and cellular oncogenes, *Biochem. J.,* 243, 313, 1987.

94. Der, C.J., Cellular oncogenes and human carcinogenesis, *Clin. Chem.,* 33, 641, 1987.

95. Willman, C.L. and Fenoglio-Preiser, C.M., Oncogenes, suppressor genes, and carcinogenesis, *Hum. Pathol.,* 18, 895, 1987.

96. Marks, F., What's new in oncogenes and growth factors?, *Pathol. Res. Pract.,* 182, 831, 1987.

97. Temin, H.M., Evolution of cancer genes as a mutation-driven process, *Cancer Res.,* 48, 1697, 1988.

98. Rowley, J.D., Identification of the constant chromosome regions involved in human hematologic malignant disease, *Science,* 216, 749, 1982.

99. Klein, G., Specific chromosomal translocations and the genesis of B-cell-derived tumors in mice and men, *Cell,* 32, 311, 1983.

100. Yunis, J.J., The chromosomal basis of human neoplasia, *Science,* 221, 227, 1983.

101. Chaganti, R.S.K., Significance of chromosome change to hematopoietic neoplasms, *Blood,* 62, 515, 1983.

102. Gilbert, F., Chromosomes, genes, and cancer: a classification of chromosome abnormalities in cancer, *J. Natl. Cancer Inst.,* 71, 1107, 1983.

103. Le Beau, M.M. and Rowley, J.D., Recurring chromosomal abnormalities in leukaemia and lymphoma, *Cancer Surv.,* 3, 371, 1984.

104. Dewald, G.W., Noel, P., Dahl, R.J., and Supurbeck, J.L., Chromosome abnormalities in malignant hematologic disorders, *Mayo Clin. Proc.,* 60, 675, 1985.

105. Popescu, N.C. and DiPaolo, J.A., Relationship of chromosomal alterations to gene expression in carcinogenesis, *Carcinogenesis,* 10, 419, 1985.

106. Le Beau, M.M. and Rowley, J.D., Chromosomal abnormalities in leukemia and lymphoma: clinical and biological significance, *Adv. Hum. Genet.,* 15, 1, 1986.

107. Bloomfield, C.D., Trent, J.M., and van den Berghe, H., Report of the committee on structural chromosome changes in neoplasia, *Cytogenet. Cell Genet.,* 46, 344, 1987.

108. Sandberg, A.A., A chromosomal hypothesis of oncogenesis, *Cancer Genet. Cytogenet.,* 8, 277, 1983.

109. Rowley, J.D., Biological implications of consistent chromosome rearrangements in leukemia and lymphoma, *Cancer Res.,* 44, 3159, 1984.

110. Klein, G., Constitutive activation of oncogenes by chromosomal translocations in B-cell derived tumors, *AIDS Res.,* 2 (Suppl. 1), 1, 1986.

111. Croce, C.M., Chromosome translocations and human cancer, *Cancer Res.,* 46, 6019, 1986.

112. Chevenix-Trench, G., The molecular genetics of human non-Hodgkin's lymphoa, *Cancer Genet. Cytogenet.,* 27, 191, 1987.

113. De Klein, A., Oncogene activation by chromosomal rearrangement in chronic myelocytic leukemia, *Mutat. Res.,* 186, 161, 1987.

114. Rosson, D. and Reddy, E.P., Activation of the *abl* oncogene and its involvement in chromosomal translocations in human leukemia, *Mutat. Res.,* 195, 231, 1988.

115. Harper, M.E. and Saunders, G.F., Localization of single copy DNA sequences on G-banded human chromosomes by *in situ* hybridization, *Chromosoma (Berlin),* 83, 431, 1981.

116. Popescu, N.C., Amsbaugh, S.C., Swan, D.C., and DiPaolo, J.A., Induction of chromosome banding by trypsin/ EDTA for gene mapping by in situ hybridization, *Cytogenet. Cell Genet.,* 39, 73, 1985.

117. Tereba, A., Chromosomal localization of protooncogenes, *Int. Rev. Cytol.,* 95, 1, 1985.

118. McAlpine, P.J., Van Cong, N., Boucheix, C., Pakstis, A.J., Doute, R.C., and Shows, T.B., The 1987 catalog of mapped genes and report of the nomenclature committee, *Cytogenet. Cell Genet.,* 46, 29, 1987.

119. Rabin, M., Watson, M., Barker, P.E., Ryan, J., Breg, W.R., and Ruddle, F.H., N-*ras* transforming gene maps to region p11-p13 on chromosome 1 by in situ hybridization, *Cytogenet. Cell Genet.,* 38, 70, 1984.

120. Popescu, N.C., Amsbaugh, S.C., DiPaolo, J.A., Tronick, S.R., Aaronson, S.A., and Swan, D.C., Chromosomal localization of three human *ras* genes by *in situ* molecular hybridization, *Somat. Cell Mol. Genet.,* 11, 149, 1985.

121. Haluska, F.G., Huebner, K., Isobe, M., Nishimura, T., Croce, C.M., and Vogt, P.K., Localization of the human *JUN* protooncogene to chromosome region 1p31-32, *Proc. Natl. Acad. Sci. U.S.A.,* 85, 2215, 1988.

122. McBride, O.W., Kirsch, I., Hollis, G., Nau, M., Battey, J., and Minna, J., Human L-*myc* (*MYCL*) proto-oncogene is on chromosome 1p32, *Cytogenet. Cell Genet.,* 40, 694, 1985.

123. Morton, C.C., Taub, R., Diamond, A., Lane, M.A., Cooper, G.M., and Leder, P., Mapping of the human *Blym*-1 transforming gene activated in Burkitt lymphomas to chromosome 1, *Science,* 223, 173, 1984.

124. Marth, J.D., Disteche, C., Pravtcheva, D., Ruddle, F., Krebs, E.G., and Perlmutter, R.M., Localization of a lymphocyte-specific protein tyrosine kinase gene (*lck*) at a site of frequent chromosomal abnormalities in human lymphomas, *Proc. Natl. Acad. Sci. U.S.A.,* 83, 7400, 1986.

125. Tronick, S.R., Popescu, N.C., Cheah, M.S.C., Swan, D.C., Amsbaugh, S.C., Lengel, C.R., DiPaolo, J.A., and Robbins, K.C., Isolation and chromosomal localization of the human *fgr* proto-oncogene, a distinct member of the tyrosine kinase gene family, *Proc. Natl. Acad. Sci. U.S.A.,* 82, 6595, 1985.

126. Chaganti, R.S.K., Balazs, I., Jhanwar, S.C., Murty, V.V.V.S., Koduru, P.R.K., Grzeschik, K.-H., and Stavnezer, E., The cellular homologue of the transforming gene of SKV avian retrovirus maps to human chromosome region 1q22-q24, *Cytogenet. Cell Genet.,* 43, 181, 1986.

127. Kruh, G.D., King, C.R., Kraus, M.H., Popescu, N.E., Amsbaugh, S.C., McBride, W.O., and Aaronson, S.A., A novel human gene closely related to the *abl* proto-oncogene, *Science,* 234, 1545, 1986.

128. Brownell, E., Fell, H.P., Tucker, P.W., Geurts van Kessel, A.H.M., Hagemeijer, A., and Rice, N.R., Regional localization of the human c-*rel* locus using translocation chromosome analysis, *Oncogene,* 2, 527, 1988.

129. Schwab, M., Varmus, H.E., Bishop, J.M., Grzeschik, K.H., Naylor, S.L., Sakaguchi, A.Y., Brodeur, G., and Trent, J., Chromosome localization in normal cells and neuroblastomas of a gene related to c-*myc*, *Nature,* 308, 288, 1984.

130. Rider, S.H., Gorman, P.A., Shipley, J.M., Moore, G., Vennstrom, B., Solomon, E., and Sheer, D., Localization of the oncogene c-*erb*A2 to human chromosome 3, *Ann. Hum. Genet.,* 51, 153, 1987.

131. Bonner, T., O'Brien, S.J., Nash, W.G., Rapp, U.R., Morton, C.C., and Leder, P., The human homologous of *raf* (*mil*) oncogene are located on human chromosomes 3 and 4, *Science,* 223, 71, 1984.

132. d'Auriol, L., Mattei, M.-G., Andre, C., and Galibert, F., Localization of the human c-*kit* protooncogene on the q11-q12 region of chromosome 4, *Hum. Genet.,* 78, 374, 1988.

133. Groffen, J., Heisterkamp, N., Spurr, N., Dana, S., Wasmuth, J.J., and Stephenson, J.R., Chromosomal localization of the human c-*fms* oncogene, *Nucleic Acids Res.,* 11, 6331, 1983.

134. Nagarajan, L., Louie, E., Tsujimoto, Y., ar-Rushdi, A., Huebner, K., and Croce, C.M., Localization of the human *pim* oncogene (*PIM*) to a region of chromosome 6 involved in translocations in acute leukemias, *Proc. Natl. Acad. Sci. U.S.A.,* 83, 2556, 1986.

135. Popescu, N.C., Kawakami, T., Matsui, T., and Robbins, K.C., Chromosomal localization of the human *fyn* gene, *Oncogene,* 1, 449, 1987.

136. Satoh, H., Yoshida, M.C., Matsushime, H., Shibuya, M., and Sasaki, M., Regional localization of the human c-*ros*-1 on 6q22 and *flt* on 13q12, *Jpn. J. Cancer Res.,* 78, 772, 1987.

137. Janssen, J.W.G., Vernole, P., de Boer, P.A.J., Oosterhuis, J.W., and Collard, J.G., Sublocalization of c-*myb* to 6q21-q23 by *in situ* hybridization and c-*myb* expression in a human teratocarcinoma with 6q rearrangements, *Cytogenet. Cell Genet.,* 41, 129, 1986.

138. Huebner, K., ar-Rushdi, A., Griffin, C.A., Isobe, M., Kozak, C., Emanuel, B.S., Nagarajan, L., Cleveland, J.L., Bonner, T.I., Goldsborough, M.D., Croce, C.M., and Rapp, U., Actively transcribed genes in the *raf* oncogene group, located on the X chromosome in mouse and human, *Proc. Natl. Acad. Sci. U.S.A.,* 83, 3934, 1986.

139. Shimizu, N., Hunts, J., Merlino, G., Wang-Peng, J., Xu, Y.-H., Yamamoto, T., Toyoshima, K., and Pastan, I., Regional mapping of the EGF receptor (EGFR)/c-*erb*B protooncogene, *Cytogenet. Cell Genet.,* 40, 743, 1985.

140. Rousseau-Merck, M.-F., Bernheim, A., Chardin, P., Miglierina, R., Tavitian, A., and Berger, R., The *ras*-related *ral* gene maps to chromosome 7p15-22, *Hum. Genet.,* 79, 132, 1988.

141. Dean, M., Park, M., Le Beau, M.M., Robins, T.S., Diaz, M.O., Rowley, J.D., Blair, D.G., and Vande Woude, G.F., The human *met* oncogene is related to the tyrosine kinase oncogenes, *Nature,* 318, 385, 1985.

142. Neel, B.G., Jhanwar, S.C., Chaganti, R.S.K., and Hayward, W.S., Two human c-*onc* genes are located on the long arm of chromosome 8, *Proc. Natl. Acad. Sci. U.S.A.,* 79, 7842, 1982.

143. Caubet, J.-F., Mathieu-Mahul, D., Bernheim, A., Larsen, C.-J., and Berger, R., Human proto-oncogene c-*mos* maps to 8q11, *EMBO J.,* 4, 2245, 1985.

144. Jhanwar, S.C., Neel, B.G., Hayward, W.S., and Chaganti, R.S.K., Localization of the cellular oncogenes ABL, SIS, and FES on human germ line chromosomes, *Cytogenet. Cell Genet.,* 38, 73, 1984.

145. Jhanwar, S.C., Neel, B.G., Hayward, W.S., and Chaganti, R.S.K., Localization of c-*ras* oncogene family on human germ-line chromosomes, *Proc. Natl. Acad. Sci. U.S.A.,* 80, 4794, 1983.

146. Casey, G., Smith, R., McGillivray, D., Peters, G., and Dickson, C., Characterization and chromosome assignment of the human homolog of *int*-2, a potential proto-oncogene, *Mol. Cell. Biol.,* 6, 502, 1986.

147. Adelaide, J., Mattei, M.-G., Marics, I., Raybaud, F., Planche, J., De Lapeyriere, O., and Birnbaum, D., Chromosomal localization of the *hst* oncogene and its co-amplification with the *int*.2 oncogene in a human melanoma, *Oncogene,* 2, 413, 1988.

148. Tsujimoto, Y., Yunis, J., Onorato-Showe, L., Erikson, J., Nowell, P.C., and Croce, C.M., Molecular cloning of the chromosomal breakpoint of B-cell lymphomas and leukemias with the t(11;14) chromosome translocation, *Science,* 224, 1403, 1984.

149. de Taisne, C., Gegonne, A., Stehelin, D., Bernheim, A., and Berger, R., Chromosomal localization of the human proto-oncogene c-*ets*, *Nature,* 310, 581, 1984.

150. Arheden, K., Mandahl, N., Strömbeck, B., Isaksson, M., and Mitelman, F., Chromosome localization of the human oncogene INT1 to 12q13 by *in situ* hybridization, *Cytogenet. Cell Genet.*, 47, 86, 1988.

151. Ekstrand, A.J. and Zech, L., Human c-*fos* proto-oncogene mapped to chromosome 14, band q24.3-q31. Possibilities for oncogene activation by chromosomal rearrangements in human neoplasms, *Exp. Cell Res.*, 169, 262, 1987.

152. Isobe, M., Emanuel, B.S., Givol, D., Oren, M., Croce, C.M., Localization of gene for human p53 tumour antigen to band 17p13, *Nature*, 320, 84, 1986.

153. Mitelman, F., Manolov, G., Manolova, Y., Billström, R., Heim, S., Kristoffersson, U., Mandahl, N., Ferro, M.T., and San Roman, C., High resolution chromosoma analysis of constitutional and acquired t(15:17) maps c-*erb*A to subband 17q11.2, *Cancer Genet. Cytogenet.*, 22, 95, 1986.

154. Schechter, A.L., Hung, M.-C., Vaidyanathan, L., Weinberg, R.A., Yang-Feng, T.L., Francke, U., Ullrich, A., and Coussens, L., The *neu* gene: an *erb*B-homologous gene distinct from and unlinked to the gene encoding the EGF receptor, *Science*, 229, 976, 1985.

155. Tsujimoto, Y., Finger, L.R., Yunis, J., Nowell, P.C., and Croce, C.M., Cloning of the chromosome breakpoint of neoplastic B cells with the t(14;18) chromosome translocation, *Science*, 226, 1097, 1984.

156. Yoshida, M.C., Sasaki, M., Mise, K., Semba, K., Nishizawa, M., Yamamoto, T., and Toyoshima, K., Regional mapping of the human proto-oncogene c-*yes*-1 to chromosome 18 at band q21.3, *Jpn. J. Cancer Res.*, 76, 559, 1985.

157. Spurr, N.K., Hughes, D., Goodfellow, P.N., Brook, J.D., and Padua, R.A., Chromosomal assignment of c-*MEL*, a human transforming oncogene, to chromosome 19 (p13.2-q13.2), *Somat. Cell Mol. Genet.*, 12, 637, 1986.

158. Quintrell, N., Lebo, R., Varmus, H., Bishop, J.M., Pettenati, M.J., Le Beau, M.M., Diaz, M.O., and Rowley, J.D., Identification of a human gene (*HCK*) that encodes a protein-tyrosine kinase and is expressed in hemopoietic cells, *Mol. Cell. Biol.*, 7, 2267, 1987.

159. Parker, R.C., Mardon, G., Lebo, R.V., Varmus, H.E., and Bishop, J.M., Isolation of duplicated human c-*src* genes located on chromosomes 1 and 20, *Mol. Cell. Biol.*, 5, 831, 1985.

160. Watson, D.K., Sacchi, N., McWilliams-Smith, M.J., O'Brien, S.J., and Papas, T.S., The avian and mammalian *ets* genes: molecular characterization, chromosome mapping, and implication in human leukemia, *Anticancer Res.*, 6, 631, 1986.

161. Noguchi, T., Mattei, M.-G., Oberlè, I., Planche, J., Imbert, J., Pelassy, C., Birg, F., and Birnbaum, D., Localization of the *mcf*.2 transforming sequence to X chromosome, *EMBO J.*, 6, 1301, 1987.

162. Sakaguchi, A.Y., Lalley, P.A., Zabel, B.U., Ellis, R.W., Scolnick, E.M., and Naylor, S.L., Chromosome assignments of four mouse cellular homologs of sarcoma and leukemia virus oncogenes, *Proc. Natl. Acad. Sci. U.S.A.*, 81, 525, 1984.

163. Blatt, C., Harper, M.E., Franchini, G., Nesbitt, M.N., and Simon, M.I., Chromosomal mapping of murine c-*fes* and c-*src* genes, *Mol. Cell. Biol.*, 4, 978, 1984.

164. Kozak, C., Gunnell, M.A., and Rapp, U.R., A new oncogene, c-*raf*, is located on mouse chromosome 6, *J. Virol.*, 49, 297, 1984.

165. Cahilly, L.A. and George, D.L., Regional mapping of cKi-*ras* proto-oncogene on mouse chromosome 6 by *in situ* hybridization, *Cytogenet. Cell Genet.*, 39, 140, 1985.

166. Martin-DeLeon, P.A. and Picciano, S.R., *In situ* localization of murine c-*Ki-ras-2* oncogene: preliminary evidence for conservation of telomeric territory of oncogenes?, *Somat. Cell Mol. Genet.*, 14, 205, 1988.

167. Kozak, C.A., Sears, J.F., and Hoggan, M.D., Genetic mapping of the mouse oncogenes c-Ha-*ras*-1 and c-*fes* to chromosome 7, *J. Virol.*, 47, 217, 1983.

168. Kozak, C.A., Sears, J.F., and Hoggan, M.D., Genetic mapping of the mouse proto-oncogene c-*sis* to chromosome 15, *Science*, 221, 867, 1983.

169. Erikson, J., Miller, D.A., Miller, O.J., Abcarian, P.W., Skurla, R.M., Mushinski, J.F., and Croce, C.M., The c-*myc* oncogene is translocated to the involved chromosome 12 in mouse plasmacytoma, *Proc. Natl. Acad. Sci. U.S.A.*, 82, 4212, 1985.

170. Huppi, K., Duncan, R., and Potter, M., *Myc-1* is centromeric to the linkage group *Ly-6—Sis—Gdc-1* on mouse chromosome 15, *Immunogenetics*, 27, 215, 1988.

171. Watson, D.K., McWilliams-Smith, M.J., Kozak, C., Reeves, R., Gearhart, J., Nunn, M.F., Nash, W., Fowle, J.R., III, Duesberg, P., Papas, T.S., and O'Brien, S.J., Conserved chromosomal positions of dual domains of the *ets* protooncogene in cats, mice, and humans, *Proc. Natl. Acad. Sci. U.S.A.*, 83, 1792, 1986.

172. Brownell, E., Kozak, C.A., Fowle, J.R., III, Modi, W.S., Rice, N.R., and O'Brien, S.J., Comparative genetic mapping of cellular *rel* sequences in man, mouse, and the domestic cat, *Am. J. Hum. Genet.*, 39, 194, 1986.

173. Searle, A.G., Peters, J., Lyon, M.F., Evans, E.P., Edwards, J.H., and Buckle, V.J., Chromosome maps of mouse and man. III, *Genomics*, 1, 3, 1987.

174. Hilkens, J., Cuypers, H.T., Selten, G., Kroezen, V., Hilgers, J., and Berns, A., Genetic mapping of *Pim-1* putative oncogene to mouse chromosome 17, *Somat. Cell Mol. Genet.*, 12, 81, 1986.

175. Nadeau, J.H. and Phillips, S.J., The putative oncogene *Pim-1* in the mouse: its linkage and variation among *t* haplotypes, *Genetics*, 117, 533, 1987.

176. Zabel, B.U., Fournier, R.E.K., Lalley, P.A., Naylor, S.A., and Sakaguchi, A.Y., Cellular homologs of the avian erythroblastosis virus *erb*-A and *erb*-B genes are syntenic in mouse but asyntenic in man, *Proc. Natl. Acad. Sci. U.S.A.,* 81, 4874, 1984.

177. Silver, J., Whitney, J.B., III, Kozak, C., Hollis, G., and Kirsch, I., *Erbb* is linked to the alpha-globin locus on mouse chromosome 11, *Mol. Cell. Biol.,* 5, 1784, 1985.

178. Ma, N.S.F., Owl monkey gene loci for c-fes and albumin are syntenic, *Cytogenet. Cell Genet.,* 43, 211, 1986.

179. Stallings, R.L., Crawford, B.D., Black, R.J., and Chang, E.H., Assignment of *RAS* proto-oncogenes in Chinese hamsters: implications for mammalian gene linkage conservation and neoplasia, *Cytogenet. Cell Genet.,* 43, 2, 1986.

180. Ingvarsson, S., Asker, C., Wirschubsky, Z., Szpirer, J., Levan, G., Klein, G., and Sümegi, J., Mapping of *Lmyc* and *Nmyc* to rat chromosomes r and 6, *Somat. Cell Mol. Genet.,* 13, 335, 1987.

181. Szpirer, J., DeFeo-Jones, D., Ellis, R.W., Levan, G., and Szpirer, C., Assignment of three rat cellular RAS oncogenes to chromosomes 1, 4 and X, *Somat. Cell. Mol. Genet.,* 11, 93, 1985.

182. Chen, H-L., Maeda, S., Takahashi, R., and Sugiyama, T., Chromosome marker and enhanced expression of c-Ha-*ras* in a DMBA-induced erythroleukemia cell line (D5A1), *Cancer Genet. Cytogenet.,* 28, 301, 1987.

183. Hameister, H. and Adolph, S., Oncogenes and the mammalian X chromosome, *Hum. Genet.,* 72, 241, 1986.

184. Uzvölgyi, E., Kiss, I., Pitt, A., Arsenian, S., Ingvarssson, S., Udvardy, M., Hamada, M., Klein, G., and Sümegi, J., *Drosophila* homolog of the murine *Int-1* protooncogene, *Proc. Natl. Acad. Sci. U.S.A.,* 85, 3034, 1988.

185. Hill, M. and Hillova, J., Production virale dans les fibroblastes de poule traités par l'acide desoxyribonucleique de cellules XC de rat transformées par le virus de Rous, *C.R. Acad. Sci. Paris,* D272, 3094, 1971.

186. Hillova, J., Goubin, G., and Hill, M., Transfection des fibroblastes de poule par l'acide desoxyribonucleique denaturé de cellules transformées de Rous, *C.R. Acad. Sci. Paris,* D274, 1070, 1972.

187. Hill, M. and Hillova, J., Virus recovery in chicken cells tested with Rous sarcoma cell DNA, *Nature New Biol.,* 237, 35, 1972.

188. Desai, L.S., Wulff, U.C., Cohen, J.L., and Foley, G.E., Human leukemic cells: biological action of exogenous human leukemic DNA, *Biochimie,* 55, 1461, 1973.

189. Graham, F.L. and van der Eb, A.J., A new technique for the assay of infectivity of human adenovirus 5 DNA, *Virology,* 52, 456, 1973.

190. Wigler, M., Silverstein, S., Lee, L.-S., Pellicer, A., Cheng, Y.-C., and Axel, R., Transfer of purified herpes virus thymidine kinase gene to cultured mouse cells, *Cell,* 11, 223, 1977.

191. Perucho, M., Hanahan, D., and Wigler, M., Genetic and physical linkage of exogenous sequences in transformed cells, *Cell,* 22, 309, 1980.

192. Shih, C., Shilo, B.Z., Goldfarb, M.P., Dannenberg, A., and Weinberg, R.A., Passage of phenotypes of chemically transformed cells via transfection of DNA and chromatin, *Proc. Natl. Acad. Sci. U.S.A.,* 76, 5714, 1979.

193. Cooper, G.M., Okenquist, S., and Silverman, L., Transforming activity of DNA of chemically transformed and normal cells, *Nature,* 284, 418, 1980.

194. Cooper, G.M. and Neiman, P.E., Transforming genes of neoplasms induced by avian lymphoid leukosis viruses, *Nature,* 287, 656, 1980.

195. Krontiris, T.G. and Cooper, G.M., Transforming activity of human tumor DNAs, *Proc. Natl. Acad. Sci. U.S.A.,* 78, 1181, 1981.

196. Shih, C., Padhy, L.C., Murray, M., and Weinberg, R.A., Transforming genes of carcinomas and neuroblastomas introduced into mouse fibroblasts, *Nature,* 290, 261, 1981.

197. Perucho, M., Goldfarb, M., Shimizu, K., Lama, C., Fogh, J., and Wigler, M., Human-tumor-derived cell lines contain common and different transforming genes, *Cell,* 27, 467, 1981.

198. Zhan, X., Culpepper, A., Reddy, M., Loveless, J., and Goldfarb, M., Human oncogenes detected by a defined medium culture assay, *Oncogene,* 1, 369, 1987.

199. Schäfer, R., Griegel, S., Dubbert, M.-A., and Willecke, K., Unstable transformation of mouse 3T3 cells by transfection with DNA from normal human lymphocytes, *EMBO J.,* 3, 659, 1984.

200. Brady, G., Funk, A., Mattern, J., Schütz, G., and Brown, R., Use of gene transfer and a novel cosmid rescue strategy to isolate transforming sequences, *EMBO J.,* 4, 2583, 1985.

201. Thorgeirsson, U.P., Turpeenniemi-Hujanen, T., Williams, J.E., Westin, E.H., Heilman, C.A., Talmadge, J.E., and Liotta, L.A., NIH/3T3 cells transfected with human tumor DNA containing activated *ras* oncogenes express the metastatic phenotype in nude mice, *Mol. Cell. Biol.,* 5, 259, 1985.

202. Bondy, G.P., Wilson, S., and Chambers, A.F., Experimental metastatic ability of H-*ras*-transformed NIH3T3 cells, *Cancer Res.,* 45, 6005, 1985.

203. Varani, J., Fligiel, S.E.G., and Wilson, B., Motility of ras^H oncogene transformed NIH-3T3 cells, *Invasion Metast.,* 6, 335, 1986.

204. Bradley, M.O., Kraynak, A.R., Storer, R.D., and Gibbs, J.B., Experimental metastasis in nude mice of NIH 3T3 cells containing various *ras* genes, *Proc. Natl. Acad. Sci. U.S.A.,* 83, 5277, 1986.

205. Jelinek, W.R., Toomey, T.P., Leinwand, L., Duncan, C.H., Biro, P.A., Choudary, P.V., Weisman, S.M., Rubin, C.M., Houck, C.M., Deininger, P.L., and Schmid, C.W., Ubiquituous, intersepersed repeated sequences in mammalian genomes, *Proc. Natl. Acad. Sci. U.S.A.,* 77, 1398, 1980.

206. Schmid, C.W. and Jelinek, W.R., The *alu* family of disperse repetitive sequences, *Science,* 216, 1065, 1982.

207. Szybalski, W., Szybalska, E.H., and Ragni, G., Genetic studies with human cell lines, *Natl. Cancer Inst. Monogr.,* 7, 75, 1962.

208. Lemoine, N.R., Wynford-Thomas, V., and Wynford-Thomas, D., Optimisation of conditions for detection of activated oncogenes by transfection of NIH 3T3 cells, *Br. J. Cancer,* 55, 639, 1987.

209. Wake, C.T., Gudewicz, T., Porter, T., White, A., and Wilson, J.H., How damaged is the biologically active subpopulation of transfected DNA?, *Mol. Cell. Biol.,* 4, 387, 1984.

210. Blair, D.G., Oskarsson, M., Wood, T.G., McClements, W.L., Fischinger, P.J., and Vande Woude, G.G., Activation of the transforming potential of a normal cell sequence: a molecular model for oncogenesis, *Science,* 212, 941, 1981.

211. Santos, E., Reddy, E.P., Pulciani, S., Feldmann, R.J., and Barbacid, M., Spontaneous activation of a human proto-oncogene, *Proc. Natl. Acad. Sci. U.S.A.,* 80, 4679, 1983.

212. Schäfer, R., Griegel, S., Schwarte, I., Geisse, S., Traub, O., and Willecke, K., Transforming activity of DNA fragments from normal human lymphocytes results from spontaneous activation of a c-Ha-*ras1* gene, *Mol. Cell. Biol.,* 5, 3617, 1985.

213. Birchmeier, C., Birnbaum, D., Waitches, G., Fasano, O., and Wigler, M., Characterization of an activated human *ros* gene, *Mol. Cell. Biol.,* 6, 3109, 1986.

214. Ishikawa, F., Takaku, F., Nagao, M., and Sugimura, T., Rat c-*raf* oncogene activation by a rearrangement that produces a fused protein, *Mol. Cell. Biol.,* 7, 1226, 1987.

215. Tahira, T., Ochiai, M., Hayashi, K., Nagao, M., and Sugimura, T., Activation of human c-*raf*-1 by replacing the N-terminal region with different sequences, *Nucleic Acids Res.,* 15, 4809, 1987.

216. Calos, M.P., Lebkowski, J.S., and Botchan, M.R., High mutation frequency in DNA transfected into mammalian cells, *Proc. Natl. Acad. Sci. U.S.A.,* 80, 3015, 1983.

217. Lebkowski, J.S., DuBridge, R.B., Antell, E.A., Greisen, K.S., and Calos, M.P., Transfected DNA is mutated in monkey, mouse, and human cells, *Mol. Cell. Biol.,* 4, 1951, 1984.

218. Nowell, P.C., Tumor progression and clonal evolution: the role of genetic instability, in *Chromosome Mutation and Neoplasia,* German, G., Ed., Alan R. Liss, New York, 1983, 413.

219. Verrelle, P., Lascaut, V., Poupon, M.-F., and Hillova, J., DNA transfection affects the metastatic capacity of tumour cells, *Anticancer Res.,* 7, 181, 1987.

220. Copeland, N.G., Jenkins, N.A., and Cooper, G.M., Integration of Rous sarcoma virus DNA during transfection, *Cell,* 23, 51, 1981.

221. Roth, D.B. and Wilson, J.H., Relative rates of homologous and nonhomologous recombination in transfected DNA, *Proc. Natl. Acad. Sci. U.S.A.,* 82, 3355, 1985.

222. Robins, D.M., Ripley, S., Henderson, A.S., and Axel, R., Transforming DNA integrates into the host chromosome, *Cell,* 23, 29, 1981.

223. Krump-Konvalinkova, V. and Angenent, G.C., Fate of biological activity of exogenous DNA sequences during serial transfections in NIH/3T3 cells, *Biochem. Biophys. Res. Commun.,* 132, 635, 1985.

224. Look, A.T., Peiper, S.C., Douglass, E.C., Trent, J.M., and Sherr, C.J., Amplification of genes encoding human myeloid membrane antigens after DNA-mediated gene transfer, *Blood,* 67, 637, 1986.

225. Müller, R. and Müller, D., Co-transfection of normal NIH/3T3 DNA and retroviral LTR sequences: a novel strategy for the detection of potential c-*onc* genes, *EMBO J.,* 3, 1121, 1984.

226. Garte, S.J., Currie, D.D., and Troll, W., Inhibition of H-*ras* oncogene transformation of NIH3T3 cells by protease inhibitors, *Cancer Res.,* 47, 3159, 1987.

227. Kato, S., Anderson, R.A., and Camerini-Otero, R.D., Foreign DNA introduced by calcium phosphate is integrated into repetitive DNA elements of the mouse L cell genome, *Mol. Cell. Biol.,* 6, 1787, 1986.

228. Strain, A.J., Inhibitors of ADP-ribosyl transferase enhance the transformation of NIH3T3 cells following transfection with SV40 DNA, *Exp. Cell Res.,* 159, 531, 1985.

229. Dotto, G.P., Parada, L.F., and Weinberg, R.A., Specific growth response of *ras*-transformed embryo fibroblasts to tumour promoters, *Nature,* 318, 472, 1985.

230. Thomas, K.R. and Capecchi, M.R., Introduction of homologous DNA sequences into mammalian cells induces mutations in the cognate gene, *Nature,* 324, 34, 1986.

231. Glanville, N., Unstable expression and amplification of a transfected oncogene in confluent and subconfluent cells, *Mol. Cell. Biol.,* 5, 1456, 1985.

232. Wiberg, F.C., Sunnerhagen, P., and Bjursell, G., New, small circular DNA in transfected mammalian cells, *Mol. Cell. Biol.,* 6, 653, 1986.

233. Buitenwerf, J., De Jong, W., Van Strien, A., and Van der Nordaa, J., Characterization of SV40-transformed human liver cells before and after passage through crisis, *Intervirology,* 17, 222, 1982.

234. Kopelovich, L., Are all normal diploid human cell strains alike? — relevance to carcinogenic mechanisms *in vitro, Exp. Cell Biol.,* 50, 266, 1982.

235. Daya-Grosjean, L., Azzarone, B., Maunoury, R., Zaech, P., Elia, G., Zaniratti, S., and Benedetto, A., SV40 immortalization of adult human mesenchymal cells from neuroretina: biological, functional and molecular characterization, *Int. J. Cancer,* 33, 319, 1984.

236. Embleton, M.J., Stibbe, A., and Butler, P.C., Transformation of NIH-3T3 fibroblasts by transfection with DNA from transplanted but not primary rat hepatomas, *Med. Sci. Res.,* 15, 1347, 1987.

237. Newbold, R.F. and Overell, R.W., Fibroblast immortality is a prerequisite for transformation by EJ c-Ha-*ras* oncogene, *Nature,* 304, 648, 1983.

238. Pereira-Smith, O.M. and Smith, J.R., Evidence for the recessive nature of cellular immortality, *Science,* 221, 964, 1983.

239. Gilden, R.V. and Rice, N.R., Oncogenes, *Carcinogenesis,* 4, 791, 1983.

240. Boone, C.W., Malignant hemangioendotheliomas produced by subcutaneous inoculation of Balb/3T3 cells attached to glass beads, *Science,* 188, 68, 1975.

241. Katz, E. and Carter, B.J., A mutant cell line derived from NIH/3T3 cells: two oncogenes required for *in vitro* transformation, *J. Natl. Cancer Inst.,* 77, 909, 1986.

242. Greig, R.G., Koestler, T.P., Trainer, D.L., Corwin, S.P., Miles, L., Kline, T., Sweet, R., Yokoyama, S., and Poste, G., Tumorigenic and metastatic properties of "normal" and *ras*-transfected NIH/3T3 cells, *Proc. Natl. Acad. Sci. U.S.A.,* 82, 3698, 1985.

243. Becker, D., Lane, M.-A., and Cooper, G.M., Transformation of NIH 3T3 cells by DNA of the MCF-7 mammary carcinoma cell line induces expression of an endogenous murine leukemia provirus, *Mol. Cell. Biol.,* 4, 2247, 1984.

244. Flatow, U., Willingham, M.C., and Rabson, A.S., Butyrate prevents Harvey sarcoma virus focus formation but permits oncogene expression, *Cancer Lett.,* 22, 203, 1984.

245. Dubois, M.-F., Vignal, M., Le Cunff, M., and Chany, C., Interferon inhibits transformation of mouse cells by exogenous cellular or viral genes, *Nature,* 303, 433, 1983.

246. Samid, D., Chang, E.H., and Friedman, R.M., Development of transformed phenotype induced by a human *ras* oncogene is inhibited by interferon, *Biochem. Biophys. Res. Commun.,* 126, 509, 1985.

247. Samid, D., Chang, E.H., and Friedman, R.M., Biochemical correlates of phenotypic reversion in interferon-treated mouse cells transformed by a human oncogene, *Biochem. Biophys. Res. Commun.,* 119, 21, 1984.

248. Perucho, M. and Esteban, M., Inhibitory effect of interferon on the genetic and oncogenic transformation by viral and cellular genes, *J. Virol.,* 54, 229, 1985.

249. Samid, D., Flessate, D.M., and Friedman, R.M., Interferon-induced revertants of *ras*-transformed cells: resistance to transformation by specific oncogenes and retransformation by 5-azacytidine, *Mol. Cell. Biol.,* 7, 2196, 1987.

250. Brouty-Boyé, D., Wybier-Franqui, J., Nardeux, P., Daya-Grosjean, L., Andeol, Y., and Suarez, H.G., Interferon-induced phenotypic changes in human tumor cells relative to the effects of interferon on c-*ras* oncogene expression, *J. Interferon Res.,* 6, 461, 1986.

251. Pitot, H.C., Contributions to our understanding of the natural history of neoplastic development in lower animals to the cause and control of human cancer, *Cancer Surv.,* 2, 519, 1983.

252. Kerbel, R.S., Waghorne, C., Man, M.S., Elliott, B., and Breitman, M.L., Alteration of the tumorigenic and metastatic properties of neoplastic cells is associated with the process of calcium phosphate-mediated DNA transfection, *Proc. Natl. Acad. Sci. U.S.A.,* 84, 1263, 1987.

253. Muschel, R.J., Williams, J.E., Lowy, D.R., and Liotta, L.A., Harvey *ras* induction of metastatic potential depends upon oncogene activation and the type of recipient cell, *Am. J. Pathol.,* 121, 1, 1985.

254. Franza, B.R., Jr., Maruyama, K., Garrels, J.I., and Ruley, H.E., *In vitro* establishment is not a sufficient prerequisite for transformation by activated ras oncogenes, *Cell,* 44, 409, 1986.

255. Persons, D.A., Wilkison, W.O., Bell, R.M., and Finn, O.J., Altered growth regulation and enhanced tumorigenicity of NIH 3T3 fibroblasts transfected with protein kinase C-I cDNA, *Cell,* 52, 447, 1988.

256. Tveit, K.M., Pettersen, E.O., Fossa, S.D., and Pihl, A., Selection of tumour cell subpopulations occurs during cultivation of human tumours in soft agar. A DNA flow cytometric study, *Br. J. Cancer,* 52, 701, 1985.

257. Hwang, L.-H.S. and Gilboa, E., Expression of genes introduced into cells by retroviral infection is more efficient than that of genes introduced into cells by DNA transfection, *J. Virol.,* 50, 417, 1984.

258. Sparrow, S., Jones, M., Billington, S., and Stace, B., The *in vivo* malignant transformation of mouse fibroblasts in the presence of human tumour xenografts, *Br. J. Cancer,* 53, 793, 1986.

259. Gupta, V., Rajaraman, S., Gadson, P., and Costanzi, J.J., Primary transfection as a mechanism for transformation of host cells byl human tumor cells implanted in nude mice, *Cancer Res.,* 47, 5194, 1987.

260. Shimizu, K., Goldfarb, M., Suard, Y., Perucho, M., Li, Y., Kamata, T., Feramisco, J., Stavnezer, E., Fogh, J., and Wigler, M.H., Three human transforming genes are related to the viral *ras* oncogenes, *Proc. Natl. Acad. Sci. U.S.A.,* 80, 2112, 1983.

261. Bos, J.L., Toksoz, D., Marshall, C.J., Verlaan-de Vries, M., Veeneman, G.H., van der Eb, A.J., van Boom, J.H., Janssen, J.W.G., and Steenvoorden, A.C.M., Amino-acid substitutions at codon 13 of the N-*ras* oncogene in human acute myeloid leukaemia, *Nature,* 315, 726, 1985.

262. Martin-Zanca, D., Hughes, S.H., and Barbacid, M., A human oncogene formed by fusion of truncated tropomyosin and protein tyrosine kinase sequences, *Nature*, 319, 743, 1986.

263. Devine, J.M., Mechanism of activation of *HuBlym*-1 gene unresolved, *Nature*, 321, 437, 1986.

264. Rogers, J., Relationship of *Blym* genes to repeated sequences, *Nature*, 320, 579, 1986.

265. Cooper, G.M., Goubin, G., Diamond, A., and Neiman, P., Relationship of *Blym* genes to repeated sequences, *Nature*, 320, 579, 1986.

266. Hung, M.-C., Schechter, A.L., Chevray, P.-Y.M., Stern, D.F., and Weinberg, R.A., Molecular cloning of the *neu* gene: absence of gross structural alteration in oncogenic alleles, *Proc. Natl. Acad. Sci. U.S.A.*, 83, 261, 1986.

267. Padua, R.A., Barrass, N., and Currie, G.A., A novel transforming gene in a human malignant melanoma cell line, *Nature*, 311, 671, 1984.

268. Hollingsworth, M.A., Rebellato, L.M., Moore, J.W., Finn, O.J., and Metzgar, R.S., Antigens expressed on NIH 3T3 cells following transformation with DNA from a human pancreatic tumor, *Cancer Res.*, 46, 2482, 1986.

269. Sakamoto, H., Mori, M., Taira, M., Yoshida, T., Matsukawa, S., Shimizu, K., Sekiguchi, M., Terada, M., and Sugimura, T., Transforming gene from human stomach cancers and a noncancerous portion of stomach mucosa, *Proc. Natl. Acad. Sci. U.S.A.*, 83, 3997, 1986.

270. Taira, M., Yoshida, T., Miyagawa, K., Sakamoto, H., Tereda, M., and Sugimura, T., cDNA sequence of human transforming gene *hst* and identification of the coding sequence required for transforming activity, *Proc. Natl. Acad. Sci. U.S.A.*, 84, 2980, 1987.

271. Yuasa, Y. and Sudo, K., Transforming genes in human hepatomas detected by a tumorigenicity assay, *Jpn. J. Cancer Res.*, 78, 1036, 1987.

272. Delli Bovi, P. and Basilico, C., Isolation of a rearranged human transforming gene following transfection of Kaposi sarcoma DNA, *Proc. Natl. Acad. Sci. U.S.A.*, 84, 5660, 1987.

273. Delli Bovi, P., Curatola, A., Kern, F.G., Greco, A., Ittmann, M., and Basilico, C., An oncogene isolated by transfection of Kaposi's sarcoma DNA encodes a growth factor that is a member of the FGF family, *Cell*, 50, 729, 1987.

274. Groner, B., The *mas* oncogene, *Trends Genet.*, 2, 250, 1986.

275. Ishizaka, Y., Ochiai, M., Ishikawa, F., Sato, S., Miura, Y., Nagao, M., and Sugimura, T., Activated N-*ras* oncogene in a transformant derived from a rat small intestinal adenocarcinoma induced by 2-aminodiyrido(1,2-*a*:3′,2′-*d*)imidazole, *Carcinogenesis*, 8, 1575, 1987.

276. Takahashi, M., Ritz, J., and Cooper, G.M., Activation of a novel human transforming gene, *ret*, by DNA rearrangement, *Cell*, 42, 581, 1985.

277. Ishikawa, F., Takaku, F., Hayashi, K., Nagao, M., and Sugimura, T., Activation of rat c-*raf* during transfection of hepatocellular carcinoma DNA, *Proc. Natl. Acad. Sci. U.S.A.*, 83, 3902, 1986.

278. Ishikawa, F., Takaku, F., Ochiai, M., Hayashi, K., Hirohashi, S., Terada, M., Takayama, S., Nagao, M., and Sugimura, T., Activated c-*raf* gene in a rat hepatocellular carcinoma induced by 2-amino-3-methylimidazo(4,5-*f*)quinoline, *Biochem. Biophys. Res. Commun.*, 132, 186, 1985.

279. Fukui, M., Yamamoto, T., Kawai, S., Mitsunobu, F., and Toyoshima, K., Molecular cloning and characterization of an activated human c-*raf*-1 gene, *Mol. Cell. Biol.*, 7, 1776, 1987.

280. Eva, A. and Aaronson, S.A., Isolation of a new human oncogene from a diffuse B-cell lymphoma, *Nature*, 316, 273, 1985.

281. Eva, A., Vecchio, G., Diamond, M., Tronick, S.R., Ron, D., Cooper, G.M., and Aaronson, S.A., Independently activated *dbl* oncogenes exhibit similar yet distinct structural alterations, *Oncogene*, 1, 355, 1987.

282. Srivastava, S.K., Wheelock, R.H.P., Aaronson, S.A., and Eva, A., Identification of the protein encoded by the human diffuse B-cell lymphoma (*dbl*) oncogene, *Proc. Natl. Acad. Sci. U.S.A.*, 83, 8868, 1986.

283. Eva, A., Vecchio, G., Rao, C.D., Tronick, S.R., and Aaronson, S.A., The predicted *DBL* oncogene product defines a distinct class of transforming proteins, *Proc. Natl. Acad. Sci. U.S.A.*, 85, 2061, 1988.

284. Janssen, J.W.G., Steenvoorden, A.C.M., Losekoot, M., and Bartram, C.R., Novel transforming sequences in human acute myelocytic leukemia cell lines, *Oncogene*, 1, 175, 1987.

285. Janssen, J.W.G., Steenvoorden, A.C.M., Schimidtberger, M., and Bartram, C.R., Activation of the mas oncogene during transfusion of monoblastic cell line DNA, *Leukemia*, 2, 318, 1988.

286. Kozma, S.C., Redmond, S.M.S., Xiao-Chang, F., Saurer, S.M., Groner, B., and Hynes, N.E., Activation of the receptor kinase domain of the *trk* oncogene by recombination with two different cellular sequences, *EMBO J.*, 7, 147, 1988.

287. Oskam, R., Coulier, F., Ernst, M., Martin-Zanca, D., and Barbacid, M., Frequent generation of oncogenes by *in vitro* recombination of *TRK* protooncogene sequences, *Proc. Natl. Acad. Sci. U.S.A.*, 85, 2964, 1988.

288. Benditt, E.P. and Benditt, J.M., Evidence for a monoclonal origin of human atherosclerotic plaques, *Proc. Natl. Acad. Sci. U.S.A.*, 70, 1753, 1973.

289. Penn, A., Garte, S.J., Warren, L., Nesta, D., and Mindich, B., Transforming gene in human atherosclerotic plaque DNA, *Proc. Natl. Acad. Sci. U.S.A.*, 83, 7951, 1986.

290. Scott, J., Oncogenes in atherosclerosis, *Nature*, 325, 574, 1987.

291. Manoharan, T.H., Burgess, J.A., Ho, D., Newell, C.L., and Fahl, W.E., Integration of a mutant c-Ha-*ras* oncogene into C3H/10T1/2 cells and its relationship to tumorigenic transformation, *Carcinogenesis,* 6, 1295, 1985.

292. Hsiao, W.-L.W., Gattoni-Celli, S., and Weinstein, I.B., Oncogene-induced transformation of C3H 10T1/2 cells is enhanced by tumor promoters, *Science,* 226, 552, 1984.

293. Lee, W.M.F., Schwab, M., Westaway, D., and Varmus, H.E., Augmented expression of normal c-*myc* is sufficient for cotransformation of rat embryo cells with a mutant *ras* gene, *Mol. Cell. Biol.,* 5, 3345, 1985.

294. Yancoupoulos, G.D., Nisen, P.D., Tesfaye, A., Kohl, N.E., Goldfarb, M.P., and Alt, F.W., N-*myc* can cooperate with *ras* to transform normal cells in culture, *Proc. Natl. Acad. Sci. U.S.A.,* 82, 5455, 1985.

295. Connan, G., Rassoulzadegan, M., and Cuzin, F., Focus formation in rat fibroblasts exposed to a tumour promoter after transfer of polyoma *plt* and *myc* oncogenes, *Nature,* 314, 277, 1985.

296. Porteous, D.J., Morten, J.E.N., Foster, M.E., Cranston, G., Weir-Thompson, E., Busuttil, A., Bostock, C.J., and Steel, C.M., HRAS1-selected, chromosome-mediated transformants vary in phenotype *in vitro* and tumorigenic potential *in vivo, Int. J. Cancer,* 38, 603, 1986.

297. Pozzatti, R., Muschel, R., Williams, J., Padmanabhan, R., Howard, B., Liotta, L., and Khoury, G. P., Primary rat embryo cells transformed by one or two oncogenes show different metastatic potentials, *Science,* 232, 223, 1986.

298. Liboi, E., Caruso, M., and Basilico, C., New rat cell line that is highly susceptible to transformation by several oncogenes, *Mol. Cell. Biol.,* 4, 2925, 1984.

299. Minden, M.D., Gusella, J.F., and Housman, D., Chromosome-mediated transfer of the malignant phenotype by human acute muelogenous leukemic cells, *Blood,* 64, 842, 1984.

300. Kurata, S., Kurata, N., and Ikawa, Y., Production of recombinant rat viruses as a method of oncogene isolation in coculture medium, *Cancer Res.,* 47, 5908, 1987.

301. Colburn, N.H., Lerman, M.I., Hegameyer, G.A., and Ginhart, T.D., A transforming activity not detected by DNA transfer to NIH 3T3 cells is detected by JB6 mouse epidermal cells, *Mol. Cell. Biol.,* 5, 890, 1985.

302. Jonak, Z.L., Braman, V., and Kennett, R.H., Production of continuous mouse plasma cell lines by transfection with human leukemia DNA, *Hybridoma,* 3, 107, 1984.

303. Hynes, N.E., Jaggi, R., Kozma, S.C., Ball, R., Muellener, D., Wetherall, N.T., Davis, B.W., and Groner, B., New acceptor cell for transfected genomic DNA: oncogene transfer into a mouse mammary epithelial cell line, *Mol. Cell. Biol.,* 5, 268, 1985.

304. Ananthaswamy, H.N., Price, J.E., Goldberg, L.H., and Bales, E.S., Simultaneous transfer of tumorigenic and metastatic phenotypes by transfection with genomic DNA from a human cutaneous squamous cell carcinoma, *J. Cell. Biochem.,* 36, 137, 1988.

305. Garcia, I., Sordat, B., Rauccio-Farinon, E., Dunand, M., Kraehenbuhl, J.-P., and Diggelmann, H., Establishment of two rabbit mammary epithelial cell lines with distinct oncogenic potential and differentiated phenotype after microinjection of transforming genes, *Mol. Cell. Biol.,* 6, 1974, 1986.

306. Hoeijmakers, J.H.J., Odijk, H., and Westerveld, A., Differences between rodent and human cell lines in the amount of integrated DNA after transfection, *Exp. Cell Res.,* 169, 111, 1987.

307. Sager, R., Tanaka, K., Lau, C.C., Ebina, Y., and Anisowicz, A., Resistance of human cells to tumorigenesis induced by cloned transforming genes, *Proc. Natl. Acad. Sci. U.S.A.,* 80, 7601, 1983.

308. Pater, A. and Pater, M.M., Transformation of primary human embryonic kidney cells to anchorage independence by a combination of BK virus DNA and the Harvey-*ras* oncogene, *J. Virol.,* 58, 680, 1986.

309. Hurlin, P.J., Fry, D.G., Maher, V.M., and McCormick, J.J., Morphological transformation, focus formation, and anchorage independence in diploid human fibroblasts by expression of a transfected H-*ras* oncogene, *Cancer Res.,* 47, 5752, 1987.

310. Sutherland, B.M. and Bennett, P.V., Transformation of human cells by DNA transfection, *Cancer Res.,* 44, 2769, 1984.

311. Sutherland, B.M., Bennett, P.V., Freeman, A.G., Moore, S.P., and Strickland, P.T., Transformation of human cells by DNAs ineffective in transformation of NIH 3T3 cells, *Proc. Natl. Acad. Sci. U.S.A.,* 82, 2399, 1985.

312. Tainsky, M.A., Shamanski, F.L., Blair, D., and Vande Woude, G., Human recipient cell for oncogene transfection studies, *Mol. Cell. Biol.,* 7, 1280, 1987.

313. Forrester, K., Almoguera, C., Han, K., Grizzle, W.E., and Perucho, M., Detection of high incidence of K-*ras* oncogenes during human colon tumorigenesis, *Nature,* 327, 298, 1987.

314. Syvänen, A.-C., Nucleic acid hybridization: from research tool to routine diagnostic method, *Med. Biol.,* 64, 313, 1986.

315. Neumann, R., Die Technik der Nukleinsäurehybridisierung und ihre Bedeutung für diagnostische Fragestellungen, *Naturwissenschaften,* 74, 125, 1987.

316. Lang, H., Ebeling, W., Reckmann, B., and Rieke, E., Gene analysis and the clinical chemist, *J. Clin. Chem. Clin. Biochem.,* 25, 123, 1987.

317. Kalsheker, N., Analytical approaches involving recombinant DNA techniques in the diagnosis of human genetic disorders, *Analyst,* 112, 1475, 1987.

318. Kafatos, F.C., Jones, C.W., and Efstratiadis, A., Determination of nucleic acid sequence homologies and relative concentrations by a dot blot hybridization procedure, *Nucleic Acids Res.,* 7, 1541, 1979.

319. Southern, E.M., Detection of specific sequences among DNA fragments separated by gel electrophoresis, *J. Mol. Biol.,* 98, 503, 1975.

320. McDonell, M.W., Simon, N.M., and Studier, F.W., Analysis of restriction fragments of T7 DNA and determination of molecular weights by electrophoresis in neutral and alkaline gels, *J. Mol. Biol.,* 110, 119, 1977.

321. Wahl, G., Stern, M., and Stark, G., Efficient transfer of large DNA fragments from agarose gels to diazobenzyloxymethyl-paper and rapid hybridization by using dextran sulfate, *Proc. Natl. Acad. Sci. U.S.A.,* 76, 3683, 1979.

322. Vandenplas, S., Wiid, I., Grobler-Rabie, A., Brebner, K., Ricketts, M., Wallis, G., Bester, A., Boyd, C., and Mathew, C., Blot hybridisation analysis of genomic DNA, *J. Med. Genet.,* 21, 164, 1984.

323. Wong-Staal, F., Dalla-Favera, R., Franchini, G., Gelmann, E.P., and Gallo, R.C., Three distinct genes in human DNA related to the transforming genes of mammalian sarcoma retroviruses, *Science,* 213, 226, 1981.

324. Goubin, G., Goldman, D.S., Luce, J., Neiman, P.E., and Cooper, G.M., Molecular cloning and nucleotide sequence of a transforming gene detected by transfection of chicken B-cell lymphoma DNA, *Nature,* 302, 114, 1983.

325. Devine, J.M., Diamond, A., Lane, M.A., and Cooper, G.M., Characterization of the B*lym*-1 transforming genes of chicken and human B-cell lymphomas, *J. Cell. Physiol.,* Suppl. 3, 193, 1984.

326. Diamond, A., Devine, J.M., and Cooper, G.M., Nucleotide sequence of a human *Blym* transforming gene activated in a Burkitt's lymphoma, *Science,* 225, 516, 1984.

327. Taparowsky, E., Shimizu, K., Goldfarb, M., and Wigler, M., Structure and activation of the human N-*ras* gene, *Cell,* 34, 581, 1983.

328. Watt, R., Stanton, L.W., Marcu, K.B., Gallo, R.C., Croce, C.M., and Rovera, G., Nucleotide sequence of cloned cDNA of human c-*myc* oncogene, *Nature,* 303, 725, 1983.

329. Collins, S., Coleman, H., and Groudine, M., Expression of *bcr* and *bcr-abl* fusion transcripts in normal and leukemic cells, *Mol. Cell. Biol.,* 7, 2870, 1987.

330. Weiss, L.M., Warnke, R.A., Sklar, J., and Cleary, M.L., Molecular analysis of the t(14;18) chromosomal translocation in malignant lymphomas, *N. Engl. J. Med.,* 317, 1185, 1987.

331. Seizinger, B.R., Martuza, R.L., and Gusella, J.F., Loss of genes on chromosome 22 in tumorigenesis of human acoustic neuroma, *Nature,* 322, 644, 1986.

332. Driyja, T.P., Rapaport, J.M., Joyce, J.M., and Petersen, R.A., Molecular detection of deletions involving band q14 of chromosome 13 in retinoblastomas, *Proc. Natl. Acad. Sci. U.S.A.,* 83, 7391, 1986.

333. Zbar, B., Brauch, H., Talmadge, C., and Linehan, M., Loss of alleles of loci on the short arm of chromosome 3 in renal cell carcinoma, *Nature,* 327, 721, 1987.

334. Seizinger, B.R., de la Monte, S., Atkins, L., Gusella, J.F., and Martuza, R.L., Molecular genetic approach to human meningioma: loss of genes on chromosome 22, *Proc. Natl. Acad. Sci. U.S.A.,* 84, 5419, 1987.

335. Benedict, W.F., Srivatsan, E.S., Mark, C., Banerjee, A., Sparkes, R.S., and Murphree, A.L., *Cancer Res.,* 47, 4189, 1987.

336. Solomon, E., Voss, R., Hall, V., Bodmer, W.F., Jass, J.R., Jeffreys, A.J., Lucibello, F.C., Patel, I., and Rider, S.H., Chromosome 5 allele loss in human colorectal carcinomas, *Nature,* 328, 616, 1987.

337. Naylor, S.L., Johnson, B.E., Minna, J.D., and Sakaguchi, A.Y., Loss of heterozygosity of chromosome 3p markers in small-cell lung cancer, *Nature,* 329, 451, 1987.

338. Kok, K., Osinga, J., Carritt, B., Davis, M.B., van der Hout, A.H., Landsvater, R.M., de Leij, L.F.M.H., Berendsen, H.H., Postmus, P.E., Poppema, S., and Buys, C.H.C.M., Deletion of a DNA sequence at the chromosomal region 3p21 in all major types of lung cancer, *Nature,* 330, 578, 1987.

339. Wildrick, D.M. and Boman, B.M., Chromosome 5 allele loss at the glucocorticoid receptor locus in human colorectal carcinomas, *Biochem. Biophys. Res. Commun.,* 150, 591, 1988.

340. Monpezat, J.-P., Delattre, O., Bernard, A., Grunwald, D., Remvikos, Y., Muleris, M., Salmon, R.J., Frelat, G., Dutrillaux, B., and Thomas, G., Loss of alleles on chromosome 18 and on the short arm of chromosome 17 in polyploid colorectal carcinomas, *Int. J. Cancer,* 41, 404, 1988.

341. Skolnick, M.H. and White, R., Strategies for detecting and characterizing restriction fragment length polymorphisms (RFLPs), *Cytogenet. Cell Genet.,* 32, 58, 1982.

342. Santos, E., Martin-Zanca, D., Reddy, E.P., Pierotti, M.A., Della Porta, G., and Barbacid, M., Malignant activation of a K-*ras* oncogene in lung carcinoma but not in normal tissue of the same patient, *Science,* 223, 661, 1984.

343. Bos, J.L., Verlaan-de Vries, M., Jansen, A.M., Veeneman, G.H., van Boom, J.H., and van der Eb, A.J., Three different mutations in codon 61 of the human N-*ras* gene detected by synthetic oligonucleotide hybridization, *Nucleic Acids Res.,* 12, 9155, 1984.

344. Valenzuela, D.M. and Groffen, J., Four human carcinoma cell lines with novel mutations in position 12 of c-K-*ras* oncogene, *Nucleic Acids Res.,* 14, 843, 1986.

345. Saiki, R.K., Scharf, S., Faloona, F., Mullis, K.B., Horn, G.T., Erlich, H.A., and Arnheim, N., Enzymatic amplification of beta-globin genomic sequences and restriction site analysis for diagnosis of sickle cell anemia, *Science,* 230, 1350, 1985.

346. Bos, J.L., The *ras* gene family and human carcinogenesis, *Mutat. Res.,* 195, 255, 1988.

347. Verlaan-de Vries, M., Bogaard, M.E., van den Elst, H., van Boom, J.H., van der Eb, A.J., and Bos, J.L., A dot-blot screening procedure for mutated *ras* oncogenes using synthetic oligodeoxynucleotides, *Gene,* 50, 313, 1986.

348. McMahon, G., Davis, E., and Wogan, G.N., Characterization of c-Ki-*ras* oncogene alleles by direct sequencing of enzymatically amplified DNA from carcinogen-induced tumors, *Proc. Natl. Acad. Sci. U.S.A.,* 84, 4974, 1987.

349. Engelke, D.R., Hoener, P.A., and Collins, F.S., Direct sequencing of enzymatically amplified human genomic DNA, *Proc. Natl. Acad. Sci. U.S.A.,* 85, 544, 1988.

350. Almoguera, C., Shibata, D., Forrester, K., Martin, J., Arnheim, N., and Perucho, M., Most human carcinomas of the exocrine pancreas contain mutant c-K-*ras* genes, *Cell,* 53, 549, 1988.

351. Inoue, H., Gushi, K., Matsuura, S., and Sakata, Y., A sensitive colofimetric detection of virus DNA and oncogene, *Biochem. Biophys. Res. Commun.,* 143, 323, 1987.

352. Thomas, P., Hybridization of denatured RNA and small DNA fragments transferred to nitrocellulose, *Proc. Natl. Acad. Sci. U.S.A.,* 77, 5201, 1980.

353. Thompson, J. and Gillespie, D., Molecular hybridization in concentrated guanidine thiocyanate solutions, *Anal. Biochem.,* 163, 281, 1987.

354. Pellegrino, M.G., Meyer, W.A., III, Lanciotti, R.S., Bhaduri-Hauck, L., Volsky, D.J., Sakai, K., Folks, T.M., and Gillespie, D., A sensitive solution hybridization technique for detecting RNA in cells: application to HIV in blood cells, *BioTechniques,* 5, 452, 1987.

355. Müller, R., Müller, D., and Guilbert, L., Differential expression of c-*fos* in hematopoietic cells: correlation with differentiation of monomyelocytic cells *in vitro, EMBO J.,* 3, 1887, 1984.

356. Gastl, G., Ward, G., and Rapp, U.R., Immunocytochemistry of oncogenes, in *Immunocytochemistry,* 2nd ed., Polak, J.M., and Van Noorden, S., Eds., Wright-PSG, Bristol, England, 1986, 273.

357. Stoner, G.D., You, M., Skouv, J., Budd, G.C., Pansky, B., and Wang, Y., Detection of oncogene mRNA sequences in cultured cells by *in situ* hybridization, *Ann. Clin. Lab. Sci.,* 17, 74, 1987.

358. Le Beau, M.M., Westbrook, C.A., Diaz, M.O., and Rowley, J.D., c-*src* is consistently conserved in the chromosomal deletion (20q) observed in myeloid disorders, *Proc. Natl. Acad. Sci. U.S.A.,* 82, 6692, 1985.

359. McKeithan, T.W., Shima, E.A., Le Beau, M.M., Minowada, J., Rowley, J.D., and Diaz, M.O., Molecular cloning of the breakpoint junction of a human chromosomal 8;14 translocation involving the T-cell receptor alpha-chain gene and sequences on the 3′ side of *MYC, Proc. Natl. Acad. Sci. U.S.A.,* 83, 6636, 1986.

360. Le Beau, M.M., Rowley, J.D., Sacchi, N., Watson, D.K., Papas, T.S., and Diaz, M.O., Hu-*ets*-2 is translocated to chromosome 8 in the t(8;21) in acute myelogenous leukemia, *Cancer Genet. Cytogenet.,* 23, 269, 1986.

361. Rosendorff, J., Bowcock, A.M., Kuyl, J.M., Mendelow, B., Pinto, M.R., and Bernstein, R., Localization of the human c-*mos* gene by *in situ* hybridization in two cases of acute nonlymphocytic leukemia type M2, *Cancer Genet. Cytogenet.,* 24, 137, 1987.

362. Winter, E., Yamamoto, F., Almoguera, C., and Perucho, M., A method to detect and characterize point mutations in transcribed genes: amplification and overexpression of the mutant c-K-*ras* allele in human tumor cells, *Proc. Natl Acad. Sci. U.S.A.,* 82, 75, 1985.

363. Forrester, K., Almoguera, C., Jordano, J., Grizzle, W.E., and Perucho, M., *J. Tumor Marker Oncol.,* 2, 113, 1987.

364. Myers, R.M., Larin, Z., and Maniatis, T., Detection of single base substitutions by ribonuclease cleavage at mismatches in RNA:DNA duplexes, *Science,* 230, 1242, 1985.

365. Papkoff, J., Hunter, T., and Beemon, K., *In vitro* translation of virion RNA from Moloney murine sarcoma virus, *Virology,* 101, 91, 1980.

366. Cremer, K., Reddy, E.P., and Aaronson, S.A., Translational products of Moloney murine sarcoma virus RNA: identification of proteins encoded by the murine sarcoma virus *src* gene, *J. Virol.,* 38, 704, 1981.

367. Feig, L.A., Bast, R.C., Jr., Knapp, R.C., and Cooper, G.M., Somatic activation of ras^k gene in human ovarian carcinoma, *Science,* 223, 698, 1984.

368. Fosslien, E., Stastny, J., and Yamashiroya, H., Advances in protein analysis of biological systems, *Surv. Synth. Pathol. Res.,* 1, 282, 1983.

369. Anderson, L. and Anderson, N., Some perspectives on two-dimensional protein mapping, *Clin. Chem.,* 30, 1898, 1984.

370. Stastny, J., Prasad, R., and Fosslien, E., Tissue proteins in breast cancer, as studied by use of two-dimensional electrophoresis, *Clin. Chem.,* 30, 1914, 1984.

371. Wirth, P.J., Rao, M.S., and Evarts, R.P., Coordinate polypeptide expression during hepatocarcinogenesis in male F-344 rats: comparison of the Solt-Farber and Reddy models, *Cancer Res.,* 47, 2839, 1987.

372. Bravo, R. and Celis, E.J., Up-dated catalogue of HeLa cell proteins: percentages and characteristics of the major cell polypeptides labeled with a mixture of 16 ^{14}C-labeled amino acids, *Clin. Chem.,* 28, 766, 1982.

373. Strand, M. and August, J.T., Polypeptides of cells transformed by RNA or DNA tumor viruses, *Proc. Natl. Acad. Sci. U.S.A.,* 74, 2729, 1977.

374. Litin, B.S. and Grimes, W.J., Two-dimensional electrophoresis of membrane proteins from normal and transformed cells, *Cancer Res.,* 39, 2595, 1979.

375. Maytin, E.V., Balduzzi, P.C., Notter, M.F.D., and Young, D.A., Changes in the synthesis and phosphorylation of cellular proteins in chick fibroblasts transformed by two avian sarcoma viruses, *J. Biol. Chem.,* 259, 12135, 1984.

376. Krebs, E.G., The phosphorylation of proteins: a major mechanism for biological regulation, *Biochem. Soc. Trans.,* 13, 813, 1985.

377. Shenolikar, S., Control of cell function by reversible protein phosphorylation, *J. Cyclic Nucleot. Protein Phosphoryl. Res.,* 11, 531, 1987.

378. Manning, D.R., DiSalvo, J., and Stull, J.T., Protein phosphorylation: quantitative analysis *in vivo* and in intact cell systems, *Mol. Cell. Endocrinol.,* 19, 1, 1980.

379. Hunter, T. and Sefton, J.A., Protein-tyrosine kinases, *Annu. Rev. Biochem.,* 54, 897, 1985.

380. Sefton, B.M., The viral tyrosine protein kinases, *Curr. Top. Microbiol. Immunol.,* 123, 39, 1986.

381. Mäkelä, T.P. and Alitalo, K., Tyrosine kinases in control of cell growth and transformation, *Med. Biol.,* 64, 325, 1986.

382. Edelman, A.M., Blumenthal, D.K., and Krebs, E.G., Protein serine/threonine kinases, *Annu. Rev. Biochem.,* 56, 567, 1987.

383. Cooper, J.A. and Hunter, T., Regulation of cell growth and transformation by tyrosine-specific protein kinases: the search for important cellular substrate proteins, *Curr. Top. Microbiol. Immunol.,* 107, 125, 1983.

384. Heldin, C.-H. and Westermark, B., Growth factors: mechanism of action and relation to oncogenes, *Cell,* 37, 9, 1984.

385. Feige, J.-J. and Chambaz, E.M., Membrane receptors with protein-tyrosine kinase activity, *Biochimie,* 69, 379, 1987.

386. Pimentel, E., *Hormones, Growth Factors, and Oncogenes,* CRC Press, Boca Raton, FL, 1987.

387. Moelling, K., Heimann, B., Beimling, P., Bepler, G., Köppler, H., Havemann, K., and Balzer, T., Analysis of oncogene proteins in human cell tumor lines, *Contr. Oncol.,* 24, 76, 1987.

388. Giallongo, A., Appella, E., Ricciardi, R., Rovera, G., and Croce, C.M., Identification of the c-*myc* oncogene product in normal and malignant B cells, *Science,* 222, 430, 1983.

389. Ramsay, G., Evan, G.I., and Bishop, J.M., The protein encoded by the human proto-oncogene c-*myc*, *Proc. Natl. Acad. Sci. U.S.A.,* 81, 7742, 1984.

390. Patchinsky, T., Walter, G., and Bister, K., Immunological analysis of v-*myc* gene products using antibodies against a *myc*-specific peptide, *Virology,* 136, 348, 1984.

391. Evan, G.I., Lewis, G.K., Ramsay, G., and Bishop, J.M., Isolation of monoclonal antibodies for the human c-*myc* proto-oncogene product, *Mol. Cell. Biol.,* 5, 3610, 1985.

392. Suzuki, T., Yanaihara, C., Hirota, M., Iwafuchi, M., Inoue, T., Mochizuki, T., Iguchi, K., Abe, K., and Yanaihara, N., Immunohistochemical demonstration of c-*myc* gene product in tumors induced in nude mice by human hepatoblastoma: a study with antiserum to a related synthetic peptide, *Biomed. Res.,* 7, 365, 1986.

393. Maly, A. and Krchnák, V., Identification of c-myb (chicken), c-myb (mouse) and v-myb (AMV) protein products by immunoprecipitation with antibodies directed against a synthetic peptide, *FEBS Lett.,* 205, 104, 1986.

394. Uchida, Y., Yamaguchi, K., Abe, K., Tsuchishashi, T., Asanuma, F., Nagasaki, K., Kimura, S., Yanaihara, N., and Track, N.S., Radioimmunoassay of c-*myc* protein, *Jpn. J. Cancer Res.,* 77, 615, 1986.

395. Bizub, D., Heimer, E.P., Felix, A., Chizzonite, R., Wood, A., and Skalka, A.M., Antisera to the variable region of *ras* oncogene proteins, and specific detection of H-*ras* expression in an experimental model of chemical carcinogenesis, *Oncogene,* 1, 131, 1987.

396. Ishihara, H., Nakagawa, H., Ono, K., and Fukuda, A., Antibodies against synthetic carboxy-terminal peptides distinguish H-*ras* and K-*ras* oncogene products p21, *J. Immunol. Methods,* 103, 131, 1987.

397. Wong, G., Arnheim, N., Clark, R., McCabe, P., Innis, M., Aldwin, L., Nitecki, D., and McCormick, F., Detection of activated M_r 21,000 product of *ras* oncogenes, using antibodies with specificity for amino acid 12, *Cancer Res.,* 46, 6029, 1986.

398. Niman, H.L., Thompson, A.M.H., Yu, A., Markman, M., Willems, J.J., Herwig, K.R., Habib, N.A., Wood, C.B., Houghten, R.A., and Lerner, R.A., Anti-peptide antibodies detect oncogene-related proteins in urine, *Proc. Natl. Acad. Sci. U.S.A.,* 82, 7924, 1985.

399. Niman, H.L., Human oncogene-related proteins in urine during pregnancy and neoplasia, *Clin. Lab. Med.,* 6, 181, 1986.

400. Stock, L.M., Brosman, S.A., Fahey, J.L., and Liu, B.C.-S., *ras* related oncogene protein as a tumor marker in transitional cell carcinoma of the bladder, *J. Urol.,* 137, 789, 1987.

401. Tanaka, T., Slamon, D.J., and Cline, M.J., Efficient generation of antibodies to oncoproteins by using synthetic peptide antigens, *Proc. Natl. Acad. Sci. U.S.A.,* 82, 3400, 1985.

402. Singh, B., Goldman, R., Hutton, L., Herzog, N.K., and Arlinghaus, R.B., The P55 protein affected by v-*mos* expression is vimentin, *J. Virol.,* 61, 3625, 1987.

403. Ward, J.M., Pardue, R.L., Junker, J.L., Takahashi, K., Shih, T.Y., and Weislow, O.S., Immunocytochemical localization of Ras^{Ha} p21 in normal and neoplastic cells in fixed tissue sections from Harvey sarcoma virus-infected mice, *Carcinogenesis,* 7, 645, 1986.

404. Hand, P.H., Thor, A., Wunderlich, D., Murarao, R., Caruso, A., and Schlom, J., Monoclonal antibodies of predefined specificity detect activated *ras* gene expression in human mammary and colon carcinomas, *Proc. Natl. Acad. Sci. U.S.A.,* 81, 5227, 1984.

405. Thor, A., Hand, P.H., Wunderlich, D., Caruso, A., Muraro, R., and Schlom, J., Monoclonal antibodies define differential *ras* gene expression in malignant and benigh colonic diseases, *Nature,* 311, 562, 1984.

406. Immunohistochemical detection of the *ras* oncogene p21 product in an experimental tumour and in human colorectal neoplasms, *Br. J. Cancer,* 52, 697, 1985.

407. Kerr, I.B., Lee, F.D., Quintanilla, M., and Balmain, A., Immunocytochemical demonstration of p21 *ras* family oncogene product in normal mucosa and in premalignant and malignant tumours of the colorectum, *Br. J. Cancer,* 52, 695, 1985.

408. Ghosh, A.K., Moore, M., and Harris, M., Immunohistochemical detection of *ras* oncogene p21 product in benign and malignant mammary tissue in man, *J. Clin. Pathol.,* 39, 428, 1986.

409. Ohuchi, N., Thor, A., Page, D.L., Hand, P.H., Halter, S.A., and Schlom, J., Expression of the 21,000 molecular weight *ras* protein in a spectrum of benign and malignant human mammary tissues, *Cancer Res.,* 46, 2511, 1986.

410. Tahara, E., Yasui, W., Taniyama, K., Ochiai, A., Yamamoto, T., Nakajo, S., and Yamamoto, M., Ha-*ras* oncogene product in human gastric carcinoma: correlation with invasiveness, metastasis or prognosis, *Jpn. J. Cancer Res.,* 77, 517, 1986.

411. Agnantis, N.J., Petraki, C., Markoulatos, P., and Spandidos, D.A., Immunohistochemical study of the *ras* oncogene expression in human breast lesions, *Anticancer Res.,* 6, 1157, 1986.

412. Candlish, W., Kerr, I.B., and Simpson, H.W., Immunocytochemical demonstration and significance of p21 *ras* family oncogene product in benign and malignant breast disease, *J. Pathol.,* 150, 163, 1986.

413. Michelasi, F., Leuthner, S., Lubienski, M., Bostwick, D., Rodgers, J., Handcock, M., and Block, G.E., Ras oncogene p21 levels parallel malignant potential of different human colonic benign conditions, *Arch. Surg.,* 122, 1414, 1987.

414. Mizukami, Y., Nomomura, A., Hashimoto, T., Terahata, S., Matsubara, F., Michigishi, T., and Noguchi, M., Immunohistochemical demonstration of *ras* p21 oncogene product in normal, benign, and malignant human thyroid tissues, *Cancer,* 61, 873, 1988.

415. Lee, I., Gould, V.E., Radosevich, J.A., Thor, A., Ma, Y., Schlom, J., and Rosen, S., and Rosen, S.T., Immunohistochemical evaluation of ras oncogene expression in pulmonary and pleural neoplasms, *Virchows Arch. B,* 53, 146, 1987.

416. Sikora, K., Evan, G., Stewart, J., and Watson, J.V., Detection of the c-*myc* oncogene product in testicular cancer, *Br. J. Cancer,* 52, 171, 1985.

417. Jack, A.S., Kerr, I.B., Evan, G., and Lee, F.D., The distribution of the c-*myc* oncogene product in malignant lymphomas and various normal tissues as demonstrated by immunocytochemistry, *Br. J. Cancer,* 53, 713, 1986.

418. Chan, S.Y.T., Evan, G.I., Ritson, A., Watson, J., Wraight, P., and Sikora, K., Localisation of lung cancer by a radiolabelled monoclonal antibody against the c-*myc* oncogene product, *Br. J. Cancer,* 54, 761, 1986.

419. Spandidos, D.A., Pintzas, A., Kakkanas, A., Yiagnisis, M., Mahera, H., Patra, E., and Agnantis, N.J., Elevated expression of the *myc* gene in human benign and malignant breast lesions compared to normal tissue, *Anticancer Res.,* 7, 1299, 1987.

420. Allum, W.H., Newbold, K.M., Macdonald, F., Russell, B., and Stokes, H., Evaluation of p62^{c-myc} in benign and malignant gastric epithelia, *Br. J. Cancer,* 56, 785, 1987.

421. Cerny, T., Barnes, D.M., Hasleton, P., Barber, P.V., Healy, K., Gullick, W., and Thatcher, N., Expression of epidermal growth factor receptor (EGF-R) in human lung tumours, *Br. J. Cancer,* 54, 265, 1986.

422. Sakai, K., Mori, S., Kawamoto, T., Taniguchi, S., Kobori, O., Morioka, Y., Kuroki, T., and Kano, K., Expression of epidermal growth factor receptors on normal human gastric epithelia and gastric carcinomas, *J. Natl. Cancer Inst.,* 77, 1047, 1986.

423. Mori, S., Akiyama, T., Morishita, Y., Shimizu, S., Sakai, K., Sudoh, K., Toyoshima, K., and Yamamoto, T., Light and electron microscopical demonstration of c-*erbB*-2 gene product-like immunoreactivity in human malignant tumors, *Virchows Arch., B,* 54, 8, 1987.

424. Gusterson, B.A., Gullick, W.J., Venter, D.J., Powles, T.J., Elliott, C., Ashley, S., Tidy, A., and Harrison, S., *Mol. Cell. Probes,* 2, 383, 1988.

425. van de Vijver, M.J., Mooi, W.J., Wisman, P., Peterse, J.L., and Nusse, R., Immunohistochemical detection of the *neu* protein in tissue sections of human breast tumors with amplified *neu* DNA, *Oncogene,* 2, 175, 1988.

426. Czerniak, B., Herz, F., Koss, L.G., and Schlom, J., *ras* oncogene p21 as a tumor marker in the cytodiagnosis of gastric and colonic carcinomas, *Cancer,* 60, 2432, 1987.

427. Moore, J.P., Hancock, D.C., Littlewood, T.D., and Evan, G.I., A sensitive and quantitative enzyme-linked immunosorbence assay for the c-*myc* and N-*myc* oncoproteins, *Oncogene Res., 2*, 65, 1987.

428. Erisman, M.D., Scott, J.K., Watt, R.A., and Astrin, S.M., The c-*myc* protein is constitutively expressed at elevated levels in colorectal carcinoma cell lines, *Oncogene, 2*, 367, 1988.

429. Watson, J.V., Stewart, J., Evan, G.I., Ritson, A., and Sikora, K., The clinical significance of flow cytometric c-*myc* oncoprotein quantitation in testicular cancer, *Br. J. Cancer, 53*, 331, 1986.

430. Hendy-Ibbs, P., Cox, H., Evan, G.I., and Watson, J.V., Flow cytometric quantitation of DNA and c-*myc* oncoprotein in archival biopsies of uterine cerviex neoplasia, *Br. J. Cancer, 55*, 275, 1987.

431. Watson, J.V., Stewart, J., Cox, H., Sikora, K., and Evan, G.I., Flow cytometric quantitation of the c-*myc* oncoprotein in archival neoplastic biopsies of the colon, *Mol. Cell. Probes, 1*, 151, 1987.

432. Bains, M.A., Hoy, T.G., Baines, P., and Jacobs, A., Nuclear c-myc protein, maturation, and cell-cycle status of human haemopoietic cells, *Br. J. Haematol., 67*, 293, 1987.

433. Young, H.A., Klein, R.A., Shih, T.Y., Morgan, A.C., Jr., and Schroff, R.W., Detection of the intracellular *ras* p21 oncogene product by flow cytometry, *Anal. Biochem., 156*, 67, 1986.

434. Strand, M., Transformation-related antigens identified by monoclonal antibodies, *Proc. Natl. Acad. Sci. U.S.A., 77*, 3234, 1980.

435. Colcher, D., Hand, P.H., Teramoto, Y.A., Wunderlich, D., and Schlom, J., Use of monoclonal antibodies to define the diversity of mammary tumor viral gene products in virions and mammary tumors of the genus *Mus*, *Cancer Res., 41*, 1451, 1981.

436. Lipsich, L.A., Lewis, A.J., and Brugge, J.S., Isolation of monoclonal antibodies that recognize the transforming proteins of avian sarcoma viruses, *J. Virol., 48*, 352, 1983.

437. Frackelton, A.R., Ross, A.H., and Eisen, H.N., Characterization and use of monoclonal antibodies for isolation of phosphotyrosyl proteins from retrovirus-transformed cells and growth factor-stimulated cells, *Mol. Cell. Biol., 3*, 1343, 1983.

438. Tanaka, T. and Kurth, R., Monoclonal antibodies specific for the avian sarcoma virus transforming protein pp60^{src}, *Virology, 133*, 202, 1984.

439. Drebin, J.A., Stern, D.F., Link, V.C., Weinberg, R.A., and Greene, M.I., Monoclonal antibodies identify a cell-surface antigen associated with an activated cellular oncogene, *Nature, 226*, 545, 1984.

440. Evan, G.I., Lewis, G.K., and Bishop, J.M., Isolation of monoclonal antibodies specific for products of avian oncogene *myb*, *Mol. Cell. Biol., 4*, 2843, 1984.

441. Tamura, T. and Bauer, H., Monoclonal antibody against the carboxy terminal peptide of pp60^{src} of Rous sarcoma virus reacts with native pp60^{src}, *EMBO J., 1*, 1479, 1982.

442. Parsons, S.J., McCarley, D.J., Ely, C.M., Benjamin, D.C., and Parsons, J.T., Monoclonal antibodies to Rous sarcoma virus pp60^{src} react with enzymatically active cellular pp60^{src} of avian and mammalian origin, *J. Virol., 51*, 272, 1984.

443. Hand, P.H., Thor, A., Wunderlich, D., Muraro, R., Caruso, A., and Schlom, J., Monoclonal antibodies of predefined specificity detect activated *ras* gene expression in human mammary and colon carcinomas, *Proc. Natl. Acad. Sci. U.S.A., 81*, 5227, 1984.

444. Furth, M.E., Davis, L.J., Fleurdelys, D., and Scolnick, E.M., Monoclonal antibodies of the p21 products of the transforming genes of Harvey murine sarcoma virus and of the cellular *ras* gene family, *J. Virol., 43*, 294, 1982.

445. Carney, W.P., Petit, D., Hamer, P., Der, C.J., Finkel, T., Cooper, G.M., Lefebvre, M., Mobtaker, H., Delellis, R., Tischler, A.S., Dayal, Y., Wolfe, H., and Rabin, H., Monoclonal antibody specific for an activated RAS protein, *Proc. Natl. Acad. Sci. U.S.A., 83*, 7485, 1986.

446. Kuzumaki, N., Oda, A., Yamagiwa, S., Taniguchi, N., Kobayashi, H., and Oikawa, T., Establishment of four mouse hybridoma cell lines producing monoclonal antibodies reactive with *ras* oncogene product p21, *J. Natl. Cancer Inst., 77*, 1273, 1986.

447. Freedman, D. and Auersperg, N., Detection of an intracellular transforming protein (v-Ki-ras p21) using flow activated cell sorter (FACS), *In Vitro Cell. Dev. Biol., 22*, 621, 1986.

448. Kanai, T., Hirohashi, S., Noguchi, M., Shimoyama, Y., Shimosato, Y., Noguchi, S., Nishimura, S., and Abe, O., Monoclonal antibody highly sensitive for the detection of *ras* p21 in immunoblotting analysis, *Jpn. J. Cancer Res., 78*, 1314, 1987.

449. Kennett, R.H., Leunk, R., Meyer, B., and Silenzio, V., Detection of *E. coli* colonies expressing the v-*sis* oncogene product with monoclonal antibodies made against synthetic peptides, *J. Immunol. Methods, 85*, 169, 1985.

450. Evan, G.I. and Hancock, D.C., Studies on the interaction of the human c-*myc* protein with cell nuclei: p62^{c-myc} as a member of a discrete subset of nuclear proteins, *Cell, 43*, 253, 1985.

451. Caruso, A., Schlom, J., Vilasi, V., Weeks, M.O., and Hand, P.H., Development of quantitative liquid competition radioimmunoassays for the *ras* oncogene and proto-oncogene p21 products, *Int. J. Cancer, 38*, 587, 1986.

452. Wong-Staal, F., Dalla-Favera, R., Franchini, G., Gelmann, E.P., and Gallo, R.C., Three distinct genes in human DNA related to the transforming genes of mammalian sarcoma retroviruses, *Science, 213*, 226, 1981.

453. Dalla Favera, R., Gelmann, E.P., Gallo, R.C., and Wong-Staal, F., A human *onc* gene homologous to the transforming gene (v-*sis*) of simian sarcoma virus, *Nature,* 292, 31, 1981.

454. Josephs, S.F., Dalla Favera, R., Gelmann, E.P., Gallo, R.C., and Wong-Staal, F., 5′ viral and human cellular sequences corresponding to the transforming gene of simian sarcoma virus, *Science,* 219, 503, 1983.

455. Josephs, S.F., Guo, C., Ratner, L., and Wong-Staal, F., Human proto-oncogene nucleotide sequences corresponding to the transforming region of simian sarcoma virus, *Science,* 223, 487, 1984.

456. Josephs, S.F., Ratner, L., Clarke, M.F., Westin, E.H., Reitz, M.S., and Wong-Staal, F., *Science,* 225, 636, 1984.

457. Ratner, L., Josephs, S.F., Jarrett, R., Reitz, M.S., Jr., and Wong-Staal, F., Nucleotide sequence of transforming human c-*sis* cDNA clones with homology to platelet-derived growth factor, *Nucleic Acids Res.,* 13, 5007, 1985.

458. Van den Ouweland, A.M.W., Roebroek, A.J.M., Schalken, J.A., Claesen, C.A.A., Bloemers, H.P.J., and Van de Ven, W.J.M., Structure and nucleotide sequence of the 5′ region of the human and feline c-*sis* proto-oncogenes, *Nucleic Acids Res.,* 14, 765, 1986.

459. Van den Ouweland, A.M.W., Van Groningen, J.J.M., Schalken, J.A., Van Neck, H.W., Bloemers, H.P.J., and Van de Ven, Genetic organization of the c-*sis* transcription unit, *Nucleic Acids Res.,* 15, 959, 1987.

460. Rao, C.D., Igarashi, H., Chiu, I.-M., Robbins, K.C., and Aaronson, S.A., Structure and sequence of the human c-*sis*/platelet-derived growth factor 2 (*SIS/PDGF2*) transcriptional unit, *Proc. Natl. Acad. Sci. U.S.A.,* 83, 2392, 1986.

461. Parker, R.C., Varmus, H.E., and Bishop, J.M., Cellular homologue (c-*src*) of the transforming gene of Rous sarcoma virus: isolation, mapping, and transcriptional analysis of c-*src* and flanking regions, *Proc. Natl. Acad. Sci. U.S.A.,* 78, 5842, 1981.

462. Gibbs, C.P., Tanaka, A., Anderson, S.K., Radul, J., Baar, J., Ridgway, A., Kung, H.-J., and Fujita, D.J., Isolation and structural mapping of a human c-*src* gene homologous to the transforming gene (v-*src*) of Rous sarcoma virus, *J. Virol.,* 53, 19, 1985.

463. Parker, R.C., Mardon, G., Lebo, R.V., Varmus, H.E., and Bishop, J.M., Isolation of duplicated human c-*src* genes located on chromosomes 1 and 20, *Mol. Cell Biol.,* 5, 831, 1985.

464. Tanaka, A., Gibbs, C.P., Arthur, R.R., Anderson, S.K., Kung, H.-J., and Fujita, D.J., DNA sequence encoding the amino-terminal region of the human c-*src* protein: implications of sequence divergence among *src*-type kinase oncogenes, *Mol. Cell. Biol.,* 7, 1978, 1987.

465. Trus, M.D., Sodroski, J.G., and Haseltine, W.A., Isolation and characterization of a human locus homologous to the transforming gene (v-*fes*) of feline sarcoma virus, *J. Biol. Chem.,* 257, 2730, 1982.

466. Groffen, J., Heisterkamp, N., Grosveld, F., Van de Ven, W., and Stephenson, J.R., Isolation of human oncogene sequences (v-*fes* homolog) from a cosmid library, *Science,* 216, 1136, 1982.

467. Roebroek, A.J.M., Schalken, J.A., Verbeek, J.S., Van den Ouweland, A.M.W., Onnekink, C., Bloemers, H.P.J., and Van de Ven, W.J.M., The structure of the human c-*fes/fps* proto-oncogene, *EMBO J.,* 4, 2897, 1985.

468. Nishizawa, M., Semba, K., Yoshida, M.C., Yamamoto, T., Sasaki, M., and Toyoshima, K., Structure, expression and chromosomal location of the human c-*fgr* gene, *Mol. Cell. Biol.,* 6, 511, 1986.

469. Inoue, K., Ikawa, S., Semba, K., Sukegawa, J., Yamamoto, T., and Toyoshima, K., Isolation and sequencing of cDNA clones homologous to the v-*fgr* oncogene from a human B lymphocyte cell line, IM-9, *Oncogene,* 1, 301, 1987.

470. Watson, R., Oskarsson, M., and Vande Woude, G.F., Human DNA sequence homologous to the transforming gene (*mos*) of Moloney murine sarcoma virus, *Proc. Natl. Acad. Sci. U.S.A.,* 79, 4078, 1982.

471. Chang, E.H., Gonda, M.A., Ellis, R.W., Scolnick, E.M., and Lowy, D.R., Human genome contains four genes homologous to transforming genes of Harvey and Kirsten murine sarcoma viruses, *Proc. Natl. Acad. Sci. U.S.A.,* 79, 4848, 1982.

472. Tabin, C.J., Bradley, S.M., Bargmann, C.I., Weinberg, R.A., Papageorge, A.G., Scolnick, E.M., Dhar, R., Lowy, D.R., and Chang, E.H., Mechanism of activation of a human oncogene, *Nature,* 300, 143, 1982.

473. Reddy, E.P., Reynolds, R.K., Santos, E., and Barbacid, M., A point mutation is responsible for the acquisition of transforming properties by the T24 human bladder carcinoma oncogene, *Nature,* 300, 149, 1982.

474. Capon, D.J., Chen, E.Y., Levinson, A.D., Seeburg, P.H., and Goeddel, D.V., Complete nucleotide sequences of the T24 human bladder carcinoma oncogene and its normal homologue, *Nature,* 301, 33, 1983.

475. Reddy, E.P., Nucleotide sequence analysis of the T24 human bladder carcinoma oncogene, *Science,* 220, 1061, 1983.

476. Shimizu, K., Birnbaum, D., Ruley, M.A., Fasano, O., Suard, Y., Edlund, L., Taparowsky, E., Goldfarb, M., and Wigler, M., Structure of the Ki-*ras* gene of the human lung carcinoma cell line Calu-1, *Nature,* 304, 497, 1983.

477. McGrath, J.P., Capon, D.J., Smith, D.H., Chen, E.Y., Seeburg, P.H., Goeddel, D.V., and Levinson, A.D., Structure and organization of the human Ki-*ras* proto-oncogene and a related processed pseudogene, *Nature,* 304, 501, 1983.

478. Taparowsky, E., Shimizu, K., Goldfarb, M., and Wigler, M., Structure and activation of the human N-*ras* gene, *Cell,* 34, 581, 1983.

479. Miyoshi, J., Kagimoto, M., Soeda, E., and Sakaki, Y., The human c-Ha-*ras*2 is a processed pseudogene inactivated by numerous base substitutions, *Nucleic Acids Res.,* 12, 1821, 1984.

480. Sekiya, T., Fushimi, M., Hori, H., Hirohashi, S., Nishimura, S., and Sugimura, T., Molecular cloning and the total nucleotide sequence of the human c-Ha-*ras*-1 gene activated in a melanoma from a Japanese patient, *Proc. Natl. Acad. Sci. U.S.A.,* 81, 4771, 1984.

481. Hall, A. and Brown, R., Human N-*ras*: cDNA cloning and gene structure, *Nucleic Acids Res.,* 13, 5255, 1985.

482. Lowe, D.G., Capon, D.J., Delwart, E., Sakaguchi, A.Y., Naylor, S.L., and Goeddel, D.V., Structure of the human murine R-*ras* genes, novel genes closely related to *ras* protein-oncogenes, *Cell,* 48, 137, 1987.

483. Honkawa, H., Masahashi, W., Hashimoto, S., and Hashimoto-Gotoh, T., Identification of the principal promoter sequence of the c-H-*ras* transforming oncogene: deletion analysis of th 5'-flanking region by focus formation assay, *Mol. Cell. Biol.,* 7, 2933, 1987.

484. Dalla Favera, R., Gelmann, E.P., Martinotti, S., Franchini, G., Papas, T.S., Gallo, R.C., and Wong-Staal, F., Cloning and characterization of the *onc* gene (v-*myc*) of avian myelocytomatosis virus (MC29), *Proc. Natl. Acad. Sci. U.S.A.,* 79, 6497, 1982.

485. Watson, D.K., Psallidopoulos, M.C., Samuel, K.P., Dalla-Favera, R., and Papas, T.S., Nucleotide sequence analysis of human c-*myc* locus, chicken homologue, and myelocytomatosis virus MC29 transforming gene reveals a highly conserved gene product, *Proc. Natl. Acad. Sci. U.S.A.,* 80, 3642, 1983.

486. Watt, R., Nishikura, K., Sorrentino, J., ar-Rushdi, A., Croce, C.M., and Rovera, G., The structure and nucleotide sequence of the 5' end of the human c-*myc* oncogene, *Proc. Natl. Acad. Sci. U.S.A.,* 80, 6307, 1983.

487. Battey, J., Moulding, C., Taub, R., Murphy, W., Stewart, T., Potter, H., Lenoir, G., and Leder, P., The human c-*myc* oncogene: structural consequences of translocation into the IgH locus in Burkitt lymphoma, *Cell,* 34, 779, 1983.

488. Gazin, C., Dupont de Dinechin, S., Hampe, A., Masson, J.-M., Martin, P., Stehelin, D., and Galibert, F., Nucleotide sequence of the human c-*myc* locus: provocative open reading frame within the first exon, *EMBO J.,* 3, 383, 1984.

489. Michitsch, R.W. and Melera, P.W., Nucleotide sequence of the 3' exon of the human N-myc gene, *Nucleic Acids Res.,* 13, 2545, 1985.

490. Kohl, N.E., Legouy, E., DePinho, R.A., Nisen, P.D., Smith, R.K., Gee, C.E., and Alt, F.W., Human N-*myc* is closely related in organization and sequence to c-*myc*, *Nature,* 319, 73, 1986.

491. Stanton, L.W., Schwab, M., and Bishop, J.M., Nucleotide sequence of the human N-*myc* gene, *Proc. Natl. Acad. Sci. U.S.A.,* 83, 1772, 1986.

492. DePinho, R.A., Hatton, K.S., Tesfaye, A., Yancopoulos, G.D., and Alt, F.W., The human *myc* gene family: structure and activity of L-*myc* and an L-*myc* pseudogene, *Genes Dev.,* 1, 1311, 1987.

493. Kaye, F., Battey, J., Nau, M., Brooks, B., Seifter, E., De Greve, J., Birrer, M., Sausville, E., and Minna, J., Structure and expression of the human L-*myc* gene reveal a complex pattern of alternative mRNA processing, *Mol. Cell. Biol.,* 8, 186, 1988.

494. Heisterkamp, N., Groffen, J., and Stephenson, J.R., The human v-*abl* cellular homologue, *J. Mol. Appl. Genet.,* 2, 57, 1983.

495. Heisterkamp, N., Stephenson, J.R., Groffen, J., Hansen, P.F., de Klein, A., Bartram, C.R., and Grosveld, G., Localization of the c-*abl* oncogene adjacent to a translocation break point in chronic myelocytic leukaemia, *Nature,* 306, 239, 1983.

496. Bernards, A., Rubin, C.M., Westbrook, C.A., Paskind, M., and Baltimore, D., The first intron in the human c-*abl* gene is at least 200 kilobases long and is a target for translocations in chronic myelogenous leukemia, *Mol. Cell. Biol.,* 7, 3231, 1987.

497. Franchini, G., Wong-Staal, F., Baluda, M.A., Lengel, C., and Tronick, S.R., Structural organization and expression of human DNA sequences related to the transforming gene of avian myeloblastosis virus, *Proc. Natl. Acad. Sci. U.S.A.,* 80, 7385, 1983.

498. Bender, T.P. and Kuehl, W.M., Murine *myb* protooncogene mRNA: cDNA sequence and evidence for 5' heterogeneity, *Proc. Natl. Acad. Sci. U.S.A.,* 83, 3204, 1986.

499. Verbeek, J.S., Roebroek, A.J.M., van den Ouweland, A.M.W., Bloemers, H.P.J., and Van de Ven, W.J.M., Human c-*fms* proto-oncogene: comparative analysis with an abnormal allele, *Mol. Cell. Biol.,* 5, 422, 1985.

500. Bonner, T.I., Kerby, S.B., Sutrave, P., Gunnell, M.A., Mark, G., and Rapp, U.R., Structure and biological activity of human homologs of the *raf/mil* oncogene, *Mol. Cell. Biol.,* 5, 1400, 1985.

501. Bonner, T.I., Opperman, H., Seeburg, P., Kerby, S.B., Gunnell, M.A., Young, A.C., and Rapp, U.R., The complete coding sequence of the human *raf* oncogene and the corresponding structure of the c-*raf*-1 gene, *Nucleic Acids Res.,* 14, 1009, 1986.

502. Beck, T.W., Huleihel, M., Gunnell, M., Bonner, T.I., and Rapp, U.R., The complete coding sequence of the human A-*raf*-1 oncogene and transforming activity of a human A-*raf* carrying virus, *Nucleic Acids Res.,* 15, 595, 1987.

503. Matsushime, H., Wang, L.-H., and Shibuya, M., Human c-*ros*-1 gene homologous to the v-*ros* sequence of UR2 sarcoma virus encodes for a membrane receptorlike molecule, *Mol. Cell. Biol.,* 6, 3000, 1986.

504. Sukegawa, J., Semba, K., Yamanashi, Y., Nishizawa, M., Miyajima, N., Yamamoto, T., and Toyoshima, K., Characterization of cDNA clones for the human c-*yes* gene, *Mol. Cell. Biol.,* 7, 41, 1987.

505. Coussens, L., Yang-Feng, T.L., Chen, Y.-C., Gray, A., McGrath, J., Seeburg, P.H., Libermann, T.A., Schlessinger, J., Francke, U., Levinson, A., and Ullrich, A., Tyrosine kinase receptor with extensive homology to EGF receptor shares chromosomal location with *neu* oncogene, *Science,* 230, 1132, 1985.

506. Tal, M., King, C.R., Kraus, M.H., Ullrich, A., Schlessinger, J., and Givol, D., Human HER2 (*neu*) promoter: evidence for multiple mechanisms for transcriptional initiation, *Mol. Cell Biol.,* 7, 2597, 1987.

507. Angel, P., Allegretto, E.A., Okino, S.T., Hattori, K., Boyle, W.J., Hunter, T., and Karin, M., Oncogene *jun* encodes a sequence-specific *trans*-activator similar to AP-1, *Nature,* 332, 166, 1988.

508. Takeya, T. and Hanafusa, H., Structure and sequence of the cellular gene homologous to the RSV *src* gene and the mechanism for generating the transforming virus, *Cell,* 32, 881, 1983.

509. Watson, D.K., Reddy, E.P., Duesberg, P.H., and Papas, T.S., Nucleotide sequence analysis of the chicken c-*myc* gene reveals homologous and unique coding regions by comparison with the transforming gene of avian myelocytomatosis virus MC29, delta*gag-myc, Proc. Natl. Acad. Sci. U.S.A.,* 80, 2146, 1983.

510. Shih, C.-K., Linial, M., Goodenow, M.M., and Hayward, W.S., Nucleotide sequence 5' of the chicken c-*myc* coding region: localization of a noncoding exon that is absent from *myc* transcripts in most avian leukosis virus-induced lymphomas, *Proc. Natl. Acad. Sci. U.S.A.,* 81, 4697, 1984.

511. Nottenburg, C. and Varmus, H.E., Features of the chicken c-*myc* gene that influence the structure of c-*myc* RNA in normal cells and bursal lymphomas, *Mol. Cell. Biol.,* 6, 2800, 1986.

512. Lee, W.-H., Phares, W., and Duesberg, P.H., Structural relationship between the chicken DNA locus, proto-*fps*, and the transforming gene of Fujinami sarcoma virus, d*gag-fps, Virology,* 129, 79, 1983.

513. Seeburg, P.H., Lee, W.-H., Nunn, M.F., and Duesberg, P.H., The 5'ends of the transforming gene of Fujinami sarcoma virus and of the cellular proto-*fps* gene are not colinear, *Virology,* 133, 460, 1984.

514. Huang, C.-C., Hammond, C., and Bishop, J.M., Nucleotide sequence and topography of chicken c-*fps*: genesis of a retroviral oncogene encoding a tyrosine-specific protein kinase, *J. Mol. Biol.,* 181, 175, 1985.

515. Jansen, H.W., Trachmann, C., and Bister, K., Structural relationship between the chicken protooncogene c-*mil* and the retroviral oncogene v-*mil, Virology,* 137, 217, 1984.

516. Jansen, H.W. and Bister, K., Nucleotide sequence analysis of the chicken c-*mil*, the progenitor of the retroviral oncogene v-*mil, Virology,* 143, 359, 1985.

517. Rosson, D. and Reddy, E.P., Nucleotide sequence of chicken c-*myb* complementary DNA and implications for *myb* oncogene activation, *Nature,* 319, 604, 1986.

518. Gerondakis, S. and Bishop, J.M., Structure of the protein encoded by the chicken proto-oncogene c-*myb, Mol. Cell. Biol.,* 6, 3677, 1986.

519. Dvořák, M., Trávnicek, M., Sulová, A., and Riman, J., Two exons specific for the *myb* proto-oncogene found upstream from the avian myeloblastosis virus-transduced *myb* sequences, *Folia Biol (Praha),* 33, 1, 1987.

520. Zahroui, A. and Cuny, G., Nucleotide sequence of the chicken proto-oncogene c-*erbA* corresponding to domain 1 of v-*erbA, Eur. J. Biochem.,* 166, 63, 1987.

521. Podell, S.B. and Sefton, B.M., Chicken proto-oncogene c-*ros* cDNA clones: identification of a c-*ros* RNA transcript and deduction of the amino acid sequence of the carboxyl terminus of the c-*ros* product, *Oncogene,* 2, 9, 1987.

522. Mölders, H., Jenuwein, T., Adamkiewicz, J., and Müller, R., Isolation and structural analysis of a biologically active chicken c-*fos* cDNA: identification of evolutionarily conserved domains in *fos* protein, *Oncogene,* 1, 377, 1987.

523. Fujiwara, K.T., Ashida, K., Nishina, H., Iba, H., Miyajima, N., Nishizawa, M., and Kawai, S., The chicken c-*fos* gene: cloning and nucleotide sequence analysis, *J. Virol.,* 61, 4012, 1987.

524. Watson, D.K., McWilliams, M.J., and Papas, T.S., Molecular organization of the chicken *ets* locus, *Virology,* 164, 99, 1988.

525. Wilhelmsen, K.C. and Temin, H.M., Structure and dimorphism of c-*rel* (turkey), the cellular homolog to the oncogene of reticuloendotheliosis virus strain T, *J. Virol.,* 49, 521, 1984.

526. Wilhelmsen, K.C., Eggleton, K., and Temin, H.M., Nucleic acid sequences of the oncogene v-*rel* in reticuloendotheliosis virus strain T and its cellular homolog, the proto-oncogene c-*rel, J. Virol.,* 52, 172, 1984.

527. Wang, J.Y.J., Ledley, F., Goff, S., Lee, R., Groner, Y., and Baltimore, D., The mouse c-*abl* locus: molecular cloning and characterization, *Cell,* 36, 349, 1984.

528. Schalken, J.A., van den Ouweland, A.M.W., Bloemers, H.P.J., and van de Ven, W.J.M., Characterization of the feline c-*abl* proto-oncogene, *Biochim. Biophys. Acta,* 824, 104, 1985.

529. van der Hoorn, F.A. and Firzlaff, J., Complete c-*mos* (rat) nucleotide sequence: presence of conserved domains in c-*mos* proteins, *Nucleic Acids Res.,* 12, 2147, 1984.

530. Bargmann, C.I., Hung, M.-C., and Weinberg, R.A., The *neu* oncogene encodes an epidermal growth factor receptor-related protein, *Nature,* 319, 226, 1986.

531. Ruta, M., Wolford, R., DeFeo-Jones, D., Ellis, R.W., and Scolnick, E.M., Nucleotide sequences of the two rat cellular *ras*^{H} genes, *Mol. Cell. Biol.,* 6, 1706, 1986.

532. Damante, G., Filetti, S., and Rapoport, B., Nucleotide sequence and characterization of the 5' flanking region of the rat Ha-*ras* protooncogene, *Proc. Natl. Acad. Sci. U.S.A.,* 84, 774, 1987.

533. Hayashi, K., Makino, R., Kawamura, H., Arisawa, A., and Yoneda, K., Characterization of rat c-*myc* and adjacent regions, *Nucleic Acids Res.,* 15, 6419, 1987.
534. Ishikawa, F., Takaku, F., Nagao, M., and Sugimura, T., Cysteine-rich regions conserved in amino-terminal halves of *raf* gene family products and protein kinase C, *Jpn. J. Cancer Res.,* 77, 1183, 1986.
535. Ishikawa, F., Takaku, F., Nagao, M., and Sugimura, T., The complete primary structure of the rat A-*raf* cDNA coding region: conservation of the putative regulatory regions present in rat c-*raf*, *Oncogene Res.,* 1, 243, 1987.
536. Gonda, T.J., Gough, N.M., Dunn, A.R., and de Blaquiere, J., Nucleotide sequence of cDNA clones of the murine *myb* proto-oncogene, *EMBO J.,* 4, 2003, 1985.
537. George, D.L., Scott, A.F., Trusko, S., Glick, B., Ford, E., and Dorney, D.J., Structure and expression of amplified cKi-*ras* gene sequences in Y1 mouse adrenal tumor cells, *EMBO J.,* 4, 1199, 1985.
538. Castle, S. and Sheiness, D., Structural organization of the mouse proto-myb gene, *Biochem. Biophys. Res. Commun.,* 132, 688, 1985.
539. DePinho, R.A., Legouy, E., Feldman, L.B., Kohl, N.E., Yancopoulos, G.D., and Alt, F.W., Structure and expression of the murine N-*myc* gene, *Proc. Natl. Acad. Sci. U.S.A.,* 83, 1827, 1986.
540. Taya, Y., Mizusawa, S., and Nishimura, S., Nucleotide sequence of the coding region of the mouse N-*myc* gene, *EMBO J.,* 5, 1215, 1986.
541. Lavu, S. and Reddy, E.P., Structural organization and nucleotide sequence of mouse c-*myb* oncogene: activation in ABPL tumors is due to viral integration in an intron which results in the deletion of the 5′ coding sequences, *Nucleic Acids Res.,* 14, 5309, 1986.
542. Legouy, E., DePinho, R., Zimmerman, K., Collum, R., Yancopoulos, G., Mitsock, L., Kriz, R., and Alt, F.W., Structure and expression of the murine L-*myc* gene, *EMBO J.,* 6, 3359, 1987.
543. Rothwell, V.M. and Rohrschneider, L.R., Murine c-*fms* cDNA: cloning, sequence analysis and retroviral expression, *Oncogene Res.,* 1, 311, 1987.
544. Doniger, J., Differential conservation of non-coding regions within human and guinea pig N-*ras* genes, *Oncogene,* 1, 331, 1987.
545. Doniger, J., Alternative splicing results in a truncated N-*ras* protein, *Oncogene,* 2, 293, 1988.
546. Soe, L.H. and Roy-Burman, P., Structure of the polymorphic feline c-*myc* oncogene locus, *Gene,* 31, 123, 1984.
547. Verbeek, J.S., de Ruyter, P., Bloemers, H.P.J., and Van de Ven, W.J.M., Molecular cloning and characterization of feline cellular genetic sequences homologous to the oncogene of the McDonough strain of feline sarcoma virus, *Virology,* 141, 322, 1985.
548. Soe, L.H., Ghosh, A.K., Maxson, R.E., Hoover, E.A., Hardy, W.D., Jr., and Roy-Burman, P., Nucleotide sequence of the 1.2-kb 3′-region and genotype distribution of two common c-*myc* alleles of the domestic cat, *Gene,* 47, 185, 1986.
549. Roebroek, A.J.M., Schalken, J.A., Onnekink, C., Bloemers, H.P.J., and Van de Ven, W.J.M., Structure of the feline c-*fes/fps* proto-oncogene: genesis of a retroviral oncogene, *J. Virol.,* 61, 2009, 1987.
550. Wadsworth, S.C., Madhavan, K., and Bilodeau, and Wentworth, D., Maternal inheritance of transcripts from three *Drosophila* src-related genes, *Nucleic Acids Res.,* 13, 2153, 1985.
551. Simon, M.A., Drees, B., Kornberg, T., and Bishop, J.M., The nucleotide sequence and the tissue-specific expression of *Drosophila* c-*src*, *Cell,* 42, 841, 1985.
552. Mark, G.E., MacIntyre, R.J., Digan, M.E., Ambrosio, L., and Perrimon, N., *Drosophila melanogaster* homologs of the *raf* oncogene, *Mol. Cell. Biol.,* 7, 2134, 1987.
553. Wiman, K.G., Clarkson, B., Hayday, A.C., Saito, H., Tonegawa, S., and Hayward, W.S., Activation of a translocated c-*myc* gene: role of structural alterations in the upstream region, *Proc. Natl. Acad. Sci. U.S.A.,* 81, 6798, 1984.
554. Krontiris, T.G., DiMartino, N.A., Colb, M., Mitcheson, H.D., and Parkinson, D.R., Human restriction fragment length polymorphisms and cancer risk assessment, *J. Cell. Biochem.,* 30, 319, 1986.
555. Larsen, C.J., Polymorphisme génétique et susceptibilité au cancer, *Nouv. Rev. Fr. Hematol.,* 30, 39, 1988.
556. Xu, D.Q., Guilhot, S., and Galibert, F., Restriction fragment length polymorphism of the human c-*fms* gene, *Proc. Natl. Acad. Sci. U.S.A.,* 82, 2862, 1985.
557. Verbeek, J.S., Roebroek, A.J.M., van den Ouweland, A.M.W., Bloemers, H.P.J., and Van de Ven, W.J.M., Human c-*fms* proto-oncogene: comparative analysis with an abnormal allele, *Mol. Cell. Biol.,* 5, 422, 1985.
558. Verbeek, J.S., van Heerikhuizen, H., de Pauw, B.E., Haanen, C., Bloemers, H.P.J., and Van de Ven, W.J.M., A hereditary abnormal c-*fms* proto-oncogene in a patient with acute lymphocytic leukaemia and congenital hypothyroidism, *Br. J. Haematol.,* 61, 135, 1985.
559. Mathieu-Mahul, D., Xu, D.Q., Saule, S., Lidereau, R., Berger, R., Mauchauffé, M., and Larsen, C.J., An EcoRI restriction fragment length polymorphism (RFLP) in the human c-erb A locus, *Hum. Genet.,* 71, 41, 1985.
560. Fung, Y.-K.T., Lewis, W.G., Crittenden, L.B., and Kung, H.-J., Activation of the cellular oncogene c-*erbB* by LTR insertion: molecular basis for induction of erythroblastosis by avian leukosis virus, *Cell,* 33, 357, 1983.
561. Raines, M.A., Lewis, W.G., Crittenden, L.B., and Kung, H.-J., c-*erbB* activation in avian leukosis virus-induced erythroblastosis: clustered integration sites and the arrangement of provirus in the c-*erbB* alleles, *Proc. Natl. Acad. Sci. U.S.A.,* 82, 2287, 1985.

562. Rider, S.H., Bailey, C.J., Voss, R., Sheer, D., Hiorns, L.R., and Solomon, E., RFLP for the human erb-A1 gene, *Nucleic Acids Res.,* 15, 863, 1987.

563. Lidereau, R., Mathieu-Mahul, D., Theillet, C., Renaud, M., Mauchauffé, M., Gest, J., and Larsen, C.-J., Presence of an allelic *Eco*RI restriction fragment of the c-*mos* locus in leukocyte and tumor cell DNAs of breast cancer patients, *Proc. Natl. Acad. Sci. U.S.A.,* 82, 7068, 1985.

564. Hollstein, M., Montesano, R., and Yamasaki, H., Presence of an EcoRI RFLP of the c-*mos* locus in normal and tumor tissue of esophageal cancer patients, *Nucleic Acids Res.,* 14, 8695, 1986.

565. Lidereau, R., Cole, S.T., Larsen, C.J., and Mathieu-Mahul, D., A single point mutation responsible for c-*mos* polymorphism in cancer patients, *Oncogene,* 1, 235, 1987.

566. Corell, B. and Zoll, B., Evidence against a tumour-specific *Eco*RI RFLP in the c-*mos* locus, *FEBS Lett.,* 230, 81, 1988.

567. Krontiris, T.G., DiMartino, N.A., Colb, M., and Parkinson, D.R., Unique allelic restriction fragments of the human Ha-*ras* locus in leukocyte and tumour DNAs of cancer patients, *Nature,* 313, 369, 1985.

568. Chandler, L.A., Ghazi, H., Jones, P.A., Boukamp, P., and Fusenig, N.E., Allele-specific methylation of the human c-Ha-*ras*-1 gene, *Cell,* 50, 711, 1987.

569. Radice, P., Pierotti, M.A., Borrello, M.G., Illeni, M.T., Rovini, D., and Dalla Porta, G., HRAS1 proto-oncogene polymorphisms in human malignant melanoma: TaqI defined alleles significantly associated with the disease, *Oncogene,* 2, 91, 1987.

570. Thein, S.L., Oscier, D.G., Flint, J., and Wainscoat, J.S., Ha-*ras* hypervariable alleles in myelodysplasia, *Nature,* 321, 84, 1986.

571. Sutherland, C., Shaw, H.M., Roberts, C., Grace, J., Stewart, M.M., McCarthy, W.H., and Kefford, R.F., Harvey-*ras* oncogene restriction fragment alleles in familial melanoma kindreds, *Br. J. Cancer,* 54, 787, 1986.

572. Gerhard, D.S., Dracopoli, N.C., Bale, S.J., Houghton, A.N., Watkins, P., Payne, C.E., Greene, M.H., and Housman, D.E., Evidence against Ha-*ras*-1 involvement in sporadic and familial melanoma, *Nature,* 325, 73, 1987.

573. Ishikawa, J., Maeda, S., Takahashi, R., Kamidono, R., and Sugiyama, T., Lack of correlation between rare Ha-*ras* alleles and urothelial cancer in Japan, *Int. J. Cancer,* 40, 474, 1987.

574. Hayward, N.K., Keegan, R., Nancarrow, D.J., Little, M.H., Smith, P.J., Gardiner, R.A., Seymour, G.J., Kidson, C., and Lavin, M.F., c-Ha-ras-1 alleles in bladder cancer, Wilms' tumour and malignant melanoma, *Hum. Genet.,* 78, 115, 1988.

575. Ryan, J., Barker, P.E., Nesbitt, M.N., and Ruddle, F.H., *KRAS2* as a genetic marker for lung tumor susceptibility in inbred mice, *J. Natl. Cancer Inst.,* 79, 1351, 1987.

576. van den Ouweland, A.M.W., Breuer, M.L., Steenbergh, P.H., Schalken, J.A., Bloemers, H.P.J., and Van de Ven, W.J.M., Comparative analysis of the human and feline c-*sis* proto-oncogenes. Identification of 5'human c-*sis* coding sequences that are not homologous to the transforming gene of simian sarcoma virus, *Biochim. Biophys. Acta,* 825, 140, 1985.

577. Xu, D.Q. and Galibert, F., Restriction fragment length polymorphism caused by a deletion within the human c-*abl* gene (*ABL*), *Proc. Natl. Acad. Sci. U.S.A.,* 83, 3447, 1986.

578. Daniel, L., Ahmed, C.M.I., Bloodgood, R.S., Kidd, J.R., Castiglione, C.M., Duttagupta, S., and Lebowitz, Polymorphism of the human c-*abl* gene: relation to incidence and couse of chronic myelogenous leukemia, *Oncogene,* 1, 193, 1987.

579. Yuasa, Y., Reddy, E.P., Rhim, J.S., Tronick, S.R., and Aaronson, S.A., Activated N-*ras* in a human rectal carcinoma cell line associated with clonal homozygosity in *myb* locus-restriction fragment polymorphism, *Jpn. J. Cancer Res.,* 77, 639, 1986.

580. Mock, B., Skurla, R., Huppi, K., D'Hoostelaere, L., Klinman, D., and Mushinsky, J.F., A restriction fragment length polymorphism at the murine c-*myb* locus, *Nucleic Acids Res.,* 15, 4700, 1987.

581. Kurosawa, H., Yamada, M., and Nagakome, Y., Restriction fragment length polymorphisms of the human N-*myc* gene: relationship to gene amplification, *Oncogene,* 2, 85, 1987.

582. Kawashima, K., Shikama, H., Imoto, K., Izawa, M., Naruke, T., Okabayashi, K., and Nishimura, S., Close correlation between restriction fragment length polymorphisms of the L-*MYC* gene and metastasis of human lung cancer to the lymph nodes and other organs, *Proc. Natl. Acad. Sci. U.S.A.,* 85, 2353, 1988.

583. Chenevix-Trench, G., Behm, F., and Westin, E., Allelic variation of the c-*raf-1* oncogene in non-Hodgkin's lymphoma, *Leukemia,* 1, 82, 1987.

584. Savage, P.D., Hanson, C.A., and Kersey, J.H., Identification of a restriction fragment length polymorphism involving the oncogene ETS-1 on chromosome 11q23, *Blood,* 70, 327, 1987.

585. Willard, H.F., Skolnick, M.H., Pearson, P.L., and Mandel, J.L., Report of the committee on human gene mapping by recombinant DNA techniques, *Cytogenet. Cell Genet.,* 40, 360, 1985.

586. Sacchi, N., Perroni, L., and Papas, T.S., A polymorphic *Sst*I site within the human ETS-1 gene in the 11q23 region, *Nucleic Acids Res.,* 14, 9545, 1986.

587. Bishop, J.M., Drees, B., Katzen, A.L., Kornberg, T.B., and Simon, M.A., Proto-oncogenes of *Drosophila melanogaster, Cold Spring Harbor Symp. Quant. Biol.,* 50, 727, 1985.

588. Wheals, A.E., Oncogene homologues in yeast, *BioEssays,* 3, 108, 1985.
589. Prakash, K. and Seligy, V.L., Oncogene related sequences in fungi: linkage of some to actin, *Biochem. Biophys. Res. Commun.,* 133, 2983, 1985.
590. Stallings, R.L., Munk, A.C., Longmire, J.L., Jett, J.H., Wilder, M.E., Siciliano, M.J., Adair, G.M., and Crawford, B.D., Oncogenic and linkage groups conservation during mammalian chromosome evolution, *Chromosoma (Berlin),* 92, 156, 1985.
591. Gojobori, T. and Yokoyama, S., Rates of evolution of the retroviral oncogene of Moloney murine sarcoma virus and of its cellular homologues, *Proc. Natl. Acad. Sci. U.S.A.,* 82, 4198, 1985.
592. Gojobori, T. and Yokoyama, S., Molecular evolutionary rates of oncogenes, *J. Mol. Evol.,* 26, 148, 1987.
593. Simon, M.A., Kornberg, T.B., and Bishop, J.M., Three loci related to the *src* oncogene and tyrosine-specific protein kinase activity in *Drosophila, Nature,* 302, 837, 1983.
594. Telford, J., Burckhardt, J., Butler, B., and Pirrotta, V., Alternative processing and developmental control of the transcripts of the *Drosophila abl* oncogene homologue, *EMBO J.,* 4, 2609, 1985.
595. Henkemeyer, M.J., Bennett, R.L., Gertler, F.B., and Hoffmann, F.M., DNA sequence, structure, and tyrosine kinase activity of the *Drosophila melanogaster* Abelson proto-oncogene homolog, *Mol. Cell. Biol.,* 8, 843, 1988.
596. Henkemeyer, M.J., Gertler, F.B., Goodman, W., and Hoffmann, F.M., The Drosophila Abelson proto-oncogene homolog: identification of mutant alleles that have pleiotropic effects late in development, *Cell,* 51, 821, 1987.
597. Kamps, M.P., Taylor, S.S., and Sefton, B.M., Direct evidence that oncogenic tyrosine kinases and cyclic AMP-dependent protein kinase have homologous ATP-binding sites, *Nature,* 310, 589, 1984.
598. Ullrich, A., Bell, J.R., Chen, E.Y., Herrera, R., Petruzzelli, L.M., Dull, T.J., Gray, A., Coussens, L., Liao, Y.-C., Tsubokawa, M., Mason, A., Seeburg, P.H., Grunfeld, C., Rosen, O.M., and Ramachandran, J., Human insulin receptor and its relationship to the tyrosine kinase family of oncogenes, *Nature,* 313, 756, 1985.
599. Lowy, D.R. and Willumsen, B.M., The *ras* gene family, *Cancer Surv.,* 5, 275, 1986.
600. Barbacid, M., *ras* genes, *Annu. Rev. Biochem.,* 56, 779, 1987.
601. Nemoto, N., Kodama, K., Tazawa, A., Masahito, P., and Ishikawa, T., Extensive sequence homology of the goldfish *ras* gene to mammalian *ras* genes, *Differentiation,* 32, 17, 1986.
602. Temeles, G.L., Gibbs, J.B., D'Alonzo, J.S., Sigal, I.S., and Scolnick, E.M., Yeast and mammalian *ras* proteins have conserved biochemical properties, *Nature,* 313, 700, 1985.
603. Mozer, B., Marlor, R., Parkhurst, S., and Corces, V., Characterization and developmental expression of a *Drosophila ras* oncogene, *Mol. Cell. Biol.,* 5, 885, 1985.
604. Müller, R. and Verma, I.M., Expression of cellular oncogenes, *Curr. Top. Microbiol. Immunol.,* 112, 73, 1984.
605. Adamson, E.D., Oncogenes in development, *Development,* 99, 449, 1987.
606. Adamson, E.D., Expression of proto-oncogenes in the placenta, *Placenta,* 8, 449, 1987.
607. Kaczmarek, L., Protooncogene expression during the cell cycle, *Lab. Invest.,* 54, 365, 1986.
608. Denhardt, D.T., Edwards, D.R., and Parfett, C.L.J., Gene expression during the mammalian cell cycle, *Biochim. Biophys. Acta,* 865, 83, 1986.
609. Ferrari, S. and Baserga, R., Oncogenes and cell cycle genes, *BioEssays,* 7, 9, 1987.
610. Rittling, S.R. and Baserga, R., Regulatory mechanisms in the expression of cell cycle dependent genes, *Anticancer Res.,* 7, 541, 1987.
611. Rowley, P.T. and Skuse, G.R., Oncogene expression in myelopoiesis, *Int. J. Cell Cloning,* 5, 255, 1987.
612. Reed, J.C., Alpers, J.D., Nowell, P.C., and Hoover, R.G., Sequential expression of protooncogenes during lectin-stimulated mitogenesis of normal human lymphocytes, *Proc. Natl. Acad. Sci. U.S.A.,* 83, 3982, 1986.
613. Calabretta, B., Kaczmarek, L., Mars, W., Ochoa, D., Gibson, C.W., Hirschhorn, R.R., and Baserga, R., Cell-cycle-specific genes differentially expressed in human leukemias, *Proc. Natl. Acad. Sci. U.S.A.,* 82, 4463, 1985.
614. Kaczmarek, L., Calabretta, B., and Baserga, R., Expression of cell-cycle-dependent genes in phytohemagglutinin-stimulated human lymphocytes, *Proc. Natl. Acad. Sci. U.S.A.,* 82, 5375, 1985.
615. Rittling, S.R., Gibson, C.W., Ferrari, S., and Baserga, R., The effect of cycloheximide on the expression of cell cycle dependent genes, *Biochem. Biophys. Res. Commun.,* 132, 327, 1985.
616. Thompson, C.B., Challoner, P.B., Neiman, P.E., and Groudine, M., Levels of c-*myc* oncogene mRNA are invariant throughout the cell cycle, *Nature,* 314, 363, 1985.
617. Hann, S.R., Thompson, C.B., and Eisenman, R.N., c-*myc* oncogene protein synthesis is independent of the cell cycle in human and avian cells, *Nature,* 314, 366, 1985.
618. Bravo, R., Burckhardt, J., and Müller, R., Persistence of the complement state in mouse fibroblasts is independent of c-*fos* and c-*myc* expression, *Exp. Cell Res.,* 160, 540, 1985.
619. Bravo, R., Burckhardt, J., Curran, T., and Müller, R., Expression of c-*fos* in NIH3T3 cells is very low but inducible throughout the cell cycle, *EMBO J.,* 5, 695, 1986.
620. Lev, Z., Kimchie, Z., Hessel, R., and Segev, O., Expression of *ras* cellular oncogenes during development of *Drosophila melanogaster, Mol. Cell. Biol.,* 5, 1540, 1985.

621. Lev, Z., Leibovitz, N., Segev, O., and Shilo, B.-Z., Expression of the *src* and *abl* cellular oncogenes during development of *Drosophila melanogaster*, *Mol. Cell. Biol.*, 4, 982, 1984.

622. Rijsewijk, F., Scheuermann, M., Wagenaar, E., Parren, P., Weigel, D., and Nusse, R., The Drosophila homolog of the mouse mammary oncogene *int*-1 is identical to the segment polarity gene *wingless*, *Cell*, 50, 649, 1987.

623. Schwab, M. and Anders, A., Carcinogenesis in *Xiphophorus* and the role of the genotype in tumor susceptibility, in *Neoplasms — Comparative Pathology of Growth in Animals, Plants, and Man*, Kaiser, H.E., Ed., Williams and Wilkins, Baltimore, 1981, 451.

624. Anders, F., Schartl, M., and Scholl, E., Evaluation of environmental and hereditary factors in carcinogenesis based on studies in *Xiphophorus*, in *Philetic Approaches to Cancer*, Dawe, C.J., Ed., Japan Scientific Society Press, Tokyo, 1981, 289.

625. Anders, F., Scholl, E., and Schartl, M., Environmental and hereditary factors in the causation of neoplasia, based on studies in the *Xiphophorus* fish melanoma system, in *Phenotypic Expression in Pigment Cells*, Seiji, M., Ed., University of Tokyo Press, Tokyo, 1981, 491.

626. Vielkind, J. and Vielkind, U., Melanoma formation in fish of the genus *Xiphophorus*: a genetically-based disorder in the determination and differentiation of a specific pigment cell, *Can. J. Genet. Cytol.*, 24, 133, 1982.

627. Ozato, K. and Wakamatsu, Y., Multi-step regulation of oncogene expression in fish hereditary melanoma, *Differentiation*, 24, 181, 1983.

628. Anders, F., Schartl, M., Barnekow, A., Schmidt, C.R., Lüke, W., Jaenel-Dess, G., and Anders, A., The genes that carcinogens act upon, *Haematol. Blood Transfusion*, 29, 228, 1985.

629. Schartl, M., Barnekow, A., Bauer, H., and Anders, F., Correlations of inheritance and expression between a tumor gene and the cellular homolog of the Rous sarcoma virus-transforming gene in *Xiphophorus*, *Cancer Res.*, 42, 4222, 1982.

630. Vielkind, J.R. and Dippel, E., Oncogene-related sequences in xiphophorin fish prone to hereditary melanoma formation, *Can. J. Genet. Cytol.*, 26, 607, 1984.

631. Mäueler, W., Raulf, F., and Schartl, M., Expression of proto-oncogenes in embryonic, adult, and transformed tissue of *Xiphophorus* (Teleostei: Poeciliidae), *Oncogene*, 2, 421, 1988.

632. Gonda, T.J., Sheiness, D.K., and Bishop, J.M., Transcripts from the cellular homologs of retroviral oncogenes: distribution among chicken tissues, *Mol. Cell. Biol.*, 2, 617, 1982.

633. Coll, J., Saule, S., Martin, P., Raes, M.B., Lagrou, C., Graf, T., Beug, H., Simon, I.E., and Stehelin, D., The cellular oncogenes c-*myc*, c-*myb* and c-*erb* are transcribed in defined types of avian hematopoietic cells, *Exp. Cell Res.*, 149, 151, 1983.

634. Gessler, M. and Barnekow, A., Differential expression of the cellular oncogenes c-*src* and c-*yes* in embryonal and adult chicken tissues, *Biosci. Rep.*, 4, 757, 1984.

635. Müller, R., Slamon, D.J., Tremblay, J.M., Cline, M.J., and Verma, I.M., Differential expression of cellular oncogenes during pre- and postnatal development of the mouse, *Nature*, 299, 640, 1982.

636. Goyette, M., Petropoulos, C.J., Shank, P.R., and Fausto, N., Expression of a cellular oncogene during liver regeneration, *Science*, 219, 510, 1983.

637. Fausto, N. and Shank, P.R., Oncogene expression in liver regeneration and hepatocarcinogenesis, *Hepatology*, 3, 1016, 1983.

638. Wang, J.Y.J. and Baltimore, D., Cellular RNA homologous to the Abelson murine leukemia virus transforming gene: expression and relationship to the viral sequence, *Mol. Cell. Endocrinol.*, 3, 773, 1983.

639. Müller, R., Slamon, D.J., Adamson, E.D., Tremblay, J.M., Müller, D., Cline, M.J., and Verma, I.M., Transcription of c-*onc* genes c-*ras*^{Ki} and c-*fms* during mouse development, *Mol. Cell. Biol.*, 3, 1062, 1986.

640. Slamon, D.J. and Cline, M.J., Expression of cellular oncogenes during embryonic and fetal development of the mouse, *Proc. Natl. Acad. Sci. U.S.A.*, 81, 7141, 1984.

641. Leon, J., Guerrero, I., and Pellicer, A., Differential expression of the *ras* gene family in mice, *Mol. Cell. Biol.*, 7, 1535, 1987.

642. Zimmerman, K.A., Yancopoulos, G.D., Collum, R.G., Smith, R.K., Kohl, N.E., Denis, K.A., Nau, M.M., Witte, O.N., Toran-Allerand, D., Gee, C.E., Minna, J.D., and Alt, F.W., Differential expression of *myc* family genes during murine development, *Nature*, 319, 780, 1986.

643. Ponzetto, C. and Wolgemuth, D.J., Haploid expression of a unique c-*abl* transcript in the mouse male germ line, *Mol. Cell. Biol.*, 5, 1791, 1985.

644. Mason, I., Murphy, D., and Hogan, B.L.M., Expression of c-fos in parietal endoderm, amnion and differentiating F9 teratocarcinoma cells, *Differentiation*, 30, 76, 1985.

645. Dony, C. and Gruss, P., Proto-oncogene c-*fos* expression in growth regions of fetal bone and mesodermal web tissue, *Nature*, 328, 711, 1987.

646. Schneider, M.D., Payne, P.A., Ueno, H., Perryman, M.B., and Roberts, R., Dissociated expression of c-*myc* and a *fos*-related competence gene during cardiac myogenesis, *Mol. Cell. Biol.*, 6, 4140, 1986.

647. Sheiness, D. and Gardinier, M., Expression of a proto-oncogene (proto-*myb*) in hemopoietic tissues of mice, *Mol. Cell. Biol.*, 4, 1206, 1984.

648. Jakobovits, A., Shackleford, G.M., Varmus, H.E., and Martin, G.R., Two proto-oncogenes implicated in mammary carcinogenesis, *int-1* and *int-2* are independently regulated during mouse development, *Proc. Natl. Acad. Sci. U.S.A.*, 83, 7806, 1986.

649. Wilkinson, D.G., Bailes, J.A., and McMahon, A.P., Expression of the proto-oncogene *int-1* is restricted to specific neural cells in the developing mouse embryo, *Cell*, 50, 79, 1987.

650. Wilkinson, D.G., Peters, G., Dickson, C., and McMahon, A.P., Expression of the FGF-related proto-oncogene *int-2* during gastrulation and neurulation in the mouse, *EMBO J.*, 7, 691, 1988.

651. Shackleford, G.M. and Varmus, H.E., Expression of the proto-oncogene *int-1* is restricted to postmeiotic male germ cells and the neural tube of mid-gestational embryos, *Cell*, 50, 89, 1987.

652. Claycomb, W.C. and Lanson, N.A., Jr., Proto-oncogene expression in proliferating and differentiating cardiac and skeletal muscle, *Biochem. J.*, 247, 701, 1987.

653. Willman, C.L., Stewart, C.C., Griffith, J.K., Stewart, S.J., and Tomasi, T.B., Differential expression and regulation of the *src* and c-*fgr* protooncogenes in myelomonocytic cells, *Proc. Natl. Acad. Sci. U.S.A.*, 84, 4480, 1987.

654. Goyette, M., Petropoulos, C.J., Shank, P.R., and Fausto, N., Regulated transcription of c-Ki-*ras* and c-*myc* during compensatory growth of rat liver, *Mol. Cell. Biol.*, 4, 1493, 1984.

655. Thompson, N.L., Mead, J.E., Braun, L., Goyette, M., Shank, P.R., and Fausto, N., Sequential protooncogene expression during rat liver regeneration, *Cancer Res.*, 46, 3111, 1986.

656. Makino, R., Hayashi, K., and Sugimura, T., c-*myc* transcript is induced in rat liver at a very early stage of regeneration or by cycloheximide treatment, *Nature*, 310, 697, 1984.

657. Zhang, X.-K., Huang, D.-P., Chiu, D.-K., and Chiu, J.-F., The expression of oncogenes in human developing liver and hepatomas, *Biochem. Biophys. Res. Commun.*, 142, 932, 1987.

658. Emilia, G., Donelli, A., Ferrari, S., Torelli, U., Selleri, L., Zucchini, P., Moretti, L., Venturelli, D., Ceccherrelli, G., and Torelli, G., Cellular levels of mRNA from c-*myc*, c-*myb* and c-*fes onc*-genes in normal myeloid and erythroid precursors of human bone marrow: an *in situ* hybridization study, *Br. J. Haematol.*, 62, 287, 1986.

659. Evinger-Hodges, M.J., Dicke, K.A., Gutterman, J.U., and Blick, M., Proto-oncogene expression in human normal bone marrow, *Leukemia*, 1, 597, 1987.

660. Jacobs, C. and Rubsamen, H., Expression of pp60[c-src] protein kinase in adult and fetal human tissue: high activities in some sarcomas and mammary carcinomas, *Cancer Res.*, 43, 1696, 1983.

661. Müller, R., Tremblay, J.M., Adamson, E.D., and Verma, I.D., Tissue and cell type-specific expression of two human c-*onc* genes, *Nature*, 304, 454, 1983.

662. Mitchell, R.L., Zokas, L., Schreiber, R.D., and Verma, I.D., Rapid induction of the expression of proto-oncogene *fos* during human monocytic differentiation, *Cell*, 40, 209, 1985.

663. Sariban, E., Mitchell, T., and Kufe, D., Expression of the c-*fms* proto-oncogene during human monocytic differentiation, *Nature*, 316, 64, 1985.

664. Pfeifer-Ohlsson, S., Goustin, A.S., Rydnert, J., Wahlstrom, T., Bjersing, L., Stehelin, D., and Ohlsson, R., Spatial and temporal pattern of cellular *myc* oncogene expression in developing human placenta: implications for embryonic cell proliferation, *Cell*, 38, 585, 1984.

665. Maruo, T. and Mochizuki, M., Immunohistochemical localization of epidermal growth factor receptor and myc oncogene product in human placenta: implication for trophoblast proliferation and differentiation, *Am. J. Obstet. Gynecol.*, 156, 721, 1987.

666. Goustin, A.S., Betsholtz, C., Pfeifer-Ohlsson, S., Persson, H., Rydnert, J., Bywater, M., Holmgren, G., Heldin, C.-H., Westermark, B., and Ohlsson, R., Coexpression of the *sis* and *myc* proto-oncogenes in developing human placenta suggests autocrine control of trophoblast growth, *Cell*, 41, 301, 1985.

667. Sarkar, S., Kacinski, B.M., Kohorn, E.I., Merino, M.J., Carter, D., and Blakemore, K.J., Demonstration of myc and ras oncogene expression by hybridization in situ in hydatiform mole and in BeWo choriocarcinoma cell line, *Am. J. Obstet. Gynecol.*, 154, 390, 1986.

668. Kelly, K., Cochran, B.H., Stiles, C.D., and Leder, P., Cell-specific regulation of the c-*myc* gene by lymphocyte mitogens and platelet-derived growth factor, *Cell*, 35, 603, 1983.

669. Campisi, J., Gray, H.E., Pardee, A.B., Dean, M., and Sonenshein, G.E., Cell-cycle control of c-*myc* but not c-*ras* expression is lost following chemical transformation, *Cell*, 36, 241, 1984.

670. McCormack, J.E., Pepe, V.H., Kent, R.B., Dean, M., Marshak-Rothstein, A., and Sonenshein, G.E., Specific regulation of c-*myc* oncogene expression in a murine B-cell lymphoma, *Proc. Natl. Acad. Sci. U.S.A.*, 81, 5546, 1984.

671. Persson, H., Hennighausen, L., Taub, R., DeGrado, W., and Leder, P., Antibodies to human c-*myc* oncogene product: evidence of an evolutionarily conserved protein induced during cell proliferation, *Science*, 225, 687, 1984.

672. Ferrari, S., Torelli, U., Selleri, L., Donelli, A., Venturelli, D., Narni, F., Moretti, L., and Torelli, G., Study of the levels of expression of two oncogenes, c-*myc* and c-*myb*, in acute and chronic leukemias of both lymphoid and myeloid lineage, *Leukemia Res.*, 9, 833, 1985.

673. Starksen, N.F., Simpson, P.C., Bishopric, N., Coughlin, S.R., Lee, W.M.F., Escobedo, J.A., and Williams, L.T., Cardiac myocyte hypertrophy is associated with c-*myc* protooncogene expression, *Proc. Natl. Acad. Sci. U.S.A.,* 83, 8348, 1986.

674. Campisi, J., Gray, H.E., Pardee, A.B., Dean, M., and Sonenshein, G.E., Cell-cycle control of c-*myc* but not c-*ras* expression is lost following chemical transformation, *Cell,* 36, 241, 1984.

675. Stewart, T.A., Bellve, A.R., and Leder, P., Transcription and promoter usage of the c-*myc* gene in normal somatic and spermatogenic cells, *Science,* 226, 707, 1984.

676. Ferrari, S., Torelli, U., Selleri, L., Donelli, A., Venturelli, D., Moretti, L., and Torelli, G., Expression of human c-*fes* *onc*-gene occurs at detectable levels in myeloid but not in lymphoid cell populations, *Br. J. Haematol.,* 59, 21, 1985.

677. Feldman, R.A., Gabrilove, J.L., Tam, J.P., Moore, M.A.S., and Hanafusa, H., Specific expression of the human cellular *fps/fes*-encoded protein NCP92 in normal and leukemic myeloid cells, *Proc. Natl. Acad. Sci. U.S.A.,* 82, 2379, 1985.

678. Ferrari, S., Torelli, U., Selleri, L., Donelli, A., Venturelli, D., Moretti, L., and Torelli, G., Expression of human c-*fes* *onc* gene occurs at detectable levels in myeloid but not in lymphoid cell populations, *Br. J. Haematol.,* 59, 21, 1985.

679. Chen, J.H., The proto-oncogene c-*ets* is preferentially expressed in lymphoid cells, *Mol. Cell. Biol.,* 5, 2993, 1985.

680. Schneider-Schaulies, J., Schimpl, A., and Wecker, E., Kinetics of cellular oncogene expression in mouse lymphocytes. II. Regulation of c-fos and c-myc gene expression, *Eur. J. Immunol.,* 17, 723, 1987.

681. Fahrlander, P.D., Piechaczyk, M., and Marcu, K.B., Chromatin structure of the murine c-*myc* locus: implications for the regulation of normal and chromosomally translocated genes, *EMBO J.,* 4, 3195, 1985.

682. Renan, M.J., Sequence homologies in the contol regions of c-*myc*, c-*fos*, HTLV and the interleukin-2 receptor, *Cancer Lett.,* 28, 69, 1985.

683. Remmers, E.F., Yang, J.-Q., and Marcu, K.B., A negative transcriptional control element located upstream of the murine c-*myc* gene, *EMBO J.,* 5, 899, 1986.

684. Sejersen, T., Björklund, H., Sümegi, J., and Ringertz, N.R., N-myc and c-src genes are differentially regulated in PCC7 embryonal carcinoma cells undergoing neuronal differentiation, *J. Cell. Physiol.,* 127, 274, 1986.

685. Wood, T.G., McGeady, M.L., Baroudy, B.M., Blair, D.G., and Vande Woude, G.F., Mouse c-*mos* oncogene activation is prevented by upstream sequences, *Proc. Natl. Acad. Sci. U.S.A.,* 81, 7817, 1984.

686. Horowitz, M., Luria, S., Rechavi, G., and Givol, D., Mechanism of activation of the mouse c-*mos* oncogene by the LTR of an intracisternal A-particle gene, *EMBO J.,* 3, 2937, 1984.

687. Riggs, A.D. and Jones, P.A., 5-methylcytosine, gene regulation, and cancer, *Adv. Cancer Res.,* 40, 1, 1983.

688. Hoffman, R.M., Altered methionine metabolism, DNA methylation and oncogene expression in carcinogenesis, *Biochim. Biophys. Acta,* 738, 49, 1984.

689. Ramsden, M., Cole, G., Smith, J., and Balmain, A., Differential methylation of the c-H-*ras* gene in normal mouse cells and during skin tumour progression, *EMBO J.,* 4, 1449, 1985.

690. Kaneko, Y., Shibuya, M., Nakayama, T., Hayashida, N., Toda, G., Endo, Y., Oka, H., and Oda, T., Hypomethylation of c-*myc* and epidermal growth factor receptor genes in human hepatocellular carcinoma and fetal liver, *Jpn. J. Cancer Res.,* 76, 1136, 1985.

691. Vorce, R.L. and Goodman, J.I., Investigation of parameters associated with activity of the Kirsten-*ras*, Harvey-*ras*, and *myc* oncogenes in normal rat liver, *Toxicol. Appl. Pharmacol.,* 90, 86, 1987.

692. Gattoni, S., Kirschmeier, P., Weinstein, I.B., Escobedo, J., and Dina, D., Cellular Moloney murine sarcoma (c-mos) sequences are hypermethylated and transcriptionally silent in normal and transformed cells, *Mol. Cell. Biol.,* 2, 42, 1982.

693. Groffen, J., Heisterkamp, N., Blennerhassett, G., and Stephenson, J.R., Regulation of viral and cellular oncogene expression by cytosine methylation, *Virology,* 127, 213, 1983.

694. Feinberg, A.P. and Vogelstein, B., Hypomethylation of *ras* oncogenes in primary human cancers, *Biochem. Biophys. Res. Commun.,* 111, 47, 1983.

695. Vorce, R.L. and Goodman, J.L., Methylation of the serum albumin gene as compared to the Kirsten-ras oncogene in hepatocytes and non-parenchymal cells of rat liver, *Biochem. Biophys. Res. Commun.,* 126, 879, 1985.

696. Cheah, M.S.C., Wallace, C.D., and Hoffman, R.M., Hypomethylation of DNA in human cancer cells: a site-specific change in the c-*myc* locus, *J. Natl. Cancer Inst.,* 73, 1057, 1984.

697. Dani, C., Blanchard, J.M., Piechaczyk, M., El Sabouty, S., Marty, L., and Jeanteur, P., Extreme instability of myc mRNA in normal and transformed human cells, *Proc. Natl. Acad. Sci. U.S.A.,* 81, 7046, 1984.

698. Darveau, A., Pelletier, J., and Sonenberg, N., Differential efficiencies of *in vitro* translation of mouse c-*myc* transcripts differing in the 5′ untranslated region, *Proc. Natl. Acad. Sci. U.S.A.,* 82, 2315, 1985.

699. Löhr, H., Löhr, G.W., Kanz, L., and Fauser, A.A., Expression of c-myc in stimulated T lymphocytes of the helper/inducer phenotype producing lymphokine(s) supporting multilineage colony formation, *Acta Haematol.,* 76, 192, 1986.

700. Gravekamp, C., van den Bulck, L.P., Vijg, J., van de Griend, R.J., and Bolhuis, R.L.H., c-myc gene expression and interleukin-2 receptor levels in cloned human CD2⁺, CD3⁺ and CD2⁺, CD3⁻ lymphocytes, *Natl. Immun. Cell Growth Regul.,* 6, 28, 1987.

701. Lipsick, J.S. and Boyle, W.J., c-*myb* protein expression is a late event during T-lymphocyte activation, *Mol. Cell. Biol.,* 7, 3358, 1987.

702. Reed, J.C., Tsujimoto, Y., Alpers, J.D., Croce, C.M., and Nowell, P.C., Regulation of *bcl*-2 proto-oncogene expression during normal human lymphocyte proliferation, *Science,* 236, 1295, 1987.

703. McNerney, R., Darling, D., and Johnstone, A., Differential control of proto-oncogene c-*myc* and c-*fos* expression in lymphocytes and fibroblasts, *Biochem. J.,* 245, 605, 1987.

704. Kujubu, D.A., Lim, R.W., Varnum, B.C., and Herschman, H.R., Induction of transiently expressed genes in PC-12 pheochromocytoma cells, *Oncogene,* 1, 257, 1987.

705. Lim, R.W., Varnum, B.C., and Herschman, H.R., Cloning of tetradecanoyl phorbol ester-induced "primary response" sequences and their expression in density-arrested Swiss 3T3 cells and a TPA non-proliferative variant, *Oncogene,* 1, 263, 1987.

706. Pompidou, A., Corral, M., Michel, P., Kruh, J., and Curran, T., La stimulation de lymphocytes humains par l'acétate de phorbol et un ionophore calcique induit une expression transitoire précoce de l'oncogène c-fos suivie de l'oncogène c-myc, *C.R. Acad. Sci. Paris,* 303, 445, 1986.

707. Pompidou, A., Corral, M., Michel, P., Defer, N., Kruh, J., and Curran, T., The effects of phorbol ester and Ca ionophore on c-fos and c-myc expression and on DNA synthesis in human lymphocytes are not directly related, *Biochem. Biophys. Res. Commun.,* 148, 435, 1987.

708. Radzioch, D., Bottazzi, B., and Varesio, L., Augmentation of c-*fos* mRNA expression by activators of protein kinase C in fresh, terminally differentiated resting macrophages, *Mol. Cell. Biol.,* 7, 595, 1987.

709. Bravo, R., Neuberg, M., Burckhardt, J., Almendral, J., Wallich, R., and Müller, R., Involvement of common and cell type-specific pathways in c-*fos* gene control: stable induction by cAMP in macrophages, *Cell,* 48, 251, 1987.

710. Ran, W., Dean, M., Levine, R.A., Henkle, C., and Campisi, J., Induction of c-*fos* and c-*myc* mRNA by epidermal growth factor or calcium ionophore is cAMP dependent, *Proc. Natl. Acad. Sci. U.S.A.,* 83, 8216, 1986.

711. Sikorska, M., Whitfield, J.F., and Walker, P.R., The regulatory and catalytic subunits of cAMP-dependent protein kinases are associated with transcriptionally active chromatin during changes in gene expression, *J. Biol. Chem.,* 263, 3005, 1988.

712. Moore, J.P., Todd, J.A., Hesketh, T.R., and Metcalfe, J.C., c-*fos* and c-*myc* gene activation, ionic signals, and DNA synthesis in thymocytes, *J. Biol. Chem.,* 261, 8158, 1986.

713. Matsui, T., Takahashi, R., Nakao, Y., Koizumi, T., Katakami, Y., Mihara, K., Sugiyama, T., and Fujita, T., 1,25-dihydroxyvitamin D₃-regulated expression of genes involved in human in human T-lymphocyte proliferation and differentiation, *Cancer Res.,* 46, 5827, 1986.

714. Introna, M., Hamilton, T.A., Kaufman, E., Adams, D.O., and Bast, R.C., Jr., Treatment of murine peritoneal macrophages with bacterial lipopolysaccharide alters expression of c-FOS and c-MYC oncogenes, *J. Immunol.,* 137, 2703, 1986.

715. Kartha, S., Sukhatme, V.P., and Toback, F.G., ADP activate protooncogene expression in renal epithelial cells, *Am. J. Physiol.,* 252, F1175, 1987.

716. Gottesman, M.M. and Fleischmann, R.D., The role of cAMP in regulating tumour cell growth, *Cancer Surv.,* 5, 291, 1986.

717. Blomhoff, H.K., Smeland, E.B., Beiske, K., Blomhoff, R., Ruud, E., Bjoro, T., Pfeifer-Ohlsson, S., Watt, R., Funderud, S., Godal, T., and Ohlsson, R., Cyclic AMP-mediated suppression of normal and neoplastic B cell proliferation is associated with regulation of *myc* and Ha-*ras* protooncogenes, *J. Cell. Physiol.,* 131, 426, 1987.

718. Dean, R., Kim, S.S., and Delgado, D., Expression of c-myc oncogene in human fibroblasts during *in vitro* senescence, *Biochem. Biophys. Res. Commun.,* 135, 105, 1986.

719. Delgado, D., Raymond, L., and Dean, R., c-ras expression decreases during *in vitro* senescence in human fibroblasts, *Biochem. Biophys. Res. Commun.,* 137, 917, 1986.

720. Matocha, M.F., Cosgrove, J.W., Atack, J.R., and Rapoport, S.I., Selective elevation of c-*myc* transcript levels in the liver of the aging Fischer-344 rat, *Biochem. Biophys. Res. Commun.,* 147, 1, 1987.

721. Ono, T., Tawa, R., Shinya, K., Hirose, S., and Okada, S., Methylation of the c-myc gene changes during aging process of mice, *Biochem. Biophys. Res. Commun.,* 139, 1299, 1986.

722. Nakamura, K.D. and Hart, R.W., Comparison of proto oncogene expression in seven primate fibroblast cultures, *Mechan. Ageing Dev.,* 39, 177, 1987.

723. Koeffler, H.P., Induction of differentiation of human acute myelogenous leukemia cells: therapeutic implications, *Blood,* 62, 709, 1983.

724. Niles, R.M., Chemical induction of tumor cell differentiation, *Surv. Synth. Pathol. Res.,* 4, 282, 1985.

725. Freshney, R.I., Induction of differentiation in neoplastic cells, *Anticancer Res.,* 5, 111, 1985.

726. Westin, E.H., Wong-Staal, F., Gelmann, E.P., Dalla Favera, R., Papas, T.S., Lautenberger, J.A., Eva, A., Reddy, E.P., Tronick, S.R., Aaronson, S.A., and Gallo, R.C., Expression of cellular homologues of retroviral *onc* genes in human hematopoietic cells, *Proc. Natl. Acad. Sci. U.S.A.,* 79, 2490, 1982.

727. Reitsma, P.H., Rothberg, P.G., Astrin, S.M., Trial, J., Bar-Shavit, Z., Hall, A., Teitelbaum, S.L., and Kahn, A.J., Regulation of *myc* expression in HL-60 leukaemia cells by a vitamin D metabolite, *Nature,* 306, 492, 1983.

728. Craig, R.W. and Bloch, A., Early decline in c-*myb* oncogene expression in the differentiation of human myeloblastic leukemia (ML-1) cells induced with 12-*O*-tetradecanoylphorbol-13-acetate, *Cancer Res.,* 44, 442, 1984.

729. Grosso, L.E. and Pitot, H.C., The expression of the *myc* proto-oncogene in a dimethylsulfoxide resistant HL-60 cell line, *Cancer Lett.,* 22, 55, 1984.

730. Grosso, L.E. and Pitot, H.C., Modulation of c-*myc* expression in the HL-60 cell line, *Biochem. Biophys. Res. Commun.,* 119, 473, 1984.

731. Filmus, J. and Buick, R.N., Relationship of c-*myc* expression to differentiation and proliferation of HL-60 cells, *Cancer Res.,* 45, 822, 1985.

732. Grosso, L.E. and Pitot, H.C., Transcriptional regulation of c-*myc* during chemically induced differentiation of HL-60 cultures, *Cancer Res.,* 45, 847, 1985.

733. Watanabe, T., Sariban, E., Mitchell, T., and Kufe, D., Human c-*myc* and N-*ras* expression during induction of HL-60 cellular differentiation, *Biochem. Biophys. Res. Commun.,* 126, 999, 1985.

734. Linevsky, J., Cohen, M.B., Hartman, K.D., Knode, M.C., and Glazer, R.I., Effect of neoplanocin A on differentiation, nucleic acid methylation, and c-*myc* mRNA expression in human promyelocytic leukemia cells, *Mol. Pharmacol.,* 28, 45, 1985.

735. de Bustros, A., Baylin, S.B., Berger, C.L., Roos, B.A., Leong, S.S., and Nelkin, B.D., Phorbol esters increase calcitonin gene transcription and decrease c-*myc* mRNA levels in cultured human medullary thyroid carcinoma, *J. Biol. Chem.,* 260, 98, 1985.

736. Thiele, C.J., Reynolds, C.P., and Israel, M.A., Decreased expression of N-*myc* precedes retinoic acid-induced morphological differentiation of human neuroblastoma, *Nature,* 313, 404, 1985.

737. Amatruda, T.T., III, Sidell, N., Ranyard, J., and Koeffler, H.P., Retinoic acid treatment of human neuroblastoma cells is associated with decreased N-*myc* expression, *Biochem. Biophys. Res. Commun.,* 126, 1189, 1985.

738. Hammerling, U., Bjelfman, C., and Pahlman, S., Different regulation of N- and c-*myc* expression during phorbol ester-induced maturation of human SH-SY5Y neuroblastoma cells, *Oncogene,* 2, 73, 1987.

739. Lee, J., Mehta, K., Blick, M.B., Gutterman, J.U., and Lopez-Berestein, G., Expression of c-*fos*, c-*myb*, and c-*myc* in human monocytes: correlation with monocytic differentiation, *Blood,* 69, 1542, 1987.

740. Benjamin, D., Magrath, I.T., Triche, T.J., Schroft, R.W., Jensen, J.P., and Korsmeyer, S.J., Induction of plasmacytoid differentiation by phorbol ester in B-cell lymphoma cell lines bearing 8;14 translocations, *Proc. Natl. Acad. Sci. U.S.A.,* 81, 3547, 1984.

741. Tsiftsoglou, A.S. and Robinson, S.H., Differentiation of leukemic cell lines: a review focusing on murine erythroleukemia and human HL-60 cells, *Int. J. Cell Cloning,* 3, 349, 1985.

742. Collins, S.J., the HL-60 promyelocytic leukemia cell line: proliferation, differentiation, and cellular oncogene expression, *Blood,* 70, 1233, 1987.

743. Leglise, M.C., Dent, G.A., Ayscue, L.H., and Ross, D.W., Leukemic cell maturation: phenotypic variability and oncogene expression in HL60 cells: a review, *Blood Cells,* 13, 319, 1988.

744. Weil, S.C., Rosner, G.L., Reid, M.S., Chisholm, R.L., Farber, N.M., Spitznagel, J.K., and Swanson, M.S., cDNA cloning of human myeloperoxidase: decrease in myeloperoxidase mRNA upon induction of HL-60 cells, *Proc. Natl. Acad. Sci. U.S.A.,* 84, 2057, 1987.

745. Tyers, M., Rachubinski, R.A., Sartori, C.S., Harley, C.B., and Haslam, R.J., Induction of the 47kDa platelet substrate of protein kinase C during differentiation of HL-60 cells, *Biochem. J.,* 243, 249, 1987.

746. Brelvi, Z.S. and Studzinski, G.P., Changes in the expression of oncogenes encoding nuclear phosphoproteins but not c-Ha-ras have a relationship to monocytic differentiation of HL 60 cells, *J. Cell Biol.,* 102, 2234, 1986.

747. Studzinski, G.P. and Brelvi, Z.S., Changes in proto-oncogene expression associated with reversal of macrophage-like differentiation of HL 60 cells, *J. Natl. Cancer Inst.,* 79, 67, 1987.

748. Mitchell, R.L., Henning-Chubb, C., Huberman, E., and Verma, I.M., c-*fos* expression is neither sufficient nor obligatory for differentiation of monocytes to macrophates, *Cell,* 45, 497, 1986.

749. Griep, A.E. and DeLuca, H.F., Decreased c-*myc* expression is an early event in retinoic acid-induced differentiation of F9 teratocarcinoma cells, *Proc. Natl. Acad. Sci. U.S.A.,* 83, 5539, 1986.

750. McCachren, S.S., Jr., Nichols, J., Kaufman, R.E., and Niedel, J.E., Dibutyryl cyclic adenosine monophosphate reduces expression of c-*myc* during HL-60 differentiation, *Blood,* 68, 412, 1986.

751. Cayre, Y., Raynal, M.-C., Darzynkiewicz, Z., and Dorner, M.H., Model for intermediate steps in monocytic differentiation: c-*myc*, c-*fms*, and ferritin as markers, *Proc. Natl. Acad. Sci. U.S.A.,* 84, 7619, 1987.

752. Yokoyama, K. and Imamoto, F., Transcriptional control of the endogenous *MYC* protooncogene by antisense RNA, *Proc. Natl. Acad. Sci. U.S.A.,* 84, 7363, 1987.

753. Yen, A. and Guernsey, D.L., Increased c-*myc* RNA levels associated with the precommitment state during HL-60 myeloid differentiation, *Cancer Res.,* 46, 4156, 1986.

754. Salehi, Z., Taylor, J.D., and Niedel, J.E., Dioctanoylglycerol and phorbol esters regulate transcription of c-*myc* in human promyelocytic leukemia cells, *J. Biol. Chem.*, 263, 1898, 1988.

755. Kraft, A.S., Baker, V.V., and May, W.S., Bryostatin induces changes in protein kinase C location and activity without altering c-*myc* gene expression in human promyelocytic leukemia cells (HL-60), *Oncogene*, 1, 111, 1987.

756. Reitsma, P.H., Rothberg, P.G., Astrin, S.M., Trial, J., Bar-Shavit, Z., Hall, A., Teitelbaum, S.L., and Kahn, A.J., Regulation of *myc* gene expression in Hl-60 leukaemia cells by a vitamin D metabolite, *Nature*, 306, 492, 1983.

757. Simpson, R.U., Hsu, T., Begley, D.A., Mitchell, B.S., and Alizadeh, B.N., Transcriptional regulation of the c-myc protooncogene by 1,25-dihydroxyvitamin D$_3$ in HL-60 promyelocytic leukemia cells, *J. Biol. Chem.*, 262, 4104, 1987.

758. Trepel, J.B., Colamonici, O.R., Kelly, K., Schwab, G., Watt, R.A., Sausville, E.A., Jaffe, E.S., and Neckers, L.M., Transcriptional inactivation of c-*myc* and the transferrin receptor in dibutyryl cyclic AMP-treated HL-60 cells, *Mol. Cell. Biol.*, 7, 2644, 1987.

759. Chapekar, M.S., Hartman, K.D., Knode, M.C., and Glazer, R.I., Synergistic effect of retinoic acid and calcium ionophore A23187 on differentiation, c-*myc* expression, and membrane tyrosine kinase activity in human promyelocytic leukemia cell line HL-60, *Mol. Pharmacol.*, 31, 140, 1987.

760. Krönke, M., Schlüter, C., and Pfizenmaier, K., Tumor necrosis factor inhibits *MYC* expression in HL-60 cells at the level of mRNA transcription, *Proc. Natl. Acad. Sci. U.S.A.*, 84, 469, 1987.

761. McAchren, S.S., Jr., Salehi, Z., Weinberg, J.B., and Niedel, J.E., Transcription interruption may be a common mechanism of c-myc regulation during HL-60 differentiation, *Biochem. Biophys. Res. Commun.*, 151, 574, 1988.

762. Hashimoto, Y., Kagechika, K., Kawachi, E., and Shudo, K., New-type inducers of differentiation of HL-60 leukemia cells suppress c-*myc* expression, *Chem. Pharm. Bull. (Tokyo)*, 35, 3190, 1987.

763. Ely, C.M., Leftwich, J.A., Chenevix-Trench, G., Hall, R.E., and Westin, E.H., Altered regulation of c-*myc* in an HL-60 differentiation resistant subclone, HL-60-1E3, *Cancer Res.*, 47, 4595, 1987.

764. Müller, R., Curran, T., Müller, D., and Guilbert, L., Induction of c-*fos* during myelomonocytic differentiation and macrophage proliferation, *Nature*, 314, 546, 1985.

765. Barzilay, J., Kushtai, G., Plaksin, D., Feldman, M., and Eisenbach, L., Expression of major histocompatibility class I genes in differentiating leukemic cells is temporally related to activation of c-*fos* proto-oncogene, *Leukemia*, 1, 198, 1987.

766. Chou, R.H., Chen, T.A., Churchill, J.R., Thompson, S.W., and Chou, K.L., Reassembly of c-*myc* and relaxation of c-*fos* nucleosomes during differentiation of human leukemic (HL-60) cells, *Biochem. Biophys. Res. Commun.*, 141, 213, 1986.

767. Pantazis, P., Sariban, E., Kufe, D., and Antoniades, H.N., Induction of c-*sis* gene expression and synthesis of platelet-derived growth factor in human myeloid leukemia cells during monocytic differentiation, *Proc. Natl. Acad. Sci. U.S.A.*, 83, 6455, 1986.

768. Horiguchi, J., Warren, M.K., Ralph, P., and Kufe, D., Expression of the macrophage specific colony-stimulating factor (CSF-1) during human monocytic differentiation, *Biochem. Biophys. Res. Commun.*, 141, 924, 1986.

769. Wakamiya, N., Horiguchi, J., and Kufe, D., Detection of c-fms and CSF-1 RNA by *in situ* hybridization, *Leukemia*, 1, 518, 1987.

770. Ghysdael, J., Gegonne, A., Pognonec, P., Boulukos, K., Leprince, D., Dernis, D., Lagrou, C., and Stehelin, D., Identification in chicken macrophages of a set of proteins related to, but distinct from the chicken cellular c-*ets*-encoded protein p54$^{c\text{-}ets}$, *EMBO J.*, 5, 2251, 1986.

771. Studzinski, G.P. and Brelvi, Z.S., Increased expression of oncogene c-*Ha-ras* during granulocytic differentiation of Hl60 cells, *Lab. Invest.*, 56, 499, 1987.

772. Barnekow, A. and Gessler, M., Activation of the pp60$^{c\text{-}src}$ kinase during differentiation of monomyelocytic cells *in vitro*, *EMBO J.*, 5, 701, 1986.

773. Gee, C.E., Griffin, J., Sastre, L., Miller, L.J., Springer, T.A., Piwnica-Worms, H., and Roberts, T.M., Differentiation of myeloid cells is accompanied by increased levels of pp60$^{c\text{-}src}$ protein and kinase activity, *Proc. Natl. Acad. Sci. U.S.A.*, 83, 5131, 1986.

774. Sariban, E., Mitchell, T., Griffin, J., and Kufe, D.W., Effects of interferon-gamma on proto-oncogene expression during induction of human monocytic differentiation, *J. Immunol.*, 138, 1954, 1987.

775. Brelvi, Z.S. and Studzinski, G.P., Inhibition of DNA synthesis by an inducer of differentiation of leukemic cells, 1-α,25 dihydroxy vitamin D$_3$, precedes down regulation of the c-myc gene, *J. Cell. Physiol.*, 128, 171, 1986.

776. Brelvi, Z.S., Christakos, S., and Studzinski, G.P., Expression of monocytic-specific oncogenes c-*fos* and c-*fms* in HL-60 cells treated with vitamin D$_3$ analogs correlates with inhibition of DNA synthesis and reduced calmodulin concentration, *Lab. Invest.*, 55, 269, 1986.

777. Collins, S. and Groudine, M., Amplification of endogenous *myc*-related DNA sequences in a human myeloid leukaemia cell line, *Nature*, 298, 679, 1982.

778. Dalla Favera, R., Wong-Staal, F., and Gallo, R.C., Oncogene amplification in promyelocytic leukaemia cell line HL-60 and primary leukaemia cells of the patient, *Nature,* 298, 61, 1982.
779. Grosso, L.E. and Pitot, H.C., Chromatin structure of the c-*myc* gene in HL-60 cells during alterations of transcriptional activity, *Cancer Res.,* 45, 5035, 1985.
780. High, K.A., Stolle, C.A., Schneider, J.W., Hu, W., and Benz, E.J., Jr., c-*myc* gene inactivation during induced maturation of HL-60 cells: transcriptional repression and loss of a specific DNAse I hypersensitive site, *J. Clin. Invest.,* 79, 93, 1987.
781. Bentley, D.L. and Groudine, M., A block to elongation is largely responsible for decreased transcription of c-*myc* in differentiated HL60 cells, *Nature,* 321, 702, 1986.
782. Eick, D. and Bornkamm, G.W., Transcriptional arrest within the first exon is a fast control mechanismn in c-myc gene expression, *Nucleic Acids Res.,* 14, 8331, 1986.
783. Todokoro, K. and Ikawa, Y., Sequential expression of proto-oncogenes during a mouse erythroleukemia cell differentiation, *Biochem. Biophys. Res. Commun.,* 135, 1112, 1986.
784. Lachman, H.M. and Skoultchi, A.I., Expression of c-*myc* changes during differentiation of mouse erythroleukaemia cells, *Nature,* 310, 592, 1984.
785. Kirsch, I.R., Bertness, V., Silver, J., and Hollis, G.F., Regulated expression of the c-*myb* and c-*myc* oncogenes during erythroid differentiation, *J. Cell. Biochem.,* 32, 11, 1986.
786. Lachman, H.M., Hatton, K.S., Skoultchi, A.I., and Schildkraut, C.L., c-*myc* mRNA levels in the cell cycle change in mouse erythroleukemia cells following inducer treatment, *Proc. Natl. Acad. Sci. U.S.A.,* 82, 5323, 1985.
787. Lachman, H.M., Cheng, G., and Skoultchi, A.I., Transfection of mouse erythroleukemia cells with *myc* sequences changes the rate of induced commitment to differentiate, *Proc. Natl. Acad. Sci. U.S.A.,* 83, 6480, 1986.
788. Coppola, J.A. and Cole, M.D., Constitutive c-*myc* oncogene expression blocks mouse erythroleukaemia cell differentiation but not commitment, *Nature,* 320, 760, 1986.
789. Prochownik, E.V. and Kukowska, J., Deregulated expression of c-*myc* by murine erythroleukaemia cells prevents differentiation, *Nature,* 322, 848, 1986.
790. Ramsay, R.G., Ikeda, K., Rifkind, R.A., and Marks, P.A., Changes in gene expression associated with induced differentiation of erythroleukemia: protooncogenes, globin genes, and cell division, *Proc. Natl. Acad. Sci. U.S.A.,* 83, 6849, 1986.
791. Jonak, G.J. and Knight, E., Jr., Selective reduction of c-*myc* mRNA in Daudi cells by human beta interferon, *Proc. Natl. Acad. Sci. U.S.A.,* 81, 1747, 1984.
792. Einat, M., Resnitzky, D., and Kimchi, A., Close link between reduction of c-*myc* expression by interferon and G_0/G_1 arrest, *Nature,* 313, 597, 1985.
793. Knight, E., Jr., Anton, E.D., Fahey, D., Friedland, B.K., and Jonak, G.J., Interferon regulates c-*myc* gene expression in Daudi cells at the post-transcriptional level, *Proc. Natl. Acad. Sci. U.S.A.,* 82, 1151, 1985.
794. Dani, C., Mechti, N., Piechaczyk, M., Lebleu, B., Jeanteur, P., and Blanchard, J.M., Increased rate of degradation of c-myc mRNA in interferon-treated Daudi cells, *Proc. Natl. Acad. Sci. U.S.A.,* 82, 4896, 1985.
795. Jonak, G.J., Friedland, B.K., Anton, E.D., and Knight, E., Jr., Regulation of c-*myc* RNA and its proteins in Daudi cells by interferon-β, *J. Interferon Res.,* 7, 41, 1987.
796. Matsui, T., Takahashi, R., Mihara, K., Nakagawa, T., Koizumi, T., Nakao, Y., Sugiyama, T., and Fujita, T., Cooperative regulation of c-*myc* expression in differentiation of human promyelocytic leukemia induced by recombinant gamma-interferon and 1,25-dihydroxyvitamin D_3, *Cancer Res.,* 45, 4366, 1985.
797. Dron, M., Modjtahedi, N., Brison, O., and Tovey, M.G., Interferon modulation of c-*myc* expression in cloned Daudi cells: relationship to the phenotype of interferon resistance, *Mol. Cell. Biol.,* 6, 1374, 1986.
798. Gambari, R., del Senno, L., Piva, R., Barbieri, R., Amelotti, F., Bernardi, F., Marchetti, G., Citarella, F., Tripodi, M., and Fantoni, A., Human leukemia K562 cells relationship between hemin-mediated erythroid induction, cell proliferation, and expression of c-*abl* and c-*myc* oncogenes, *Biochem. Biophys. Res. Commun.,* 125, 90, 1984.
799. Bianchi Scarra, G.L., Romani, M., Coviello, D.A., Garrè, C., Ravazzolo, R., Vidali, G., and Ajmar, F., Terminal erythroid differentiation in the K-562 cell line by 1-beta-D-arabinofuranosylcytosine: accompaniment by c-*myc* messenger RNA decrease, *Cancer Res.,* 46, 6327, 1986.
800. Colamonici, O.R., Trepel, J.B., Vidal, C.A., and Neckers, L.M., Phorbol ester induces c-*sis* gene transcription in stem cell line K-562, *Mol. Cell. Biol.,* 6, 1847, 1986.
801. Levine, R.A., McCormack, J.E., Buckler, A., and Sonenshein, G.E., Transcriptional and posttranscriptional control of c-*myc* gene expression in WEHI 231 cells, *Mol. Cell. Biol.,* 6, 4112, 1986.
802. Gonda, T.J. and Metcalf, D., Expression of *myb, myc,* and *fos* proto-oncogenes during the differentiation of a murine myeloid leukaemia, *Nature,* 310, 249, 1984.
803. Larsson, L.-G., Gray, H.E., Tötterman, T., Pettersson, U., and Nilsson, K., Drastically increased expression of *MYC* and *FOS* protooncogenes during *in vitro* differentiation of chronic lymphocytic leukemia cells, *Proc. Natl. Acad. Sci. U.S.A.,* 84, 223, 1987.

804. Shen-Ong, G.L.C., Holmes, K.L., and Morse, H.C., III, Phorbol ester-induced growth arrest of murine myelomonocytic leukemic cells with virus-disrupted *myb* locus is not accompanied by decreased *myc* and *myb* expression, *Proc. Natl. Acad. Sci. U.S.A.,* 84, 199, 1987.

805. Lockett, T.J. and Sleigh, M.J., Oncogene expression in differentiating F9 mouse embryonal carcinoma cells, *Exp. Cell Res.,* 173, 370, 1987.

806. Dean, M., Levine, R.A., and Campisi, J., c-*myc* regulation during retinoic acid-induced differentiation of F9 cells is post-transcriptonal and associated with growth arrest, *Mol. Cell. Biol.,* 6, 518, 1986.

807. Schofield, P.N., Engstrom, W., Lee, A.J., Biddle, C., and Graham, C.F., Expression of c-*myc* during differentiation of the human teratocarcinoma cell line Tera-2, *J. Cell Sci.,* 88, 57, 1987.

808. Augenlicht, L.H., Augeron, C., Yander, G., and Laboisse, C., Overexpression of *ras* in mucus-secreting human colon carcinoma cells of low tumorigenicity, *Cancer Res.,* 47, 3763, 1987.

809. Greene, L.A. and Shooter, E.M., The nerve growth factor: biochemistry, synthesis, and mechanism of action, *Annu. Rev. Neurosci.,* 3, 353, 1980.

810. Curran, T. and Morgan, J.I., Superinduction of c-*fos* by nerve growth factor in the presence of peripherally active benzodiazepines, *Science,* 229, 1265, 1985.

811. Kruijer, W., Schubert, D., and Verma, I.M., Induction of the proto-oncogene *fos* by nerve growth factor, *Proc. Natl. Acad. Sci. U.S.A.,* 82, 7330, 1985.

812. Greenberg, M.E., Greene, L.A., and Ziff, E.B., Nerve growth factor and epidermal growth factor induce rapid transient changes in proto-oncogene transcription in PC12 cells, *J. Biol. Chem.,* 260, 14101, 1985.

813. Milbrandt, J., Nerve growth factor rapidly induces c-fos mRNA in PC12 rat pheochromocytoma cells, *Proc. Natl. Acad. Sci. U.S.A.,* 83, 4789, 1986.

814. Guerrero, I., Pellicer, A., and Burstein, D.E., Dissociation of c-fos from ODC expression and neuronal differentiation in a PC12 subline stably transfected with an inducible N-ras oncogene, *Biochem. Biophys. Res. Commun.,* 150, 1185, 1988.

815. Hagag, N., Halegoua, S., and Viola, M., Inhibition of growth factor-induced differentiation of PC12 cells by microinjection of antibody to *ras* p21, *Nature,* 319, 680, 1986.

816. Francis, G.E., Mufti, G.J., Knowles, S.M., Berney, J.J., Guimaraes, J.E.T., Secker-Walker, L.M., and Hamblin, T.J., Differentiation induction in myelodysplasia and acute myeloid leukaemia: use of synergistic drug combinations, *Leukemia Res.,* 11, 971, 1987.

817. Koller, C.A., Campbell, V.W., Polansky, D.A., Mulhern, A., and Miller, D.M., *In vivo* differentiation of blast-phase chronic granulocytic leukemia — expression of c-*myc* and c-*abl* proto-oncogenes, *J. Clin. Invest.,* 76, 365, 1985.

818. Jetten, A.M., Barrett, J.C., and Gilmer, T.M., Differential response to retinoic acid of Syrian hamster embryo fibroblasts expressing v-*src* or v-Ha-*ras* oncogenes, *Mol. Cell. Biol.,* 6, 3341, 1986.

LIST OF ABBREVIATIONS

AAF	2-Acetylamino-fluorene
AAV	Adeno-associated virus
ABR	Abnormally banded region
ADP	Adenosine diphosphate
ADPRT	ADP-ribosyl transferase
AEV	Avian erythroblastosis virus
AFP	α-Fetoprotein
AIDS	Acquired immune deficiency syndrome
AILA	Angioimmunoblastic lymphadenopathy
ALV	Avian leukemia virus
AMCV	Avian myelocytomatosis virus
AML	Acute myelocytic leukemia
AMML	Acute myelomonocytic leukemia
AMOL	Acute monocytic leukemia
AMP	Adenosine 3':5'-monophosphate
AMV	Avian myeloblastosis virus
ANLL	Acute nonlymphocytic leukemia
APML	Acute promyelocytic leukemia
ARV	Avian reticuloendothelial virus
ASV	Avian sarcoma virus
ATL	Adult T-cell leukemia
ATLV	Adult T-cell leukemia virus
ATPase	Adenosine triphosphatase
ATP	Adenosine triphosphate
AV	Avian virus
AWTA	Aniridia-Wilms' tumor association
Ab	Antibody
Ag	Antigen
BCGF	B-cell growth factor
BEVI	Baboon endogenous viral infection
BHK	Baby hamster kidney
BKV	BK virus
BLV	Bovine leukemia virus
BMK	Baby mouse kidney
BP	Benzo-*a*-pyrene
BPV	Bovine papilloma virus
BSF	B-cell stimulating factor
BaEV	Baboon endogenous virus
bp	Base pairs
cAMP	Cyclic AMP
cDNA	Complementary DNA
CEA	Carcinoembryonic antigen
CEF	Chick embryo fibroblasts
cGMP	Cyclic GMP
CHO	Chinese hamster ovary
CLL	Chronic lymphocytic leukemia
CML	Chronic myelogenous leukemia
CMP	Cytosine monophosphate
CMV	Cytomegalovirus

CSF	Colony stimulating factor
CTVT	Canine transmissible venereal tumor
cs	Cold sensitive
DENA	Diethylnitrosamine
DES	Diethylstilbestrol
DIA	Differentiation-inducing activity
DIF	Differentiation-inducing factor
DMBA	7,12-Dimethylbenz(*a*)anthracene
DMSO	Dimethylsulfoxide
DM	Double minute chromosome
DNA	Deoxyribonucleic acid
DNase	Deoxyribonuclease
EA	Eary antigen
EBNA	EBV-associated nuclear antigen
EBV	Epstein-Barr virus
EF	Elongation factor
EGF	Epidermal growth factor
ELISA	Enzyme-linked immune sorbance assay
E1	Early region 1
ENU	1-Ethyl-1-nitrosourea
EPBF	Embryonal promoter-binding factor
ERV	Endogenous retrovirus
FAIDS	Feline AIDS
FBJ-MuSV	Finkel-Biskis-Jenkins MuSV
FGF	Fibroblast growth factor
FSBA	*p*-Fluorosulfonylbenzoyl 5′-adenosine
FSH	Follicle-stimulating hormone
FSV	Fujinami avian sarcoma virus
FeLV	Feline leukemia virus
FeSV	Feline sarcoma virus
F-MuLV	Friend murine leukemia virus
GA	Gardner-Arnstein strain
GABA	γ-Aminobutyric acid
GAD	Glutamic acid decarboxylase
GC	Guanosine-cytosine
GDP	Guanosine diphosphate
GMP	Guanosine monophosphate
GM-CSF	Granulocyte-macrophage colony stimulating factor
GPDH	Glucose-6-phosphate dehydrogenase
GR	Gardner-Rasheed strain
GRE	Glucocorticoid regulatory element
GTPase	Guanosine triphosphatase
GTP	Guanosine triphosphate
GaLV	Gibbon ape leukemia virus
HBLV	Human B-lymphotropic virus
HBV	Hepatitis B virus
HBsAg	Hepatitis B virus surface antigen
HCMV	Human cytomegalovirus
HEK	Human embryo kidney
HIV	Human immunodeficiency virus
HLA	Human leukocyte antigen

HMBA	Hexamethylene bisacetamide
HMG	High mobility group
HPRT	Hypoxanthine phosphoribosyl transferase
HPV	Human papilloma virus
HRE	Hormone regulatory element
HSP	Heat shock protein
HSR	Homogeneously staining region
HSV	Herpes simplex virus
HTLV	Human T-cell lymphotropic virus
HVT	Herpes virus of turkeys
HZ	Hardy-Zuckerman strain
HuERS	Human endogenous retroviruses
IAP	Intracisternal A particle
IDF	Inhibitory diffusible factor
IFN	Interferon
IGF	Insulin-like growth factor
IL	Interleukin
IS	Insertion sequence
ITR	Inverted terminal repeat sequence
Ig	Immunoglobulin
kDa	Kilodalton
K-MuLV	Kirsten murine leukemia virus
K-MuSV	Kirsten murine sarcoma virus
kb	Kilobase
kbp	Kilobase pair
LAS	Lymphadenopathy syndrome
LAV	Lymphadenopathy-associated virus
LDH	Lactate dehydrogenase
LDL	Low-density lipoprotein
LINE	Long interspersed repetitive sequence
LMP	Latent membrane protein
LPS	Lipopolysaccharide
LPV	Lymphotropic papovavirus
LTR	Long terminal repeat
MA	Membrane antigen
MCA	3-Methyl-cholanthrene
MCF	Mink cell focus
MCFV	Mink cell focus virus
MCMV	Mouse cytomegalovirus
MDCK	Madin-Darby canine kidney
MDV	Marek's disease virus
MEL	Mouse erythroleukemia
MEN	Multiple endocrine neoplasia
MGI	Macrophage-granulocyte inducer
MHC	Major histocompatibility complex
MHSV	Malignant histiocytosis virus
MMTV	Mouse mammary tumor virus
MNNG	N-Methyl-N'-nitroso-guanidine
MPF	Maturation-promoting factor
MPLV	Myeloproliferative leukemia virus
MPMV	Mason-Pfizer monkey virus

MPO	Myeloperoxidase
mRNA	Messenger RNA
mol wt	Molecular weight
MuLV	Murine leukemia virus
MuSV	Murine sarcoma virus
NAD	Nicotinamide adenine dinucleotide
NGF	Nerve growth factor
NHBE	Normal human bronchial epithelial cells
NK	Natural killer
NMU	Nitrosomethylurea (*N*-methyl-*N*-nitrosourea)
NRK	Normal rat kidney
ODC	Ornithine decarboxylase
ORF	Open reading frame
PCNA	Proliferating cell nuclear antigen
PCR	Polymerase chain reaction
PDGF	Platelet-derived growth factor
PFK	Phosphofructokinase
PGE	Prostaglandin E
PHA	Phytohemagglutinin
PHC	Primary hepatocellular carcinoma
PI-FeSV	Parodi-Irgens FeSV
PMA	Phorbol 12-myristate 13-acetate
PTH	Parathyroid hormone
Rad-MuLV	Radiation murine leukemia virus
RAV	RSV-associated virus
REF	Rat embryo fibroblasts
REV	Reticuloendotheliosis virus
RFLP	Restriction fragment length polymorphism
RNA	Ribonucleic acid
RNAse	Ribonuclease
RNP	Ribonucleoprotein
rRNA	Ribosomal RNA
RSV	Rous sarcoma virus
RadLV	Radiation leukemia virus
SAIDS	Simian AIDS
SCE	Sister chromatid exchange
SDS	Sodium dodecyl sulfate
SFFV	Spleen focus-forming virus
SFV	Shope fibroma virus
SINE	Short interspersed repetitive sequence
SIV	Simian immunodeficiency virus
SLE	Systemic lupus erythrematosus
SMRV	Squirrel monkey retrovirus
SM	Susan McDonough strain
SNV	Spleen necrosis virus
SRV	Simian AIDS retrovirus
SSAV	Simian sarcoma-associated virus
SSV	Simian sarcoma virus
STLV	Simian T-cell leukemia virus
ST	Snyder-Theilen strain
SV-40	Simian virus 40

TAA	Tumor associated antigen
TGF	Transforming growth factor
TNF	Tumor necrosis factor
TPA	12-*O*-Tetradecanoyl-phorbol 13-acetate
tRNA	Transfer RNA
TSA	Tumor surface antigen
TSH	Thyroid-stimulating factor
TSTA	Tumor-specific transplantation antigen
ts	Temperature sensitive
UMS	Upstream mouse sequence
UV	Ultraviolet
VCA	Viral capsid antigen
VTR	Variable tandem repeat
VVGF	Vaccinia virus growth factor
WHV	Woodchuck hepatitis virus

INDEX

A

I